# The Impact of Early Life Trauma on Health and Disease

## The Hidden Epidemic

# The Impact of Early Life Trauma on Health and Disease

## The Hidden Epidemic

Edited by

**Ruth A. Lanius**
Associate Professor, University of Western Ontario, Canada

**Eric Vermetten**
Associate Professor, University Medical Center and Military Mental Health, Central Military Hospital, Utrecht, the Netherlands

**Clare Pain**
Associate Professor, University of Toronto, Canada

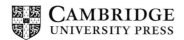

CAMBRIDGE UNIVERSITY PRESS
Cambridge, New York, Melbourne, Madrid, Cape Town, Singapore,
São Paulo, Delhi, Dubai, Tokyo, Mexico City

Cambridge University Press
The Edinburgh Building, Cambridge CB2 8RU, UK

Published in the United States of America by Cambridge University Press, New York

www.cambridge.org
Information on this title: www.cambridge.org/9780521880268

First published 2010
Reprinted with corrections 2010

Printed in the United Kingdom at the University Press, Cambridge

*A catalogue record for this publication is available from the British Library*

*Library of Congress Cataloguing in Publication data*
The impact of early life trauma on health and disease : the hidden epidemic / [edited by]
    Ruth A. Lanius, Eric Vermetten, Clare Pain.
        p. ; cm.
    Includes bibliographical references and index.
    ISBN 978-0-521-88026-8 (hardback)
    1. Post-traumatic stress disorder in children–Complications.    2. Psychic trauma in children–
    Complications.    3. Adult child abuse victims–Mental health.    4. Adult child abuse victims–Health
    and hygiene.    I. Lanius, Ruth A., 1968–    II. Vermetten, Eric, 1961–    III. Pain, Clare.    IV. Title.
    [DNLM: 1. Stress Disorders, Post-Traumatic–complications.    2. Adult Survivors of Child
    Abuse–psychology.    3. Mental Disorders–etiology.    WM 170 I335 2010]
    RJ506.P55I47 2010
    618.92′8521–dc22        2010016394

ISBN 978-0-521-88026-8 Hardback

# Contents

List of contributors    *page* vii
*Foreword*    xiii
Vincent J. Felitti
*Acknowledgements*    xvii

## Section 1 Early life trauma: impact on health and disease

**Part 1 Childhood trauma: epidemiology and historical themes    3**

1   The history of early life trauma and abuse from the 1850s to the current time: how the past influences the present    3
    Martin J. Dorahy, Onno van der Hart and Warwick Middleton

2   The epidemiology of early childhood trauma    13
    Karestan C. Koenen, Andrea L. Roberts, Deborah M. Stone and Erin C. Dunn

3   Historical themes in the study of recovered and false memories of trauma    25
    Constance J. Dalenberg and Kelsey L. Paulson

4   Early trauma, later outcome: results from longitudinal studies and clinical observations    33
    Nathan Szajnberg, Amit Goldenberg and Udi Harari

    Part 1 synopsis    43
    Alexander McFarlane

**Part 2 The effects of life trauma: mental and physical health    48**

5   Attachment dysregulation as hidden trauma in infancy: early stress, maternal buffering and psychiatric morbidity in young adulthood    48
    Jean-François Bureau, Jodi Martin and Karlen Lyons-Ruth

6   Towards a developmental trauma disorder diagnosis for childhood interpersonal trauma    57
    Bessel A. van der Kolk and Wendy d' Andrea

7   Complex adult sequelae of early life exposure to psychological trauma    69
    Julian D. Ford

8   The relationship of adverse childhood experiences to adult medical disease, psychiatric disorders and sexual behavior: implications for healthcare    77
    Vincent J. Felitti and Robert F. Anda

    Part 2 synopsis    88
    Alicia F. Lieberman

## Section 2 Biological approaches to early life trauma

**Part 3 The impact of early life trauma: psychobiological sequelae in children    95**

9   Juvenile stress as an animal model of childhood trauma    95
    Gal Richter-Levin and Shlomit Jacobson-Pick

10  Lateral asymmetries in infants' regulatory and communicative gestures    103
    Rosario Montirosso, Renato Borgatti and Ed Tronick

11  Neurobiology of childhood trauma and adversity    112
    Martin H. Teicher, Keren Rabi, Yi-Shin Sheu, Sally B. Seraphin, Susan L. Andersen, Carl M. Anderson, Jeewook Choi and Akemi Tomoda

12  The neurobiology of child neglect    123
    Michael D. De Bellis

13  Early life stress as a risk factor for disease in adulthood    133
    Philip A. Fisher and Megan Gunnar

    Part 3 synopsis    142
    Allan N. Schore

**Part 4 The impact of childhood trauma: psychobiological sequelae in adults** 148

14 Early life stress and psychiatric risk/resilience: the importance of a developmental neurobiological model in understanding gene by environment interactions 148
Kelly Skelton, Tamara Weiss and Bekh Bradley

15 The neuroendocrine effects of early life trauma 157
Jamie L. LaPrairie, Christine M. Heim and Charles B. Nemeroff

16 Long-lasting effects of childhood abuse on neurobiology 166
J. Douglas Bremner, Eric Vermetten and Ruth A. Lanius

17 Biological framework for traumatic dissociation related to early life trauma 178
Christian Schmahl, Ruth A. Lanius, Clare Pain and Eric Vermetten

18 Neurobiological factors underlying psychosocial moderators of childhood stress and trauma 189
Fatih Ozbay, Vansh Sharma, Joan Kaufman, Bruce McEwen, Dennis Charney and Steven Southwick

Part 4 synopsis 200
Sonia J. Lupien

## Section 3 Clinical perspectives: assessment and treatment of trauma spectrum disorders

**Part 5 Assessment of the impact of early life trauma: clinical science and societal effects** 207

19 Assessing the effects of early and later childhood trauma in adults 207
John Briere and Monica Hodges

20 Memory and trauma: examining disruptions in implicit, explicit and autobiographical memory 217
Melody D. Combs and Anne P. DePrince

21 Scientific progress and methodological issues in the study of recovered and false memories of trauma 225
Constance J. Dalenberg and Oxana G. Palesh

22 The psychosocial consequences of organized violence on children 234
Felicia Heidenreich, Mónica Ruiz-Casares and Cécile Rousseau

Part 5 synopsis 242
David Spiegel

**Part 6 Strategies to reduce the impact: clinical treatment** 247

23 The role of mentalizing in treating attachment trauma 247
Jon G. Allen, Peter Fonagy and Anthony Bateman

24 Pragmatic approaches to stage-oriented treatment for early life trauma-related complex post-traumatic stress and dissociative disorders 257
Richard J. Loewenstein and Victor Welzant

25 Cognitive-behavioral treatments for post-traumatic stress disorder 268
Kathleen M. Chard and Amy F. Buckley

26 Emotions and emotion regulation in the process of trauma recovery: implications for the treatment of post-traumatic stress disorder 278
Anthony Charuvastra and Marylene Cloitre

27 Psychodynamic psychotherapy: adaptations for the treatment of patients with chronic complex post-traumatic stress disorder 286
Clare Pain, Ruth A. Lanius, Pat Ogden and Eric Vermetten

Part 6 synopsis 295
Tal Astrachan, Carla Bernardes and Judith Herman

*Epilogue* 300
*Index* 303

Color plates are situated between pages 108 and 109.

# Contributors

**Jon G. Allen, PhD**
The Menninger Clinic
Houston, TX, USA

**Robert F Anda, MD, MS**
Carter Consulting Inc.
Atlanta, GA, USA

**Susan L. Andersen, PhD**
Department of Psychiatry
Harvard Medical School
Laboratory of Developmental
Neuropharmacology
McLean Hospital
Belmont, MA, USA

**Carl M. Anderson, PhD**
Department of Psychiatry
Harvard Medical School
Brain Imaging Center and
Developmental Biopsychiatry
Research Program
McLean Hospital
Belmont, MA, USA

**Wendy d' Andrea**
Trauma Center
Brookline, MA, USA

**Tal Astrachan, PsyD**
Victims of Violence Program
Department of Psychiatry
Cambridge Health Alliance
Harvard Medical School
Cambridge, MA, USA

**Anthony W. Bateman, MA, FRCPsych**
St. Ann's Hospital, Halliwick Unit
London, UK

**Carla Bernardes, PhD**
Department of Psychology
Victims of Violence Program
Cambridge Health Alliance
Harvard Medical School
Cambridge, MA, USA

**Renato Borgatti**
Department of Child and
Adolescent Neurology and Psychiatry
Scientific Institute
"E. Medea"
Lecco, Italy

**Bekh Bradley, PhD**
Atlanta VA Medical Center
Decatur, GA, USA

**J. Douglas Bremner, MD**
Departments of Psychiatry and Radiology
Emory University School of Medicine
Clinical Neuroscience Research Unit, Psychiatry &
Behavioral Science
Atlanta VAMC,
Atlanta, GA, USA

**John Briere, PhD**
Departments of Psychiatry and Psychology
Psychological Trauma Program
Keck School of Medicine
University of Southern California
Los Angeles, CA, USA

**Amy F. Buckley, Phd**
PTSD and Anxiety Disorders Division
Cincinnati VA Medical Center
Cincinnati, OH, USA

**Jean-Francois Bureau, PhD**
School of Psychology
University of Ottawa
Ottawa, ON, Canada

**Kathleen M. Chard**
PTSD and Anxiety
Disorders Division
Cincinnati VA Medical Center
Cincinnati, OH, USA

**Dennis Charney, MD**
Mount Sinai School of Medicine
Department of Psychiatry
New York, NY, USA

**Anthony Charuvastra, MD**
NYU Child Study Center Trauma and Resilience
Research Program
Nathan S. Kline Institute for Psychiatric Research
NYU Child Study Center
New York, NY, USA

**Jeewook Choi, MD, PhD**
Department of Psychiatry
The Catholic University of Korea
Daejeon St. Mary's Hospital
Jung-gu, Daejeon, Korea

**Marylene Cloitre, PhD**
Trauma and Resilience Research Program, Child
Study Center
Department of Psychiatry
New York University School of Medicine
NY, USA

**Melody D. Combs, PhD**
The Kempe Center for the Prevention and Treatment
of Child Abuse and Neglect
The Gary Pavilion at The Children's Hospital
Anschutz Medical Campus
Aurora, CO, USA

**Constance J. Dalenberg PhD**
Trauma Research Institute,
Alliant International University
San Diego, CA, USA

**Martin J. Dorahy PhD, DClinPsych**
Department of Psychology
University of Canterbury
Christchurch, New Zealand

**Michael D. De Bellis MD, MPH**
Healthy Childhood
Brain Development and Developmental
Traumatology Research Program
Department of Psychiatry and
Behavioral Sciences
Duke University Medical Center
Durham, NC, USA

**Anne P. DePrince, PhD**
University of Denver
Psychology Department
Denver, CO, USA

**Erin C. Dunn, MPH**
Harvard School of Public Health
Department of Society, Human Development, and
Health, Boston, MA, USA

**Vincent J. Felitti, MD**
Kaiser Permanente Medical Care
Program, andUniversity of California School of
Medicine
San Diego, CA, USA

**Philip A. Fisher, PhD**
Department of Psychology, University of Oregon
Senior Research Scientist, Oregon
Social Learning Center
Eugene, OR, USA

**Peter Fonagy, PhD**
The Anna Freud Centre
London, UK

**Julian D. Ford, PhD**
Department of Psychiatry
University of Connecticut
School of Medicine,
Farmington, CT, USA

**Amit Goldenberg**
Hebrew University
Mount Scopus, Jerusalem, Israel

**Megan R. Gunnar, PhD**
Institute of Child Development
University of Minnesota
Minneapolis, MN, USA

**Udi Harari**
Hebrew University
Mount Scopus, Jerusalem, Israel

**Felicia Heidenreich**
Transcultural Research and
Intervention Team (TRIT)
CSSS de la Montagne
Montréal, QC, Canada

**Christine Heim PhD**
Department of Psychiatry &
Behavioral Sciences
Emory University School of Medicine
Atlanta, GA, USA

**Judith Herman MD**
Victims of Violence Program
Department of Psychiatry
Cambridge Health Alliance
Cambridge, MA, USA

**Monica Hodges, PhD**
Department of Psychology
California State University
Long Beach CA, USA

**Shlomit Jacobson-Pick, PhD**
Institute of Neuroscience
Carleton University, Ottawa, Canada.

**Joan Kaufman, PhD**
Yale University School of Medicine
Department of Psychiatry
Yale University New Haven, CT, USA

**Karestan C. Koenen, PhD**
Harvard School of Public Health
Departments of Society, Human Development, and
Health & Epidemiology
Boston, MA, USA

**Ruth A. Lanius, MD, PhD**
Harris-Woodman Chair
Department of Psychiatry
The University of Western Ontario
London, Ontario, Canada

**Jamie L. LaPrairie MS PhD**
Emory University Department of Psychology
Women's Mental Health Program
Emory University School of Medicine
Atlanta, GA, USA

**Alicia F. Lieberman, PhD**
Department of Psychiatry
University of California San Francisco, and
Child Trauma Research Program
San Francisco General Hospital
San Francisco, CA, USA

**Richard J. Loewenstein, MD**
The Trauma Disorders Program
Sheppard Pratt Health System
Department of Psychiatry
University of Maryland School of Medicine
Baltimore, MD, USA

**Sonia J. Lupien MD**
Hôpital Louis-H. Lafontaine
Centre d'études sur le stress humain
Montréal QC, Canada

**Karlen Lyons-Ruth, PhD**
Department of Psychology
Harvard Medical School
Department of Psychiatry
Cambridge Health Alliance
Cambridge, MA, USA

**Jodi Martin, BA**
School of Psychology
University of Ottawa
Ottawa, ON, Canada

**Bruce McEwen, PhD**
The Rockefeller University
Harold and Margaret Milliken
Hatch Laboratory of Neuroendocrinology
New York, NY, USA

**Alexander C. McFarlane MB BS (Hons), MD, FRANZCP, Dip Psychotherapy**
Department of Psychiatry
CMVH University of Adelaide Node
Department of MEAO DHSP studies
The Centre for Military and
Veteransé Health
The University of Adelaide
Adelaide, Australia

**Warwick Middleton MBBS FRANZCP, MD**
School of Public Health,
La Trade University
Trauma and Dissociation Unit
Belmont Hospital, Bristane
Queensland, Australia

**Rosario Montirosso**
Department of Child and Adolescent
Neurology and Psychiatry
Scientific Institute
"E. Medea," Lecco, Italy

**Charles B. Nemeroff, PhD**
Department of Psychiatry &
Behavioral Sciences
Emory University School of Medicine
Atlanta, GA, USA

**Pat Ogden, PhD**
Sensorimotor Psychotherapy Institute
Boulder, CO, USA

**Fatih Ozbay, MD**
Mount Sinai School of Medicine
Department of Psychiatry
New York, NY, USA

**Clare Pain MD, MSc, FRCPC**
Department of Psychiatry, University of Toronto
Psychological Trauma Program, Mount Sinai
Hospital, Toronto Addis Ababa Psychiatry Project
(TAAPP), Toronto Addis Ababa
Academic Collaboration (TAAAC) Mount Sinai
Hospital, Joseph and Wolf Lebovic Health Complex
room 934,Toronto, ON, Canada

**Kelsey Paulson**
Alliant International University
San Diego, CA, USA

**Oxana G. Palesh, PhD, MPH**
Department of Radiation Oncology and
Department of Psychiatry
University of Rochester Medical Center
James P. Wilmot Cancer Center
Rochester, NY, USA

**Ms. Keren Rabi**
Massachusetts School of Professional Psychology
Child and Adolescent Program
McLean Hospital
Belmont, MA,USA

**Gal Richter-Levin, PhD**
Department of Neurobiology and Ethology and
Department of Psychology University of Haifa, Haifa
31905 Israel

**Andrea L. Roberts, PhD**
Harvard School of Public Health
Department of Society,
Human Development, and Health
Boston, MA, USA

**Cécile Rousseau, MD**
Department of Psychiatry
McGill University
Montréal, QC, Canada

**Cécile Rousseau, MD**
Division of Social and Cultural Psychiatry
McGill University
Transcultural Research and
Intervention Team (TRIT)
Youth Mental Health
CSSS de la Montagne
Montréal, QC, Canada

**Monica Ruiz-Casares**
Transcultural Research and
Intervention Team (TRIT)
CSSS de la Montagne
Montréal, QC, Canada

**Christian Schmahl, MD**
Department of Psychosomatic Medicine and
Psychotherapy, Central Institute of Mental Health
Mannheim, Germany

**Allan N. Schore, PhD**
Department of Psychiatry and
Biobehavioral Sciences
University of California at Los Angeles
David Geffen School of Medicine
Northridge, CA, USA

**Sally B. Seraphin, PhD**
Developmental Biopsychiatry Research Program
McLean Hospital
Belmont, MA, USA

**Vansh Sharma, MD**
Mount Sinai School of Medicine
Department of Psychiatry
New York, NY, USA

**Yi-Shin Sheu, BS**
Psychological and Brain Sciences Program
The Johns Hopkins University
Baltimore, MD,USA

**Kelly Skelton, MD, PhD**
Atlanta VA Medical Center
Decatur, GA, USA

**Steven Southwick, MD**
Yale University School of Medicine
Department of Psychiatry
New Haven, CT, USA

**David Spiegel, MD**
Department of Psychiatry &
Behavioral Sciences
Stanford University School of Medicine
Stanford, CA, USA

**Deborah M. Stone, ScD, MSW, MPH**
Harvard School of Public Health
Department of Society, Human
Development, and Health
Boston, MA, USA

**Nathan Szajnberg, MD**
Hebrew University
Mount Scopus, Jerusalem, Israel

**Martin H. Teicher, MD, PhD**
Department of Psychiatry
Harvard Medical School
Developmental Biopsychiatry Research Program
McLean Hospital
Belmont, MA, USA

**Akemi Tomoda, MD, PhD**
Department of Child Development
Faculty of Life Sciences
Kumamoto University, Japan

**Ed Tronick, PhD**
Child Development Unit
Children's Hospital Boston
Boston, MA, USA

**Onno van der Hart, PhD**
Department of Clinical and
Health Psychology
Utrecht University, Utrecht
Netherlands

**Bessel A. van der Kolk, MD**
Department of Psychiatry
Boston University School of Medicine
Trauma Center, Brookline, MA, USA

**Eric Vermetten, MD, PhD**
Research Military Mental Health
Central Military Hospital
UMC Utrecht, Rudolf Magnus Institute of
Neuroscience
Utrecht, Netherlands

**Tamara Weiss, MD**
Department of Psychiatry and
Behavioral Sciences
Emory University School of Medicine
Atlanta, GA, USA

**Victor Welzant, PsyD**
Private Practice
Towson, MD, USA

# Foreword

*In my beginning is my end.*

T. S. Eliot, *Four Quartets*

If you were given a newborn infant with all his or her extraordinary potential, and were directed to turn that infant into a school shooter in 15 years, or a mainlining addict in 20, how would you do that? In spite of distaste for the question, obviously at some level we know how to do that. A more general and less disturbing question is *how* do we get to be who we are as human beings – and as patients? That general question has been with us since ancient times. Gods and fate were our explanation throughout most of history. The answer has been refined in relatively recent times, actually coextensive with the quite recent time line of the germ theory, first by poets and then by psychoanalysts, who helped us to see how human development is powerfully influenced by emotionally traumatic early life experiences. More recently still, epidemiologists and neurobiologists have led the explorations.

Traumatic events of the earliest years of infancy and childhood are not lost but, like a child's footprints in wet cement, are often preserved lifelong. Time does not heal the wounds that occur in those earliest years; time conceals them. They are not lost; they are embodied. Only in recent decades has the magnitude of the problem of developmentally damaged humans begun to be recognized and understood. The limits of that understanding, and the resistance to it, are captured well in this book's title, *The Hidden Epidemic*. There is in those words the obvious implication of something causing a serious and widespread threat to health and well-being, but they also offer a paradox, subtly leading us to wonder *why* an epidemic would be hidden, and how? Compared with the questions asked during most of human history, and even those asked today by physicians in their medical histories, the questions of *The Hidden Epidemic* are extraordinary and bold.

*The Impact of Early Life Trauma on Health and Disease: The Hidden Epidemic* summarizes our current approaches to understanding how we get to be the people we are: not only as biological entities, but also as truly human beings with an outer persona and an inner soul. Just as we observe how a leg damaged in childhood sometimes does not grow to its full potential, this book asks *how* does a persona or a soul become damaged? Why are we all not perfect, or at least similar? Why are only some of us suicides, or addicts, or obese, or criminals? Why do some of us die early while others live long? What is the nature of the scream on the other side of silence? What does it mean that some memories are unspeakable, forgotten or lost in amnesia – and does it matter? Is there a hidden price being paid for this comfort of remaining unaware? What are the basic causes of these phenomena, and what are the mechanisms by which they occur? Do our current ways of medical understanding limit us as physicians? Are they actually a part of the problem? One of the authors proposes a new diagnostic strategy that involves considering the very earliest external influences, certainly including parenting, a role of enormous power whether by its presence, absence or dysfunctional performance. Other authors provide evidence that some of our most common problems in biomedicine and mental health are the result of unconsciously attempted solutions to problems dating back to the earliest years, but hidden by time, by shame, by secrecy and by social taboos against exploring certain areas of life experience. It is becoming evident that traumatic life experiences during childhood and adolescence are far more common than usually recognized, are complexly inter-related and are associated decades later in a strong and proportionate manner to outcomes that are important to medical practice, public health and the social fabric of a nation.

Biomedical researchers have helped us to recognize that childhood events, specifically abuse and emotional trauma even in the earliest years, have profound and enduring effects on the neuroregulatory systems mediating medical illness as well as social behavior from childhood into adult life. Our understanding of the connection between emotional trauma in childhood and the pathways to biomedical and psychopathology in adulthood is still being formed as neuroscientists begin to describe the changes that take place on the molecular level as a result of events or ongoing states of life that occurred hours, months or decades earlier.

The editors have paid attention to all parts of our enquiry into the significance of the earliest years of human development: to the roles of abuse and attachment, to genetics and to the epigenetic effects of parenting and other experiences of early life that lead to phenotypic plasticity, to the distinctly partial process of resiliency, and to diagnosis and treatment. The chapter authors, a mix of the internationally distinguished and those on a clearly rising trajectory, provide a blend of clinical observation and highly specific technical information in this bold attempt to bring together what is becoming known by clinical study and by sophisticated technical approaches such as functional imaging. They help us to see how neuroscience and biological psychiatry are now identifying the intermediary mechanisms by which clinical states manifest themselves. The turning point in modern understanding of the role of trauma in medical and psychiatric pathology is commonly credited to Freud, who lived within the lifetimes of many of us, as did Rene Spitz and Harry Harlow with their groundbreaking work on maternal deprivation. Would that they had lived a bit longer to see where we are taking their work.

We are beginning to have remarkable insight into how we become what we are as individuals and as a nation. This understanding is important medically, socially and economically. Indeed, it has given us reason to reconsider the very structure of medical, public health, and social services practice in the USA. We are even beginning to see some of our diagnoses as medical constructs, artifacts resulting from medical blindness to the social realities of life experiences, especially those of infancy and early childhood.

One hopes we will do ourselves proud in these years following the "decade of the brain." But, as with any major advance in knowledge, there is risk of misunderstanding and misuse. T. S. Eliot described this risk in his lines from *The Rock*:

Where is the wisdom we have lost in knowledge?
Where is the knowledge we have lost in information?

As physicians, we typically focus our attention on tertiary consequences, far downstream, while primary causes are well protected by time, by social convention and by taboo. We have often limited ourselves to the smallest part of the problem, that part in which we are erudite and comfortable as mere prescribers of medication, or users of impressive technologies. The hidden epidemic is a problem not only for psychiatry,

but also for medicine and for society in general. Perhaps greater than the risk of misunderstanding or misusing what we are learning is the risk of comfortably not using it at all. Integration of these new discoveries into everyday medical practice is our next big step. Accomplishing that will broaden our experience base sufficiently to allow the beginning of primary prevention for much of physical and mental illness. One already suspects from some of the chapters in this volume that improving parenting skills will be a core feature of primary prevention in the future of medicine and psychiatry.

To the degree that we do not figure out how to integrate this knowledge into everyday clinical practice, we contribute to the problem by authenticating as biomedical disease that which is actually the somatic inscription of life experience on to the human body and brain. The influence of childhood experience, including often-unrecognized traumatic events, is as powerful as Freud and his colleagues originally described it to be. That influence is long lasting, and the researchers in this volume are now describing the intermediary mechanisms, the neural pathways, that these stressors activate for their clinical manifestation. Unfortunately, and in spite of these findings, the biopsychosocial model and the biomedical models of psychiatry remain largely at odds rather than taking advantage of the new discoveries to reinforce each other.

Many of our most intractable public health problems are the result of compensatory behaviors such as smoking, overeating, promiscuity, and alcohol and drug use, which provide immediate partial relief from emotional problems caused by traumatic childhood experiences. That relationship is straightforward: early trauma to depression or anxiety, to obesity, to diabetes, to heart disease; trauma to smoking, to emphysema or lung cancer. But, apart from various common compensatory actions, the chronic life stress of the underlying developmental life experiences is generally unrecognized and hence unappreciated as a second and separate etiological mechanism underlying many biomedical diseases.

In a convincing call for a new theory, *The Hidden Epidemic* provides the credible basis for a new paradigm of medical, public health, and social service practice that would start with comprehensive biopsychosocial evaluation of all patients. It has been demonstrated that this approach is acceptable to patients, can be affordable, and is beneficial in multiple ways. The potential gain is huge, and is of major significance at a time when there is great political interest in the cost and processes of medical care. Also huge is the likelihood of clinician and institutional resistance to this change. Actualizing the benefits of this paradigm shift will depend on first identifying and resolving the various bases for resistance to it. In reality, this will require far more planning than would be needed to introduce a purely intellectual or technical advance. However, our experience suggests that it can be done. Doing so will likely be the major public health advance of our time.

Vincent J. Felitti
Kaiser Permanente Medical Care Program,
San Diego
Clinical Professor of Medicine,
University of California

# Acknowledgements

We began working on this book in the spring of 2006 after a memorable lunch in New York. For some years, the three of us had been attending conferences, where we listened to and met senior colleagues in the fields of developmental psychology, epidemiology, genetics, attachment theory, clinical psychiatry, sociology, and neuroscience. Their commitment to the study and research of early life trauma inspired us to capture and integrate it in this edited book. We have tried to present our author's material in a new manner that organizes and simplifies the content areas to be reader friendly. The book has three sections, and each section is divided into two parts. After each part there is a synopsis, each written by senior authors who have reviewed, commented, and reflected on the respective chapters in each section. These synopses serve as "salt and pepper" for the book.

We would like to acknowledge and thank our colleagues for their generous mentoring, teaching, and research. Many of them kindly submitted a chapter for the book. We thank Douglas Bremner for his phrase "the hidden epidemic" which we have included in the title. We also thank Cambridge University Press who trusted us to provide them with a book to print. Special thanks also to the staff at Cambridge University Press, including Pauline Graham, Betty Fulford, Laura Wood, Joanna Souter, Mark Boyd, Jane Ward, and Joanna Endell-Cooper, who, at various stages of the production process, provided their expertise and assistance. We are much indebted to Richard Marley who allowed us a significant increase in the word allowance which gives this volume the weight it now has. A very special thanks goes to Nancy Mazza for her superb assistance in the various stages of the project, and to Gabriel Shapiro who kindly and expertly worked on the first round of edits.

We also want to recognize our own students who have taught us to be better teachers, and most importantly, we acknowledge our patients to whom this book is dedicated. They have inspired us with their courage in the face of suffering and their perseverance towards recovery.

It is our hope that this book will go toward improving the recognition, assessment, treatment, pedagogy, ongoing research, and public health response to the prevention of early life trauma and reduce the deleterious effects of this hidden epidemic.

London, Utrecht, Toronto
May 14, 2010
Ruth Lanius
Eric Vermetten
Clare Pain

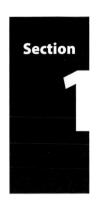

**Section**

**1**

# Early life trauma: impact on health and disease

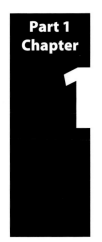
# The history of early life trauma and abuse from the 1850s to the current time: how the past influences the present

Martin J. Dorahy, Onno van der Hart and Warwick Middleton

…there are few topics in modern life that are more repugnant to consider than the abuse of a child by the very persons entrusted with his care

K. B. Oettinger (1968, p. v) [1]

While the etiological significance of early trauma and abuse for mental health difficulties has long been on the periphery of psychological thought, it has rarely taken center stage. On those occasions where it has drawn interest (e.g., the 1890s), the importance of early trauma and abuse has been resisted, rebuked and recanted, leaving its prominence to dwindle. Understanding the history of early trauma and abuse requires an appreciation of the social and political processes that govern society [2]. To limit early trauma and abuse of children to enactments by adults seeking satisfaction for perverse desires de-emphasizes societal attitudes and decrees responsible for much of the harsh and brutal treatment of children [3]. Dispute and disbelief often follow suggestions that violence within society perpetrated by those ordained to protect has a lasting impact.

Noting the resistance that acceptance of child maltreatment and its enduring effects have, this chapter outlines the history of child abuse and neglect in the medical and mental health fields. It is noteworthy that Tardieu's initial concern with physical abuse in the mid 1800s [4,5] gave way to a greater focus on child sexual abuse in the late 1800s, and that Caffey's and Kempe's work on physical maltreatment in the mid 1900s [6–10] led to much greater attention on sexual abuse in the 1980s and early 1990s. The focus on sexual abuse has been supplanted by an enhanced appreciation of multiple forms of abuse and neglect and their potentially deleterious effects on physical and mental health.

Despite progress in social awareness and scientific understanding, acknowledgement of the existence and impact of child maltreatment is continually threatened by a propensity to deny and disavow [11,12], an historical theme that recurs repeatedly in the literature reviewed in this chapter.

## From the 1850s to publications about sexual abuse

In reviewing the history of childhood, DeMause [13] outlined six modes of childrearing that he believes have characterized the association between parenting and abuse. He argued that these have evolved from the "infanticidal" mode to the "socialization" mode. The "infanticidal" mode is characterized by extreme inhumane treatment, where children were socially sanctioned as sexual and sacrificial objects. The "socialization" mode, the mode currently most dominant, sees children still exposed to considerable levels of violence, but within the home there is a greater level of socialization rather than brutality in their education. DeMause suggested that future generations will evolve to the final mode of 'helping', where the parents support the children to reach their own rather than the parents' goals. The fledgling nature of more humane parental practices in the 1800s may have led clinicians in their private practices to become aware of the pathological outcomes of trauma, even if some shied away from causal explanations.

In 1860, Ambroise Tardieu published the first paper directly related to the abuse of children, entitled "Étude Médico-Légale sur les Sévices et Mauvais Traitements Exercés sur des Enfants" (Medico-legal studies on cruelty and ill-treatment upon infants) [4]. He noted (p. 361; quoted by Masson in 1984, p. 18 [14]):

> [a]mong the numerous and very diverse facts which make up the medico-legal history of blows and wounds, there is one that forms a group completely separate from the rest. These facts, which until now have remained in total obscurity, deserve, for more than one reason, to be brought to the light of day. I am speaking of the facts of cruelty and brutal treatment of which children are particularly the victims and which derive from their parents, their teachers, from those, in a word, who exercise more or less direct authority over them.

He outlined in this work 32 cases, the majority of which were children under 10 and had the parent as the primary perpetrator. This paper identified forms of what would now be described as childhood physical abuse, as well as outlining childhood physical neglect, including starvation and other types of deprivation. Tardieu graphically presented cases of brutality and torture including severe and persistent beatings with various implements (e.g., whips, batons) and burns resulting from red-hot irons and corrosive substances. Abuses chronicled by Tardieu had led to death in over half the cases presented. Tardieu indicated that abusive parents often attempt to explain away their child's injuries as the results of an accident sustained during play or in some other innocuous way. Knight [15] has argued that Tardieu's paper contains most of the features accepted as part of the spectrum of child abuse present today.

While Tardieu focused heavily on the physical abuse of children in his 1860 paper [4], he was not ignorant of the existence, frequency and brutality of child sexual abuse, as indicated in other works. As Masson [14] outlined in some detail, Tardieu's book *Étude Médico-légale sur les Attentats aux Moeurs* (*A Medico-legal Study of Assaults on Decency*), published in its seventh and final edition in 1878 [5], details the sexual abuse of children, primarily by their fathers. Many of the cases referred to very young girls from the first few years of life to middle childhood. In early editions of the book (e.g., 4th edition, 1862), he outlined several hundred cases of child sexual abuse. Cunningham [2] pointed out that Tardieu "was the first to investigate and publish his findings on intrafamilial sexual abuse of children" (p. 346). Masson [14] suggested that, while the topic of sexual abuse was unpopular and evoked theories regarding "simulation" and children pretending to be abused for secondary gain, some French physicians from the second half of the nineteenth century accepted

the child's testament of what had been inflicted upon them, as well as the supportive physical evidence that was often present.

Around the time of Tardieu's early work on abuse, Paul Briquet [16] challenged a belief that had persisted for two and a half millennia: hysteria affected only women and resulted from the uterus, or toxins from the uterus, periodically travelling to the brain [17]. Unlike the medico-legal perspective that was the focus for Tardieu and his predecessors and that charted the physical injuries of those abused, Briquet was more interested in psychopathology.[1] The description of the disorder which subsequently bore his name is filled with anecdotal references to domestic violence and child abuse, hinting at their etiological significance for mental ill-health [16]. Of the 87 cases of hysteria in children under the age of 12, Briquet stated that one-third had been "habitually maltreated or held constantly in fear, or had been directed harshly by their parents" [16]. In another 10%, the children's symptoms were attributed to traumatic experiences other than parental abuse. Briquet came to the conclusion that hysteria was caused by "the effect of violent emotions, protracted sorrows, family conflicts, and frustrated love, upon predisposed and hypersensitive persons" (Ellenberger, 1970, p. 142 [18]). In 501 hysterical patients, he found traumatic childhood experiences, often sexual abuse, in just over 75% [19].

Jean Martin Charcot (1825–1893) accepted Briquet's findings that hysteria did not have its origins in the unfulfilled sexual needs of women but fell short of attributing early trauma as etiologically important in hysteria [20]. As Masson [14] discovered, Charcot accepted the existence of childhood sexual abuse and co-authored a little-known paper [21] that focused on the psychopathology of perpetrators. While Charcot largely avoided exploring the impact of childhood trauma on victims, he recognized that traumatizing events, including child abuse in women and work-related accidents in men, were evident in many of his hysteria patients. For example, he noted childhood sexual abuse in his patient Augustine, who re-enacted experiences of rape during hysterical "attacks," but he

---

[1] Cunningham [2] made it clear that while Tardieu was interested in the physical consequences of abuse he also realized that abuse could occur without identifiable physical repercussion and abuse broadly could have a significant impact on psychological functioning, with the residue including feelings of shame and terror.

gave it no etiological significance [20–23]. He maintained that the primary reason for their condition was constitutional weakness. He considered work-related traumatization an "agent provocateur for constitutional vulnerabilities" in males suffering from so-called traumatic hysteria [22].

Pierre Janet (1859–1947) also included constitutional factors in his view on the development of hysteria, but he regarded traumatic experiences – and, therefore, the existence of traumatic memories – as a major etiological factor. In 1925, he wrote: "Directly or indirectly, [the traumatic memory] was the cause of some of the symptoms of the disease" (p. 590), in both hysteria and psychasthenia (the other broad class of mental disorders that Janet distinguished). Of the 591 cases described in Janet's first four major clinical works, 257 involved some degree of traumatization [19]. The traumas experienced by Janet's patients included traumatic loss, witnessing violent death, incest, rape, physical abuse in childhood and traffic accidents. His publications do not show a specific interest in child abuse and neglect, and he may actually have overlooked this background in some of his patients. However, he regarded inadequate childrearing practices, either in combination with traumatic experiences or in their own right, as factors that may contribute to the development of mental disorders [24].

Such was the power of Freud's conviction in the role of incestuous childhood trauma (a view shared by Binet and other French luminaries) that in an 1896 paper [25] which represented a synopsis of the ideas expanded shortly after in "The aetiology of hysteria," he noted the nature and timing of sexual childhood trauma required for later psychological difficulties, namely hysteria. He stated, *"…sexual traumas must have occurred in early childhood (before puberty), and their content must consist of an actual irritation of the genitals (of processes resembling copulation)"* (p. 163, italics in original). In "The aetiology of hysteria," Freud [26] further specified that sexual trauma between the ages of 1 and 8 years is required for hysterical symptoms to develop (i.e., sexual experiences "date … back, into the third or fourth, or even second year of life … a person who has not had sexual experiences … [before 8] can no longer become disposed to hysteria…" p. 212). In the 18 cases (6 men, 12 women) that form the data for the childhood sexual experience theory of hysteria, Freud outlined the origin and characteristics of three different trauma types associated with eventual symptom development. The first is an isolated

sexual assault committed by a relative stranger. The second grouping is sexual experiences at the hands of carers, including "close relatives"[2] (p. 208), and which were generally more chronic in nature. Finally, he noted sexual relationships between two children, often brother and sister, and often being the direct result of the brother re-enacting his own sexual abuse experiences on his sister [26].

Two years after "The aetiology of hysteria," Freud hinted at doubts about the early sexual etiology of hysteria in a letter to Fliess in August 1897 [28], and further articulated them in a follow-up letter a little over a month later [27]. However, Freud never fully recanted his belief that real child sexual abuse by the father was not etiologically related to later psychological difficulties.[3] For example, in a footnote added in 1924 to his 1896 paper [31], "Further remarks on the neuropsychosis of defence," Freud notes:

> This section is dominated by an error which I have since repeatedly acknowledged and corrected. At that time [1896] I was not yet able to distinguish between my patients' phantasies about their childhood years and their real recollections. As a result, I attributed to the aetiological factor of seduction a significance and universality which it does not possess … Nevertheless, we need not reject everything written in the text above. *Seduction retains a certain aetiological importance, and even today I think some of these psychological comments are to the point* (p. 168, italics added).

Freud's dwindling faith from 1897 in the role of sexual trauma in psychopathology development, along with his growing theoretical formulations concerning oedipal fantasy, shifted focus away from the impact of child abuse. It provided one framework for professionals and society at large to distance themselves from the reality and shame of adults' exploitative actions towards children. Interestingly, while around the turn of the century Freud's belief in the impact of childhood sexual abuse had greatly diminished, interest in other forms of child maltreatment remained.

---

[2] Freud did not explicitly state the father here, though seemingly had this in mind, as evidenced in his quoted correspondence with Fliess in 1897 [27].

[3] Kris [29] was later to term as the "seduction theory" Freud's belief in the etiological significance of child sexual abuse for hysteria. The use of the term "seduction," which Freud himself used, seems to curiously understate child sexual abuse by an adult when associated with terms such as "win over" or "attract" but more fully captures the power differential and cruel maltreatment when associated with terms such a "betrayal" "corrupt" and "dishonour" [30].

In 1899, the Vienna newspapers focused increasingly on cases of parents who had murdered or tortured their children [32]. Socially, child physical abuse was in the foreground, but this largely failed to ignite professional interest in the psychological sequalae of such maltreatment:

- initial focus on harsh childrearing practices and physical maltreatment preceded significant psychological interest in child sexual abuse
- the traumatic etiology of hysteria was largely replaced by fantasy.

## From 1900 to publications about physical abuse

Psychoanalysis' emphasis on fantasy did not go completely unchallenged by analysts. Perhaps most famously, Ferenczi in 1949 [33] espoused the frequency and reality of child sexual abuse as a central etiological factor in the development of neurosis. His paper "Confusion of tongues between adults and the child" was originally presented at the 1932 International Psycho-Analytic Congress, and Ferenczi implored those present to be open not only to the reality of sexual abuse narratives in their patients but also to ways in which they (the analysts) inadvertently suppressed such narratives. Yet the cultural tension within the analytic movement created by such suggestions meant that Ferenczi's paper was initially withheld from publication by Freud's intellectual guardian, Ernest Jones [34].

With psychoanalysis dominating clinical psychological thought for much of the first half of the twentieth century, the etiological significance of early trauma was largely confined to a footnote. In some areas of psychiatry, the effects of childhood trauma, such as those pertaining to what was then called multiple personality, were not entirely forgotten. Janet was very mindful of the effects of early trauma in many of his dissociative patients [35,36]. Moreover, Barresi [37] proposed that Prince's case work shows that childhood traumas other than sexual and physical abuse could have profound effects on psychological functioning. He explored in depth Prince's second case of multiple personality (BCA) and indicated the traumatic experience that laid the foundations for later psychological problems. He also noted that others have suggested that the etiological foundations for severe problems in Prince's first case of multiple personality (Miss Beauchamp [38]) was the loss of a brother in childhood. Modern theory might speculate on the nature of disrupted attachment associated with such loss. These historical accounts highlight the importance of not limiting the potentially damaging effects of childhood trauma to sexual and physical victimization at the hands of caregivers.

After Freud's shift away from seduction and prior to the mid 1900s, the little interest that psychological trauma generated as an etiological variable was dominated by the horrors of war, given the human cost of World Wars I and II [39,40]. Yet, even these massive traumas failed to capture the collective minds of psychological scientists and the general population. This may have been partially because of the dominance of Freud's intrapsychic fantasy model, Babinski's "simulation" model (which promoted suggestibility rather than trauma as a cause of hysterical disturbance) and the German emphasis on secondary gain (e.g., compensation) in the creation and maintenance of combat-related difficulties [12].

It took pediatric interest in the medically unexplainable physical injuries of children to revive awareness of child maltreatment. Growing medical attention to the phenomenon and cause of pediatric subdural hematomas (e.g., Ingraham & Heyl [41] and Sherwood [42]) lead Caffey [6, 7] to profile the histories and physical injuries in such cases. In the six case reports he presented, all had multiple fractures to large bones in the arms and legs. Perhaps understandably reticent at that point to go beyond the data he had, Caffey suggested that all fractures seemed to be the result of physical trauma, but that the origin and "causal mechanism remain obscure" (p. 173). He suspected child physical abuse in all cases, noting that new fractures appeared shortly after the child was discharged from hospital and returned home. However, in only one case did he more explicitly state parental "intentional ill-treatment" (p. 172). Caffey's work continued to focus on trauma as an origin for these grave physical injuries [7]. However, his attention was not on sadistic, brutal and wilful parenting practices, such as direct, aggressive and powerful physical blows to the infant's body. Rather, he was concerned with what he saw as the very common practice of shaking infants and engaging in other physical practices, deemed by parents and physicians at that time as relatively innocuous, but which were responsible for death, physical injury and severe abnormal neurological development in many cases [8]. The 1960s brought with it a greater focus on direct and intentional child maltreatment, courtesy of changes at a social level:

- while psychoanalytic thinking was largely focused on sexual fantasy, several key figures and those studying multiple personality continued to see the etiological relevance of child trauma
- interest in the physical impact of brutal parenting was re-awoken by pediatric investigators.

## From 1960 to publications about child abuse and neglect

The 1960s saw an increase in social awareness of child maltreatment conforming with the plea of Fontana et al. [43] in 1963 that "[s]ociety must acknowledge that the problem of child abuse and neglect does exist" (p. 1393). The breaking through into social consciousness of the reality of childhood trauma was largely linked to social changes arising from more professionals working with children and families, and to the liberation of women from the domestic realm, with their movement into occupations providing insights and perspectives that had been largely missing from social influence [44]. These social changes, according to Finkelhor [44], brought with them moral changes that impacted on child maltreatment and included the idea that love, not strict and harsh discipline, was more effective for socialization and emotional development.

While the occurrence of child maltreatment had been evident in the medical literature prior to the mid 1900s, Parton [45] argued that it was not until this time that it was considered a social problem. This view originally arose in the USA and then expanded to other parts of the world. Parton believed that the discovery of child abuse as a social problem was dependent on the development of diagnostic radiology in pediatric medicine. Knight [15] has provided a case published by West in 1888 [46] of several children from one family showing injuries that were consistent with severe physical abuse, but for which the medical professionals developed other theories, including rickets and syphilis. Knight suggested that child abuse would have been brought into the diagnostic frame if radiological equipment had of been available at that time. From the publications of Caffey [6,8] onwards, the structural damage resulting from physical assaults by caregivers could be clearly seen, as noted by Kempe et al. [10]: "To the informed physician, the bones tell a story the child is too young or too frightened to tell" (p. 18).

Kempe and colleagues [10] put child physical abuse on the medical radar by proposing the term battered child syndrome. They defined it as "… a clinical condition in young children [usually younger than 3] who have received serious physical abuse, generally from a parent or foster parent" (p. 17). The term captured the extant literature on physical abuse at that time and indicated the primary dominance of physical abuse as a focus for child maltreatment investigation. Finkelhor [44] noted, "What the Kempe work signalled … was that influential medical professionals had joined the ranks of those advocating for child protection and were prepared to lead a new social movement to greatly expand governmental activity in this area" (p. xii). To define a more inclusive range of maltreatment and neglect types, the term battered child[4] or battered baby, as it became known in the UK [45], was eventually changed to "child abuse and neglect." This term stressed the pervasive and perhaps permanent adverse effects on emotional well-being and psychological and physical development [47].

The emphasis on child sexual abuse so prominent in the late 1800s was largely absent from discussion by the pioneers of child physical abuse during the mid 1900s. Various forms of physical abuse and neglect were described, and emotional neglect was even in the frame. Yet, sexual abuse tended to be excluded from the list of events described under child maltreatment. Fontana et al. [43] perhaps best captured this omission when they note, "[t]he neglect and abuse of children denotes a situation ranging from the deprivation of food, clothing, shelter and parental love to incidents in which children are physically abused and mistreated by an adult, resulting in obvious physical trauma to the child, and, unfortunately, often leading to death" (p. 1389). While professionals and society may have been more readily open to believing that parents could physically and emotionally maltreat their children, greater change was required before the existence and effects of sexual abuse could be revisited. Even key psychiatric texts in the mid 1970s grossly underestimated the prevalence of incest and trivialized its malignant impact on the victims (e.g., Freeman et al. [48]).

Following the impetus created in the 1960s, a string of influential publications in the 1970s and early 1980s ensured that child abuse and neglect became serious topics of professional and academic endeavor, and

[4] Various terms were proposed around this time to describe physical injury in children from caregivers, including not only the battered child syndrome [10], but maltreatment syndrome in children [43] and parent–infant stress syndrome [8]. The use of the term syndrome indicated the medicalization of the experience of child physical abuse and neglect.

further raised social awareness of their presence and impact [9,49–54]. Amongst these were scholarly papers on child sexual abuse, some of which became prominent in the literature thanks partly to the influence of the women's liberation movement on social attitudes and awareness of the victimization of women [11]. The 1980s to early 1990s saw both increased reporting and increased interest in child sexual abuse (e.g., Berliner & Elliott [55]).

The renewed interest in a professional sexual abuse literature has so far survived attempts to undermine it. These include challenges put forward by such organizations as the False Memory Syndrome Foundation. As society in the 1980s began to grapple with the real extent of child abuse, and child sexual abuse in particular, it was perhaps inevitable that society's resistance became more organized. In the early to mid 1990s, societal counter-transference responses to childhood trauma began to encompass two extremes: those who denied it, minimized it, or who as perpetrators had vested interests in discrediting its investigation; and those who so strongly identified with abuse victims that they progressively lost objectivity. Polarized views on the existence and effect of child abuse have now shifted to a more middle ground.

Interestingly, the relatively selective focus on child sexual abuse in the 1980s and 1990s has not yet given way to disinterest and paradigm shift as it did in the late 1880s, nor has it further increased polarized perspective taking. Rather, it has created a greater appreciation and investigation of other forms of abuse and neglect. For example, the study of emotional abuse, emotional neglect and exposure to domestic violence as particular forms of trauma warranting investigation in their own rights has become more prominent [56,57].

With the tide of interest still high, contemporary studies of the incidence and prevalence of various forms of childhood abuse have become more sophisticated in an attempt to determine the scale of the problem with greater accuracy [58–60]. For example, in coalescing 16 studies of non-clinical participants, primarily on child sexual abuse in adults, Gorey and Leslie [61] found a prevalence of 14.5% in women and 7.2% in men. These figures were derived after excluding the amplifying effects of low response rate and a broad definition of abuse (e.g., non-contact, exhibitionism). Using a very large nationally representative sample, with tightly defined definitions of abuse, Cappelleri *et al.* [62] found an incidence rate over a 3 month period in 1986 of 2.11 per 1000 for child sexual abuse

and 4.95 per 1000 for child physical abuse. Numerous studies dating from the early 1980s have demonstrated that from 40% to over 70% of psychiatric inpatients will give a history of childhood sexual and/or physical abuse when enquiry is made [63–66]. Similar trends have been reported with psychiatric outpatients.

In addition to effects to achieve more accurate determination of the epidemiology of child abuse, research is documenting the psychological and physical effects of early trauma. DeMause [67] provided a relatively comprehensive list of difficulties found to be associated with early abuse, including: "Severe somatic reactions, depersonalisation, self-hatred, hysterical seizures, depression, borderline personality formation, promiscuity, sexual dysfunction, suicide, self-mutilation, night terrors and flashbacks, multiple personalities [i.e., dissociative identities], post-traumatic stress disorders, delinquency, bulimia, and the overall stunting of feelings and capacities" (p.140). More recently, explanatory frameworks have been offered for the etiological role of early trauma in a range of psychological difficulties [68–70]. Research has also expanded beyond mental health, implicating child maltreatment and early trauma as etiologically significant in a range of physical health problems, including liver and heart disease (Ch. 8).

Just as developments in technology from the 1940s assisted the identification of physical abuse, various technological advances in observing and analyzing the brain have allowed the structural and functional effects of child abuse to be examined. Various chapters in this volume have reviewed this work (e.g., Chs. 11 and 12):

- physical abuse dominated clinical interest in the mid 1900s
- sexual abuse dominated clinical interest in the late 1990s
- a broad interest in various forms of child maltreatment is now evident.

# The tenuous existence of child maltreatment

As Herman [11] observed, the recognition and interest in trauma broadly and child abuse specifically have always fought powerful social and psychological forces aimed at suppressing them: "The knowledge of horrible events periodically intrudes into public awareness but is rarely retained for long. Denial, repression and dissociation operate on a social as well as an individual level" (p. 2). DeMause [71] has chronicled the professional resistance and personal attacks aimed at him by colleagues in various academic disciplines for developing a theoretical framework and accruing supporting evidence suggesting that the history of childhood is less than rosy, with trauma and abuse the norm rather than exception. Kempe and colleagues [10] noted the reluctance of professionals to acknowledge physical abuse as a cause of injury, despite radiological evidence.

As a result, the proliferation of research on child maltreatment since the 1960s should not be interpreted as the end of professional skepticism regarding the significant effects of child relational trauma. The drive to ignore or attack the importance of current and past child maltreatment remains evident in many areas of mental health practice. For example, while biological factors undoubtedly play a significant role in many cases of psychosis, there is an abundance of evidence supporting the impact of early trauma on the development of psychosis (see Read *et al.* [72]), yet biological accounts in isolation still dominate treatment and teaching on the etiology of psychosis [73]. Early abuse and trauma, if implicated at all, are seen as secondary to biological factors, rather than as primary enablers for psychotic disturbance. Just as the research findings do not support childhood abuse and neglect as the only pathway to psychosis, there is no compelling evidence to suggest that biological models satisfactorily account for all psychosis (e.g., Ross [73]). Acceptance and acknowledgement of explanations more consistent with empirical findings needs to overcome what societal attention to child abuse and neglect has always had to overcome: society's desire for minimization and denial.

- the existence and effect of child maltreatment is perpetually fighting for acceptance against powerful psychological and social processes set to deny, ignore or undermining it

## Summary and conclusion

References to childhood trauma from Tardieu's early work focused on physical abuse in the mid 1800s. Later that century, and with a shift from the physical to psychological consequences of early trauma, the literature was dominated by a central etiological focus on sexual abuse. A similar pattern occurred in the mid 1900s. The literature, which refocused attention on the importance of childhood trauma and set the trajectory for a greater appreciation and acceptance of childhood

adversity in health and mental health problems, was dominated by accounts of physical abuse [74]. The role of sexual childhood trauma began to dominate thinking again from the late 1970s and characterized the bulk of interest throughout the 1980s and early 1990s [64,74]. Not only did changing social pressures (e.g., the women's liberation movement) and the weight of evidence force an acceptance of the reality of child sexual abuse, but also the long held belief that incest was a universal cultural taboo was persuasively debunked [67]. The focus on early sexual abuse gave way to a greater and broader investment in the role of various forms of childhood trauma, abuse and neglect in adverse effects on psychological and physical development, as well as on health and mental health functioning. The renewed interested in child abuse has yet to follow in the footsteps of its last dominant foray into consciousness by being turned away from and ignored. This may be in part because child abuse and neglect now fit with the "psychosocial conception of reality," which was not the case in the mid–late 1800s (Cunningham, p. 350 [2]).

Yet, as Radbill [3] noted, "[a]buse of children has excited periodic waves of sympathy, each rising to a high pitch, and then curiously subsiding until the next period of excitation" (p. 15). Rather than accept the traumatic consequence that one human's malevolent and maltreating actions can have on another, it is seemingly easier to deny that it happened at all, to deny the extent of its impact, to blame its victims, or to relabel its manifestations as caused by things other than ourselves [11,75]. If history has a lesson, it may be that the current significance given to childhood abuse and trauma for health and mental health outcomes rests on unsolid foundations. These foundations appear dependent on society's ability to tolerate and take responsibility for adults' maltreatment of children. The ability to accept such a proposition rests in part on accepting that one of the single most pathogenic factors in the causation of mental illness, and some physical health problems, is humans themselves.

## References

1. Oettinger, K. B. (1968). Foreword. In R. E. Helfer and C. H. Kempe (eds.), *The battered child* (p. v). Chicago, IL: University of Chicago Press.

2. Cunningham, J. L. (1988). Contributions to the history of psychology: French historical views on the acceptability of evidence regarding child sexual abuse. *Psychological Reports*, **63**, 343–353.

3. Radbill, S. X. (1968). A history of child abuse and infanticide. In R. E. Helfer and C. H. Kempe (eds.), *The battered child* (pp. 3–17). Chicago, IL: University of Chicago Press.

4. Tardieu, A. (1860). Étude médico-légale sur les sévices et mauvais traitements exercés sur des enfants. *Annales de Hygiene Publique et Médicine Légale*, **13**, 361–398.

5. Tardieu, A. (1878). *Étude médico-légale sur les attentats aux moeurs,* 7th edn. Paris: Baillière.

6. Caffey, J. (1946). Multiple fractures in the long bones of infants suffering from chronic subdural hematoma. *American Journal of Roentgenology*, **56**, 163–173.

7. Caffey, J. (1965). Significance of the history in the diagnosis of traumatic injury to children. *Journal of Pediatrics*, **67**, 1000–1014.

8. Caffey, J. (1972). On the theory and practice of shaking infants: Its potential residual effects of permanent brain damage and mental retardation. *American Journal of Diseases of Children*, **124**, 161–169.

9. Kempe, C. H. (1978). Sexual abuse: Another hidden pediatric problem. *Pediatrics*, **62**, 382–389.

10. Kempe, C. H ., Silverman, F. N ., Steele, B. F., Droegemueller, W. and Silver, H. K. (1962). The battered-child syndrome. *Journal of the American Medical Association*, **181**, 17–24.

11. Herman, J. L. (1992). *Trauma and recovery: The aftermath of violence: From domestic abuse to political terror.* New York: Basic Books.

12. van der Kolk, B. A ., Weisaeth, L. and van der Hart, O. (1996). The history of trauma in psychiatry. In B. A. van der Kolk, A. C. McFarlane and L. Weisaeth (eds.), *Traumatic stress: The effects of overwhelming experience on mind, body, and society* (pp. 47–74). New York: Guilford.

13. DeMause, L. (1998). The history of child abuse. *Journal of Psychohistory*, **25**, 216–236.

14. Masson, J. M. (1984). *The assault on truth: Freud's suppression of the seduction theory.* London: Faber & Faber.

15. Knight, B. (1986). The history of child abuse. *Forensic Science International,* **30**, 135–141.

16. Briquet, P. (1859). *Traité clinique et thérapeutique de l'hystérie.* Paris: Baillière.

17. Stone, M. H. (1998). *Healing the mind: A history of psychiatry from antiquity to the present.* London: Norton.

18. Ellenberger, H. (1970). *The discovery of the unconscious: The history and evolution of dynamic psychiatry.* New York: Basic Books.

19. Crocq, L. and De Verbizier, J. (1989). Le traumatisme psychologique dans l'oeuvre de Pierre Janet. *Annales Médico-Psychologiques*, **147**, 983–987.

20. De Marneffe, D. (1991). Looking and listening: The construction of clinical knowledge in Charcot and Freud. *Signs: Journal of Women in Culture and Society*, **17**, 71–111.

21. Charcot, J. M. and Magnan, V. (1882). Inversion du sens génital et autres perversions sexuelles. *Archives de Neurologie*, **7**, 296–322.

22. Micale, M. S. (2001). Jean-Martin Charcot and *les névroses traumatiques*: From medicine to culture in French trauma theory of the late nineteenth century. In M. S. Micale and P. Lerner (eds.), *Traumatic pasts* (pp. 115–139). Cambridge, UK: Cambridge University Press.

23. Van der Hart, O. (2008). Charcot, Jean-Martin (1825–1893). In G. Reyes, J. D. Elhai and J. Ford (eds.), *The encyclopedia of trauma* (pp. 111–112). New York: Wiley.

24. Janet, P. (1919). *Les médications psychologiques.* Paris: Félix Alcan. [English edition: *Psychological healing.* New York: Macmillan, 1925.]

25. Freud, S. (1896). Further remarks on the neuro-psychosis of defence. In J. Strachey (ed.), *The standard edition of the complete psychological works of Sigmund Freud*, Vol. 3. London: Vintage, 2001.

26. Freud, S. (1896). The aetiology of hysteria. In J. Strachey (ed.), *The standard edition of the complete psychological works of Sigmund Freud*, Vol. 3. London: Vintage, 2001.

27. Freud, S. (1897). Letter to Fliess (letter 69). In J. Strachey (ed.), *The standard edition of the complete psychological works of Sigmund Freud*, Vol. 1. London: Vintage, 2001.

28. Freud, S. (1897). Letter to Fliess (letter 67). In J. Strachey (ed.), *The standard edition of the complete psychological works of Sigmund Freud*, Vol. 1. London: Vintage, 2001.

29. Kris, E. (1954). *The origins of psychoanalysis.* New York: Basic Books.

30. *Collins dictionary and thesaurus* (1991). Glasgow: HarperCollins.

31. Freud, S. (2001). Early psycho-analytic publications. In J. Strachey (ed.), *The standard edition of the complete psychological works of Sigmund Freud*, Vol. 3. London: Vintage.

32. Wolff, L. (1988). *Postcards from the end of the world: Child abuse in Freud's Vienna.* New York: Atheneum.

33. Ferenczi, S. (1949). Confusion of tongues between adults and the child. *International Journal of Psycho-analysis*, **30**, 225–231. [Original presented to the International Psycho-Analytic Congress in 1932.]

34. Hoffer, A. (2003). Images in psychiatry: Sandor Ferenczi, MD, 1873–1933. *American Journal of Psychiatry*, **160**, 1937.

35. Dorahy, M. J. and van der Hart, O. (2007). Relationship between trauma and dissociation. In E. Vermetten, M. J. Dorahy and D. Spiegel (eds.), *Traumatic dissociation: Neurobiology and treatment* (pp. 3–30). Arlington, VA: American Psychiatric Press.

36. van der Hart, O. and Friedman, B. (1989). A reader's guide to Pierre Janet on dissociation: A neglected intellectual heritage. *Dissociation*, **2**, 3–16.

37. Barresi, J. (1994). Morton Prince and B.C.A.: A historical footnote on the confrontation between dissociation theory and Freudian psychology in a case of multiple personality. In R. M. Klein and B. K. Doane (eds.), *Psychological concept and dissociative disorders* (pp. 85–129). Hillsdale, NJ: Lawrence Erlbaum.

38. Prince, M. (1905). *The Dissociation of a Personality*. New York: Longmans, Green & Co.

39. Kardiner, A. (1941). *The traumatic neuroses of war*. New York: Hoeber.

40. Myers, C. S. (1915). A contribution to the study of shell shock. *Lancet*, **i**, 316–320.

41. Ingraham, F. D. and Heyl, H. L. (1939). Subdural hematoma in infancy and childhood. *Journal of the American Medical Association*, **112**, 198–204.

42. Sherwood, D. (1930). Chronic subdural hematoma in infants. *American Journal of Diseases of Children*, **39**, 980–1021.

43. Fontana, V. J., Donovan, D. and Wong, R. J. (1963). The "maltreatment syndrome" in children. *New England Journal of Medicine*, **269**, 1389–1394.

44. Finkelhor, D. (2002). Introduction. In J. E. B. Myers, L. Berliner, J. Briere *et al.* (eds.), *The APSAC handbook on child maltreatment,* 2nd edn (pp. xi–xvi). London: Sage.

45. Parton, N. (2004). The natural history of child abuse: A study in social problem definition. *British Journal of Social Work*, **9**, 431–451.

46. West, S. (1888). Acute periosteal swellings in several young infants of the same family, probably rickety in nature. *British Medical Journal*, **i**, 856.

47. Helfer, R. E. and Kempe, C. H. (1976). *Child abuse and neglect: The family and the community*. Cambridge, MA: Ballinger.

48. Freeman, A. M., Kaplan, H. I. and Sadock, B. J. (1976). *Modern synopsis of comprehensive psychiatry*. Baltimore, MD: Williams & Wilkins.

49. Garbarino, J. (1978). The elusive 'crime' of emotional abuse. *Child Abuse & Neglect*, **2**, 89–99.

50. Gil, D. A. (1975). Unraveling child abuse. *American Journal of Orthopsychiatry*, **45**, 346–356.

51. Herman, J. L. (1981). *Father–daughter incest*. Cambridge, MA: Harvard University Press.

52. Meadow, R. (1977). Munchausen syndrome by proxy. The hinterland of child abuse. *Lancet*, **ii**, 343–345.

53. Pelton, L. H. (1978). Child abuse and neglect: The myth of classlessness. *American Journal of Orthopsychiatry*, **48**, 608–617.

54. Summit, R. (1983). The child sexual abuse accommodation syndrome. *Child Abuse and Neglect*, **7**, 177–193.

55. Berliner, L. and Elliott, D. M. (2002). Sexual abuse of children. In J. E. B. Myers *et al.* (eds.), *The APSAC handbook on child maltreatment,* 2nd edn (pp. 55–78). London: Sage.

56. Erickson, M. F. and Egeland, B. (2002). Child neglect. In J. E. B. Myers, L. Berliner, J. Briere, *et al.* (eds.), *The APSAC handbook on child maltreatment*, 2nd edn (pp. 3–20). London: Sage.

57. Iwaniec, D., Larkin, E. and Higgins, S. (2006). Research review: Risk and resilience in cases of emotional abuse. *Child and Family Social Work*, **11**, 73–82.

58. Finkelhor, D., Hotaling, G., Lewis, I. A. and Smith, C. (1990). Sexual abuse in a national survey of adult men and women: Prevalence, characteristics and risk factors. *Child Abuse & Neglect*, **14**, 19–28.

59. National Center on Child Abuse and Neglect (1988). *Study findings: Study of the National incidence and prevalence of child abuse and neglect*. Washington, DC: US Department of Health and Human Services.

60. Pilkington, B. and Kremer, J. (1995). A review of the epidemiological research on child sexual abuse: Community and college student samples. *Child Abuse Review*, **4**, 84–98.

61. Gorey, K. M. and Leslie, D. R. (1997). The prevalence of child sexual abuse: Integrative review adjustment for potential response and measurement biases. *Child Abuse and Neglect*, **21**, 391–398.

62. Cappelleri, J. C., Eckenrode, J. and Powers, J. L. (1993). The epidemiology of child abuse: Findings from the Second National Incidence and Prevalence Study of Child Abuse and Neglect. *American Journal of Public Health*, **83**, 1622–1624.

63. Bryer, J. B., Nelson, B. A., Miller, J. B. *et al.* (1987). Childhood sexual and physical abuse as factors in adult psychiatric illness. *American Journal of Psychiatry*, **144**, 1426–1430.

64. Craine, L. S., Hensen, C. E., Colliver, J. A. and MacLean, D. C. (1988). Prevalence of a history of sexual abuse among female psychiatric patients in a state hospital system. *Hospital and Community Psychiatry*, **39**, 300–304.

65. Enslie, G. D. and Rosenfeld, A. (1983). Incest reported by children and adolescents hospitalised for severe psychiatric problems. *American Journal of Psychiatry*, **140**, 708–711.

66. Jacobson, A. and Richardson, B. (1987). Assault experiences of 100 psychiatric inpatients: Evidence of the need for routine inquiry. *American Journal of Psychiatry*, **144**, 908–913.

67. DeMause, L. (1991). The universality of incest. *Journal of Psychohistory*, **19**, 123–164.

68. Bremner, J. D. (2002). *Does stress damage the brain: Understanding trauma-related disorders from a mind–body perspective*. New York: Norton.

69. Ross, C. A. (2000). *The trauma model: A solution to the problem of comorbidity in psychiatry*. Richardson, TX: Manitou Communications.

70. van der Hart, O., Nijenhuis, E. R. S. and Steele, K. (2006). *The haunted self: Structural dissociation and the treatment of chronic traumatization.* New York: Norton.

71. DeMause, L. (1988). On writing childhood history. *Journal of Psychohistory,* 16, 135–171.

72. Read, J., Fink, P. J., Rudegeair, T., Felitti, V. and Whitfield, C. L. (2008). Child maltreatment and psychosis: A return to a genuinely integrated bio-psycho-social model.

*Clinical Schizophrenia and Related Psychosis, October,* 235–254.

73. Ross, C. A. (2004). *Schizophrenia: Innovations in diagnosis and treatment.* New York: Haworth.

74. Oates, R. K. and Donnelly, A. C. (1997). Influential papers in child abuse. *Child Abuse & Neglect,* **21**, 319–326.

75. Middleton, W. (2004). Dissociative disorders: A personal "work in progress." *Australasian Psychiatry,* **12**, 245–252.

# Chapter 2

# The epidemiology of early childhood trauma

Karestan C. Koenen, Andrea L. Roberts, Deborah M. Stone and Erin C. Dunn

## Introduction

The word trauma is the Greek word for wound and for damage and defeat. In medicine, trauma refers to a critical bodily injury, wound or shock that overwhelms the body's natural defenses and requires medical assistance for healing. Similarly, psychological trauma is "a circumstance in which an event overwhelms or exceeds a person's capacity to protect his or her psychic well-being and integrity" [1]. Consequently, the very definition of psychological trauma is complex, involving both characteristics of the event itself and subjective aspects of the individual's response. This complexity is reflected in the definition of psychological trauma presented in the *Diagnostic and Statistical Manual of Mental Disorders* (DSM-IV) for post-traumatic stress disorder (PTSD) [2]. To be considered a qualifying trauma, an event must meet both the objective A(1) criterion: "the person experienced, witnessed, or was confronted with an event or events that involved actual or threatened death or serious injury or a threat to the physical integrity of self or others" and the subjective A(2) criterion: "the person's response involved intense fear, helplessness or horror" [2]. The subjective aspect of this definition presents a challenge for epidemiologists interested in quantifying the prevalence of childhood trauma. In this chapter, we will focus on the epidemiology of potentially traumatic events in childhood, that is, events that meet the A(1) criterion for PTSD, whether or not the A(2) criterion has been evaluated. It will be up to the authors of later chapters to discuss the consequences of such events and determine whether and what type of such events actually traumatize the individuals experiencing them.

This chapter has three sections. In the first, we describe the prevalence of early childhood trauma in the general population of the USA using data from the National Comorbidity Study – Replication (NCS-R)

[3]. In the second section, we discuss some of the methodological issues around assessing the prevalence of childhood trauma, focusing on estimates of child maltreatment as a specific example. Finally, in the third section, we discuss risk factors for childhood trauma.

## Prevalence of early childhood trauma

In order to determine the prevalence of early childhood trauma, data publically available from the NCS-R were analyzed [3]. The NCS-R is a nationally representative household survey of English speakers 18 years and older in the 48 coterminous states of the USA [4,5]. (Non-English speakers were not included in the NCS-R because they were the focus of two parallel surveys of Hispanic and Asian American individuals.) Exposure to potentially traumatic events was assessed as part of the PTSD interview in Part 2 of the survey (5692 participants) via the World Mental Health Composite International Diagnostic Interview [6]. The interview queries 26 specific traumatic events and offers interviewees the opportunity to provide information about an event not specifically queried. If the interviewee endorses a specific event, he or she is then asked what age they were when the event first occurred. Childhood events were all those events occurring before the age of 13. Table 2.1 presents the prevalence of specific traumatic events by sex; Table 2.2 presents the same information stratified by race; and Table 2.3 presents these data by the highest level of education completed by the participant's caregiver with the highest educational attainment. These traumas are categorized into assaultive violence and other injuries and shocking experiences, in keeping with current trauma research [7]. The NCS-R data were weighted to account for differential probability of selection of respondents within households, differential non-response, and to adjust for residual differences between the sample and the US

**Table 2.1** Exposure to traumatic events prior to 13 years of age by sex reported by respondents in the National Comorbidity Study – Replication Survey[a]

| Traumatic experiences | Total (n = 5692) | | Male (n = 2673) | | Female (n = 3019) | | χ² value[c] | OR (95% CI)[d] |
|---|---|---|---|---|---|---|---|---|
| | No. | % (SE)[b] | No. | % (SE)[b] | No. | % (SE)[b] | | |
| Any traumatic experience | 2190 | 38.48 (1.02) | 1001 | 37.59 (1.38) | 1189 | 39.37 (1.29) | 1.20 | 0.92 (0.80–1.07) |
| Any assaultive violence | 1290 | 22.66 (0.82) | 519 | 19.41 (1.12) | 771 | 25.53 (1.05) | 16.17*** | 0.70 (0.59–0.83) |
| Any other injury or shocking experience | 1308 | 22.99 (0.69) | 672 | 25.15 (1.11) | 636 | 21.07 (0.90) | 7.78** | 1.26 (1.07–1.48) |
| Assaultive violence | | | | | | | | |
| Any sexual violence | 490 | 8.62 (0.45) | 96 | 3.57 (0.46) | 395 | 13.09 (0.64) | 123.36*** | 0.25 (0.19–0.32) |
| Raped | 219 | 3.82 (0.27) | 43 | 1.65 (0.26) | 175 | 5.88 (0.41) | 79.11*** | 0.26 (0.19–0.36) |
| Sexually assaulted/molested | 363 | 6.39 (0.40) | 67 | 2.52 (0.36) | 296 | 9.83 (0.60) | 109.69*** | 0.24 (0.18–0.31) |
| Witness physical fights at home | 693 | 12.31 (0.59) | 292 | 11.06 (0.94) | 400 | 13.43 (0.68) | 4.48* | 0.80 (0.65–0.99) |
| Badly beaten as a child | 295 | 5.22 (0.26) | 132 | 5.0 (0.49) | 162 | 5.41 (0.30) | 0.47 | 0.92 (0.72–1.17) |
| Beaten by anyone else | 121 | 2.13 (0.23) | 102 | 3.82 (0.52) | 19 | 0.63 (0.11) | 61.64*** | 6.26 (3.80–10.32) |
| Mugged/threatened with weapon | 73 | 1.29 (0.19) | 49 | 1.85 (0.32) | 24 | 0.79 (0.15) | 13.03*** | 2.38 (1.59–3.57) |
| Stalked | 23 | 0.41 (0.09) | 3 | 0.13 (0.05) | 20 | 0.66 (0.14) | 16.61*** | 0.19 (0.09–0.42) |
| Kidnapped/held captive | 22 | 0.39 (0.09) | 9 | 0.35 (0.13) | 13 | 0.43 (0.09) | 0.37 | 0.82 (0.42–1.62) |
| Unarmed civilian in war | 33 | 0.58 (0.17) | 15 | 0.57 (0.23) | 18 | 0.59 (0.20) | 0.008 | 0.96 (0.38–2.2) |
| Civilian in ongoing terror | 24 | 0.42 (0.09) | 10 | 0.39 (0.10) | 14 | 0.45 (0.13) | 0.17 | 0.85 (0.40–1.83) |
| Refugee | 17 | 0.30 (0.15) | 6 | 0.21 (0.11) | 12 | 0.39 (0.20) | 1.39 | 0.54 (0.24–1.23) |
| Other injury or shocking experience | | | | | | | | |
| Had someone close die unexpectedly | 447 | 7.90 (0.46) | 219 | 8.23 (0.80) | 229 | 7.60 (0.41) | 0.55 | 1.09 (0.87–1.36) |
| Experienced other life-threatening accident | 100 | 1.77 (0.20) | 52 | 1.94 (0.26) | 49 | 1.61 (0.32) | 0.58 | 1.21 (0.73–2.01) |

| | Total N | Total % (SE) | Male N | Male % (SE) | Female N | Female % (SE) | $\chi^2$ | OR (CI) |
|---|---|---|---|---|---|---|---|---|
| Experienced natural or manmade disaster | 393 | 6.90 (0.51) | 200 | 7.49 (0.83) | 193 | 6.38 (0.49) | 1.61 | 1.19 (0.92–1.53) |
| Had life-threatening illness | 206 | 3.63 (0.37) | 101 | 3.79 (0.59) | 105 | 3.48 (0.40) | 0.21 | 1.09 (0.76–1.58) |
| Learned about trauma to someone close | 86 | 1.52 (0.18) | 36 | 1.37 (0.25) | 49 | 1.65 (0.27) | 0.61 | 0.83 (0.51–1.34) |
| Saw someone injured/killed | 342 | 6.0 (0.36) | 211 | 7.88 (0.61) | 131 | 4.35 (0.43) | 20.10*** | 1.89 (1.45–2.47) |
| Saw atrocities/carnage | 26 | 0.45 (0.10) | 15 | 0.58 (0.18) | 10 | 0.34 (0.12) | 1.14 | 1.73 (0.65–4.57) |
| Seriously injured/killed another person | 9 | 0.16 (0.06) | 9 | 0.34 (0.13) | – | – | – | – |
| Exposed to toxic chemicals | 19 | 0.33 (0.08) | 14 | 0.53 (0.17) | 5 | 0.15 (0.03) | 4.60* | 3.44 (1.74–6.80) |
| Contributed to serious injury/death of another person | 6 | 0.11 (0.04) | 4 | 0.15 (0.06) | 2 | 0.08 (0.04) | 1.15 | 1.94 (0.64–5.90) |

OR, odds ratio; CI, confidence interval; SE, standard error.

[a]Sample distributions (cell entries) reflect the weighted number of respondents rounded to the nearest whole number (some cell entries for the total are not exactly equal to the sum of the male and female entries as a result of rounding).

[b]Percentages were derived from the total sample (respondents were not preserved in the denominator if they were missing data or refused to respond to a particular question).

[c]Chi-square values are based on the Wald chi-square test.

[d]Unadjusted OR was derived by estimating the odds of experiencing each event prior to age 13 (versus never experiencing the event or experiencing the event at age 13 or afterwards) among males (coded as 1) and females (coded as 0).

*$p < 0.05$; **$p < 0.01$; ***$p < 0.001$.

**Table 2.2** Exposure to traumatic events prior to 13 years of age by race reported by respondents in the National Comorbidity Study – Replication Survey[a]

| Traumatic experiences | Non-Hispanic white (n = 4141) | | Non-Hispanic black (n = 704) | | Hispanic (n = 630) | | Other (n = 217) | | χ² value[b] |
|---|---|---|---|---|---|---|---|---|---|
| | No. | % (SE)[b] | No. | % (SE)[b] | No. | % (SE)[b] | No. | % (SE)[b] | |
| Any traumatic experience | 1539 | 37.17 (1.11) | 289 | 41.03 (2.77) | 266 | 42.2 (2.42) | 96 | 44.27 (5.83) | 8.16~ |
| Any assaultive violence | 841 | 20.31 (0.94) | 189 | 26.92 (2.76) | 193 | 30.65 (2.04) | 66 | 30.35 (4.67) | 24.33*** |
| Any other injury/shocking experience | 942 | 22.74 (0.80) | 177 | 25.16 (2.46) | 138 | 21.85 (2.08) | 52 | 23.99 (3.76) | 1.29 |
| **Assaultive violence** | | | | | | | | | |
| Any sexual violence | 327 | 7.89 (0.46) | 67 | 9.47 (1.47) | 69 | 10.98 (1.51) | 28 | 12.88 (3.57) | 6.29 |
| Raped | 134 | 3.28 (0.30) | 36 | 5.19 (0.99) | 34 | 5.38 (0.84) | 15 | 7.06 (3.86) | 6.60~ |
| Sexually assaulted/molested | 249 | 6.04 (0.40) | 45 | 6.34 (1.05) | 52 | 8.34 (1.24) | 16 | 7.60 (1.93) | 3.94 |
| Witness physical fights at home | 430 | 10.51 (0.58) | 111 | 15.84 (2.02) | 120 | 19.40 (2.06) | 32 | 14.65 (2.39) | 30.65*** |
| Badly beaten as a child | 198 | 4.81 (0.28) | 25 | 3.60 (0.84) | 43 | 6.85 (0.86) | 29 | 13.47 (3.34) | 16.48** |
| Beaten by anyone else | 91 | 2.19 (0.28) | 9 | 1.36 (0.57) | 16 | 2.56 (0.57) | 5 | 2.29 (1.04) | 2.23 |
| Mugged/threatened with weapon | 46 | 1.11 (0.19) | 14 | 2.05 (0.58) | 9 | 1.46 (0.72) | 3 | 1.60 (0.30) | 4.87 |
| Stalked | 12 | 0.30 (0.07) | 2 | 0.23 (0.14) | 8 | 1.28 (0.55) | 1 | 0.63 (0.34) | 4.84 |
| Kidnapped/held captive | 15 | 0.36 (0.09) | 1 | 0.16 (0.06) | 4 | 0.65 (0.46) | 2 | 1.07 (0.64) | 5.33 |
| Unarmed civilian in war | 23 | 0.57 (0.19) | 6 | 0.80 (0.75) | 3 | 0.55 (0.25) | 0 | 0.17 (0.17) | 3.43 |
| Civilian in ongoing terror | 14 | 0.35 (0.11) | 5 | 0.74 (0.27) | 4 | 0.56 (0.35) | 1 | 0.39 (0.28) | 2.00 |
| Refugee | 5 | 0.13 (0.07) | 2 | 0.34 (0.25) | 8 | 1.22 (0.96) | 2 | 0.76 (0.77) | 3.23 |
| **Other injury or shocking experience** | | | | | | | | | |
| Had someone close die unexpectedly | 310 | 7.48 (0.58) | 69 | 9.74 (1.46) | 49 | 7.76 (1.52) | 20 | 9.36 (2.80) | 2.42 |
| Experienced other life-threatening accident | 79 | 1.91 (0.28) | 8 | 1.07 (0.63) | 9 | 1.42 (0.43) | 5 | 2.30 (1.27) | 1.76 |
| Experienced natural or manmade disaster | 270 | 6.52 (0.61) | 45 | 6.32 (1.17) | 64 | 10.16 (1.64) | 14 | 6.60 (1.51) | 7.80~ |
| Had life-threatening illness | 169 | 4.10 (0.50) | 12 | 1.72 (0.46) | 19 | 2.99 (0.58) | 6 | 2.69 (1.50) | 11.31* |
| Learned about trauma to someone close | 52 | 1.25 (0.17) | 20 | 2.79 (0.80) | 11 | 1.77 (0.70) | 4 | 1.74 (0.80) | 4.48 |
| Saw someone injured/killed | 221 | 5.35 (0.38) | 69 | 9.82 (1.63) | 36 | 5.73 (1.36) | 16 | 7.22 (2.41) | 7.19~ |
| Saw atrocities/carnage | 20 | 0.49 (0.14) | 1 | 0.13 (0.10) | 1 | 0.21 (0.17) | 3 | 1.37 (0.43) | 10.67* |
| Seriously injured/killed another person | 4 | 0.09 (0.04) | 1 | 0.21 (0.21) | 4 | 0.62 (0.50) | – | – | – |
| Exposed to toxic chemicals | 14 | 0.34 (0.10) | – | – | 5 | 0.74 (0.46) | – | – | – |
| Contributed to serious injury/death of another person | 3 | 0.07 (0.03) | 2 | 0.31 (0.16) | 0 | 0.08 (0.08) | 1 | 0.26 (0.26) | 2.92 |

[a] Percentages were derived from the total sample (respondents were preserved in the denominator if they were missing data or refused to respond to a particular question).

[b] Chi-square values are based on Wald chi-square test.

~p < 0.10; *p < 0.05; **p < 0.01; ***p < 0.001.

**Table 2.3** Exposure to traumatic events prior to 13 years of age by highest level of caregiver education reported by respondents in the National Comorbidity Study – Replication Survey[a]

| Traumatic experiences | Less than high school (n = 1377) No. | % (SE) | High school (n = 1782) No. | % (SE) | Some college (n = 1403) No. | % (SE) | College education and greater (n = 518) No. | % (SE) | $\chi^2$ value[b] |
|---|---|---|---|---|---|---|---|---|---|
| Any traumatic experience | 508 | 36.89 (1.91) | 704 | 39.50 (1.63) | 590 | 42.05 (1.63) | 207 | 39.97 (2.36) | 4.38 |
| Any assaultive violence | 322 | 23.42 (1.67) | 418 | 23.47 (1.16) | 320 | 22.78 (1.48) | 91 | 17.48 (1.68) | 9.45** |
| Any other injury/shocking experience | 297 | 21.59 (1.56) | 404 | 22.69 (1.28) | 390 | 27.78 (1.84) | 140 | 27.07 (2.42) | 7.50* |
| Assaultive violence | | | | | | | | | |
| Any sexual violence | 109 | 7.91 (0.78) | 165 | 9.29 (0.78) | 133 | 9.46 (0.96) | 36 | 7.00 (1.10) | 5.33 |
| Raped | 59 | 4.31 (0.53) | 77 | 4.36 (0.47) | 52 | 3.70 (0.50) | 13 | 2.58 (0.71) | 5.86 |
| Sexually assaulted/molested | 71 | 5.20 (0.57) | 124 | 6.99 (0.58) | 108 | 7.70 (0.80) | 28 | 5.37 (0.93) | 10.55** |
| Witness physical fights at home | 197 | 14.23 (1.16) | 217 | 12.33 (0.83) | 165 | 11.82 (1.13) | 34 | 6.61 (1.31) | 17.86*** |
| Badly beaten as a child | 70 | 5.10 (0.47) | 97 | 5.50 (0.52) | 65 | 4.67 (0.66) | 20 | 3.89 (0.82) | 2.55 |
| Beaten by anyone else | 24 | 1.77 (0.47) | 36 | 2.04 (0.35) | 39 | 2.80 (0.58) | 15 | 2.80 (0.74) | 3.44 |
| Mugged/threatened with weapon | 15 | 1.09 (0.32) | 22 | 1.23 (0.25) | 26 | 1.85 (0.39) | 8 | 1.55 (0.55) | 3.77 |
| Stalked | 10 | 0.74 (0.26) | 6 | 0.34 (0.13) | 4 | 0.32 (0.16) | 2 | 0.33 (0.19) | 4.06 |
| Kidnapped/held captive | 3 | 0.25 (0.10) | 5 | 0.30 (0.14) | 10 | 0.71 (0.26) | 1 | 0.23 (0.17) | 2.55 |
| Unarmed civilian in war | 10 | 0.73 (0.42) | 11 | 0.64 (0.35) | 4 | 0.30 (0.20) | 3 | 0.54 (0.28) | 1.65 |
| Civilian in ongoing terror | 6 | 0.42 (0.15) | 4 | 0.25 (0.11) | 8 | 0.59 (0.16) | 3 | 0.50 (0.44) | 2.90 |
| Refugee | 7 | 0.49 (0.30) | 2 | 0.12 (0.08) | 4 | 0.32 (0.20) | 3 | 0.52 (0.45) | 3.85 |
| Other injury or shocking experience | | | | | | | | | |
| Had someone close die unexpectedly | 105 | 7.69 (0.79) | 151 | 8.50 (1.02) | 127 | 9.10 (0.97) | 40 | 7.72 (1.48) | 1.55 |
| Experienced other life-threatening accident | 15 | 1.06 (0.23) | 20 | 1.12 (0.23) | 51 | 3.67 (0.67) | 11 | 2.18 (0.73) | 11.19** |
| Experienced natural or manmade disaster | 80 | 5.82 (0.77) | 123 | 6.89 (0.77) | 112 | 8.02 (1.38) | 50 | 9.59 (1.34) | 6.85* |
| Had life-threatening illness | 64 | 4.69 (0.67) | 52 | 2.95 (0.45) | 68 | 4.86 (0.60) | 12 | 2.28 (0.92) | 9.98** |
| Learned about trauma to someone close | 19 | 1.35 (0.34) | 32 | 1.80 (0.34) | 21 | 1.50 (0.46) | 5 | 1.06 (0.41) | 1.42 |
| Saw someone injured/killed | 77 | 5.63 (0.69) | 90 | 5.05 (0.78) | 111 | 7.95 (1.13) | 40 | 7.73 (1.74) | 4.25 |
| Saw atrocities/carnage | 11 | 0.82 (0.30) | 6 | 0.33 (0.18) | 5 | 0.39 (0.19) | 2 | 0.40 (0.26) | 2.07 |
| Seriously injured/killed another person | 1 | 0.05 (0.06) | 0 | 0.03 (0.03) | 7 | 0.50 (0.25) | – | – | – |
| Exposed to toxic chemicals | 2 | 0.17 (0.11) | 5 | 0.30 (0.12) | 9 | 0.68 (0.24) | 1 | 0.16 (0.11) | 4.31 |
| Contributed to serious injury/death of another person | 0 | 0.03 (0.03) | 2 | 0.12 (0.06) | 1 | 0.04 (0.04) | 2 | 0.42 (0.22) | 5.92 |

[a]Percentages were derived from the total sample (respondents were not preserved in the denominator if they were missing data or refused to respond to a particular question).
[b]Chi-square values are based on the Wald chi-square test.
*$p < 0.10$; **$p < 0.05$; ***$p < 0.01$.

population on selected sociodemographic characteristics [4]. The SAS procedures for analyzing data from complex sample surveys (e.g., *PROCSURVEYFREQ*) were used to produce accurate statistical estimates (e.g., point estimates, variances) [8].

Table 2.1 demonstrates that exposure to potentially traumatic events is common in childhood; when events are collapsed across categories, almost 40% of adults in the general population report having experienced at least one event by age 13. Even more striking is the prevalence of assaultive violence in childhood. Almost 20% of males and over 25% of females report having directly experienced or witnessed violence by the age of 13; females were significantly more likely to experience assaultive violence than males ($p < 0.001$). Sex differences were apparent in the types of violence experienced. For example, the most common types of assaultive violence reported by males was witnessing physical fights at home (11%), being badly beaten as a child by a parent or caregiver (5%) and being beaten by anyone else (4%). For females, the most common types of assaultive violence reported were witnessing physical fights at home (13%) and sexual violence (13%), followed by being badly beaten as a child by a parent or caregiver (5%). Males had a higher overall prevalence in terms of other types of trauma (other injury or shocking experience; $p = 0.004$).

Table 2.2 presents the prevalence of exposure to potentially traumatic events before the age of 13 by race/ethnicity. The prevalence of exposure to any traumatic event, to any other injury or shocking experience and for most specific event types did not significantly differ by race. However, significant race differences were found for exposure to assaultive violence. Compared with white participants, Hispanics (odds ratio [OR], 1.73; 95% confidence interval [CI], 1.39–2.17; $p < 0.0001$), blacks (OR, 1.45; 95% CI, 1.07–1.94; $p = 0.02$) and participants from other racial groups (OR, 1.7; 95% CI, 1.12–2.62; $p = 0.01$) had increased odds of being exposed to any assaultive violence prior to age 13. Specifically, race/ethnic differences (comparing whites with all other ethic groups) were found for being badly beaten as a child by parents or caregivers (Hispanics, OR 1.46; 95% CI, 1.06–2.003; $p = 0.02$; other race/ethnic groups, OR, 3.08; 95% CI, 1.74–5.45; $p = 0.0001$) and witnessing physical fights at home (Hispanics, OR, 2.05; 95% CI, 1.61–2.62; $p < 0.0001$; blacks, OR, 1.60; 95% CI, 1.17–2.21; $p = 0.004$; other race/ethnic groups, OR, 1.46; CI, 0.99–2.16; $p = 0.057$). Although these racial/ethnic groupings most likely fail to fully capture

the complexity of race and trauma risk, the results suggest that children of color may experience a greater burden of certain types of trauma in childhood, particularly assaultive violence within the home.

Table 2.3 presents the prevalence of exposure to potentially traumatic events before the age of 13 by level of caregiver education. The prevalence of exposure to any traumatic event did not differ by caregiver education. However, individuals whose parents had less than a college degree were at increased risk of experiencing assaultive violence. In terms of specific types of violence, individuals whose parents had a less than a high school education were at increased risk of witnessing physical fights at home. It is worth noting that exposure to the vast majority of the traumas queried was not significantly more common among individuals whose parents had less education.

# Methodological issues

The data presented from the NCS-R give a sense of the overwhelming burden of childhood trauma in the general population of the USA. However, data on childhood trauma from the NCS-R and other epidemiological studies need to be viewed within the context of the many methodological challenges to estimating the burden of childhood trauma. These challenges lead to large disparities in estimates from study to study in the prevalence of certain traumas.

In order to illustrate these methodological challenges and how they impact prevalence estimates, prevalence estimates of one particular trauma type, child maltreatment, was examined in detail. Estimates for child maltreatment through neglect and emotional, physical or sexual abuse vary substantially from study to study. For example, in his review of international studies, Finkelhor [9] found a range of reported sexual abuse from 7% to 36% for males and 3% to 29% for females. Some of the methodological reasons for the variation are discussed below.

## Definitions and measures used

Definitions vary based on the types of activity qualifying as abuse or neglect, and the minimum age difference required between the victim and perpetrator for an act to be considered abuse. Official records also depend on whether the harm or endangerment standard is applied, with the latter being more broadly defined. The number of questions asked of respondents also affects estimates, with more questions being considered more reliable than fewer questions. For example, in a prevalence study, Finkelhor *et al.* [10] asked four questions to assess child sexual abuse including questions about exhibitionism, touching/grabbing, oral/anal sex and sexual intercourse. A positive response to any of these four acts determined a history of child sexual abuse; 27% of females responded affirmatively to at least one question [10]. In contrast, in the National Violence Against Women Survey, sexual abuse was defined as simply attempted or completed rape. Based on this definition, only 6.3% of those aged 12–17 years responded affirmatively [11].

## Response rates

The prevalence of child abuse appears to be inversely related to survey response rates, such that lower response rates appear to be associated with higher prevalence rates of sexual abuse across 25 studies (results not shown). Among females, for example, surveys of sexual abuse with response rates lower than 60% found an aggregate prevalence of 27.8%, compared with prevalence estimates of 16.8% in surveys with response rates greater than 60% [12].

## Age, period and cohort effects

Memories may fade over time, resulting in lower reported prevalences of abuse in older cohorts. Younger cohorts, on the one hand, may also be more likely to report abuse, given the lessening of stigma or greater recognition of abuse as a societal problem. On the other hand, younger cohorts may report lower prevalences of abuse if prevention efforts have led to actual declines in abuse (period effect) [13]. For a discussion of recent declines in child sexual abuse see Jones and Finkelhor [14].

## Retrospective versus prospective reporting

The reliability of retrospective recall of child abuse and neglect is controversial. Retrospective reports may be considered unreliable with regard to childhood experiences because memories fade[15]. Moreover, events that occurred before the age of 5 may not be recalled as a result of infantile amnesia [16]. Also of concern is mood-dependent recall, in which participants are more likely to recall events consistent with their current mood – individuals who are depressed may be more likely to recall negative life events [17]. Consequently, retrospective reports of abuse are most concerning for studies correlating self-reports of abuse with current mental state (e.g., psychiatric disorders). Problems with recall are illustrated by prospective studies of

substantiated abuse cases. For example, Widom and Morris [18] found that only 41–67% of females with court-documented abuse histories recalled their abuse experiences when interviewed in young adulthood.

## Population sampled

Prevalence estimates appear to differ widely depending on the population sampled. For example, in the Adverse Childhood Experiences Study, a population of adults within a large health maintenance organization reported a prevalence estimate of child sexual abuse of 20.7%, whereas adults in the NCS-R were found to report a prevalence of 11% [3,19].

## Official versus self-report data

Although minimum standards do exist for the definition of abuse and neglect, set forth in Federal law 42 U.S.C.A. 5106g, the Child Abuse Prevention and Treatment Act of 1988 (amended by the Keeping Children and Families Safe Act of 2003), each state in the USA sets its own definitions of abuse and neglect [20]. The Child Abuse Prevention and Treatment Act also set up a national data collection and analysis program. However, not all states have reported rates of maltreatment consistently over time. All states have mandatory reporters (e.g., therapists and teachers); however, these vary across states, the District of Columbia and US territories. Mandatory reporters also vary in their willingness to report abuse. Finkelhor *et al.* [21] found that data from official sources reflect large social class and ethnic biases compared with data collected via population surveys. Various official figures are also often contradictory. Cases compiled from state agencies do not always match criminal records.

## Data collection methods

Face-to-face interviews may yield different prevalence estimates of abuse and neglect than telephone, self-administered or computer-assisted surveys. Data from the redesign of the National Crime Victims Survey suggest that participants reveal more information about victimization experiences on the phone than face to face [22].

## Risk factors for trauma exposure in childhood

Despite the methodological challenges to establishing childhood trauma, as detailed above, extant research has come to some consensus as to risk and protective factors. As is demonstrated in this analysis of the NCS-R data, childhood trauma is not randomly distributed in the population. Factors associated with greater risk of childhood trauma occur at the individual, family, neighborhood, local, regional and national level; the bulk of research focuses on individual and family factors. (Very few studies cited here are limited to children 12 years old or younger. Many studies of lifetime exposure in childhood are retrospective from late adolescence [age 17] or early adulthood, while studies of recent exposures are primarily of teenagers.)

## Individual factors

Individual factors associated with risk of childhood trauma include demographic descriptors such as sex, age and race/ethnicity, as well as health and behavioral characteristics, including mental health, substance use, sexuality and prior traumatization.

### Sex

Male sex is strongly associated with assaultive and physical trauma. For instance, in a US nationally representative sample of children aged 10–16, boys reported significantly higher lifetime violent victimization, such as physical assault, than girls (57.6% vs. 44.8%) [23]. In US regional studies, boys report nearly twice the rate of assaultive violence than girls (62.6% vs. 33.7% in one urban study) [24,25], twice the rate of witnessing violence or injury as girls [24] and are twice as likely to report *causing* severe harm or death to another person [26]. International studies have found that boys are more likely than girls to receive threats of being beaten and to have had a friend or relative be assaulted [27]. Boys are also at greater risk being hit by cars [28], being injured on a playground [29] and witnessing a shocking event [25]. In contrast to boys' higher risk of physical assault and injury, girls are at greater risk of sexual assault. For example, in a US representative sample, girls had higher rates of sexual victimization involving contact than boys (3.2% vs. 0.6%) [23]. Studies of specific urban and rural localities in the US report similar findings [24–26], as do multiple international studies [30,31].

### Age

Children of different ages are at risk for different types of trauma. Children younger than 5 years are at elevated risk of witnessing domestic abuse [32] and near drowning [33]. In middle childhood, the risk of pedestrian traffic accidents peaks [28], as does the incidence of parental physical abuse [34]. In contrast,

teenagers are more likely to experience sexual abuse than younger children [30]. Although the risk for certain traumas is greater in early childhood, a review of the literature suggests that overall risk of experiencing a trauma increases with age during childhood [35].

### Race/ethnicity

Trauma rates have been observed to vary according to the race/ethnicity of the child, with US rates for non-whites being higher than those for whites for many trauma types. National data show that Native American boys experience higher rates of multiple physical or sexual assault [36], and regional studies indicated that black children experience higher rates of violent assault [25] and that non-white children are more likely to witness domestic violence [37,38]. Among non-assaultive injuries, rates of drowning or near-drowning in children older than 4 years are more than twice as high for blacks than for whites [33], and asthma hospitalization rates are three times greater among black children [39]. Looking at mortality data as an indicator of non-fatal trauma, black and American Indian/Alaskan Native children in all age groups experience higher rates of mortality than whites [40].

### Behavioral and health characteristics

Individual behavioral and health characteristics predict trauma exposure in children. Additionally, teenagers and young adults reporting minority sexualities (homosexual, bisexual or mostly heterosexual) report higher rates of childhood sexual and physical abuse than respondents with 100% heterosexual orientation [41,42]. Children with physical disabilities such as blindness or deafness, or cognitive impairments, are at greater risk of sexual abuse [43]. Hearing loss is a risk factor for serious injury in childhood [44], while epilepsy increases risk of submersion injury in children [33]. Low birthweight is a risk factor for infant injury [45]. Substance use [46,47] and risky sexual behaviors [47] predict being victimized by subsequent trauma.

Several longitudinal studies have found that childhood mental health problems predict subsequent traumatic events. Internalizing problems, including anxiety disorders and rising emotional distress, have been linked prospectively to increased trauma risk [47]. Early childhood externalizing, aggressive and disruptive problems have also been linked to subsequent exposure to assaultive violence [24,48], while early conduct problems have been associated with increased lifetime trauma prevalence [49].

## Prior trauma

Prior trauma, age at trauma and stressful life events are associated with higher probability of subsequent trauma exposure in several national studies. Children who experienced four or more victimizations in the baseline year of a longitudinal study were five times more likely than other children to be multiply victimized the subsequent year [50]. Earlier age of first victimization was associated with increased likelihood of multiple physical or sexual victimizations among US adolescents [36] .

## Protective individual factors

Individual traits that are protective have also been identified in prospective studies, including high early childhood intelligence quotient [24], high first-grade reading scores [48] and having many good friends [50].

## Family risk factors

Certain family characteristics are associated with higher risk of trauma in children, including demographic factors, family functioning and parental traits and behaviors. Low household income, low maternal education and single-parenthood are associated with increased risk of childhood trauma, and tend to cluster in families. In the USA, these traits often occur in non-white families living in urban areas; therefore, disentangling potential causal relationships of each factor with trauma is difficult [23–26,32,38].

## Income

In a US nationally representative sample of children aged 2 to 17, annual household income under $20 000 was found to be associated with higher rates of assault with a weapon, attempted assault, multiple peer assault, completed or attempted rape, emotional abuse and witnessing violence, but it was not significantly related to rates of physical assault, sexual victimization or property victimization [51]. In a longitudinal US study, parental unemployment and family homelessness, both related to poverty, also predicted subsequent traumatization [50]. In the US, children without private health insurance, who tend to be poor, have higher rates of hospitalization for physical and mental illness, are more severely ill at admission and have higher mortality than children with private insurance [52]. Worldwide, children living in lower-income households are at higher risk of traffic injury [53,54], including pedestrian injury [28].

## Maternal education

Low maternal education appears to be associated with an increased prevalence of injury and death, beginning in infancy [45,55]. One US study found that the risk of experiencing any type of trauma increased for each reduction in the mother's educational attainment, peaking at 5.5 times greater (95% CI, 2.7–10.9) for children whose mother had less than high school education, compared with those whose mother had a college education [24].

## Family composition

In US and international studies, residence in a single-parent or step-parent household is associated with higher trauma rates. Rates of assaultive trauma are higher, including more robbery or theft, more threats of beating [25], more suicide attempts, more childhood physical and sexual abuse [56], and higher rates of multiple victimizations in a single year [24,57]. Rates of non-assaultive traumas are also higher, including more traffic and other serious accidents, more illnesses and more near-drownings [56,57].

## Parental mental health

Parents' health and well-being have been linked to risk of trauma in children. Studies have found that parental psychopathology puts children at increased risk for trauma [26,49], as does imprisonment [26,50]. In US national samples, family alcohol and substance problems were associated with children's victimization [36,50], although regional studies have found contradictory results [26,49]. Poor family functioning, including parental fighting [50] and poor communication [26], has been associated with children's subsequent traumatization.

## Protective factors

Although few studies of trauma explore protective factors at the family level, one study in the city of Chicago found that, after adjusting for many family and neighborhood factors, social support to parents was strongly associated with reduced likelihood of parent-to-child physical aggression [34].

# Community-level factors

Risk for childhood trauma varies by locality, country and world region. For example, in the USA, different regions have significantly different rates of violent victimization, with the mountain region having the highest rate (64.6%), and the east north central region the lowest rate (46.4%) [23]. Urban areas also report higher rates of victimization, with 59.6% of children in large cities reporting victimization, while suburban (53.6%) and rural children (46.3%) report somewhat lower rates [23]. Studies of single urban areas have found that rates of assaultive violence vary by neighborhood [25]. Specific neighborhood traits are also associated with child trauma. For example, concentrated poverty in a neighborhood is associated with increased risk of parent-to-child physical aggression [34] and injury among children aged 5 to 14 years [58]. In localities with poor housing stock, children are exposed to environmental hazards, including mold, allergens, pollutants [59] and endotoxins [60], which cause asthma attacks.

Not surprisingly, children in different countries also experience different rates of trauma. In general, children in poorer countries are at much higher risk of trauma than children in wealthier countries. Although we could find few national prevalence estimates for early childhood traumatic events in low-income countries, mortality risk data can also provide an indication of risk for non-fatal injury. The probability of a child dying before the age of 5 in 2005 averaged 15.3% in least-developed countries, 8.3% in developing countries and 0.6% in industrialized countries [61]. Similarly, the probability of a child dying before the age of 15 ranges enormously by world region, from 22.0% in sub-Saharan Africa to 1.1% in the developed countries [62].

In the developing world, undernutrition associated with poverty is a primary risk factor for childhood mortality, underlying more than half of all deaths in children under age 5 [63]. Therefore, poor nutrition can be presumed to be a causal factor in many sibling bereavements and serious but non-fatal childhood illnesses. Road traffic accidents are another major cause of injury and death, and a global review found that death rates among children under 14 years were six times higher in low- and middle-income countries than in high-income countries [64]. Children in poor countries are also at far greater risk of parental bereavement than children elsewhere: 99% of worldwide maternal deaths from pregnancy complications and childbirth occur in low-income countries, leaving orphaned children at high risk for further trauma [61].

## Conclusions

Epidemiological data suggest that childhood trauma (before the age of 13 years) is highly prevalent both in the USA and internationally. In fact, the public health burden of childhood trauma may be greatest in the developing world, particularly in places that are experiencing ongoing conflict and violence. Despite the methodological challenges to estimating the prevalence of specific types of childhood trauma, such as abuse and neglect, extant research has come to some consensus as to the individual, family and community-level factors that increase risk of childhood trauma. It is our hope that knowledge of such factors will inform future efforts to prevent and ultimately reduce the public health burden of childhood trauma.

## References

1. Cloitre, M., Cohen, L. R. and Koenen, K. C. (2006). *Treating the trauma of childhood abuse: Therapy for the interrupted life*. New York: Guilford.

2. American Psychiatric Association (2000). *Diagnostic and statistical manual of mental disorders*, 4th edn. Washington, DC: American Psychiatric Press.

3. Interuniversity Consortium for Political and Social Research. *The National Comorbidity Study – Replication. Public Use Data Set*. http://www.icpsr.umich.edu/CPES/ (accessed January 2010).

4. Kessler, R. C., Berglund, P., Chiu, W. T. *et al.* (2004). The US National Comorbidity Survey Replication (NCS-R): design and field procedures. *International Journal of Methods in Psychiatric Research*, **13**, 69–92.

5. Kessler, R. C., Bergland, P., Demier, O. *et al.* (1994). Lifetime prevalence and age-of-onset distributions of DSM-IV disorders in the National Comorbidity Survey Replication. *Archives of General Psychiatry*, **62**, 593–602.

6. Kessler, R. C. and Ustun, T. B. (2004). The World Mental Health (WMH) Survey Initiative Version of the World Health Organization (WHO) Composite International Diagnostic Interview (CIDI). *International Journal of Methods in Psychiatric Research*, **13**, 93–121.

7. Breslau, N., Peterson, E. L., Poisson, L. M., Schultz, L. R. and Lucia, V. C. (2004). Estimating post-traumatic stress disorder in the community: Lifetime perspective and the impact of typical traumatic events. *Psychological Medicine*, **34**, 889–898.

8. SAS Institute. *PROCSURVEYFREQ*. Cary, NC: SAS Institute.

9. Finkelhor, D. (1994). The international epidemiology of child sexual abuse. *Child Abuse & Neglect*, **18**, 409–417.

10. Finkelhor, D., Hotaling, G., Lewis, I. A. and Smith, C. *et al.* (1990). Sexual abuse in a national survey of adult men and women: Prevalence, characteristics, and risk factors. *Child Abuse & Neglect*, **14**, 19–28.

11. Tjaden, P. and Thoennes, N. (2006). *Extent, nature, and consequences of rape victimization: Findings from the national violence against women survey*. Washington,

DC: National Institute of Justice & Centers for Disease Control and Prevention.

12. Gorey, K. M. and Leslie, D. R. (1997). The prevalence of child sexual abuse: Integrative review adjustment for potential response and measurement biases. *Child Abuse & Neglect*, **21**, 391–398.

13. Briere, J. (1992). Methodological issues in the study of sexual abuse effects. *Journal of Consulting and Clinical Psychology,* **60**, 196–203.

14. Jones, L. M. and Finkelhor, D. (2003). Putting together evidence on declining trends in sexual abuse: A complex puzzle. *Child Abuse & Neglect*, **27**, 133–135.

15. Hardt, J. and Rutter, M. (2004). Validity of adult retrospective reports of adverse childhood experiences: Review of the evidence. *Journal Child Psychology and Psychiatry,* **45**, 260–273.

16. Lewis, M. (1995). Memory and psychoanalysis: A new look at infantile amnesia and transference. *Journal of the American Academy of Child and Adolescent Psychiatry*, **34**, 405–417.

17. McFarland, C. and Buehler, R. (1998). The impact of negative affect on autobiographical memory: The role of self-focused attention to moods. *Journal of Personality and Social Psychology*, **75**, 1424–1440.

18. Widom, C. S. and Morris, S. (1997). Accuracy of adult recollections of childhood victimization Part II: Childhood sexual abuse. *Psychological Assessment*, **9**, 34–46.

19. Dong, M., Anda, R. F., Felitti, V. J. *et al.* (2004). The interrelatedness of multiple forms of childhood abuse, neglect, and household dysfunction. *Child Abuse & Neglect*, **28**, 771–784.

20. Child Abuse Prevention and Treatment Act 1974. P.L. 93–247, in 42 U.S.C. 5101 et seq; 42 U.S.C. 5116 et seq. 1974.

21. Finkelhor, D., Hambly, S. L., Ormrod, R. and Turner, H. (2005). The Juvenile Victimization Questionnaire: Reliability, validity, and national norms. *Child Abuse & Neglect*, **29**, 383–412.

22. Kindermann, C., Lynch, J. and Cantor, D. (1997). *National Crime Victimization Survey: The Effects of the redesign on victimization estimates* (pp. 1–7). Washington, DC: US Department of Justice, Office of Justice Programs.

23. Finkelhor, D. and Dziuba-Leatherman, J. (1994). Children as victims of violence: A national survey. *Pediatrics*, **94**, 413–420.

24. Breslau, N., Lucia, V. C. and Alvarado, G. F. (2006). Intelligence and other predisposing factors in exposure to trauma and posttraumatic stress disorder: A follow-up study at age 17 years. *Archives of General Psychiatry,* **63**, 1238–1245.

25. Breslau, N., Wilcox, H. C., Storr, C. L., Lucia, V. C. and Anthony, J. C. (2004). Trauma exposure and posttraumatic stress disorder: A study of youths in urban America. *Journal of Urban Health*, **81**, 530–544.

26. Costello, E. J., Erkanli, A., Fairbank, J. A. and Angold, A. (2002). The prevalence of potentially traumatic events in childhood and adolescence. *Journal of Trauma and Stress,* **15**, 99–112.

27. Bodvarsdottir, I. and Elklit, A. (2007). Victimization and PTSD-like states in an Icelandic youth probability sample. *BMC Psychiatry*, **7**, 51.

28. Malek, M., Guyer, B. and Lescohier, I. (1990). The epidemiology and prevention of child pedestrian injury. *Advances in Neurology,* **22**, 301–313.

29. Tan, N. C., Ang, A., Heng, D., Chen, J. and Wong, H. B. (2007). Evaluation of playground injuries based on ICD, E codes, international classification of external cause of injury codes (ICECI), and abbreviated injury scale coding systems. *Asia-Pacific Journal of Public Health*, **19**, 18–27.

30. Edgardh, K. and Ormstad, K. (2000). Prevalence and characteristics of sexual abuse in a national sample of Swedish seventeen-year-old boys and girls. *Acta Paediatrica*, **89**, 310–319.

31. Walker, J. L., Carey, P. D., Mohr, N., Stein, D. J. and Seedat, S. (2004). Gender differences in the prevalence of childhood sexual abuse and in the development of pediatric PTSD. *Archives in Women's Mental Health*, **7**, 111–121.

32. Fantuzzo, J., Boruch, R., Beriama, A., Atkins, M. and Marcus, S. (1997). Domestic violence and children: Prevalence and risk in five major U.S. cities. *Journal of the American Academy of Child and Adolescent Psychiatry*, **36**, 116–122.

33. Ibsen, L. M. and Koch, T. (2002). Submersion and asphyxial injury. *Critical Care Medicine*, **30** (Suppl.), S402–S408.

34. Molnar, B. E., Buka, S. L., Brennan, R. T., Holton, J. K. and Earls, F. (2003). A multilevel study of neighborhoods and parent-to-child physical aggression: Results from the project on human development in Chicago neighborhoods. *Child Maltreatment*, **8**, 84–97.

35. Feldman, B. J., Conger, R. D. and Burzette, R. G. (2004). Traumatic events, psychiatric disorders, and pathways of risk and resilience during the transition to adulthood. *Research in Human Development*, **1**, 259–290.

36. Stevens, T. N., Ruggiero, K. J., Kilpatrick, D. G., Resnick, H. S. and Saunders, B. E. (2005). Variables differentiating singly and multiply victimized youth: Results from the National Survey of Adolescents and implications for secondary prevention. *Child Maltreatment,* **10**, 211–223.

37. Fantuzzo, J. and Fusco, R. (2007). Children's direct sensory exposure to substantiated domestic violence crimes. *Violence and Victims*, **22**, 158–171.

38. Fantuzzo, J. W., Fusco, R. A., Mohr, W. K. and Perry, M. A. (2007). Domestic violence and children's presence: A population-based study of law enforcement surveillance

of domestic violence. *Journal of Family Violence*, **22**, 331–340.

39. Akinbami, L. J. and Schoendorf, K. C. (2002). Trends in childhood asthma: Prevalence, health care utilization, and mortality. *Pediatrics*, **110**, 315–322.

40. Bernard, S. J., Paulozzi, L. J. and Wallace, D. L. (2007). Fatal injuries among children by race and ethnicity: United States, 1999–2002. *MMWR Surveillance Summaries*, **56**, 1–16.

41. Austin, S. B., Roberts, A. L., Corliss, H. L. and Molnar, B. E. (2008). Sexual violence victimization history and sexual risk indicators in a community-based urban cohort of "mostly heterosexual" and heterosexual young women. *American Journal of Public Health*, **98**, 1015–1020.

42. Saewyc, E. M., Pettingell, S. L. and Skay, C. L. (2006). Hazards of stigma: The sexual and physical abuse of gay, lesbian, and bisexual adolescents in the United States and Canada. *Child Welfare*, **85**, 195–213.

43. Putnam, F. W. (2003). Ten-year research update review: Child sexual abuse. *Journal of the American Academy of Child and Adolescent Psychiatry*, **42**, 269–278.

44. Mannw, J. R., Zhou, L., McKee, M. and McDermott, S. (2007). Children with hearing loss and increased risk of injury. *Annals of Family Medicine*, **5**, 528–533.

45. Scholer, S. J., Hickson, G. B. and Ray, W. A. (1999). Sociodemographic factors identify US infants at high risk of injury mortality. *Pediatrics*, **103**, 1183–1188.

46. Stein, M. B., Hofler, M., Perkonigg, A. *et al.* (2002). Patterns of incidence and psychiatric risk factors for traumatic events. *International Journal of Methods in Psychiatric Research*, **11**, 143–153.

47. Raghavan, R., Bogart, L. M., Elliott, M. N., Vestal, K. D. and Schuster, M. A. (2004). Sexual victimization among a national probability sample of adolescent women. *Perspectives on Sexual and Reproductive Health*, **36**, 225–232.

48. Storr, C. L., Ialongo, N. S., Anthony, J. C. and Breslau, N. (2007). Childhood antecedents of exposure to traumatic events and posttraumatic stress disorder. *American Journal of Psychiatry*, **164**, 119–125.

49. Breslau, N., Davis, G. C., Andreski, P. and Peterson, E. (1991). Traumatic events and posttraumatic stress disorder in an urban population of young adults. *Archives of General Psychiatry*, **48**, 216–222.

50. Finkelhor, D., Ormrod, R. K. and Turner, H. A. (2007). Re-victimization patterns in a national longitudinal sample of children and youth. *Child Abuse & Neglect*, **31**, 479–502.

51. Finkelhor, D., Ormrod, R., Turner, H. and Hamby, S. L. (2005). The victimization of children and youth: A comprehensive, national survey. *Child Maltreatment*, **10**, 5–25.

52. Todd, J., Armon, C., Griggs, A., Poole, S. and Berman, S. (2006). Increased rates of morbidity, mortality, and charges for hospitalized children with public or no health insurance as compared with children with private insurance in Colorado and the United States. *Pediatrics*, **118**, 577–585.

53. Hasselberg, M., Laflamme, L. and Weitoft, G. R. (2001). Socioeconomic differences in road traffic injuries during childhood and youth: A closer look at different kinds of road user. *Journal of Epidemiology and Community Health*, **55**, 858–862.

54. Laflamme, L. and Diderichsen, F. (2000). Social differences in traffic injury risks in childhood and youth: A literature review and a research agenda. *Injury Prevention*, **6**, 293–298.

55. Scholer, S. J., Mitchel, Jr., E. F. and Ray, W. A. (1997). Predictors of injury mortality in early childhood. *Pediatrics*, **100**, 342–347.

56. Elklit, A. (2002). Victimization and PTSD in a Danish national youth probability sample. *Journal of the American Academy of Child and Adolescent Psychiatry*, **41**, 174–181.

57. Finkelhor, D., Ormrod, R. K. and Turner, H. A. (2007). Polyvictimization and trauma in a national longitudinal cohort. *Developmental Psychopathology*, **19**, 149–166.

58. Haynes, R., Reading, R. and Gale, S. (2003). Household and neighbourhood risks for injury to 5–14 year old children. *Social Science & Medicine*, **57**, 625–636.

59. Lanphear, B. P., Aligne, C. A., Auinger, P., Weitzman, M. and Byrd, R. S. (2001). Residential exposures associated with asthma in US children. *Pediatrics*, **107**, 505–511.

60. Thorne, P. S., Kulhankova, K., Yin, M. *et al.* (2005). Endotoxin exposure is a risk factor for asthma: The national survey of endotoxin in United States housing. *American Journal of Respiration and Critical Care Medicine*, **172**, 1371–1377.

61. United Nations Children's Fund. (2007). *State of the world's children 2007*. New York: United Nations Children Fund.

62. Murray, C. J. and Lopez, A. D. (1997). Mortality by cause for eight regions of the world: Global Burden of Disease Study. *Lancet*, **349**, 1269–1276.

63. Bryce, J., Boschi-Pinto, C., Shibuya, K. and Black, R. E. (2005). WHO estimates of the causes of death in children. *Lancet*, **365**, 1147–1152.

64. Nantulya, V. M. and Reich, M. R. (2003). Equity dimensions of road traffic injuries in low- and middle-income countries. *Injury Control and Safety Promotion*, **10**, 13–20.

# Chapter 3

# Historical themes in the study of recovered and false memories of trauma

Constance J. Dalenberg and Kelsey L. Paulson

The knowledge that memory does not always conform to the true record of the past is probably as old as human social communication. "You are remembering your actions the way you want to remember them," we tell our intimates during an argument. Similarly, "you don't remember because you don't want to remember," or the more ubiquitous accusation – "you have a very convenient memory" – acknowledge widespread awareness of motivated memory failure and memory distortion. Nietzsche made one the best known statements in this vein in 1886 [1]: "'I have done that,' says my memory. 'I cannot have done that,' says my pride, and remains inexorable. At last, memory yields." So why is the loss and recovery of trauma memory now considered by some to be controversial? What are the historical themes that maintain or exacerbate the controversy?

## Professional consensus

The first answer to the question of why recovered memory of trauma is controversial would be that for the most part, it is not. The American Psychological Association (APA) [2], American Psychiatric Association [3], International Society for Traumatic Stress Studies [4] and many other groups have taken public stands that therapists should not assume the truth or falsity of recovered memory. Both recovered memory and false memory (FM) are possible, these organizations assert, and therapists should focus on the short- and long-term consequences of the memories (e.g., depression, post-traumatic stress disorder, etc.), rather than attempt to make claims as to knowledge of truth value. The International Society of Traumatic Stress Studies, the premier research organization representing all expert factions within the research and clinical professional communities, concludes that there is an *international consensus* across scientists in North America, Europe, Australia and New Zealand [4] that

"(1) traumatic events are usually remembered in part or in whole; (2) traumatic memories may be forgotten, then remembered at some later time; and (3) illusory memories can also occur" (p. 15).

In an effort to quell voices of extremism on both sides, consensus papers have appeared in scientific journals, at times written jointly by clinical researchers and non-clinical cognitive researchers (e.g., Berliner & Loftus, 1992 [5]). After the 1996 NATO meeting on trauma and memory in Port de Bourgenay, France, cognitive psychologist Stephen Lindsay joined with clinical researcher John Briere to publish a consensus paper [6], concluding that (p. 639):

> [T]here is no doubt that people can and do experience the recovery of memories of previously nonremembered childhood sexual abuse. It is likely that in some such cases the recollections are essentially veridical and that in some cases they are essentially false, and both of us agree that, barring exposure to suggestive influences, the former are probably much more common.

Similarly, Knapp and VandeCreek [7], after reviewing the extant literature, concluded that there was a "professional consensus" that "some memories of past traumas can be lost and later recovered" and "false memories can be created" (p. 366). Those who "deny the authenticity of all repressed memories," and those who "would accept them all as true" were defined by Loftus [8] (p. 524) and by most researchers today as holding "extreme positions."

Large-scale surveys also showed that a strong majority of clinical psychologists (over 90%), including the majority of researcher clinicians (88%), holds the position that accurate recovered memories are possible [9]. Pope and Tabachnick [10] found that over 70% of clinical psychologists had personally treated a recovered memory survivor, and Polusny and Follette [11] found that 28% had seen such a case in the last year.

*The Impact of Early Life Trauma on Health and Disease: The Hidden Epidemic,* ed. Ruth A. Lanius, Eric Vermetten and Clare Pain. Published by Cambridge University Press. Copyright © Cambridge University Press 2010.

## The impact of the "zealots"

Before detailing a few of the historical sources of the "zealotry," it is worth emphasizing that extremity is quite obviously in the eye of the beholder. Robyn Dawes, a key supporter of FM positions in the debate, has conducted key research on this point. Dawes *et al.* [12] found that when undergraduates were asked to state opinions held by those with whom they agreed and disagreed, they wrote much more extreme statements to put into the mouths of their opponents. Importantly, the members of the opposing faction also saw these items as extreme and did not endorse them. In line with this perhaps-unwitting use of straw-person arguments, an important tactic in the recovered memory debate has been to identify extreme and offensive statements made by key opposition (typically marginal members), and to equate these statements with the view of the opposing side. Thus, highly complex differences between groups have been presented as insurmountable differences in values (e.g., "I value science and you don't"; "I value children and you don't") that can be used to entirely discount the arguments of opposing researchers.

Within any field, the reader will find horror stories of doctors who see the need for their chosen specialty everywhere (bipolar children, attention-deficit hyperactivity disorder, fibromyalgia, post-traumatic stress disorder), and those who entirely dismiss an accepted concept. Elizabeth Loftus [8] presented a compelling example of a private investigator, hired by a father who had been accused of molestation, who confronts the paradigmatic overzealous therapist. According to the account, the therapist told the private investigator (pretending to be a patient) that the investigator's vague symptoms were clearly body memories from a repressed trauma, disclosing that she (the therapist) too was an incest survivor. If accurately presented, this therapist is an extremist. Similarly, FM researcher Ralph Underwager, who suggested in his interview with *Paidika*, a European journal, that focus on child sexual abuse was the results of efforts by radical feminists and lesbians who were jealous of the closeness and intimacy of sexuality between man and boy [13], also represents an extreme position.

## Who values science?

The communication problems among researchers in the recovered memory field begin with overuse of such examples. It is no doubt true that the average researcher specializing in child trauma has a higher estimate of the likelihood of trauma than does the average researcher specializing in FM (just as the reverse is likely true for estimates on FM). However, in discussions that C. Dalenberg has had with virtually all the mainstream FM researchers, few have ever expressed agreement with the statement of Wakefield and Underwager [14] about pedophilia. Similarly, the practice of diagnosing repressed trauma from vague symptoms after a few sessions has been repeatedly denounced by trauma specialists. In fact, virtually all are on record denouncing this practice (e.g., Bowman [15], Briere [16], Courtois [17]). The picture becomes muddier when such practices are equated with more subtle statements, such as Loftus's example of a therapist who tells a patient that many people struggling with relevant problems have experienced painful childhood events such as physical or sexual abuse, and asks if "anything like that ever happened to you?" [8]. The first example is unacceptable therapeutic work. The second is leading, but may allow a reluctant client to divulge a shamed past. The merits of such an intervention deserve debate and complex clinical discussion. Collapsing the range of actual clinical behaviors (i.e., equating general trauma questioning with pressured inquisition) has hidden the truly controversial behaviors from the view of the debaters, leaving memory researchers with the impression that trauma researchers at times accept browbeating clients, and leaving trauma researchers with the impression that memory researchers do not understand the importance of screening for trauma history.

Attacks on the uncritical acceptance shown by therapists almost invariably cite Bass and Davis's workbook (*Courage to Heal* [18]), a text of advice, poetry and victim accounts, and E. Sue Blume's *Secret Survivors* [19]. Both texts grew out of the grassroots movement on prevention and treatment of child abuse that predated the professional interest in the problem, and both appeal more to the lay reader than to the scientist-practitioner. Both texts also were widely used in the therapist community, particularly in the early 1990s, and have been praised by survivors as helpful to their recovery.

Specific sentences are repeatedly cited from Bass and Davis's 495-page text (e.g., "If you are unable to remember any specific instances like the ones mentioned above but still have a feeling that something abusive happened to you, it probably did," cited by Loftus [8], p. 21) that clearly go beyond the data available on the validity of suspicion as an indicator of lost memory. These sentences, however, should be understood in the context of the time, very early in the understanding of sexual abuse dynamics. The first feminist writers on sexual abuse (e.g., Armstrong [20]) faced strong resistance, both in the media and in the professional community, that has been largely forgotten in the more recent debate. Armstrong's book, reviewed in the *New York Times* Book Review [21], was described as "pornography masquerading as science," with victim accounts dismissed as "wallowing in [the topic of incest] for the sake of titillation." *Time* magazine (1980) quoted Wardell Pomeroy, coauthor of the Kinsey reports, as stating that it was time to declare that incest was not necessarily a perversion, and might at times be beneficial. The 1979 *SIECUS Report* of the US Sex Information and Education Council questioned whether the incest taboo should be considered similar to the masturbation taboo [22]. In such an atmosphere, also considering the widespread belief that incest memories were commonly fantasies of women who had Oedipal desires for their fathers (cf. [23]), convictions among therapists that the pressure not to remember outweighed the pressure to disclose might have been more warranted than is true today.

Both trauma researcher and memory researcher groups have been uncomfortable with fully acknowledging the contribution of the influential lay groups who ally with them. For the trauma researcher, this would mean the admission that a large subset of practicing therapists are not trained in critical analysis of psychological literature, testing or statistics. These groups are trained in the prevalence and negative effects of child trauma, and they have been critical to the development and maintenance of more appropriate societal responses to the problem of child abuse. In developing their understanding of abuse, they had little help from either mainstream trauma research or from mainstream cognitive research. In fact, when Browne and Finkelhor [24] conducted an extensive review of the literature on child sexual abuse just prior to the publication of *Courage to Heal* [18]; they cited only 49 references, 19 of which were manuals, government reports or unpublished papers and dissertations and 16 were books and chapters. Only 15 relevant peer-reviewed articles were located. Karen Meiselman's text on incest [25], one of the first scientific treatises in modern child abuse research, identified 47 studies in the entire world literature on the subject, 25 of which documented results for fewer than 10 survivors. Child

abuse research is a relatively new field, and all admit that there is much to learn. This understanding should not undermine attempts to deepen scientific theory and research in the area, but should stem ill-conceived efforts to attack those who first drew our attention to the problem.

## Who values children?

As FM researchers accuse trauma researchers of exaggerating the effects of child abuse for political purposes, and trauma researchers accuse FM researchers of underestimating these same effects, also postulating a hidden agenda, we see a theme of the equation of FM advocacy and dismissal of the seriousness of child abuse. McNally [26] rightly noted a substantial overlap between the positions of researchers on the recovered memory issue and those held on the Rind controversy, a vociferous discussion of a *Psychological Bulletin* article by Rind *et al.* [27]. This controversy is worth a brief review.

Rind *et al.* [27] published a meta-analysis on the effects of child sexual abuse on adjustment in college samples. After finding a small overall effect size, the authors concluded that lasting psychological harm through child sexual abuse was uncommon. They suggested that child sexual abuse might be akin to masturbation, in that value-laden terms for the behavior were once used. A more "value-neutral" science would eliminate the term abuse (substituting child–adult sex) if, for instance, the child participated "willingly" and did not show "negative reactions" (p. 46). Pedophile groups immediately picked up the study for dissemination, praising the APA for "having the courage" to publish a study showing that "the current war on boy-lovers has no basis in science." Attorneys began attempting to use the study to support pedophile clients, arguing that the behaviors of their clients were not harmful (e.g., Harker [28]), and the study's conclusions began to appear in amicus briefs written by the False Memory Syndrome Foundation.

On July 30, 1999, the Rind meta-analysis became the first scientific study to be formally denounced by the US Congress. The APA took a stance ultimately satisfactory to no one. Ray Fowler, then President of APA, wrote a letter to Congress [29] that the Rind *et al.* review "included opinions of the authors that are inconsistent with APA's stated and deeply held positions" (p. 1), and announced a procedure whereby APA would expect journals to "consider the social policy implications of articles on controversial topics"

(p. 2). The latter vague statement understandably worried many academics studying controversial topics.

Trauma and FM-affiliated scientists responded quite differently to the Rind study. Trauma researchers criticized the methods and conclusions of the work in multiple ways, reminding readers that estimates of psychopathology based on college samples are likely to be skewed, criticizing the use and interpretation of the correlation coefficient as the measure of effect size, objecting to biases in sampling that they believed were present, and criticizing the conclusion of "no harm" when only specific harms were assessed [30–33]. Further, they disagreed with suggestion by Rind and colleagues that the label "child sexual abuse" should be reserved for those children who were showing present symptoms and who did not "consent," typically arguing that it is not meaningful to speak of a "willing" 5-year-old child in the context of sexual activity or to attempt "value-neutral" discussion of child abuse sexuality [31,32]. In addition to the scientific criticisms, prior speeches or articles by Rind and colleagues that appeared to be pro-pedophilia were cited. The FM scientists (e.g., Lillienfeld [34]) pointed out the logical fallacy of arguing against Rind *et al.* [27] by disparaging the authors. Often (as in Lillienfeld [34]), they then disparaged the critics; the scientific issues went largely undebated.

Just as all scientists must acknowledge that the typical non-scientific and overzealous child advocates would throw in their lot with the trauma research group, so must we acknowledge that pedophile groups will ally with the FM position. This does not equate trauma research with anti-scientific thinking or FM research with support for pedophilia. It does, I believe, place a special burden on trauma researchers to teach and champion scientific thinking, and an equal burden on FM researchers to craft their statements about what they are and are not saying about the seriousness of child sexual abuse more carefully. Many researchers on both sides of the argument meet that burden. But just as FM scientists will cite inadequate response to *Courage to Heal* [18] as an example of failure of trauma research scientists to meet their obligation to the field, trauma scientists are concerned with the discussion of children as "willing" sexual partners in the Rind *et al.* approach [27] and question the lack of skepticism applied to the Rind findings.

It is now normative in recovered memory discussions for FM researchers to frame the debate in terms of "scientists" (themselves) versus "clinicians" (the researchers who disagree with them on the recovered memory issue, many of whom also treat patients). Alternatively, FM scientists self-label as "skeptics" with the opposing researchers labeled as "advocates." The history of the debate reviewed above, however, suggests that the groups disagree on many scientific issues (methodology, statistics and the interpretation of group differences) *as scientists*. Further, both groups contain skeptics, but FM groups are said to lack skepticism regarding the claims of perpetrators, while trauma researchers are said to overvalue the claims of victims. It stultifies debate to assume that all who disagree with one's position must be motivated by nefarious or ignominious motives (e.g., their unscientific prior biases, their wishes to protect their forensic or clinical pocketbooks, or their lack of compassion for abused children or falsely accused parents). If both groups wish to claim the high ground of science, as they do, then that ground is best claimed by engaging the best evidence and the best arguments of the opposition.

## The firewall

Admittedly, however, both groups of central theoreticians tend to comment on the partially scientific or non-scientific (moral or political) issues that are informed by the debate. The following is an example.

**Question 1.** Can a child truly consent to sexuality with an adult?

**Question 2.** Should sexual activity between a 50-year-old man and a "willing" 12-year-old girl be called abuse?

**Question 3.** As society acknowledges that both false accusation and child sexual abuse are problems to be avoided, but must make real-world decisions without 100% certainty, how should the lines of evidence be drawn? Does "better ten guilty men be acquitted than one innocent man be jailed" equate in scientific studies to "better ten true recovered memory victims be rejected as mistaken/lying than one false memory be seen as accurate"?

**Question 4.** What is the nature of the "proof" we should require for a specific mechanism of recovered memory or FM accounts before we declare that each are probably legitimate phenomena?

**Question 5.** Should we assume one mechanism (typically the mechanism this investigator studies) in the absence of proof of another, or should we begin each investigation on more even ground?

**Question 6.** Is a well-documented case example part of that proof?

Answers to such questions provide a window into the investigator's guiding philosophy of science or morality, but they are not science in and of themselves. These questions, and assumed "right" or "scientific" answers to these questions, lurk behind the pronouncements that there is "no evidence" for the opposition scientist's opinion. Disagreements between Rind and Spiegel about whether fondling of a child (who later shows few if any symptoms) is "abuse" are informed in each case by the author's scientific knowledge, but the answers do not and will not come entirely from science. The "firewall" that McNally [26] urges between science and politics cannot reasonably manifest itself either in value-free scientists or even in scientists who do not disclose their value systems through their writings. It can manifest itself, however, in greater willingness to recognize that (a) the contamination or confounding of the opposition's science by their values will be more obvious to us than the same contamination occurring in our own work, and (b) science contaminated or confounded by values differing from our own may still be science, and may still contain useful information about the real world.

## Is it repression?

The historical connection between the concept of repression and the phenomenon of recovered memory has been a central impediment to movement in the debate. Interestingly, both groups argue that repression is unlikely to be the mechanism behind accurate recovered memory, with some of the more vociferous critics being psychoanalytic writers who believe that the concept has been misapplied in the debate [35,36]. Mechanism evidence is discussed in Chs. 4 and 27 of this volume. Here it is simply noted that the evidence for or against the viability of a mechanism in the laboratory has little bearing on whether the phenomenon itself exists. That is, if we were to find tomorrow that *Helicobacter pylori* is not in fact important in causing ulcers, no one would argue that medical professionals should then decide that ulcers themselves are nonexistent. Similarly, although the question of whether traumatic amnesia can be caused by repression is interesting and relevant, the answer to the question does not decide the issue of the validity of recovered memory.

Complicating the issue, of course, is our lack of agreement on what we mean by "repression." Holmes [37], the most well-known critic of repression, requires that any experimental demonstration shows that the mechanism itself is unconscious. Thus it is not repression, but suppression, if the individual consciously

withdraws his attention from a memory, actively pushing the memory out of mind until the memory trace weakens and disappears from everyday conscious awareness. But repression as it is defined by Holmes, Loftus and other critics of FM, is not the mechanism described by recovered memory theorists, or even by ardent psychoanalytic theorists. The latter point out that Freud himself referred to pressure from the conscious and pull from the unconscious to account for repression, and Freud used the term suppression and repression interchangeably in his writings [36]. Consequently, early writers on recovered memory were using the term "repression" to mean motivated amnesia and were not necessarily arguing that the unconscious reached and snatched the memory from conscious awareness.

The early attacks on the repression concept [8, 37,38] were a positive impetus for trauma scientists to be more careful about language. This, in fact, occurred. In the years before the publication of the APA Task Force statements (1997 and earlier), approximately 24% of those publishing from a trauma perspective used repressed memory in their title rather than labeling the phenomenon in a way that did not imply mechanism (recovered memory). In publications from 1998 to 2006, that number fell to 14%. However, for those publishing from a FM perspective, the number using the term repressed memory remained high (36% in both time periods). If one believed strongly that there is no evidence for repression, why use the term to describe a phenomenon that may be multidetermined, particularly when this is not the term of choice for those whom one opposes? It seems likely that the answer again reflects the historical antagonism of the players in the debate. Just as those championing a "right to choose" in the abortion debate refer to their opponents as anti-choice, while their opposition speaks of "right to life" and "pro-abortion," so FM advocates framed the language of the debate in a way that creates significant obstacles for their colleagues in trauma research. Trauma researchers have in part begun to turn the tables, arguing that the words "false memory" have been overused [39].

## Extreme belief or extreme circumstances?

A final theme that underlies some of the misunderstanding is the focus on the extreme case. At times, this focus likely reflects the compelling nature of these cases – the popular priest who rapes dozens of children, warning them that God will punish any disclosure; the naive young woman drawn into a paranoid web of supposition about her Satanic past authored by her therapist. These episodes, memory researchers argue, are too implausible to believe or too extreme to be "forgotten."

The extreme memory – multiple episodes of an unusual type of abuse – is a common target for FM theorists. As many theorists point out, dozens of investigations show that repeated events are more difficult to forget, as common sense would affirm, although details may become confused between incidents (e.g., Powell *et al.* [40]). Thus, FM scientists argue that victims asserting such events must be presenting a memory that is false. However, research and common sense again coalesce in confirming that extreme, repeated, and implausible false events are also more difficult to implant as FMs [41]. That is, you could perhaps convince each of us, with putative false information from a parent, that we had once been taken to Minnesota for a vacation. However, the false belief that we journeyed there monthly to participate in cannibalistic feasts would be (we believe) resisted.

Given the evidence discussed above, *both* FMs of extreme events *and* recovered memories of extreme events should be rare. To the extent that the events recalled are extreme and unusual, the present state of research thus suggests that scientists should expect to find a constellation of more unusual features. For example, FM theorists might expect particularly strong suggestive influences rather than simply evidence that the individual had read *Courage to Heal*. Perhaps interrogatory suggestion procedures took place over time with an individual who can be shown to respond strongly to suggestion (unlike most patients with recovered memory [42]). Recovered memory theorists might expect to find that an individual with an extreme event account was abused by a figure who had major control and influence over his or her experience [43], was a survivor showing character traits of particularly high emotional and cognitive avoidance [44], and reported a more spontaneous recovery within safe circumstances in response to a highly salient cue [45,46]. In situations in which neither of these sets of descriptors is clearly present, the evaluator would have strong reason to suspect the alternative hypothesis of a false statement made in response to social demand or malingering. Neither FM researchers nor recovered memory researchers have paid sufficient research attention to the power of social demand to lead

an individual to consciously present himself or herself falsely in abuse-focused therapy (or in forensic settings that follow).

## The bubble of acrimony

The themes discussed above led to much misunderstanding between researchers in the early to mid 1990s. For a brief period, name-calling and (often thinly veiled) accusations of incompetence or lack of character replaced an evaluation of theory and data. Today such articles are more rare, and we see few authors publicly wondering whether FM is a myth generated by pedophiles or suggesting that recovered memory is a fad promulgated by incompetent therapists. It was, therefore, a surprise to see one recent article representing a return to the bad old days [47], recalling the name-calling ("persistence of folly," "brief bubble of fashion") of earlier years. Pope *et al.* [47] argue that because articles using the term "repressed memory" rose to a high of 107 publications in 1997, declining to a mean of 25 publications per year in 2001–2003 (a fall of more than 75%), the field does not inspire serious scientific interest.

The reader will no doubt immediately recognize a few of the many problems with this argument (see also Dalenberg *et al.* [48]). Pope *et al.* [47] assessed the occurrence of publications in *PsycINFO* that mentioned both FM and trauma (more precisely, child abuse or sexual abuse). The publications reduce from a high of 101 in 1997 to a mean in 2001–2003 of 14.33 (a reduction of 86%). Does this invalidate the concept of FM, and reflect that FM of abuse was a concept briefly in fashion but with no scientific support? Alternatively, does it reflect the intense period of discussion that erupted during the years in which professional organizations were developing position statements on the topic? In considering these possibilities, it should be noted that 68 chapters reviewing the controversy were written in the period 1996–1999, compared with seven in the 4 years before, and nine in the 4 years after.

The acrimony in the initial stages of the debate also reflects reactions by and to the members of the False Memory Syndrome Foundation. This organization, formed in 1992, was developed with the aid of Underwager, Wakefield and the Freyds (a couple accused of sexually abusing their daughter) and became a lightning rod for debate. Individual Foundation Board members took positions that were controversial in the clinical community (e.g., Harold

Lief's decision to serve on the board with the Freyds after disclosing that he had functioned as their personal psychiatrist [43]). Books, chapters and articles written by members of the Foundation (e.g., Ofshe & Watters [49]) at times were extreme and offensive in content, and appeared to exaggerate the scientific case for FM syndrome. Ofshe and Watters's book contained references to therapists as "the-rapists," repeated references to "hysteria" and highly selective and distorted descriptions of court cases. In one such case, a child's suicide note was rewritten to support Ofshe and Watters's point of view [49]. These behaviors and opinions led to strong denunciation by a former chair of the APA ethics committee [50], as well as to concern among the "middle ground" theorists in the debate as to why others on the Foundation's Board did not publicly object to some of these activities (as the Board recommended that clinicians do when confronted with overzealous therapists). As of now, however, even the False Memory Syndrome Foundation officially states on its website (www.fmsfonline.org) that recovered memories of abuse may be accurate as well as inaccurate.

## Conclusions

The acrimony that has fueled the debate on recovered memory has abated in most arenas, clearing the way for scientific research that has clearly established the reality of the phenomena of both FM and accurate recovered memory. Further work will benefit from a clearer distinction between the study of phenomena (both recovered and false memory) and their mechanisms (suggestion, repression, dissociation), direct and forthright debate about the nature and weight of types of evidence (existence proof, laboratory analogue, clinical research), recognition of the effect of perspective and personal value system on the design and interpretation of research, collaboration across disciplines to create meaningful and valid paradigms and a more committed effort to entertain alternative hypotheses in recovered memory and FM research.

## References

1. Nietzsche, F. (1886/2001). *Beyond good and evil.* Cambridge, UK: Cambridge University Press.
2. American Psychological Association. (1996). Final conclusions of the American Psychological Association Working Group on Investigation of Memories of Childhood Abuse. *Psychology, Public Policy and Law*, **4**, 933–940.
3. American Psychiatric Association. (1993). *Statement of memories of sexual abuse.* Washington, DC: American Psychiatric Press.
4. International Society for Traumatic Stress Studies. (1998). *Childhood trauma remembered: A report on the current scientific knowledge base and its applications.* Deerfield, IL: International Society for Traumatic Stress Studies.
5. Berliner, L. and Loftus, E. (1992). Sexual abuse accusations: Desperately seeking reconciliation. *Journal of Interpersonal Violence*, **7**, 570–578.
6. Lindsay, S. and Briere, J. (1997). The controversy regarding recovered memories of childhood sexual abuse: Pitfalls, bridges, and future directions. *Journal of Interpersonal Violence*, **12**, 631–647.
7. Knapp, S. and VandeCreek, L. (2000). Recovered memories of childhood abuse: Is there an underlying professional consensus? *Professional Psychology: Research and Practice*, **31**, 365–371.
8. Loftus, E. (1993). The reality of repressed memories. *American Psychologist*, **48**, 518–537.
9. Dammeyer, M., Nightengale, N. and McCoy, M. (1997). Repressed memory and other controversial origins of sexual abuse allegations: Beliefs among psychologists and clinical social workers. *Child Maltreatment*, **2**, 252–263.
10. Pope, K. and Tabachnick, B. (1995). Recovered memories of abuse among therapy patients: A national survey. *Ethics and Behavior*, **5**, 237–248.
11. Polusny, M. and Follette, V. (1996). Remembering childhood sexual abuse: A national survey of psychologists' clinical practices, beliefs, and personal experiences. *Professional Psychology: Research and Practice*, **27**, 41–52.
12. Dawes, R., Singer, D. and Lemon, F. (1972). An experimental analysis of the contrast effect and its implications for intergroup communication and the indirect assessment of attitude. *Journal of Personality and Social Psychology*, **21**, 281–295.
13. Lightfoot, L. (1993). Child abuse experts says paedophilia part of "God's will" – Dr Ralph Underwager. *Sunday Times,* December 19, 1993.
14. Wakefield, H. and Underwager, R. (1995). *Return of the furies: An investigation into recovered memory therapy.* Chicago, IL: Open Court.
15. Bowman, E. (1996). Delayed memories of child abuse: Part I. An overview of research findings on forgetting, remembering, and corroborating trauma. *Dissociation*, **9**, 221–243.
16. Briere, J. (1996). *Therapy for adults molested as children.* New York: Springer.
17. Courtois, C. (1997). Guidelines for the treatment of adults abused or possibly abused as children (with attention to issues of delayed/recovered memory). *American Journal of Psychotherapy*, **51**, 497–510.

31

18. Bass, E. and Davis, L. (1988). *Courage to heal: A guide for women survivors of child sexual abuse*. New York: Harper Row.

19. Blume, E. S. (1990). *Secret survivors: Uncovering incest and its after effects in women*. New York: Ballantine.

20. Armstrong, L. (1978). *Kiss Daddy goodnight: A speakout on incest*. New York: Pocket Books.

21. Sokolov, R. (1978). Nonfiction in brief. *New York Times Book Review*. August 6, 1978, 16, 20.

22. Ramay, J. (1979). *Report of the Sexuality Information and Education Council of the USA, 7*, No. 5. New York: SIECUS.

23. Masson, J. (1984). *Assault on truth: Freud's suppression of the seduction theory*. New York: Farrar, Straus and Giroux.

24. Browne, A. and Finkelhor, D. (1986). Impact of child sexual abuse: A review of the research. *Psychological Bulletin*, **99**, 66–77.

25. Meiselman, K. (1978). *Incest*. San Francisco: Jossey-Bass.

26. McNally, R. (2003). Progress and controversy in the study of posttraumatic stress disorder. *Annual Review of Psychology*, **54**, 229–252.

27. Rind, B., Tromovitch, P. and Bauserman, R. (1998). A meta-analytic examination of assume properties of child sexual abuse using college samples. *Psychological Bulletin*, **124**, 22–53.

28. Harker, V. (1999). Former gym teacher gets 88 years in molestation case. *Arizona Republic*, October 21, p. A15.

29. Fowler, R. (1999, June 9). *APA letter to the Honorable Rep. DeLay (R-Tx)*. Washington, DC: American Psychiatric Association; http://www.apa.org/releases/delay.html (accessed April 10, 2008).

30. Dallam, S., Gleaves, D., Cepeda-Benito, A. *et al.* (2001). The effects of child sexual abuse: Comment on Rind, Tromovitch and Bauserman (1998). *Psychological Bulletin*, **127**, 715–733.

31. Ondersma, S., Chaffin, M., Berliner, L. *et al.* (2001). Sex with children is abuse: Comment on Rind, Tromovitch, and Bauserman (1998). *Psychological Bulletin*, **127**, 707–714.

32. Spiegel, D. (2001). Who is in procrustes' bed? *Sexuality and Culture*, **5**, 79–86.

33. Whittenburg, J., Tice, P., Baker, G. and Lemmey, D. (2001). A critical appraisal of the 1998 meta-analytic review of child sexual aubse outcomes reported to Rind, Tromovitch and Bauserman. *Journal of Child Sexual Abuse*, 135–155.

34. Lillienfeld, S. (2002). When worlds collide: social science, politics, and the Rind *et al.* (1998) child sexual abuse meta-analysis. *American Psychologist*, **57**, 176–188.

35. Boag, S. (2006). Freudian repression, the common view, and pathological science. *Review of General Psychology*, **10**, 74–86.

36. Erdelyi, M. (2006). The unified theory of repression. *Behavioral and Brain Sciences*, **29**, 499–551.

37. Holmes, D. (1995). The evidence for repression: An examination of sixty years of research. In J. Singer (ed.), *Repression and dissociation: Implications for personality theory, psychopathology and health* (pp. 85–102). Chicago, IL: University of Chicago Press.

38. Loftus, E. and Ketcham, K. (1994). *The myth of repressed memory*. New York: St. Martin's Press.

39. Pezdek, K. and Lam, S. (2007). What research paradigms have cognitive psychologists used to study "false memory," and what are the implications of these choices? *Consciousness and Cognition*, **16**, 2–17.

40. Powell, M., Roberts, K., Ceci, S. and Hembrooke, H. (1999). The effects of repeated experience on children's suggestibility. *Developmental Psychology*, **35**, 1462–1477.

41. Pezdek, K., Finger, K. and Hodge, D. (1997). Planting false childhood memories: The role of event plausibility. *Psychological Science*, **8**, 437–441.

42. Leavitt, F. (1997). False attribution of suggestibility to explain recovered memory of childhood sexual abuse following extended amnesia. *Child Abuse & Neglect*, **21**, 265–272.

43. Freyd, J. (1996). *Betrayal trauma: the logical of forgetting childhood abuse*. Cambridge, MA: Harvard University Press.

44. Dalenberg, C. (2006). Recovered memory and the Daubert criteria: Recovered memory as professionally tested, peer reviewed, and accepted in the relevant scientific community. *Trauma, Violence and Abuse*, 7, 274–310.

45. Dalenberg, C. (1996). Accuracy, timing, and circumstances of disclosure in therapy of recovered and continuous memories of abuse. *Journal of Psychiatry and Law*, **24**, 229–275.

46. Geraerts, E., Schooler, J., Merckelbach, H. *et al.* (2007). The reality of recovered memories: Corroborating continuous and discontinuous memories of childhood sexual abuse. *Psychological Science*, **18**, 564–568.

47. Pope, H., Barry, S., Bodkin, A. and Hudson, J. (2006). Tracking scientific interest in the dissociative disorders: A study of scientific publication output 1984–2003. *Psychotherapy and Psychosomatics*, **75**, 19–24.

48. Dalenberg, C., Loewenstein, R., Spiegel, D. *et al.* (2007). Scientific study of the dissociative disorders. *Psychotherapy and Psychosomatics*, **76**, 400–401.

49. Ofshe, R. and Watters, E. (1994). *Making monsters: False memories, psychotherapy, and sexual hysteria*. New York: Charles Scribners' Sons.

50. Pope, K. (1996) Memory, abuse and science: Questioning claims about the false memory syndrome epidemic. *American Psychologist*, **51**, 957–974.

# Early trauma, later outcome: results from longitudinal studies and clinical observations

Nathan Szajnberg, Amit Goldenberg and Udi Harari

## Introduction

This chapter explores the effects of early adverse experiences by reporting on long-term outcomes of childhood trauma. We will review two major prospective studies, then present clinical vignettes to give life to the research findings, and discuss the implications of types of childhood trauma for later outcome. We learn that children abused by their parents continue to re-experience forms of suffering, either predominately internally, even after those children have grown up and are liberated from abuse, or in some cases, seek out external adversity. Massie and Szajnberg's *Lives Across Time* study [1] commenced with the studies of Brody and colleagues [2–4] with married couples, primarily working and middle class with their first children. The Minnesota study, *The Development of the Person*, began in 1974 [5] and followed indigent mothers (61% unmarried and 50% of whom were teenagers at their first child's birth) and their infants.

Trauma in this chapter refers to child abuse by the parent. The literature on childhood trauma is voluminous: we refer the reader to such classics as the studies of Anna Freud and Burlingham of children during V-bombing of London and of orphan survivors from Nazi Theresienstadt [6]; Terr's sensitive and elegant study of kidnappings (Chowchilla) [7]; Pynoos and colleagues' studies of children after earthquakes, war (Kuwait) and sniper killings (LA) [8]; Laor and colleagues' study of children after Iraqi SCUD bombings (Israel) [9]; and Jungmeen and Cicchetti's study of child abuse and neglect [10]. Further, Bowlby broadened the definition of childhood trauma as any events that seriously threatened the attachment relationship, which could include parental death, divorce, psychoses and such [11]. More subtly, Khan articulated "strain trauma" as differing from discrete traumata,

referring to matters such as the chronic day-to-day demeaning of a child or an ongoing parent conflict [12]. This chapter, however, will focus primarily on physical abuse by the child's parent: this is legally defined in the USA and must be reported. Physical abuse is easier to discover and study than many other types of abuse.

Other types of abuse are not dismissed. The current account is restricted for greater certitude, and perhaps to cover a more psychologically severe form of abuse: attacks by someone from whom the dependent child expects protection and caring.

## Repetition compulsion?

Freud postulated that the repetition compulsion is an attempt, an inherent process, to actively master what was once passively experienced [13]. The repetition compulsion compelled Freud to revise his thinking, to understand why someone would actively seek to redo, reexperience the adversities of life. Discovering the repetition compulsion response became one of Freud's significant contributions to our knowledge of our nature, along with repression, ambivalence, transference, sexuality and unlocking the elegant constructions of dream life.

In 1977, Winnicott [14] described an apparently different inherent process, something that drives development: normal, healthy young children's maturational process towards optimal growth. This process is similar to Piaget's concept of the inherent driving force behind good cognitive development [15]. This inherent driving force may be related to Bowlby's adaptation of "ethnology" [11,16,17]; there are (healthy) inherent drives/processes in each juvenile that can be released by a good-enough caring adult – in Bowlby's framework, these are working models to optimize attachment. Winnicott, Piaget and Bowlby used different terms for a common phenomenon: qualities of a potentiality within the young organism, ready to sprout with decent caring. This process (unlike Freud's idea of repetition compulsion) is not initiated by adversity; rather it comes naturally, something closer to Dylan Thomas's, "The force that through the green fuse drives the flower" [18].

Giovacchini [19] revisited Freud's concept of repetition compulsion and integrates it with Winnicott's maturational processes to explain why psychoanalysis works. If we generalize the repetition compulsion to include both conflictual and structural internal adversities – that is, neurotic internal conflicts or deficits/distortions in character structure – then the transferential recreation of neurotic (internalized) relationships occurs because of the inherence of the repetition compulsion. Yet, following Winnicott [14], along with the attempted wish for mastery of adverse experiences, there is a "healthy" hopeful maturational drive to repair what was hurt, a concept captured by Searles, "Patient as therapist to his therapist," discussed by Flarsheim [20]. That is, the patient's attempt to "cure" the therapist's errors is a transference repetition of the child's hope to cure his parents' ailments or inadequacies so that the parent will better care for the child. In Giovacchini's sense [19], the repetition compulsion is a specific form of the general phenomenon of this inherent maturational drive.

## Discussion of *Lives Across Time*

The *Lives Across Time* study [1] is described briefly; the accounts therein are further discussed in Massie and Szajnberg's *My Life is a Longing* [21]. Brody and colleagues [2–4] recruited 132 full-term healthy infants among married couples in 1964–1965. The mothers and infants were observed during the first year, including filming play and feeding. Based on observations, the mothering care was classified as more and less effective according to the three criteria: empathy, organization and efficiency. The children were followed until six years old and were then met again at 18 years. Massie and Szajnberg [21] performed the 30-year assessments of 76 subjects who were found, using a lengthy semi-structured interview that included elements of the SCL-90 [22], the Adult Attachment Interview [23] and life history particularly from their last follow-up at 18 years to age 30. Outcomes used were Adult Attachment Interview, the *Diagnostic and Statistical Manual* (DSM) [24] and its Global Assessment of Functioning (GAF),

Eriksonian stages and Vallaint's Defense Mechanism hierarchy.

## Physical abuse

Five of the seventy-six – all boys – were physically abused by their fathers. In each case, this was revealed only at the 30 year follow-up. Despite home visits and close observation in the first 7 years and interviews and testing at 18 years, the physical abuse was unknown to the original investigators, although in one case, the researchers were concerned enough (about what we would now consider ancillary signs) to refer the family for evaluation.

A brief example of the abuse gives flesh to this study. We learned both from "Johnny" – and independently from his sister (also in the study) – that their father had an explosive and terrifying temper, although he only beat his son. Both parents worked in a small family business until late at night. The children arrived home alone, made dinner, did their homework and went to bed. One evening, father came home and "blew-up" because he believed someone had eaten his ice cream sandwich. He yanked Johnny out of bed, screaming and beating him to confess. Another time, when his father thought Johnny was not practicing his oboe well enough, he whipped the 7 year-old with his belt buckle until the child bled and was brought to the emergency room (where the boy said he had fallen down the steps).

The following section will compare the outcomes at 30 years of abused children with the non-abused children. All abused children had histories of, or current, psychiatric diagnoses (vs. 32% of the overall group with current psychiatric diagnoses) such as dysthymia, major depression, alcohol abuse, narcissistic personality, somatizations, anxiety and, in at least three cases, multiple "accidents" with physical injuries. The latter exemplifies Freud's repetition compulsion; that is, the history and prevalence of recurrent accidents in these few subjects suggest that the passively experienced childhood abuse is transformed into an attempt to actively master the experience of physical abuse and the hope for surviving this (see the case of Ted later in this chapter). The average GAF score was 68.6 in these five subjects (versus 84 for the overall group). In addition, on record review, Massie and Szajnberg found a progression of symptom transformation [21]. At 1 year of age, two out of the five abused boys showed anxiety, sadness, developmental delay, overt anger and autoerotism. By 7 years of age, all but one showed symptoms that included fears, developmental delay, enuresis, insomnia, anxiety, overcompliance, impulsivity, head banging and rocking. By 18 years of age, all showed symptom pictures that included anxiety, self-doubts, self-criticism, perfectionism, compulsivity, tension, feeling physically vulnerable, poor self-esteem, uneven concentration, depression, longings for tenderness, emotional restriction, passivity, lack of direction, suspiciousness and impulsivity.

Massie and Szajnberg looked at five additional children from the 76 who were emotionally neglected or verbally abused [21]. Sample sizes are too small for statistical analysis. However, three were female, and while this group's average GAF was 69.6, there was a wider range in scores (60–80) than in the five physically abused boys. All had developed psychiatric diagnoses such as dysthymia, major depression, anorexia, alcohol abuse, somatizations, schizoid personality and obesity. Their symptomatic pictures began at 1 year with evidence of distress including uneven development, anaclitic depression, anxiety, hyperactivity and poor frustration tolerance. By 7 years, mood difficulties predominated, and by 18 years, the symptom pictures cloud these teenagers with anxiety, inhibitions, depression, anhedonia, counter-phobia, grandiosity, oppositionality, constriction, longing for care, meekness, emptiness, schizoptypy and loneliness.

All 10 children (physically abused plus emotionally abused) had psychiatric diagnoses by 30 years, in contrast to a 32% prevalence for the overall sample. Emotional defenses were in the primitive range, such as denial, passive aggression, identification with the aggressor apathetic withdrawal.

Here is a vignette from the study. At 30, "Ted" was affable even jovial, although his chain-smoking and nail-biting suggested tension. It was clear in infancy that his mother was awkward, lacked intimacy and soothed poorly. Only when Ted was 30 years of age was the extent of his father's abuse apparent. He describes what happened when he was 8 years old.

> My father asked me to get wood for the stove, but when I came back with only one log because they were heavy, he started beating me. An eight-year-old kid, can you imagine! My mother attacked him to get him away from me and she took the beating instead [he starts sobbing]. This came over me like a wave. I didn't cry as a kid, not like I'm crying now. My father would say, 'I'll give you something to cry about. I'll give you a shot in the head!' I lived in fear of him and his criticism and wanted to please him. I respected him because he was smart and well-read. Strong as an ox physically. Sometimes he'd call me chump

> when he felt good about me, but if I didn't do something like throw a ball well, he'd call me chump. He'd say I'd thrown the ball like a girl. But he wouldn't take time to teach me how to throw a ball. My parents divorced when I was ten, and when they sat us down to tell us they were breaking up, my sister cried, but I thought it was the greatest thing in the world. He saw us a little after that and then just disappeared.

After his father's disappearance, Ted dropped out of high school, used hallucinogens and alcohol. Ultimately, he became a skilled machinist, but he continues to drink, sky-dive and motorcycle race to "calm" himself. He has had suicidal thoughts but denies a link between these and his (counter-phobic) dangerous sports. The vignette brings into bas-relief the abusive treatment by his father: even after his father left, this boy engaged in self-abusive or self-defeating activity. Further, he calms himself with high-risk "sports."

## Development of the person

In Minnesota, Sroufe and colleagues [5] recruited 180 primiparous, impoverished mothers; 110 (61%) were unmarried and 90 (50%) were adolescents at their first child's birth. The children were followed for two decades. The study began in 1974 and the measures were rigorous and included assessment of attachment. Here, we focus on abuse and refer the reader to their book for other aspects.

Seventy-two (40%) of the mothers abused as children were observed to maltreat their children; a further 54 (30%) provided borderline childcare. The remaining 54 of those who reported they had been abused as children provided adequate care for their own children. In contrast, all but one of the mothers who reported supportive and loving parental care provided adequate care for their children.

Three protective factors interrupted the perpetuating abuse by the mothers: (a) childhood emotional support from an alternative adult, (b) psychotherapy for at least 6 months or (c) a contemporary adult supportive and satisfying relationship. Toddlers who were abused showed lower levels of persistence and enthusiasm and higher levels of inattention and negative affect. All maltreated children showed more anger, frustration and non-compliance than those who received adequate care, as was found by Massie and Szajnberg [1].

By the age of 17, 90% of the maltreated children qualified for at least one psychiatric diagnosis. Severity of physical abuse and neglect (measured by legally defined criteria in the USA) were both significantly related to total behavior problems. Of those teenagers who were relatively well adjusted, factors differentiating these children include an early history of support and competence, an alternative available caregiver, a good school and an organized home environment. ([5] pp. 189–190). Temperament did not account for differences ([5] p. 113). Sroufe *et al.* [5] concluded: "the cumulative history of care is a more powerful predictor of outcome than quality of attachment alone" (p. 112). This study is a monumental contribution and this chapter has focused on one tragic aspect: when children are beaten by their caretakers, the children suffer, perhaps in varying ways, but throughout development. Yet, some human factors can alleviate that misery: mothers' childhood or contemporary support.

## The family mosaic: hidden fractures

The following vignette comes from the principal author's experiences as medical director of the Family Mosaic Program (FMP) in San Francisco. This gives flesh to the prospective studies cited above. The FMP was established as one of seven innovative sites in the USA initially funded by the Robert Wood Johnson Foundation to treat indigent, severely emotionally disturbed institutionalized children and their families. A primary goal was to return these children to their families (or surrogates) from mental health or penal institutions.

The program in San Francisco accepted the 200 most emotionally disturbed children, primarily those from black or Hispanic neighborhoods. For instance, while less than 10% of the population in San Francisco was black, almost 90% of the denizens of the Youth Guidance Center (the jail) were black. When accepting a child, we treated all members of the immediate family. Our offices were in the Hunter's Point/Bayview (black) neighborhood, but our workers spent most of their time in the communities – this also included the Western Addition (black) and the Mission (Hispanic, mostly Central American). Half our staff was black, half Hispanic, predominately Central American.

Of the black population, most children were being raised by a grandmother, occasionally an "auntie," who were generally in their forties or fifties. These family members received special child welfare payments as well as low-fee housing to care for these children. In some cases, the substitute "mothers" had five or six children from several of their daughters and sons and were paid by child welfare: for most, this was the primary source of income; the children knew this. The biological mothers often worked Third Street (in the neighborhood) as prostitutes and many were also crack addicts; many of the fathers were in prison for felonies, some of them in Pelican Bay, a notorious prison for multiple murderers.

Of our Hispanic population, we had refugees, including from Nicaragua, some of whose fathers were killed in the wars. The rates of teenage pregnancy were very high in both populations, although we learned that the fathers often remained involved in the Hispanic population, but secretly so as not to jeopardize child welfare payments. For the black population, we found that our teenage girls became pregnant (often with intent) by 14 or 15 years. Histories of domestic violence were the norm in these young women, as was formally reported child abuse of their children, particularly in the black population. Many families were referred to FMP because of severe child abuse.

Because of space limitations, a single vignette is presented to demonstrate (a) how avidly some families hid abuse or neglect, (b) the challenge of a continuum from abuse through neglect, (c) the "normative" quality of abuse within the extended family and (d) the generational transmission of abuse and neglect in response to the wider societal racism.

This vignette shows the insidious and complex family process of secrecy and complicity, even deceit, in the abuse/neglect of a child, and the child's readiness to stay with the abusive/neglectful family, perhaps because the child was anxious about the possibility of being moved out of the family completely. To the degree that these two processes are internalized by the child – family deceit about abuse and the child's anxiety about losing even an abusive attachment figure – we begin to get some hints of how nefarious mentalized abuse/neglect relationships complicate the later treatment of such children, and how as a society we continue to be complicit in enabling these situations.

## Abuse or not abuse: is that the question?

Fourteen-year-old "Tanetia's" pediatricians called us; they were certain that she would soon die of her repeated diabetic comas without more help. A juvenile diabetic for the last few years, she lived with her 55-year-old great grandmother, "Grams," who had been selected "foster mother of the month" some 10 years earlier. She still had the yellowed, crumbling news article tacked to her entrance hall. Tanetia's grandmother lived elsewhere and her mother was a well-known crack addict and prostitute on Third Street. Grams also cared for five other children from several of her children and received welfare payments for all. She insisted that she gave Tanetia her insulin regularly and watched her diet. Because of her mother's crack addiction and history of abuse and neglect, not only were her children removed, but also the court placed a 500 yard restriction on the mother approaching the home. This restriction was more often honored in the breach; for instance, her older son, a local cocaine dealer who lived in the home, complained to our social worker that not only did his mother come to the house to steal his money, but also his drugs. Grams called him a liar.

Tanetia had so many frequent visits to the emergency room that her friends had recently begun to swing through the circular driveway, deposit her and drive off. Besides her acute comas, the pediatricians found that she had the blood vessels of a woman decades older: Tanetia could die of kidney or heart problems soon if we could not help. What we learned is how well a family can dissemble a form of neglect that could have fatal consequences.

"Asha," our case worker, was a capable and experienced professional woman who had worked in Bayview for years; she knew the area well and understood its culture. We visited the home. Teenagers entered and exited throughout our talk with Grams, who looked disheveled: gray wig askew, toothless, in a formless tent dress, shuffling in grimy slippers. (In a few weeks, when we saw her in court, she had transformed herself.) She took down her ancient *San Francisco Chronicle* article as foster mother of the month to show us. She took us to the refrigerator to see the insulin bottle. She confessed that, a while ago, Tanetia's mother and others would feed her candies to "quiet her down." (Hyperglycemic stupor and coma will quiet a child.) She complained mildly that her children and grandchildren kept having babies and bringing them to her to care for; sometimes she did not even get their welfare check – could Asha get the money?

Asha said she would help her to get the extra payments and also promised that she would come by daily until Tanetia was stabilized. I noticed that when Grams and I returned to the living room, Asha had lingered by the refrigerator; she had measured and marked the level of insulin. Within a week, Tanetia was hospitalized again. On Asha's home visit, she pointed out to Grams that none of the insulin had been used, showing her the mark on the bottle. Grams' response: she had

used a different bottle of insulin, which she had tossed. And, by the way, she couldn't keep Tanetia from going out for pizza and beer with her friends, could she? And when was Asha going to get her the extra child welfare payments?

Within a month, Asha had Tanetia's case documented and placed before the court, requesting either closer supervision or Tanetia's placement in another home. Here, the case got stranger. Grams entered Court with Tanetia. Grams was elegantly dressed, laid-out, well groomed, hair coiffed, teeth in. The university's director of pediatric endocrinology presented Tanetia's severe illness and the raft of tests that they had done to rule-out other causes for her uncontrolled diabetes to prove that this was caused by poor monitoring and care. His team anticipated that Tanetia would die within the year from acute illness, or within the next few years from secondary vascular damage resulting from poor control of her diabetes.

Then Grams took the stand. Dramatically, she unrolled a computerized list of rare causes of hyperglycemia that church members had found on the Internet. She argued that the doctors were malfeasant for neglecting to test for these problems. How – she turned to the judge – how could they take away her little girl whom she had raised from infancy? She unfolded the yellowed news article with her photo as she reminded the judge that the City of San Francisco had named her foster mother of the month just 10 years ago. She hinted at a suit for malpractice. Tanetia was called up. She said that she loved her Grams. She said that she knew that Grams needed the money. Tanetia almost whispered, "I don't want to live elsewhere." The judge being a judge, courts being courts, and this being San Francisco, insisted that Grams be given another 6 months with Tanetia and scolded FMP to work harder to help Grams to take care of this girl. At least for the next year that the psychoanalyst remained at FMP, Tanetia didn't die, nor did she leave that home.

For the reader, we raise the complexity of how societal racial discrimination becomes translated to within-family trauma; legally, the judge decided, this case did not qualify as "abuse," although it did as neglect. But, clinically, this matter is tragic. The family's collusion hid the severe, life-threatening neglect; Grams was sophisticated enough to play on the Court's reluctance to "take away" a black child from her family. She had already hired a malpractice attorney to explore whether the university's world-renown pediatric endocrinologist had erred in not pursuing very rare causes of ketoacidosis: nothing came of that; only little more came from our efforts.

This vignette gives substance to the theories of perpetuation and transmission of abuse presented in the first section of this paper, in society, transmitted to the family and individual: the phrase "repetition compulsion as a manner of active mastery of previously passive experiences," may sound abstract and, intellectualized, but if we leave the reader to imagine how this girl may internalize the abuse/neglect (such as not being given life-saving medications; fed sugar candies to induce stupor/coma to "calm" her), the family's deceit of outsiders trying to protect the child and the strength of attachment to an abusive/neglectful figure (likely insecure anxious ambivalent/resistant attachment from clinical observations). If we add to this the broader societal racial context, we get a more flesh and blood portrayal of the internal circumstances of such children.

## Discussion

What can we learn from the painful lives of these children? How can we use their experiences to improve children's lives? How can it be related to the psychoanalytic theory cited above? Narrowly, we know from *Lives Across Time* that childhood physical abuse and also emotional abuse or neglect results in an adulthood with lower social/psychological functioning (GAF) and more primitive defense mechanisms, psychiatric diagnoses and impoverished transition through Eriksonian stages. In these childhoods, fathers beat sons; mothers were less effective caregivers from their child's infancy onwards. Symptoms in childhood evolved and changed with time from, starting with early signs of distress and difficulties and changing into more complex and organized disorders: anaclitic depression, "hyperactivity," anxiety and such. In a more complex manner, some children had achieved secure attachment, indicating perhaps other more positive influences, which ameliorated in part the vicissitudes of parental abuse.

Adding complexity, in *Lives Across Time*, Bowlby's broader definition of trauma was used [11,16,17]: events that significantly threatened the attachment relationship. Looking at the overall population of 76, a child who had two or more such traumatic experiences showed a level of functioning in adulthood (GAF) that was precipitously reduced.

The GAF is a relatively coarse measure of functioning. However, a brief vignette from *Lives Across Time*

may help to elaborate how a child's inner life is affected, and how a threatened attachment can affects this child as an adult. One of the highest-functioning women in the set described her parents' "amicable" divorce. While to the outer world their divided households appeared civil, this woman described the exquisite pain she underwent at each holiday: with whom would she spend that celebration? She decided in adolescence that she would never get divorced. While she was happily married, with a child and is successful professionally at 30 years, at moments, her interview carried a somber tone. She stated with clarity that she compromised her meteoric career path in order to have more time with her family. This woman's vignette suggests that even with phenomenologically high-functioning healthy adults, the strain of threatened attachment disruption (let alone more severe overt abuse or neglect cited in the studies above), per Bowlby, has enduring adverse effects.

Another bright, professionally successful young woman, whose mother took her away from the father and moved to a different state when the girl was 6 years old, announced when she was 14 that she would never marry: as of young adulthood, she had kept her word. This returns us to Bowlby's concept of trauma as any phenomenon that the child experiences as threatening disrupted attachment. While this chapter focuses on overt abuse and severe neglect, we do not want to ignore or discount lesser versions of psychological adversity, which nevertheless have enduring effects. We do not suggest with this too-brief vignette that a parent should stay with a spouse under all circumstances. Although, as we found in *Lives Across Time*, despite the prevalence of divorce, a child may experience parental divorce as equivalent to the loss of a parent through death or drug abuse, with both intrapsychic and phenomenological manifestations subsequently. Therefore, we suggest that parents should take their children's distress into account when considering divorce. In *Lives Across Time*, we found that while one trauma did not seem to adversely affect adulthood – as measured by GAF – two or more such trauma significantly affected the adult adversely. While it may be difficult to protect children from attachment disruptions such as parental death or parental alcohol/drug abuse, it is divorce that is more under the parents' control, and its possible effects should be taken into account when considering the best interests of the child. In this chapter, we have focused on parental physical abuse as the trauma. But, as an obligation both to the reader and to the thoughtfulness of our subjects, we feel it necessary to mention that any experiences that threatens attachment – including the almost epidemic rate of divorce – may dampen a child's life course: whether this is seen as the decision not to marry or the feeling of an aching pain and vulnerability because of the parents' difficult divorce. This suffering may not fulfill nor "show up" in an assessment checklist, but we believe it deleteriously affects or dampens down a child's emotional life and development.

The later, methodologically rigorous study of Sroufe *et al.* [5] confirms and expands the conclusions reached from *Lives Across Time*: abuse results in adverse outcome. In summary, Sroufe *et al.* identified three ameliorative factors against abuse: (a) childhood emotionally supportive alternative caregivers (one of our children, at age seven, cited her dog as the best person in the family – an example of both an emotionally supportive alternative "caregiver" and a child's imaginative capacity to use her dog to provide some kind of attachment substitute), (b) psychotherapy for at least 6 months and (c), in adulthood, a supportive mate.

*Lives Across Time* and *Development of the Person* [1,5] are prospective normative studies in which abuse was found incidentally. In another series of studies, Cicchetti and colleagues [25] focused on known abuse and violence and found, for instance, that interparent violence had adverse consequences for children over and above direct child abuse: a significant number of children who lived among violent parents developed depression, anxieties and other adjustment problems. Nevertheless, the majority of the children who were maltreated or witnessed interparent violence did not develop clinically significant psychopathology. Further, manifestation of symptoms varied, waxing and waning with development. That is, witnessing domestic violence has overt adverse effects on the child, even though some of these effects are manifested subclinically.

What do we make of these findings that attachment trauma and abuse cause no overt symptoms in some children and that psychopathology symptoms vary across time? There are several explanations. The symptom-checklist nature of the DSM or similar measures (e.g., the Child Behavior Checklist) require symptoms to cross a certain threshold to make diagnoses. This approach fails to take account of significant but sub-threshold suffering and gives short shrift to plain subjective misery (which may lie below an arbitrary cut-off point) and a child's inner life. There are also various definitions of "normal" and "resilience." We resume

discussion of "resilience" after addressing DSM results and attachment.

Rather than give exhaustive details on the numerous studies on abused children by Cicchetti and colleagues, we wish to focus on two findings: that observing abuse between parents is disruptive to the child and that some children who see this do not manifest clinical symptoms in childhood/adolescence. (The sample described by Davies *et al.* [25] has not yet been followed into adulthood; the *Lives Across Times* study found "sleeper effects," and variable expression of clinical difficulties across time.)

The issue of using DSM checklists is relatively straightforward. Beginning some four decades ago, phenomenological psychiatrists tried to base diagnoses on both manifest symptoms and signs and something closer to what might be found in a statistical distribution of health–illness continuum. The same is true for other psychological instruments such as the Child Behavior Checklist: they are constructed to select for some proportion of the population outside of a range of "normal."

What is the nature of what we call "normal"? Offer and Sabshin wrote in *Normality* [26] that with regard to mental health/illness we have at least four definitions of "normal," two of which are almost diametrically opposing. Two understandings of normal are statistical and optimal. The statistical definition of normal is derived from a statistically normal distribution: anything that is two standard deviations from the mean can be defined as "normal." In this case, the two "tails" of the curve would have 2.5% of the population each: "superhealthy" and "abnormals." By statistical or epidemiological definition, 2.5% at the bottom end of the tail would be outliers [19]. In contrast, when psychoanalysts refer to "normal" they mean optimal functioning; Freud emphasized that even a good analysis could only promise to restore someone to face the everyday difficulties of life [27]. In a certain utopian sense, psychoanalysts try to phase-shift the population curve upwards, toward improved emotional health, at least for an individual.

Researchers on attachment face a similar dilemma. The first studies described three working types of attachment: secure (roughly two-thirds) and insecure avoidant or resistant/ambivalent (one-third). Some early academic researchers were careful not to call the one-third abnormal – in a strictly statistical sense, this was an expected distribution. While distribution is dependent on the population measured, attachment has been studied across thousands of children in many different cultures, but also even these children still had some "strategy" of approach/contact maintenance (E. Waters, personal communication 2009). In fact, in the more recently described disorganized attachment, the child appears to have no working model of approach/contact maintenance with the attachment figure and may be "abnormal." This small group (perhaps 4–5% in a general population) is more likely to demonstrate more overt psychopathology than other attachment groups. However, psychoanalytically informed researchers on attachment [28,29] write as if the one-third of insecurely attached children have less than optimal working models of attachment; more specifically, these children show evidence of the anxiety associated with insecure attachment.

Most well-reasoned predictions about groups yield some false positives and some false negatives. "Resilient" and "vulnerable" are acceptable as post hoc descriptions of those who did better and worse than predicted. But they are necessarily post hoc and simply describe the state of affairs. They are not predictive and do not comprise any information other than the facts they attempt to account for. Thus they cannot have any explanatory power.

If it is hypothesized that a child had a particularly strong ego or a particularly well-buffered autonomic nervous system, then this is a description of a characteristic of a child that might have explanatory power. In which case, the child could be described as high on ego strength or autonomic buffering. To describe it as "resilient" is to lose sight of the specific characteristics of interest and the distinction, in Hempel and Oppenheim's terms, between the explanans and the explanandum [30]. Further "resilient" can be misused by social Darwinians to suggest that some children are more robust, and since some children function adequately after trauma, then trauma is not so deleterious and may even build character.

The latter is a misuse of the concept of resilience, when a term like "surviving" (or as Saul Bellow said in *Mr. Sammler's Planet* [31], "lasting,") might be a more accurate description. Our study shows both "resilience" and enduring suffering extend into adulthood from childhood abuse. While some of our abused (and neglected) subjects support themselves, find intimacy, raise children and may be creative, they both suffer (subjectively) and fall short of their peers (objectively). As we summarized [1]: "… the concept of resilience is an oversimplification if it is used too

blithely." Even titles of thorough, informative studies, such as *Vulnerable But Invincible: A Study of Resilient Children* [32] or the classic *The Vulnerable Child* [33] may lead some to conclude that things can work out OK after abuse and so: maybe it is not that bad, or some children are inherently tougher than others. For instance, Wallerstein and colleagues [34] have shown that divorce affects children for decades.

Resilience is more problematic conceptually. We have a substantive literature on childhood resilience, defined operationally as positive adaptation to previous adversities. One can define adaptation, as in the case of "normal" above, as lack of diagnoses, or as reasonably good functioning vocationally or personally. Anthony [35,36], Werner and Smith [37] and Luther *et al.* [38] point to the roles of "sound physical health and external influences such as one adequate parent, supportive figures outside of the nuclear family and freedom from poverty…" According to McFarlane and Yehuda [39] and Caspi *et al.* [40], constitution or genetic endowment, along with personality traits, support systems and past experiences, may determine vulnerability/resilience.

The danger of focusing on "resilience" or "invincibility" is that it may keep us from listening empathically and respectfully to the inner lives of those who suffer. We appeal that listening should be more specific to the possible characteristics of children who suffer through trauma such as abuse yet seem to appear outwardly less affected. If one is going to use the concept resilience (as a post hoc term), then one should use it only when the person "consistently performs better than the average person under disadvantageous circumstances. Consistency is important here to distinguish resilience from one of good luck" (E. Waters, personal communication, 2009).

A further dilemma with "resilience" begs the question as to why a child should have to be resilient, particularly with regard to abuse from those who should be caring for children. Winnicott, a heroic champion of treating severely disturbed people, remarked that it is better never to have been so ill in the first place [14].

## Conclusions

We have restricted most of our chapter to child abuse by a parent as trauma. We have referred the reader to others who have explored trauma in different manifestations, such as war, earthquakes, kidnapping or sniper attacks. We have also skirted the matter of sexual abuse by a relative, a particularly nefarious, perverse and destructive form of attack upon the child, usually a girl by her father, as the Whitings have shown across cultures [41]. Here, not only is the body invaded but also the mind may be involved with "seduction." Cohler [42] described the complex inner reasoning of a girl treated residentially who, after many years of treatment, could realize and articulate why she never told anyone about the rapes by her father. In brief, she felt that during the rape/sex, her father, who was demeaning of her mother, was bestial and demeaned; she told no one, in part, as she thought and felt (psychotically) that this was a way of "getting back" at her father and also helping her mother feel better. In another case, a girl did not tell her parents that her great uncle was raping her from age 7 to 17: he was the "Don" of the family (he had been arrested several times on suspicion of murder and gone free) and had bought her family's home next door to his; she feared for her mother should she tell her. In psychoanalysis, she realized that she also felt that she was "paying the rent" for their house next door in this fancy neighborhood [25]. Such complexity as incestuous abuse deserves more time than this chapter can cover.

Developmental stage and trauma also deserve more thought than can be covered here. Pynoos and colleagues have developed an elaborate model for childhood traumas that takes into account developmental age, spatial proximity, familial structure and subsequent aggravating or alleviating events. While this model goes beyond childhood abuse by a parent, it is helpful to set this within a conceptual framework. One of the debates that Brymer *et al.* [43] engage is that between Anna Freud's observation that a child's reaction to trauma is determined by his mother's reactions [6] and Terr's observation [7] that certain events – such as the Chowchilla kidnapping and burial alive of a school bus of children – are sufficiently powerful that they are traumatic in and of themselves. The model put forward by Pynoos and colleagues [43] takes both these views into account and develops them further. While this work takes us beyond the limits of this chapter, it may lead the reader to further concepts of prevention and postvention.

Parental physical abuse in a normative population is more prevalent than we know: in the *Lives Across Time* study [1], none of the abused children was reported to appropriate agencies as the abuse was not even discovered by the researchers, who did in-home assessments. Abuse may involve a parent incompetent at caregiving, or too troubled to provide protective and sensitive childrearing. Its symptomatic effects vary with developmental age, but, invariably, abuse diminishes the more optimal possibilities of the child well into adulthood. While adverse effects may be ameliorated by protective factors such as an alternative protective adult or psychotherapy, we repeat Winnicott's comment [14]: better not to have this happen to our children. Yet, when the abused child comes to us, we can return to the issues outlined at the beginning of this chapter. Giovacchini [19] integrated the repetition compulsion with Winnicott's maturational process [14], clarifying that the transference neurosis includes not only representations of what may have gone badly but also the hopeful fantasies the child had of what could have gone well. We can greet the traumatized child by fostering the child's hopeful yearnings with our clinical knowledge, dedication and efforts.

# References

1. Massie, H. and Szajnberg, N. M. (2008). *Lives across time/growing up: Paths to emotional health and emotional illness from birth to age 30 in 76 people*, 2nd edn. London: Karnac.

2. Brody, S. and Axelrad, S. (1970). *Anxiety and ego formation in infancy*. New York: International University Press.

3. Brody, S. and Axelrad, S. (1978). *Mothers, fathers and children: Explorations in the formation of character in the first seven years*. New York: International University Press.

4. Brody, S. and Siegel, M. (1992). *The evolution of character: Birth to 18 years*. New York: International University Press.

5. Sroufe, L. A., Egeland, B., Carlson, E. and Collins, W. A. (2005). *The development of the person: The Minnesota Study of risk and adaptation from birth to adulthood*. New York: Guilford Press.

6. Freud, A. and Burlingham, D. T. (1944). *War and children*. New York: International Universities Press.

7. Terr, L. C. (1979). Children of Chowchilla: A study of psychic trauma. *Psychoanalytic Study of the Child*, **34**, 547–623.

8. Steinberg, A. M., Brymer, M. J., Decker, M. K. and Pynoos, R. S. (2004). *The University of California at Los Angeles Post-traumatic Stress Disorder Reaction Index*. Berkley, CA: University of California Press.

9. Laor, N., Wolmer, L., Wiener, Z. *et al.* (1999). Image control and symptom expression in posttraumatic stress disorder. *Journal of Nervous and Mental Disease*, **187**, 673–679.

10. Jungmeen, K. and Cicchetti, D. (2004). A longitudinal study of child maltreatment, mother–child relationship

quality and maladjustment: The role of self-esteem and social competence. *Journal of Abnormal Child Psychology,* **32**, 341–354.

11. Bowlby, J. (1973). *Attachment and loss–separation: Anxiety and anger,* Vol. 2. New York: Basic Books.

12. Khan, M. (1995). The concept of cumulative trauma. *Journal of the American Academy of Child and Adolescent Psychiatry,* **34**, 541–565.

13. Freud, S. (1914). Remembering, repeating and working-through. In S. James (ed.), *The standard edition of the complete psychological works of Sigmund Freud,* Vol. 7. New York: Norton.

14. Winnicott, D. W. (1977). *The maturational process and the facilitating environment.* London: Karnac Books.

15. Piaget, J. (1952). *The origins of intelligence in children.* New York: International Universities Press.

16. Bowlby, J. (1969). *Attachment and loss: Attachment,* Vol. 1. New York: Basic Books.

17. Bowlby, J. (1980). *Attachment and loss: Loss,* Vol. 3. New York: Basic Books.

18. Thomas, D. (1971). The force that through the green fuse drives the flower. In D. Jones (ed.), *The poems of Dylan Thomas* (p. 77). New York: New Directions.

19. Giovacchini, P. (ed.). (1972). *Tactics and techniques in psychoanalytic therapy,* Vol. 1. New York: Jason Aronson.

20. Flarsheim, A. (1972). Treatability. In P. Giovacchini (ed.), *Tactics and techniques in psychoanalytic therapy,* Vol. 1 (pp. 113–131). New York: Jason Aronson.

21. Massie, H. and Szajnberg, N. M. (2006). My life is a longing: Child abuse and its adult sequelae – results of the Brody Longitudinal Study from birth to age 30. *International Journal of Psycho-analysis,* **87**, 471–496.

22. Derogatis, L. R., Lipman, R. S. and Covi, L. (1973). The SCL-90: An outpatient psychiatric rating scale. *Psychopharmacology Bulletin,* **9**, 13–28.

23. George, C., Kaplan, N. and Main, M. (1985). *Adult attachment interview.* Berkeley, CA: University of California.

24. American Psychiatric Association. (1994). *Diagnostic and statistical manual of mental disorders,* 4th edn (DSM-IV). Washington, DC: American Psychiatric Association.

25. Davies, P. T., Sturge-Apple, M. L., Cicchetti, D. and Cummings, E. M. (2007). The role of child adrenocortical functioning in pathways between interparental conflict and child maladjustment. *Developmental Psychology,* **43**, 918–930.

26. Offer, D. and Sabshin, M. (1974). *Normality.* New York: Basic Books.

27. Freud, S. (1914). Introductory lectures on psychoanalysis. In S. James (ed.), *The standard edition of the complete psychological works of Sigmund Freud,* Vol. 16. London: The Hogarth Press and the Institute of Psycho-Analysis.

28. Szajnberg, N. M. and Crittenden, P. M. (1997). The transference refracted through the lens of attachment. *Journal of the American Academy of Psychoanalysis & Dynamic Psychiatry,* **25**, 409–438.

29. Bretherton, I. and Waters, E. (1985). Growing points in attachment theory and research. *Monographs of the Society for Research in Child Development,* Vol. 50. Chicago, IL: University of Chicago Press.

30. Hempel, C. G. and Oppenheim, P. (1948). Studies in the logic of explanation. *Philosophy of Science,* **15**, 135–175.

31. Bellow, S. (1972). *Sammler's planet.* London: Penguin.

32. Werner, E. E. and Smith, R. S. (1982). *Vulnerable but invincible: A study of resilient children (p. 229).* New York: McGraw-Hill.

33. Anthony, E. J. and Cohler, B. (1987). *The vulnerable child* (p. 432). New York: Guilford.

34. Wallerstein, J., Lewis, J. and Blakeslee, S. (2000). *The unexpected legacy of divorce.* New York: Hyperion.

35. Anthony, E. J. (1987). Risk, vulnerability, and resilience: An overview. In E. J. Anthony and Cohler B. (eds.), *The invulnerable child* (pp. 3–48). New York: Guilford.

36. Anthony, E. J. (1987). Children at high risk for psychosis growing up successfully. In E. J. Anthony and B. Cohler (eds.), *The invulnerable child* (pp. 147–184). New York: Guilford.

37. Werner, E. E. and Smith, R. S. (1992). *Overcoming the odds: High-risk children from birth to adulthood.* Ithaca: Cornell University Press.

38. Luther, S., Cicchetti, D. and Becker, B. (2000). The concept of resilience: A critical evaluation and guidelines for future work. *Child Development,* **71**, 543–562.

39. McFarlane, A. and Yehuda, R. (1996). Resilience, vulnerability, and the course of post-traumatic creations. In B. van der Kolk, A. McFarlane and L. Weisaeth (eds.), *Traumatic stress: The overwhelming effects of experience on mind, body and society* (pp. 182–213). New York: Guilford.

40. Caspi, A., McClay, J., Moffitt, T. *et al.* (2002). Role of genotype in the cycle of violence in maltreated children. *Science,* **297**, 851–854.

41. Whiting, B. B. and Whiting, J. W. M. (1975). *Children of six cultures: A psycho-cultural analysis.* Boston, MA: Harvard University Press.

42. Cohler, B. J. (1975). The residential treatment of anorexia nervosa. In P. Giovacchini (ed.), *Tactics and techniques in psychoanalytic therapy,* Vol. 2: *Countertransference* (pp. 385–398). New York: Aronson.

43. Brymer, M. J., Steinberg, A. M., Sornborger, J. *et al.* (2008). Acute interventions for refugee children and families. *Child and Adolescent Psychiatric Clinics of North America,* **17**, 625–640.

# Part 1 synopsis

Alexander McFarlane

There are few issues that better define the moral and social fabric of a society than the way that it cares for and protects children. In the nineteenth century, as the rates of infant mortality dropped [1], allowing more highly valued attachments without fear of loss, the rights of the child progressively became an underpinning characteristic of society. The enlightenment's ideals were embodied in the belief in free education for all children. The need for special safeguards for children was recognized in the Geneva *Declaration of the Rights of the Child* of 1924 [2], which were further enunciated in the *Universal Declaration of Human Rights* after World War II [3].

However, there is a stark difference between the articulation of these principles and their implementation. One of the greatest challenges in ensuring the protection of children is to acknowledge the brutality, neglect and exploitation that children can be subject to, even in the modern world. The idealized life of middle class society is in contrast to the dark and silent social underbelly of childhood abuse, whether it be physical or sexual.

Ironically, one of the great challenges of improving the protection of children has been the conflict of interest of many of the most esteemed social institutions. For example, the Christian churches, independent of denomination, as part of their socially benevolent philosophies have set up schools and orphanages. The value of the child and the child's future are the values that have implicitly underpinned their establishment. Yet it is within these institutions that some of the most endemic forms of abuse have existed, and these have emerged in their true reality in the spate of litigation in the early 1990s. This reality highlights the complexity

of describing, highlighting and implementing systems that better protect children. For this to occur, societies must confront the dark undercurrents of perversity and exploitation that do not quickly dissipate from civilized societies.

## Overview

### The barriers to recognition of abuse

In Ch. 2 Dorahy *et al.* have summarized the torturous thread of how the etiological significance of early trauma and abuse have progressively become a more established part of the fabric of a central etiological issue in psychopathology. They have highlighted the resistance and rebuke that met the clinicians who showed an emerging interest in childhood sexual abuse in the 1890s. This hostility led Freud to recant the importance of these ideas [4]. The significance of childhood neglect and abuse was then allowed to dissipate from the mainstream of thinking.

The centrality of this struggle in moulding Freud's theory of infantile sexuality is perhaps one of the most intriguing issues in the history of psychiatry. Masson's unravelling of this matter [5] highlights how Freud [4] battled to accept and deal with the reality of what he observed in the face of the social pressure and disquiet his observations created. His desire for professional acceptance led him to modify his earlier views and embody the idea that childhood fantasy explained a number of the accounts he was hearing. The failure of Freud's struggle to believe and advocate what he had initially observed is indicative of the challenging position in which professionals often find themselves. They are destined to see and document behaviors that are not contemplated by the broader body of society, and the exposure of these behaviors is met with dismay and denial. The articulation of these observations and the capacity and willingness of the broader community to acknowledge these unsavoury observations places the professional in a very challenging position. Evidence can be circumstantial and distressed individuals can give accounts that are subject to error, issues that can encourage and sustain disbelief.

This history is a challenging one for professions to address [6]. Most clinicians would like to believe that their primary skills of observation and their desire to provide optimal care for their patients mean that they observe and report their patient's predicament. However, the reported prevalence of incest in a major text of psychiatry in 1976 [7] was neglible is a testament and to the millions of patients whose stories were told but not believed, being dismissed as oedipal fantasies. This history highlights how in many ways clinicians' capacities for observation and description of patients' predicaments are more determined by the models of psychopathology they adhere to than the history presented to them by the patient. Ultimately, the ability of a clinician to see and understand what a patient describes is as determined by the imposed attitudes and beliefs from the broader society as it is by the reality of what the patient tells. Hence, clinicians work in an environment where prevailing professional practice can blind their observation.

The reluctance of medicine, psychology and psychiatry to embrace the significance of childhood abuse is part of a broader denial of the significance of psychological trauma. The spectre of suggestion has always loomed large in this field, and Babinski, Charcot's successor, repudiated his mentors' views on the basis of this argument. The general suspicion played a significant role in the formulation and understanding of the trauma of World War I [8]. The reluctance of the mental health community to embrace the potent destructiveness of the trauma of war on the psychological well-being of soldiers is in many ways akin to the reluctance of the professional community to accept the facts about the prevalence and destructiveness of childhood abuse. The terrible death and destruction brought by World War I on the minds of a generation should not be ignored in this broader discussion. The profession struggled to find a coherent narrative and model of psychopathology to understand the effects of psychological trauma. As Kardiner and Spiegel summed up in 1947 [9] (p. 1).

Subject to neurotic disturbance consequent upon war has, in the past 25 years, been submitted to a good deal of capriciousness in public interest and psychiatric whims. The public does not sustain its interest which was very great after World War I and neither does psychiatry. Hence, these conditions are not subject to continuous study ... but only to periodic efforts which cannot be characterised as very diligent ... though not true in psychiatry generally, it is a deplorable fact that each investigator who undertakes to study these conditions considers it his sacred obligation to start from scratch and work at the problem as if no one had ever done anything with it before.

Just as there was not a continuous narrative or exploration of the effects of childhood abuse, so was the case with the psychological effects of war. While these might seem diametrically opposed bodies of knowledge, underpinning them is a central understanding of how traumatic events can play a central role in undermining an individual's adjustment and mental health. As Glass summarized in 1974 in reference to World War I [10]: "The ability to cope with combat was deemed the result of faulty personality development and thus conformed the psycho-analytic model of the psychoneuroses and was so generally diagnosed" (p. 802).

With reference to World War II, Glass noted that "Military psychiatry, like civil psychiatry, ignored the lessons of wartime experience. Instead attention *was focused in the then prevalent psycho-analytic concepts and practice*" (p. 804). It was as though mental health professionals did not want to accept and articulate the destructiveness of two world wars on the generations that had been brutalized by their conduct. One suspects that societies could only face the reality of waging war if they denied the impact on the people who had to prosecute the carnage.

In this context, it is difficult to see how the reality of childhood abuse and neglect could have been embraced by the mental health community at this time.

Importantly, Dorahy *et al.* in Ch. 1 highlight the careful and systematic observation of a generation of pediatricians in the middle years of the twentieth century to document the reality of non-accidental injury and pediatric subdural haematoma, which allowed the factual reality to began to emerge. In some regards, focusing on the reality of the physical injuries posed an undeniable reality in contrast to the psychological impacts of these events. Slowly progress was made up to the present day.

# The important role of epidemiology

In the same way we owe much to the emerging discipline of epidemiology in the field of traumatic stress, there is no denying that the introduction of post-traumatic stress disorder into the *Diagnostic and Statistical Manual* of *Mental Disorders* (DSM) in 1980 [11] was a turning point in the history of the better understanding of the effects of childhood abuse and neglect. This third edition, DSM-III, adopted the definition of a traumatic event as a psychologically distressing event that is "outside the range of usual human experience" (p. 247), but even in the fourth edition (DSM-IV [12]), the associated text makes little reference to the issue of child abuse.

Careful definition of the stressor criterion has provided a benchmark for conducting epidemiological research. Population-based research has identified a surprisingly high frequency of the types of event qualifying as traumatic [13], and with more detailed questioning, the lifetime rates may be as high as 90% [14]. This finding challenges the original notion that these are events outside the range of usual human experience. Hence, the observations have created an environment where it is difficult to deny the reality of the abuse of children and the reality of their sexual violation.

Mental health professionals are constantly being confronted with the fact that the more they ask and the more carefully they ask, the more they find. The prevalence of post-traumatic stress disorder measured in the epidemiological studies in Australia has demonstrated an increase in the prevalence from 1.3% in 2001 [15] to 4.4% in 2007 [16]. What has been shown is that the way that the questions are asked about traumatic exposures significantly increases and changes the reported rates.

Chapter 2 highlights many of the ongoing challenges about the measurement of early childhood trauma. The applicability of the stressor criterion to child abuse is not the least of these problems. Particularly, the DSM-IV stressor criterion does not capture closely the essence of childhood abuse, particularly of a sexual nature, a matter that needs to be better addressed in DSM-V [13]. In their careful analysis of the data from the National Comorbidity Study–Replication Survey, Koenen *et al.* summarized the widespread nature and the complexity of childhood abuse in the US community. They point out the challenge of the retrospective nature of this reporting and how this recall is in part mood dependent, where individuals who are depressed have a greater probability of recalling negative life events. They also highlighted how Widom and

Morris [17] found that 41% and 67% of females with court-documented abuse histories failed to record these histories when interviewed in young adulthood. Hence, the findings of epidemiological studies must be seen as approximations. The central issue, however, is that this does not invalidate the broader importance and prevalence of these phenomena. Rather, researchers and clinicians alike need to confront the complexity and challenge of the history-taking process in these situations.

As Dalenberg and Paulson highlight in Ch. 3, the controversial study by Rind and colleagues [18] demonstrates how the negative effects of abuse can be distorted by studying these phenomena in certain populations such as college students. By definition, college students have been sufficiently developmentally functional to get to this point of their education, which excludes all those who have been more substantially damaged. This chapter highlights the importance of not making generalizations from specific populations without extensive caveats.

Another important reality is that prospective studies and longitudinal studies (as referred to in Chs. 2 and 4) cannot occur in children in the isolation of intervention. The mandatory reporting requirements in many legal systems mean that any child who is identified as being subject to abuse or neglect must be notified to the relevant authorities. As a consequence, any longitudinal study will as much be a documentation of the impact of intervention as of the longitudinal effects and adverse health outcomes. If longitudinal studies are made of populations at risk, it is highly probable if these are recruited through intervention services that these children will be an atypical and in a more severely affected group. Similarly, longitudinal studies of healthy childhood development are unable to make uncontaminated observations about severe abuse and neglect as any children at risk will inevitably be removed from the study environment and mandated interventions provided.

As highlighted in Ch. 4, there are intense social collusions against the accurate depiction of the predicament of children, with both the child and the caregivers minimizing the neglect. This emphasizes the challenging and problematic nature of research in this field.

## The polarizing effect of the law

Inevitably, legal systems impinge dramatically on child protection services. As has already been highlighted in this part, there are many subtleties and complexities about documenting and defining the nature of the impact of childhood abuse and neglect.

The first issue is to establish the veracity and the nature of these complaints. The risk of inaccurate recall and recovered memories is a veritable minefield at the best of times (Ch. 3). The adversarial nature of many legal systems has had a dramatic effect on the discussion and debate between mental health professionals. Inevitably, the advocacy system leads to a polarity of views and the potential exaggeration of controversy and divergence of opinion. Notorious legal cases are often widely reported in the media. These cases only serve to fuel the flames of debate and, at times, appear to diminish professionals' apparent reliability to articulate these issues of public concern systematically and carefully .

Dalenberg and Paulson in Ch. 3 highlight the challenges and risks for professional organizations who get embroiled in these debates. They further highlight how science becomes a pawn and can be diminished by the potential for selective quoting and bias. Professional societies have to struggle with the broad cathedral of memberships, where individuals can take seemingly diametrically opposed views as indicated by the sides they are engaged by in legal matters. The reputation of practitioners is further complicated by practices of some, where presumptions are made about the existence of abuse on the basis of the patterns of unusual patterns of physical and psychological symptoms. The resulting hunt for a memory of abuse is fraught with the risk of suggestion. This fertile field is where the false memory debate erupted in the mid 1990s.

The veracity of the accounts of sexual abuse victims is sometimes attacked as being merely motivated by a desire for revenge or distortion introduced by poor clinical practice. One of the critical issues about traumatic events is the problem of creating coherent verbal narratives of such events. Some of the greatest novelists of all times have been intensely preoccupied by this issue. For example, the introduction to Tolstoy's *The Sebastopol Sketches* [19] states "The hero of his story, he says is truth and truth is not at all lovely and not at all reconcilable with the military communiqués of war correspondence. The truth is that war is not what people think it is. It is not as people describe it. Everything is unreal. Nobody knows what is happening or will happen" (p. 38).

Tolstoy explores this theme of the individual narrative against the broader historical account through his epic novel *War and Peace* [20]. He highlights through the character of Rostrov recalling a cavalry charge the challenge of creating an accurate narrative. "He began with the intention of relating everything exactly as it happened, but imperceptibly, consciously, and inevitably he slipped into falsehood" (p. 298). Tolstoy went on to describe how Rostrov believed that if he had told the story of what really had happened, nobody would have believed him. This account highlights the distortion of memory in the retelling of real events and that this is not indicative necessarily of false memory.

Recent neuropsychological and neuroimaging research [21] has highlighted how traumatic events disrupt the capacity for word formulation and has impact on the areas of the brain involved in expressive language [22]. Hence, it is not surprising that the memories of childhood abuse that have been encoded at a different developmental stage may be subject to significant difficulties when subject to retrospective recall.

# Conclusions

Polarization of the argument around the recall of childhood abuse because of an imperative of certainty imposed by the courts has disrupted the careful discussion and investigation of the complexity of the issues. This general domain highlights how clinicians and researchers do not sit in a vacuum. They are pulled and pushed by the broad challenges and tensions within society. The demand for idealization and social harmony erodes a willingness within the community at large to acknowledge and understand the brutality and exploitation that can sit behind the tidy gardens of suburbia. There is probably no other field that more challenges the reluctance of individuals to have their illusions shattered and face the capacity for inhumanity that pervades many people's lives than the area of childhood abuse.

This unpleasant truth is even more confronting when the institutions that have argued and articulated moral principles and issues, namely the churches, come to be found amongst some of the most institutionalized perpetrators. This dialectic creates a more intense frame around the importance of discussing the unresolved moral questions raised in Ch. 3.

Ultimately however, we cannot remove ourselves from the need for an understanding of the clinicians' dilemmas in dealing with these children. As Szajnerg *et al.* highlight in Ch. 4, the most dedicated professional attempting to stand up and protect children can be left unsupported and attacked through the legal process as a result of a complex collusion of interests . Hence, this is not a field where professionals can function without examining their values, allegiances and potential for denial. This domain is likely to continue to affect psychology and psychiatry, challenging, extending and dividing those in research and clinical practice alike.

# References

1. Daugherty, H. G. and Kammeyer, K. C . (1995). *An introduction to population,* 2nd edn. New York: Guilford.

2. United Nations (1924). *Declaration of the rights of the child.* New York: United Nations.

3. United Nations (1948). *Universal declaration of human rights.* New York: United Nations.

4. Freud, S. (1896). The aetiology of hysteria. In J. Strackey (ed.), *The standard edition of the complete psychological works of Sigmund Freud,* Vol. 3. London: Vintage.

5. Masson, J. M. (1984). *The assault on truth: Freud's suppression of the seduction theory.* London: Faber & Faber.

6. McFarlane, A. C. (2000). On the social denial of trauma and the problem of knowing the past. In A. Y. Shalev, R. Yehuda and A. C. McFarlane (eds.), *International handbook of human response to trauma* (pp. 11–26). Dordrecht, Netherlands: Kluwer Academic.

7. Freeman, A. M. , Kaplan, H. I. and Sadock, B. J. (1976). *Modern synopsis of comprehensive psychiatry.* Baltimore, MD: Williams & Wilkins.

8. Bailey, P. (1918). War neuroses, shell shock and nervousness. *Journal of the American Medical Association,* **71,** 17–21.

9. Kardiner, A. and Spiegel, H. (1947). *War, stress and neurotic illness.* New York: Paul Hoeber.

10. Glass, A. J. (1974). Mental health programs in the armed forces. In S. Arieti (ed.), *American handbook of psychiatry,* 2nd edn. New York: Basic Books.

11. American Psychiatric Association (1980). *Diagnostic and statistical manual of mental disorders,* 3rd edn. Washington, DC: American Psychiatric Press.

12. American Psychiatric Association (1994). *Diagnostic and statistical manual of mental disorders,* 4th edn. Washington, DC: American Psychiatric Association.

13. Kessler, R. C., Bergland, P., Demier, O. *et al.* (2005). Lifetime prevalence and age-of-onset distributions of DSM-IV disorders in the National Comorbidity Survey Replication. *Archives of General Psychiatry,* **62,** 593–602.

14. Breslau, N . and Kessler, R . (2001). The stressor criterion in DSM-IV posttraumatic stress disorder: An empirical investigation. *Biological Psychiatry,* **50,** 699–704.

15. Creamer, M., Burgess, P. M. and McFarlane, A. C. (2001). Post traumatic stress disorder: Findings from the Australian National Survey of Mental Health and Wellbeing. *Psychological Medicine,* **31,** 1237–1247.

16. Australian Bureau of Statistics (2007). *National survey of mental health and wellbeing.* Canberra: Australian Bureau of Statitics. www.abs.gov.au (accessed January 22, 2010).

17. Widom, C. S. and Morris, S. (1997). Accuracy of adult recollections of childhood victimization Part II: Childhood sexual abuse. *Psychological Assessment,* **9,** 34–46.

18. Rind, B. , Tromovitch, P. and Bauserman, R. (1998). A meta-analytic examination of assume properties of child sexual abuse using college samples. *Psychological Bulletin,* **124,** 22–53.

19. Tolstoy, L. (1986). *The Sebastopol sketches.* Harmondsworth, UK: Penguin.

20. Tolstoy, L. (1979). *War and peace.* Harmondsworth, UK: Penguin.

21. Moores, K. A. , Clark, C. R., McFarlane, A. C. *et al.* (2008). Abnormal recruitment of working memory updating networks during maintenance of trauma-neutral information in post-traumatic stress disorder. *Psychiatry Research,* **163,** 156–170.

22. Johnsen, G. E . and Asbjørnsen, A. E. (2009). Verbal learning and memory impairments in posttraumatic stress disorder: The role of encoding strategies. *Psychiatry Research,* **165,** 68–77.

# The effects of life trauma: mental and physical health

# Attachment dysregulation as hidden trauma in infancy: early stress, maternal buffering and psychiatric morbidity in young adulthood

Jean-François Bureau, Jodi Martin and Karlen Lyons-Ruth

When considering childhood trauma, it is common to think of physical or sexual abuse, or of other traumatic events involving a threat to the subject's physical integrity, as described in the *Diagnostic and Statistical Manual of Mental Disorders*; 4th edn. (DSM-IV-TR) [1]. However, the experience of threat is very different during infancy, as infants cannot evaluate the threat posed by various life events, including physical injury. This chapter argues that injury from abuse is a potent risk factor for psychiatric morbidity because it is a marker for more pervasive and enduring deviations in care within primary attachment relationships. Infants are pre-adapted to rely on the availability of responsive parental care for protection from external threats, for regulation of emotions and for normalizing physiological reactions to stressors. Therefore, during early life, a *hidden trauma* can occur, resulting not from physical assault but from the unavailability of a responsive attachment figure to comfort and regulate the stress of the fear-evoking events that are a daily part of the infant's experience [2].

This chapter will focus first on the immediate outcomes of unresponsive early care during infancy, including the development of non-optimal physiological stress reactions and disorganized attachment behavior. It will then discuss long-term consequences associated with early unresponsive care, including increased dissociation, depression and the self-damaging behaviors characteristic of borderline personality disorder. Recent literature from prospective longitudinal studies beginning in infancy allows evaluation of the contribution of unresponsive early care independent from the effects of childhood abuse. The chapter concludes with a review of recent research pointing to

interaction between caregiving environment and gene expression in the dopaminergic and serotonergic systems, as these effects relate to maladaptation in childhood and psychiatric morbidity in adulthood.

## Infancy as a sensitive period?

Infancy is a developmental period of rapidly growing neurological, physical and emotional systems. Infants also develop attachment bonds in the first months of life; the attachment figure, in turn, provides regulation of the infant's stressful arousal [3,4]. Cummings and Cicchetti [5] have also suggested that early attachment relationships contribute to a child's internal representation of self, critical in the development of healthy self-esteem. According to this theory, if early parenting care contributes to an insecure attachment relationship, the detrimental effects of insecure attachment may continue after parenting risk has remitted. Further, Denham [6] has speculated that attachment figures have a greater role in the socialization of emotion regulation and expression during the first 2 years of life compared with later developmental periods. For example, children may be less vulnerable to an onset of maternal depression occurring later in the child's development, as they have already developed effective internalized emotion regulation and coping strategies and a larger network of support figures (e.g., neighbours, friends and teachers). Empirical evidence for the particular importance of stressors during the first years of life is beginning to accrue. For example, both Dearing and colleagues [7] and Brook-Gunn and colleagues [8] have found that poverty in the first 5 years of life is associated with more deleterious long-term outcomes than poverty later in childhood. More directly,

Bureau *et al.* [9] have shown that maternal depression in the first 2 years of a child's life is a better predictor of offspring depressive symptoms at age 8 and 19 years than concurrent maternal depression when a child is 8 or 19 years, or than chronicity of maternal depression over the same period of time.

# Infant security of attachment and parental care during infancy

Attachment theory [3,10] posits that children are born with an attachment system that is activated when the child is in or perceives distress. When activated, this system leads to proximity-seeking behaviors (e.g., crying) toward the caregiver who is most likely to provide comfort and protection. Furthermore, George and Solomon [11] pointed out that adults have caregiving systems that are activated when children signal distress; activation of these systems, in turn, triggers sensitive behaviors toward the child. However, the caregiving system could be affected by many stressors, including poverty, parental depression and past experiences of abuse, which could lead to unresponsive parenting.

The quality of parenting exerts critical influence on children's social-affective development, especially in the first year of life, as suggested by research from multiple sources. For example, maternal sensitivity, usually defined as the mother's ability to recognize her infant's needs and to respond accordingly, is significantly associated with infant's security of attachment [12]. In contrast, maternal insensitivity has been linked with both insecure and disorganized attachment behaviors in the second year of life [13]. Other studies have shown that a sensitive rearing environment can help to regulate infants' expressions of negative affect in the first year of life [14]. Additionally, animal and human models have demonstrated that responsive parenting behaviors can positively influence the offspring's physiological arousal to stressors [15,16].

Attachment theorists propose that a child develops an attachment bond with a primary caregiver (attachment figure) based on generalization of this caregiver's daily reactions to the child's proximity- and comfort-seeking behaviors. From these reactions, the child develops internal working models of the attachment relationship. This model allows the child to interpret and predict the caregiver's behavior, and to regulate his or her own reactions, thoughts and feelings toward the attachment figure [17]. Thus, infants and young children gradually develop consistent patterns of attachment behaviors toward the primary caregiver that are expected to reflect the child's internal working model of this particular relationship.

In their landmark study, Ainsworth and colleagues [12] described three patterns of infant attachment behaviors in the strange situation procedure, which involves brief separations and reunions between a caregiver and infant. Ainsworth and colleagues further identified that each of these patterns was associated with a particular pattern of maternal sensitivity. Children of consistently sensitive and responsive mothers were able to derive comfort from their mothers upon reunion and then return to exploring the playroom, and were more often classified as *securely attached.* Children of mothers who were uncomfortable with physical contact and lacked sensitivity minimized their expressions of distress in the strange situation, and were classified as *insecure-avoidant.* Children of mothers who were unpredictable in their sensitivity exaggerated their expressions of distress and were never fully comforted, to the detriment of exploration; these children were classified as *insecure-ambivalent.* Although not optimal, the two insecure patterns of attachment are considered adaptive secondary strategies to compensate for the mother's lack of sensitivity.

A fourth attachment classification, labeled "disorganized" was later identified [18]. Disorganized attachment is conceptualized as a breakdown in attachment strategy, such that disorganized children show no coherent attachment pattern toward the parent, instead exhibiting contradictory behaviors or fearful reactions in response to reunion with the parent in the strange situation. Disorganization is thought to originate from maladaptive parental interactive behaviors, which hinder the infant's ability to develop consistent ways of approaching the parent for comfort, perhaps through the infant's perception of the mother as a source of both comfort and fear [19]. Additional research has associated infant disorganization with parental maltreatment, parental psychopathology and disturbed parent–infant interactions [20,21], further suggesting that the child's inability to form comprehensible attachment behaviors may be influenced by parental characteristics related to unpredictable and aversive patterns of early care. The association between disorganization in infancy and frightened, frightening or disrupted maternal behaviors has been confirmed in several independent samples (for meta-analysis, see Madigan, *et al.* [20]).

# Parental care and infant physiological stress reactions

Research using animal and human models has identified associations between characteristics of the early caregiving environment and infant physiological responsiveness to stressors [22–24]. Particularly implicated is the hypothalamic–pituitary–adrenal (HPA) axis system, which participates in managing perceived threats to safety and is integral in maintaining internal equilibrium and coordinating adaptive responses to these threats [25,26]. Cortisol (corticosterone in non-primates), the end-product of the HPA system, provides a physiological indicator of HPA axis activity and follows a distinct pattern of production in normally developing offspring. Variations in production patterns are indicative of non-normative HPA system functioning and have been repeatedly linked with exposure to trauma in later childhood and adulthood [27].

Research indicates that poor parental care in infancy can similarly result in HPA axis dysregulation, and that such effects are especially strong within the first year of life [27]. Toddlers raised in Romanian or Russian orphanages, which epitomized grossly deprived, understimulating care [28], failed to demonstrate expected patterns of daily cortisol production compared with home-reared children [29,30]. Furthermore, Romanian orphans adopted into a family environment showed patterns of cortisol production 6 years later that were closer to normal, though these patterns still differed from those in Romanian children adopted sooner after birth, and from those in children raised in family environments since birth [31]. Similar results have been found in infants from family environments characterized by observed neglect [32].

Additional links have been identified between dysregulated HPA responsivity and attachment classification in infancy. Infants classified as securely attached show no prolonged elevations in cortisol levels during separation in the strange situation, while those with disorganized attachment status demonstrate elevated cortisol levels, and insecure infants have intermediate levels of cortisol when faced with separation [16,33]. Disorganized infants show the greatest reactivity to stress in these studies and are the slowest to return to baseline cortisol levels following the strange situation. Associations have also been found between dysregulated cortisol patterns and both maternal depression in early infancy [34] and lack of maternal sensitivity [35].

Animal models confirm links between quality of maternal care and infant HPA axis regulation. For example, separating rodent pups from their dams for extended time periods leads to patterns of heightened responsivity and poorer regulation of the HPA axis, which are maintained into adulthood [36–38]. Observed changes in HPA axis functioning in rat pups are particularly notable if separation interrupts routine maternal behaviors such as licking and grooming. Similarly, maternally deprived rhesus monkeys, raised either with cloth surrogates or with peers only, exhibit larger and prolonged cortisol elevations in response to stressful contexts [39]. Likewise, the rhesus mother's presence provides a protective factor against excessive cortisol reactivity to common stressors, including capture, separation and handling, even if physical contact between the infant and mother rhesus is not possible [40]. Disrupting the mother–infant interaction in other ways (e.g., altering expected availability of maternal food supply to create maternal anxiety) also leads to increased corticotrophin-releasing hormone levels in the infant lasting into adulthood [41]. Finally, Francis et al. [42] found that cross-fostering rat pups from low- to high-nurturing mothers (and vice versa) resulted in reduced corticosterune reactivity to stressors, less fearful behavior and greater neurogenesis in the hippocampus among rat pups with more nurturing mothers, regardless of genetic background. Further work documented that maternal nurturance in the first week of postnatal life altered the expression of more than 1000 genes related to neurogenesis [43].

In combination, these findings suggest that sensitivity, responsiveness and attention from primary caregivers in infancy are essential in regulating cortisol reactivity and ensuring proper HPA axis functions in response to stressors, and that a lack of available and sensitive caregiving during this period may result in dysregulated cortisol levels.

# Psychiatric morbidity in adulthood: contributions of early maternal care, infant disorganized attachment and childhood maltreatment

Disorganized attachment patterns in infancy have been associated with childhood onset of aggressive behavior problems (for meta-analysis, see van Ijzendoorn et al. [21]) and with psychopathology in young adulthood [44,45]. Because of the links between early caregiving environments and disorganized infant attachment behaviors, it is theorized that the effect of poor-quality early care on long-term outcomes would be mediated by attachment disorganization. However, research to date has not supported this theory. The literature shows instead that infant disorganization and quality of early care each contribute independently to long-term psychological adaptation, and that quality of early care has a more powerful influence overall on negative outcomes than infant attachment disorganization. For example, results from a longitudinal study by the US National Institute of Child Health and Human Development Early Child Care Research Network [46] indicates that quality of caregiver interaction provides greater prediction of later child adjustment than infant attachment behavior itself.

In several recent longitudinal studies, quality of early care and maltreatment experiences were assessed prospectively (as well as by young adult self-report) so that the contribution of quality of early care in infancy on later psychiatric morbidity could be examined separately from experiences of abuse. In the first investigation, Ogawa and colleagues [45] demonstrated that the occurrence of physical or sexual abuse during childhood was not associated with the extent of dissociation in young adulthood after controlling for parental psychological unavailability during the first 2 years of life. Instead, psychological unavailability of the parent in infancy and, to a lesser extent, infant disorganized attachment were the two strongest predictors of dissociation in young adulthood.

A more recent investigation [47] confirmed these findings and identified specific aspects of quality of care in infancy, including disrupted maternal communication, maternal flatness of affect and lack of maternal responsive involvement as significant predictors of young adult dissociation, independent of prediction from abuse experiences. Notably, this early care cluster accounted for half of the variance in dissociation after controlling for gender and demographic risk. In addition, with quality of early care controlled, only verbal abuse added to the prediction of dissociation in young adulthood, despite a high rate of sexual or physical abuse in the sample (29%). Infant disorganization was not a significant predictor of dissociative symptoms in this sample. Other non-prospective investigations separately assessing family environment by self-report have also found that history of physical abuse was associated with dissociation only in families characterized by low positive affect [48] or in individuals who perceived limited social support networks [49].

Quality of early care and infant disorganization have been similarly implicated in the development of depressive symptoms in childhood and young adulthood [9]. Maternal hostility assessed during infancy uniquely predicted depressive symptoms in both childhood and young adulthood, and low maternal involvement added to the prediction of such symptoms in young adulthood. Maternal depression during a child's infancy was also a unique predictor of young adult depressive symptoms, as noted above. Finally, disorganized attachment in infancy independently predicted depressive symptoms in childhood. Abuse experiences were not evaluated as possible contributors to depressive symptoms. Additional studies have shown that quality of parenting independently predicts depressive symptoms in offspring, rather than mediating the transmission of depressive symptomatology from depressed mother to child [50–52]. Results from these investigations confirm the long-term prediction possible from careful assessments of quality of early parent–infant interactions, and also indicate that different aspects of early parenting may contribute to different types of later psychiatric symptomatology.

A third prospective study [53] assessed the contributions of attachment, early care and childhood abuse to the extent of impulsive, self-damaging borderline features exhibited in young adulthood. In these analyses, both the caregiver's withdrawal from the child's attachment overtures in infancy and the young adult's self-reported experiences of childhood maltreatment were independent, additive predictors of borderline features. Maternal withdrawing behaviors in infancy were characterized by limited provision of dialogue and parental structuring within interactions, distanced interactions with the infant, highly limited physical contact and using toys rather than physical holding and interaction to soothe the infant. These findings converge with work by Hooley and Hiller [54], who found that relapse among patients with borderline personality disorder was associated with *less* parental expressed emotion (i.e., criticism and overinvolvement), in contrast to findings among other diagnostic groups where relapse is associated with *more* parental criticism and overinvolvement. Taken together, these findings suggest that parental withdrawal may be particularly problematic for those vulnerable to borderline personality disorder from a point early in development.

## "Maternal buffering": does quality of early care moderate the expression of child genetic predisposition?

Inadequate early care is an important risk factor in human development for multiple later psychopathologies. Results from animal models are now supporting the concept of *phenotypic plasticity*, where offspring phenotypes are seen to vary as a function of environmental context, despite similar genotypes [55]. Studies from Meaney and colleagues have repeatedly demonstrated that maternal care behaviors in rats, such as pup licking and grooming, foster enduring alterations of offspring gene expression [43,56]. Changes in genetic expression associated with decreased maternal care are evident as early as during the first week of the pup's life, and they can last through to adulthood. These findings provide support for a theoretical critical period model, in which adequate maternal care during the critical period activates various pathways of genetic development to express phenotypes that are optimally adaptive for the offspring.

Studies using human subjects have also indicated that quality of care in infancy can moderate the expression of genetic characteristics in the development of psychiatric symptomatology [57,58]. Particularly relevant here, Suomi [59] has advanced the notion of "maternal buffering" in which responsive early care buffers the otherwise genetically vulnerable offspring from the development of high stress reactivity and later maladaptive behavior.

Gene–environment interaction is also being explored in developmental studies involving quality of early care and disorganized infant attachment. Recent evidence has suggested a gene–environment interaction effect in the development of disorganized attachment, such that some infants are more susceptible to the quality of maternal regulation than others. In initial work investigating genetic main effects on infant attachment behavior, Lakatos and colleagues [60] found that infants carrying the *DRD4* seven-repeat allele were four times more likely to exhibit disorganized attachment behaviors in the strange situation. Attempts to replicate this finding have both failed [61] and succeeded [62].

In a further extension of this work, the low social risk sample of Lakatos and colleagues [60] was combined with the high social risk sample of Lyons-Ruth *et al.* [53] to create greater environmental variability within the sample. The interaction between maternal disrupted communication with the infant and the infant's *DRD4* seven-repeat allele was assessed to account for infant disorganized attachment behavior [63]; the seven-repeat allele has previously been associated with less efficient functioning of the dopamine system. The authors found that quality of mother–infant communication was strongly related to disorganized attachment status among infants without the seven-repeat allele. However, infants carrying the seven-repeat allele showed no relation between maternal disrupted communication and infant disorganized attachment status. These results indicate that infants without the seven-repeat *DRD4* genotype are highly sensitive to the regulatory effects of maternal behavior, showing organized attachment in the context of sensitive maternal regulation and disorganized attachment in the context of disrupted maternal regulation. In contrast, infants with the seven-repeat allele displayed elevated rates of disorganized behavior independent of the quality of maternal regulation. The authors suggested that the efficiency of the dopamine reward system might create differential reward value for maternal affective cues and hence confer differential sensitivity to the quality of maternal care.

Polymorphisms in the serotonin transporter gene (*5-HTTLPR*) have also been implicated in gene–environment interactions in studies of infant behavior. Barry and colleagues [64] have demonstrated that, for infants with the short allele of *5-HTTLPR* (the allele that confers less efficient serotonin function in the synapse) high maternal responsiveness at 9 months was associated with attachment security at 15 months, while low maternal responsiveness predicted a heightened risk for insecure attachment behaviors. Among infants homozygous for the more efficient long allele, there was a high rate of secure attachment regardless of maternal responsiveness. Therefore, in the case of the serotonin transporter, the data support a maternal buffering model rather than a differential susceptibility model. In a maternal buffering model, maternal responsiveness buffers the risk for increased stress response associated with the short allele, while maternal buffering is not necessary for infants with only long alleles, who were presumably already protected against the experience of stressful arousal. Additional support for a buffering role for the quality of maternal care on *5-HTTLPR* gene expression comes from research on infants' experiences of fear and negative emotionality [65], as well as from work on the development of toddlers' self-regulating behaviors [66].

Because human infants in the first few years of life are most reliant upon caregivers for comfort, regulation of fearful arousal and development of adaptive social behaviors, environmental moderation of genetic effects may have a critical window for maximum effect, as suggested by recent animal models. Further research is needed to replicate these findings, to assess whether there is a critical period for such moderation of genetic expression by maternal care and to assess the presence of a developmental window for reversing the effects of poor early regulation on the potentiation of negative genetic vulnerabilities, as suggested by animal models [65].

## Conclusions

Parents have a lifelong influence on their offspring. However, the impact of early caregiving is stronger during the first years of life. During this time, the infant is highly dependent upon attachment figures, looking to them for basic needs such as protection, nurturance and regulation of fearful emotions. A child whose parent fails to meet these needs, even if the parent is not deemed abusive or neglectful by societal standards, may develop increased physiological reactivity to stressors and may also display the lack of an effective, organized behavioral strategy for seeking comfort from attachment figures in the face of such arousal.

This chapter proposes that the risk for both physiological and behavioral dysregulation as a result of poor early care in infancy constitutes a *hidden trauma*. Current prospective longitudinal evidence indicates that this hidden trauma is likely to have equal or greater impact on the development of later morbidity than maltreatment events that are more easily observed and reported. Given the importance of early care, more work is needed in human populations to disentangle the effects of early timing of poor care from the effects of chronic poor care between infancy and adulthood. Regardless, the effects of quality of early care over a 20-year period in recent prospective studies are robust, clearly establishing that subtle aspects of early care make substantial contributions to adult psychiatric morbidities. Randomized controlled trials to evaluate models for influencing early disrupted parenting behavior, in combination with long-term follow-up studies to better map developmental trajectories toward child and adult disorder, could make a substantial impact on reducing the long-term mental health costs to families and to society related to these morbidities.

## References

1. American Psychiatric Association (2000). *Diagnostic and statistical manual of mental disorders,* 4th edn. revised. Washington, DC: American Psychiatric Press.

2. Schuder, M. and Lyons-Ruth, K. (2004). "Hidden trauma" in infancy: Attachment, fearful arousal, and early dysfunction of the stress response system. In J. Osofsky (ed.), *Trauma in infancy and early childhood* (pp. 69–104). New York: Guilford.

3. Bowlby, J. (1980). *Attachment and loss. Vol. 3. Loss, sadness, and depression.* New York: Basic Books.

4. Essex, M. J., Klein, M. H., Meich, R. and Smider, N. (2001). Timing of initial exposure to maternal major depression and children's mental health symptoms in kindergarten. *British Journal of Psychiatry,* **179**, 151–156.

5. Cummings, E. M. and Cicchetti, D. (1990). Toward a transactional model of relations between attachment and depression. In M. T. Greenberg, D. Cicchetti and E. M. Cummings (eds.), *Attachment in the preschool years: Theory, research and intervention* (pp. 339–372). Chicago, IL: University of Chicago Press.

6. Denham, S. A. (1998). *Emotional development in young children.* New York: Guilford.

7. Dearing, E., McCartney, K. and Taylor, B. A. (2006). Within-child associations between family income and externalizing and internalizing problems. *Developmental Psychology,* **42**, 237–252.

8. Brook-Gunn, J., Linver, M. R. and Fauth, R. C. (2005). Children's competence and socioeconomic status in the family and the neighbourhood. In A. J. Elliot and C. S. Dweck (eds.), *Handbook of competence and motivation* (pp. 414–435). New York: Guilford.

9. Bureau, J-F., Easterbrooks, A. and Lyons-Ruth, K. (2009). Maternal depressive symptoms in infancy: Unique contributions to children's depressive symptoms in childhood and adolescence? *Development and Psychopathology,* **21**, 519–537.

10. Bowlby, J. (1969). *Attachment and loss, Vol. 1: Attachment.* New York: Basic Books.

11. George, C. and Solomon, J. (1999). Attachment and caregiving: The caregiving behavioral system. In J. Cassidy and P. R. Shaver (eds.), *Handbook of attachment: Theory, research and clinical applications* (pp. 649–670). New York: Guilford.

12. Ainsworth, M. D. S., Blehar, M. C., Waters, E. and Wall, S. (1978). *Patterns of attachment: A psychological study of the strange situation.* Hillsdale, NJ: Erlbaum.

13. Atkinson, L., Niccols, A., Paglia, A. *et al.* (2000). A meta-analysis of time between maternal sensitivity and attachment assessment: Implications for internal working models in infancy/toddlerhood. *Journal of Social and Personal Relationships,* **17**, 791–810.

14. Belsky, J., Fish, M. and Isabella, R. (1991). Continuity and discontinuity in infant negative and positive

emotionality: Family and attachment consequences. *Developmental Psychology*, **27**, 421–431.

15. Meaney, M. J. (2001). Maternal care, gene expression, and the transmission of individual differences in stress reactivity across generations. *Annual Review of Neuroscience*, **24**, 1161–1192.

16. Spangler, G. and Grossmann, K. E. (1999). Individual and physiological correlates of attachment disorganization in infancy. In J. Solomon and C. George (eds.), *Attachment disorganization* (pp. 95–124). New York: Guilford.

17. Bretherton, I. and Munholland, K. A. (2008). Internal working models in attachment relationships: Elaborating a central construct in attachment theory. In J. Cassidy and P. R. Shaver (eds.), *Handbook of attachment: Theory, research, and clinical applications*, 2nd edn. (pp. 102–128). New York: Guilford.

18. Main, M. and Solomon, J. (1990). Procedures for identifying infants as disorganized/disoriented during the Ainsworth Strange Situation. In M. Greenberg, D. Cicchetti and E. M. Cummings (eds.), *Attachment in the preschool years: Theory, research and intervention* (pp. 121–160). Chicago, IL: University of Chicago Press.

19. Main, M. and Hesse, E. (1990). Parents' unresolved traumatic experiences are related to infant disorganized attachment status: Is frightened and/or frightening parental behaviour the linking mechanism? In M. Greenberg, D. Cicchetti and E. M. Cummings (eds.), *Attachment in the preschool years: Theory, research and intervention* (pp. 161–184). Chicago, IL: University of Chicago Press.

20. Madigan, S., Bakers-Kranenburg, M., van Ijzendoorn, M. *et al.* (2006). Unresolved states of mind, anomalous parent behaviour, and disorganized attachment: A review and meta-analysis of a transmission gap. *Attachment and Human Development*, **8**, 89–111.

21. van Ijzendoorn, M., Schuengel, C. and Bakermans-Kranenburg, M. (1999). Disorganized attachment in early childhood: Meta-analysis of precursors, concomitants, and sequelae. *Development and Psychopathology*, **11**, 225–249.

22. Fish, E. W., Shahrock, D., Bagot, R. *et al.* (2004). Epigenetic programming of stress responses through variations in maternal care. *Annals of the New York Academy of Sciences*, **1036**, 167–180.

23. Gunnar, M. (2005). Attachment and stress in early development. In C. S. Carter, L. Ahnert, K. E. Grossman *et al.* (eds.), *Attachment and bonding: A new synthesis* (pp. 245–255). Cambridge, MA: MIT Press.

24. Spangler, G., Schieche, U., Ilg, U., Maier, U. and Ackermann, C. (1994). Maternal sensitivity as an external organizer for biobehavioural regulation in infancy. *Developmental Psychobiology*, **27**, 425–437.

25. Stratakis, C. A. and Gold, G. P. (1995). Neuro-endocrinology and pathophysiology of the stress system. *Annals of the New York Academy of Sciences*, **771**, 1–18.

26. Chrousos, G. P. and Gold, P. W. (1992). The concepts of stress and stress system disorders: Overview of physical and behavioural homeostasis. *Journal of the American Medical Association*, **267**, 1244–1252.

27. Gunnar, M. R. and Donzella, B. (2001). Social regulation of the cortisol levels in early human development. *Psychoneuroendocrinology*, **27**, 199–220.

28. Ames, E. W. (1990). Spitz revisited: A trip to Romanian "orphanages." Canadian Psychological Association Newsletter, *Developmental Psychology Section*, **9**, 8–11.

29. Carlson, M. and Earls, F. (1997). Psychological and neuroendocrinological sequelae of early social deprivation in institutionalized children in Romania. *Annals of the New York Academy of Sciences*, **807**, 419–428.

30. Kroupina, M., Gunnar, M. R. and Johnson, D. E. (1997). *Report on salivary cortisol levels in a Russian baby home.* Minneapolis, MN: Institute of Child Development, University of Minnesota.

31. Gunnar, M. and Vasquez, D. (2001). Low cortisol and a flattening of expected daytime rhythm: Potential indices of risk in human development. *Development and Psychopathology*, **13**, 515–538.

32. Gilles, E. E., Berntson, G. G., Zipf, W. B. and Gunnar, M. R. (2000, July). Neglect is associated with a blunting of behavioural and biological stress responses in human infants. In *Proceedings of the International Conference on Infant Studies*, Brighton, UK.

33. Hertsgaard, L., Gunnar, M., Erickson, M. F. and Nachmias, M. (1995). Adrenocortical responses to the strange situation in infants with disorganized/disoriented attachment relationships. *Child Development*, **66**, 1100–1106.

34. Ashman, S. B. and Dawson, G. (2002). Maternal depression, infant psychobiological development, and risk for depression. In S. H. Goodman and I. H. Gotlib (eds.), *Children of depressed parents: Mechanisms of risk and implications for treatment* (pp. 37–58). Washington, DC: American Psychological Association.

35. Sethre-Hofstad, L., Stansbury, K. and Rice, M. (2002). Attunement of maternal and child adrenocortical response to child challenge. *Psychoneuroendocrinology*, **27**, 731–748.

36. Caldji, C., Tannenbaum, B., Sharma, S. *et al.* (1998). Maternal care during infancy regulates the development of neural systems mediating the expression of fearfulness in the rat. *Proceedings of the National Academy of Sciences USA*, **95**, 5445–5340.

37. Levine, S. (1994). The ontogeny of the hypothalamic–pituitary–adrenal axis: The influence of maternal factors. *Annals of the New York Academy of Sciences*, **746**, 275–288.

38. Plotsky, P. M. and Meaney, M. J. (1993). Early, postnatal experience alters hypothalamic corticotropin-releasing factor (CRF) mRNA, median eminence CRF content and stress-induced release in adult rats. *Molecular Brain Research*, **18**, 195–200.

39. Higley, J. D., Suomi, S. J. and Linnoila, M. (1992). A longitudinal study of CSF monoamine metabolite and plasma cortisol concentrations in young rhesus monkeys: Effects of early experience, age, sex, and stress on continuity of individual differences. *Biological Psychiatry*, **32**, 127–145.

40. Bayart, F., Hayashi, K. T., Faull, K. F., Barchas, J. D. and Levine, S. (1990). Influence of maternal proximity on behavioural and psychological responses to separation in infant rhesus monkeys (Macaca mulatta). *Behavioural Neuroscience*, **104**, 98–107.

41. Coplan, J. D., Andrews, M. W., Owens, M. J. *et al.* (1996). Persistent elevations of cerebrospinal fluid concentrations of corticotropin-releasing factor in adult nonhuman primates exposed to early-life stressors: Implications for the pathophysiology of mood and anxiety disorders. *Proceedings of the National Academy of Sciences USA*, **93**, 1619–1623.

42. Francis, D., Diorio, J., Liu, D. and Meaney, M. (1999). Nongenomic transmission across generations of maternal behaviour and stress responses in the rat. *Science*, **286**, 1155–1158.

43. Szyf, M., Weaver, I. and Meaney, M. J. (2007). Maternal care, the epigenome, and phenotypic differences in behaviour. *Reproductive Toxicology*, **24**, 9–19.

44. Carlson, E. A. (1998). A prospective longitudinal study of attachment disorganization/disorientation. *Child Development*, **69**, 1107–1128.

45. Ogawa, J. R., Sroufe, L. A., Weinfeld, N. S., Carlson, E. A. and Egeland, B. (1997). Development and the fragmented self: Longitudinal study of dissociative symptomatology in a non-clinical sample. *Development and Psychopathology*, **9**, 855–879.

46. National Institute of Child Health and Human Development Early Child Care Research Network (2006). Infant–mother attachment classification: Risk and protection in relation to changing maternal caregiving quality. *Developmental Psychology*, **42**, 38–58.

47. Dutra, L., Bureau, J-F., Holmes, B., Lyubchik, A. and Lyons-Ruth, K. (2009). Quality of early care and childhood trauma: A prospective study of developmental pathways to dissociation. *Journal of Nervous and Mental Disease*, **197**, 383–390.

48. Narang, D. S. and Contreras, J. M. (2005). The relationship of dissociation and affective family environment with the intergenerational cycle of child abuse. *Child Abuse & Neglect*, **29**, 683–699.

49. Carlson, V., Dalenberg, C., Armstrong, J. *et al.* (2001). Multivariate prediction of posttraumatic symptoms in psychiatric inpatients. *Journal of Traumatic Stress*, **14**, 549–567.

50. Burt, K. B., Van Dulmen, M. H. M., Carlivati, J. *et al.* (2005). Mediating links between maternal depression and offspring psychopathology: The importance of independent data. *Journal of Child Psychology and Psychiatry*, **46**, 490–499.

51. Garber, J. and Flynn, C. (2001). Predictors of depressive cognitions in young adolescents. *Cognitive Therapy and Research*, **25**, 353–376.

52. Nelson, D. R., Hammen, C., Brennan, P. A. and Ullman, J. B. (2003). The impact of maternal depression on adolescent adjustment: The role of expressed emotion. *Journal of Consulting and Clinical Psychology*, 935–944.

53. Lyons-Ruth, K., Bureau, J-F., Hennighausen, K. H., Holmes, B. M. and Easterbrooks, A. (2009). Parental helplessness and adolescent role-reversal as correlates of borderline features and self-injury. In J.-F. Bureau and K. Lyons-Ruth (Chairs), *Relational predictors of self-damaging behaviour in adolescence: Multiwave longitudinal analyses*. Symposium *at The Annual Meeting of the Society for Research in Child Development* (p. 242), Denver, CO.

54. Hooley, J. M. and Hiller, J. B. (2000). Personality and expressed emotion. *Journal of Abnormal Psychology*, **109**, 40–44.

55. Zhang, T-Y., Parent, C., Weaver, I. and Meaney, M. J. (2004). Maternal programming of individual differences in defensive responses in the rat. *Annals of the New York Academy of Sciences*, **1032**, 85–103.

56. Weaver, I., Cervoni, N., Champagne, F. A. *et al.* (2004). Epigenetic programming by maternal behaviour. *Nature Neuroscience*, **7**, 847–854.

57. Caspi, A., McClay, J., Moffitt, T. E. *et al.* (2002). Role of genotype in the cycle of violence in maltreated children. *Science*, **297**, 851–854.

58. Kaufman, J., Yang, B., Douglas-Palumberi, H. *et al.* (2004). Social supports and serotonin transporter gene moderate depression in maltreated children. *Proceedings of the National Academy of Sciences USA*, **101**, 17316–17321.

59. Suomi, S. J. (2005). How gene–environment interactions shape the development of impulsive aggression in rhesus monkeys. In D. M. Stoff and E. J. Susman (eds.), *Developmental psychobiology of aggression* (pp. 252–268). New York: Cambridge University Press.

60. Lakatos, K., Toth, I., Nemoda, Z. *et al.* (2000). Dopamine D4 receptor (DRD4) gene polymorphism is associated with attachment disorganization. *Molecular Psychiatry*, **5**, 633–637.

61. Bakermans-Kranenburg, M. J. and van Ijzendoorn, M. H. (2004). No association of dopamine D4 receptor (DRD4) and –521C/T promoter polymorphisms with

infant attachment disorganization. *Attachment and Human Development*, **6**, 211–218.

62. Gervai, J., Nemoda, Z., Lakatos, K. *et al.* (2005). Transmission disequilibrium tests confirm the link between DRD4 gene polymorphism and infant attachment. *American Journal of Medical Genetics, Part B*, **132B**, 126–130.

63. Gervai, J., Novak, A., Lakatos, K. *et al.* (2007). Infant genotype may moderate sensitivity to maternal affective communications: Attachment disorganization, quality of care, and the DRD4 polymorphism. *Social Neuroscience*, **2**, 307–319.

64. Barry, R. A., Kochanska, G. and Philibert, R. A. (2008). G × E interaction in the organization of attachment: Mother's responsiveness as a moderator of child's genotypes. *Journal of Child Psychology and Psychiatry*, **49**, 1313–1320.

65. Pauli-Pott, U., Friedl, S., Hinney, A. and Hebebrand, J. (2009). Serotonin transporter gene polymorphism (5HTTLPR), environmental conditions, and developing negative emotionality and fear in early childhood. *Journal of Neural Transmission*, **116**, 503–512.

66. Kochanska, G., Philibert, R. A. and Barry, R. A. (2009). Interplay of genes and early mother–child relationship in the development of self-regulation from toddler to preschool-age. *Journal of Child Psychology and Psychiatry*, **50**, 1331–1338.

# Chapter 6

# Towards a developmental trauma disorder diagnosis for childhood interpersonal trauma

Bessel A. van der Kolk and Wendy d'Andrea

## Introduction

The diagnostic system that was in place in the 1970s had no room to accommodate the pathology of hundreds of thousands returning Vietnam veterans. The recognition that, without a diagnosis, there is little chance to develop effective treatments led to the formulation and the incorporation of post-traumatic stress disorder (PTSD) in the *Diagnostic and Statistical Manual* (DSM) third edition [1]. The introduction of the diagnosis into the psychiatric classification system led to extensive scientific studies of the syndrome, which turned out to be relevant to victims of a range of traumatic events, including rape, torture and motor vehicle accidents.

However, during the subsequent three decades, it has become increasingly obvious that the current diagnostic system is similarly grossly inadequate to serve chronically traumatized children. Despite the fact that research has repeatedly demonstrated that human beings who are exposed to betrayal, abandonment and abuse by their caretakers suffer from vastly more complex psychobiological disturbances than human beings who are victims of earthquakes and motor vehicle accidents (e.g., van der Kolk *et al.* [2]), our diagnostic system continues to lump all trauma-related symptomatology under the category of "PTSD."

Since the formulation of the PTSD diagnosis, there has been an independent and parallel emergence of the field of developmental psychopathology [3,4]. Another significant development has been the increasing documentation of the effects of adverse early life experiences on brain development [5,6], neuroendocrinology [7,8] and immunology [4,9].

Two-thirds of adults in the USA report having suffered some form of interpersonal trauma as children. As demonstrated in Ch. 8, childhood interpersonal trauma is a root cause of many major public health problems. Currently, children and adults with histories of interpersonal trauma seeking psychological intervention are given one or more of a wide variety of heterogeneous diagnoses that do not reflect the contributions of life experience on mind, brain and or body. This chapter delineates the developmental trauma disorder (DTD) diagnosis proposed by the National Child Traumatic Stress DSM-V Taskforce.[1] Because it specifically captures the symptoms suffered by victims of childhood interpersonal trauma, the use of a DTD diagnosis can be expected to lead to a better understanding and more effective treatment of individuals exposed to these types of trauma.

Given the cultural taboos against confronting the realities surrounding child abuse and neglect, it is not surprising that research in this field has often been difficult to fund and execute. Yet, hundreds of studies over the past three decades have documented the impact of childhood interpersonal trauma on the development of affect regulation, attention, cognition, perception and interpersonal relationships. None of this research has yet been translated into changes in our diagnostic system, which continues to rely on the diagnosis of PTSD, which was originally formulated in 1978 to capture the psychopathology of

[1] This Taksforce is co-chaired by Bessel van der Kolk and Robert Pynoos and includes Bradley Stolbach, Julian Ford, Joseph Spinazzola, Marilyn Cloitre, Alicia Lieberman, Glenn Saxe, Frank Putnam, Dante Cicchetti, Martin Teicher and Wendy 'd Andrea.

Vietnam veterans and has not changed substantially since then.

The numerous clinical expressions of the damage resulting from childhood interpersonal trauma are currently relegated to a whole variety of seemingly unrelated comorbidities, such as conduct disorder, attention-deficit hyperactivity disorder (ADHD), bipolar disorder, phobic anxiety, reactive attachment disorder and separation anxiety. In fact, multiple studies show that the majority meet criteria for multiple DSM diagnoses. In one study of 364 abused children [10], 58% had the primary diagnosis of separation anxiety/overanxious disorders, 36% phobic disorders, 35% PTSD, 22% ADHD and 22% oppositional defiant disorder.

## Background

In Freedman and Kaplan's *Comprehensive Textbook of Psychiatry* [11] in 1974, Henderson [12] stated, "incest is extremely rare, and does not occur in more than 1 out of 1.1 million people" (p. 1536). Furthermore, this leading textbook of psychiatry went on to extol the possible *benefits* to a child of incest. During the 1970s, case reports of sexual abuse and incest started to appear in the medical literature, and today we know that 3 million children in the USA are reported to Child Protective Services each year for concerns of child abuse and neglect. Early adverse experiences have been conclusively linked with a range of individual and public health problems including depression, substance abuse, self-destructive activities, poor interpersonal relationships, medical illnesses and healthcare expenditure.

In the 1980s, Arthur Green and Dorothy Otnow Lewis wrote the first papers that documented that many abused children suffered neurological damage, even when there were no reports of head injury [13]. In a study of 22 sexually abused patients, 77% had abnormal brain waves and 36% had seizures [14]. This was the first concrete evidence that human abuse and neglect affect the development of vulnerable brain regions. Subsequent research by Martin Teicher, Michael DeBellis, Ruth Lanius, Paul Plotsky and many others has begun to delineate a constellation of brain abnormalities associated with childhood abuse and neglect. The results are quite consistent across studies: being in a persistent low-level fear state affects development of the primary information-processing areas of the brain [15].

Ironically, as we have become more and more technically proficient and knowledgeable about epidemiology and brain development, we seem to have lost track of the context in which humans develop and thrive. It is remarkable that even though research has shown that the majority of psychiatric inpatients have histories of childhood molestation, abuse or abandonment by caregivers, and despite the fact that the consequences of adverse childhood experiences constitute the single largest public health problem in the USA [16] and likely worldwide, there is enormous resistance to placing the care of developing humans where it belongs: at the forefront of our attention. There continues to be vastly more funding for studying the genetic components of mental illness, and for relatively obscure disorders such as obsessive-compulsive disorder, than for preventing and treating the long-term effects of child abuse and neglect [17]. Studies of both child and adult populations over the last 25 years have established that traumatic stress in childhood does not occur in isolation in the majority of trauma-exposed individuals, but rather it is characterized by co-occurring, often chronic, types of victimization and other adverse experiences [2,18–20].

The recognition of the profound difference between adult-onset PTSD and the clinical effects of interpersonal violence on children and the need to develop effective treatments for these children were the principal reasons for the establishment of the National Child Traumatic Stress Network in 2001. During the intervening decade, it became evident that the current diagnostic classification system is inadequate for the tens of thousands of traumatized children receiving psychiatric care for trauma-related difficulties.

A survey of 1699 children receiving trauma-focused treatment across 25 network sites of the National Child Traumatic Stress Network [20] showed that the vast majority (78%) were exposed to multiple and/or prolonged interpersonal trauma, with a modal 3 trauma exposure types; less than 25% met diagnostic criteria for PTSD. Less than 10% were exposed to serious accidents or medical illness. Most children exhibited post-traumatic sequelae not captured by PTSD: at least 50% had significant disturbances in affect regulation; attention and concentration; negative self-image; impulse control; and aggression and risk taking [20]. These findings are in line with the voluminous epidemiological, biological and psychological research on the impact of childhood interpersonal trauma that has been published since the mid 1980s, which includes effects on tens of thousands of children. Hence, it is critical to find a way out of this morass of multiple comorbid diagnoses and to identify a new diagnostic category that captures the profusion of symptoms in these children.

# Effects of childhood interpersonal trauma on brain activity, self-awareness and social functioning

## Brain activity

Alarm states erase people's sense of time: in brain scans, one can observe decreased activation of these cortical areas when subjects are exposed to reminders of their traumatic experiences [21,22]. Cut adrift from the internal regulating capabilities of the cortex, subcortical structures promote behavior that reacts reflexively, impulsively and aggressively to any perceived threat. Alarm states interfere with contemplation of the consequences of one's behavior. Because the brain areas responsible for executive functioning go off-line under threat, frightened people lose touch with the flow of time and get stuck in a terrifying, seemingly never-ending present. As a result, their responses are directed toward their desperate need for immediate relief, and delayed gratification is difficult, if not impossible. The documentation of these abnormalities explains why traumatized individuals usually have little understanding of what upsets them and little control over their reactions.

Traumatized individuals have more selective development of non-verbal cognitive capacities. People raised by unresponsive, abusive or chaotic caregivers have learned that non-verbal information is more critical for survival than words. Lanius and colleagues [21,22] have shown that chronically traumatized individuals have decreased activation in the dorsolateral and medial prefrontal brain regions, particularly when under stress. These are the areas of the brain that are associated with executive functioning and the capacity to think and contextualize the self in the world with continuity over time.

## Self-experience and social functioning

The foundation of self-experience is grounded in the capacity to identify and utilize physical sensations [23]. When infants have upsetting sensations, they use their facial expressions, body movements and vocal cords to ensure attention from their caregiver. Most caregiving interactions are geared toward changing the child's sensations and restoring their inner balance. And the child learns that he or she can rely on the caregiver. When squirming and crying fail to elicit a caring response, children change their strategy. Crittenden [24] and Fosha [25] have used attachment theory to describe three ways in which children learn to cope with consistently unresponsive caregivers.

One way is "feeling but not dealing": an elaboration of anxious/preoccupied attachment where the individual gets stuck in a continuous alarm or defeat response that does not significantly change even when people around them seem to respond appropriately. No amount of care seems to be able to provide a sense of safety and comfort. These children seem to be stuck in a continuous state of alarm, which becomes independent from actual threat.

The second adaptation is "dealing but not feeling," an elaboration of avoidant/dismissive attachment, where the child copes by appearing to retain equilibrium without caregiver assistance. When this occurs, the person continues to be able to function despite inadequate caregiving by learning to ignore their own physical sensations and warning signs. They develop "alexithymia," in which they are plagued by unpleasant physical sensations that are disconnected from emotional experience; emotions lose their function as warning signals. These individuals cannot use their feelings to adjust how they relate to other people, and they are prone to respond to stress with somatic problems. The third form of coping has been called "neither feeling nor dealing," the sort of disorganized response that is most common in abused and neglected children who are raised by frightened or frightening caregivers. These children often manifest psychiatric symptoms as adults and require chronic psychiatric care.

## The need for a new diagnosis

In spite of valiant efforts to integrate the complexity of the impact of trauma on mind and brain into diagnosis in the DSM-IV [26] (and attempts to do this again for the DSM-V under the rubric of Developmental Trauma Disorder [27]), these patients currently do not have a diagnostic home; consequently, it is impossible for organized psychiatry and psychology to study complexly traumatized people in a coherent fashion. The urgent need for a developmentally sensitive interpersonal trauma diagnosis is provisionally covered by DTD (Box 6.1).

# Box 6.1. Consensus proposed criteria for developmental trauma disorder

There are five criteria (A–E), each with specific features of which some or all must be observed.

## A. Exposure

The child or adolescent has experienced or witnessed multiple or prolonged adverse events over a period of at least 1 year beginning in childhood or early adolescence, including *both*:

- direct experience or witnessing of repeated and severe episodes of interpersonal violence *and*

- significant disruptions of protective caregiving as the result of repeated changes in primary caregiver, repeated separation from the primary caregiver, or exposure to severe and persistent emotional abuse.

## B. Affective and physiological dysregulation

The child exhibits impaired normative developmental competencies related to arousal regulation, including at least *two* of the following:

- inability to modulate, tolerate or recover from extreme affect states (e.g., fear, anger, shame), including prolonged and extreme tantrums, or immobilization

- disturbances in regulation in bodily functions (e.g., persistent disturbances in sleeping, eating and elimination; overreactivity or underreactivity to touch and sounds; disorganization during routine transitions)

- diminished awareness/dissociation of sensations, emotions and bodily states

- impaired capacity to describe emotions or bodily states.

## C. Attentional and behavioral dysregulation

The child exhibits impaired normative developmental competencies related to sustained attention, learning or coping with stress, including at least *three* of the following:

- preoccupation with threat or impaired capacity to perceive threat, including misreading of safety and danger cues

- impaired capacity for self-protection, including extreme risk taking or thrill seeking

- maladaptive attempts at self-soothing (e.g., rocking and other rhythmical movements, compulsive masturbation)

- habitual (intentional or automatic) or reactive self-harm

- inability to initiate or sustain goal-directed behavior.

## D. Self- and relational dysregulation

The child exhibits impaired normative developmental competencies in their sense of personal identity and involvement in relationships, including at least *three* of the following:

- intense preoccupation with safety of the caregiver or other loved ones (including precocious caregiving) or difficulty tolerating reunion with them after separation

- persistent negative sense of self, including self-loathing, helplessness, worthlessness, ineffectiveness or defectiveness

- extreme and persistent distrust, defiance or lack of reciprocal behavior in close relationships with adults or peers

- reactive physical or verbal aggression toward peers, caregivers or other adults

- inappropriate (excessive or promiscuous) attempts to get intimate contact (including but not limited to sexual or physical intimacy) or excessive reliance on peers or adults for safety and reassurance

- impaired capacity to regulate empathic arousal, as evidenced by lack of empathy for, or intolerance of, expressions of distress of others, or excessive responsiveness to the distress of others.

## E. Duration of disturbance

Symptoms in criteria B, C and D, above, for at least 6 months.

## F. Functional impairment

The disturbance causes clinically significant distress or impairment in at least two of the following areas of functioning:

- scholastic: underperformance, non-attendance, disciplinary problems, dropout, failure to complete degree/credential(s), conflict with school personnel, learning disabilities or intellectual impairment that cannot be accounted for by neurological or other factors
- familial: conflict, avoidance/passivity, running away, detachment and surrogate replacements, attempts to physically or emotionally hurt family members, non-fulfillment of responsibilities within the family
- peer group: isolation, deviant affiliations, persistent physical or emotional conflict, avoidance/passivity, involvement in violence or unsafe acts, age-inappropriate affiliations or style of interaction
- legal: arrests/recidivism, detention, convictions, incarceration, violation of probation or other court orders, increasingly severe offenses, crimes against other persons, disregard or contempt for the law or for conventional moral standards
- health: physical illness or problems that cannot be fully accounted for by physical injury or degeneration, involving the digestive, neurological (including conversion symptoms and analgesia), sexual, immune, cardiopulmonary, proprioceptive or sensory systems; severe headaches (including migraine); chronic pain or fatigue
- vocational (for youth involved in, seeking or referred for employment, volunteer work or job training): disinterest in work/vocation, inability to get or keep jobs, persistent conflict with coworkers or supervisors, underemployment in relation to abilities, failure to achieve expectable advancements.

These chronic and severe coexisting problems (emotion regulation, impulse control, attention and cognition, dissociation, interpersonal relationships, and self and relational schemas) are best understood as a single coherent pathology. However, in absence of a developmentally sensitive trauma-specific diagnosis for children, these children are instead diagnosed with an average of 3–8 comorbid axis I and II disorders [28]. Although various psychiatric diagnoses have overlapping symptoms with other diagnoses (e.g., anxiety and depression may both feature psychomotor agitation), the purpose of a diagnosis is to capture a relatively unique constellation of symptoms. Some symptoms of DTD may overlap with existing diagnoses but its conceptual specificity distinguishes it from existing diagnoses and represents an advance in the current state of diagnostic nomenclature. The continued practice of applying multiple distinct comorbid diagnoses to traumatized children has grave consequences: it defies parsimony, obscures etiological clarity and runs the danger of relegating treatment and intervention to a small aspect of the child's psychopathology, rather than promoting a comprehensive treatment approach.

## Rationale and characteristics of the developmental trauma disorder diagnosis

The epidemiological and biological data on child trauma outcomes compel the scientific community to consider whether the spectrum of symptoms experienced by abused children represents (a) multiple distinct psychiatric diagnoses or (b) the disruption of interconnected developmental competencies, resulting in a diverse but consistent set of symptoms. In order to examine the validity of DTD, the evidence supporting the following facets of the DTD diagnosis are reviewed below: (a) childhood interpersonal trauma results in a coherent set of symptoms (DTD); (b) these symptoms have specificity; (c) the symptoms are not accounted for by any existing single DSM-IV diagnosis, including PTSD; (d) research on the biological development of systems disrupted by childhood trauma is consistent with DTD symptoms; and (e) the application of non-specific diagnoses to maltreated children is likely to lead to poor treatment outcomes, while interventions that comprehensively address the spectrum of problems of children exposed to interpersonal trauma are likely to improve treatment outcome.

# Symptomatology arising from childhood interpersonal trauma

Numerous studies have documented that exposure to interpersonal trauma during childhood is associated with increased incidence of affect and impulse dysregulation, alterations in attention and consciousness, disturbances of self-perception and systems of meaning, interpersonal difficulties and somatization. Moreover, these symptoms most frequently co-occur with each other following childhood interpersonal trauma. We propose that DTD is made up of post-trauma adaptations across these five domains.

## Affect and impulse dysregulation

Approximately 700 studies have documented the increased disturbance of affect and impulse regulation following childhood interpersonal trauma [29]. Dysregulation of affect and impulse control following exposure to interpersonal trauma is manifested in a broad spectrum of symptoms. Affect dysregulation can include lability, explosive anger, self-destructive behavior, psychic numbing and social withdrawal, dysphoria, depression and loss of motivation. Impulse dysregulation is associated with self-injury, risk-taking, aggression, eating disorders, substance use, oppositional behavior and reenactment of trauma. Affect dysregulation and impulse dysregulation are interwoven problems: impulsive behavior represents a failure of affect regulation, while self-injury, substance abuse and eating disorders can be understood as ill-fated attempts at self-regulation. Affect and impulse dysregulation include not only overt disruptive behaviors but also behavioral and emotional "shutting down" in the face of overwhelming stress. Furthermore, the triggers for such dysregulation may be broad and only subtly reminiscent of trauma stimuli.

## Disturbances of attention, cognition and consciousness

Disturbances of attention, cognition and consciousness are manifested as dissociation, depersonalization, memory disturbance, inability to concentrate (regardless of whether the task evokes trauma reminders), poor executive functioning, lack of curiosity, learning difficulties, problems with space and time orientation and poor language development. Over 400 studies have documented the association between childhood victimization and dissociative symptoms (e.g., Kaplow et al. [30] and Neumann et al. [31]). Using neuropsychological paradigms, an additional 400 studies have documented that maltreated children selectively attend to negative stimuli, have broad difficulties with attention, concentration and memory, and have response inhibition deficits. Furthermore, these deficits have been documented in children regardless of diagnosed psychopathology.

## Distortions in self-perception and systems of meaning

Distortions in self-perception and systems of meaning include poor self-worth and self-esteem, poor body image, poor sense of separateness, shame and guilt, learned helplessness, expectations of victimization and lack of sense of meaning and belief system. Over 50 studies document the occurrence of distorted self-perception resulting from childhood trauma (e.g., Sachs-Ericsson et al. [32]). Recent meta-analyses have demonstrated that distorted self-perception is a significant source of distress in children exposed to interpersonal trauma, and not merely an "associated feature" [31,33]. Evidence supports similar conclusions for post-abuse shame and guilt from over 100 quantitative studies.

## Interpersonal difficulties

Interpersonal difficulties in children following abuse and neglect include disrupted attachment styles, difficulties with trust, low interpersonal effectiveness, adulthood sexual problems, re-victimization, poor social skills and poor boundaries [34,35]. Nearly 1000 studies have documented interpersonal difficulties after childhood interpersonal trauma, and a meta-analysis of 38 studies found that childhood interpersonal trauma significantly predicted interpersonal difficulties in adulthood [31].

## Somatization and biological dysregulation

Somatization and biological dysregulation include digestive distress, migraines, conversion symptoms, sexual symptoms, chronic pain, poor energy, cardiopulmonary symptoms, analgesia, poor balance and proprioception, and sensory integration difficulties. Increased somatization and biological dysregulation have been documented in maltreated children and in adults who had been maltreated as children in at least 100 quantitative studies (e.g., Ehlert et al. [36]).

## Co-occurring symptoms

Symptoms of DTD arise from interference in the development of broad-reaching neurobiological regulatory systems. Numerous studies have documented a variety of developmental disruptions following childhood exposure to interpersonal trauma; the symptoms captured in the DTD diagnosis are related to severity of exposure to trauma, as well as to exposure to multiple forms of interpersonal trauma.

Equally pertinent to a complex trauma diagnosis are studies that document the co-occurrence of the symptoms discussed above, particularly in the aftermath of interpersonal trauma. The DSM-IV field trials were the initial foray into examining the inter-related symptoms affected by childhood trauma exposure. In a sample of 525 adults, early life interpersonal trauma was significantly associated with a spectrum of symptoms, which included disruptions consistent with DTD [2]. This study showed that childhood interpersonal trauma exposure results in very different symptom constellations than childhood non-interpersonal trauma and adult trauma exposure.

## Childhood interpersonal trauma as the source of developmental trauma disorder

Several large-sample studies have examined the causal relationship between childhood interpersonal trauma and DTD symptoms. These studies have documented the correlations of age of first trauma exposure, trauma severity and duration of exposure with DTD symptoms [37,38] .

## The issue of comorbidity following childhood interpersonal trauma exposure

The relationship of childhood trauma and multiple psychiatric diagnoses is a testament to the pervasive impact of childhood victimization on multiple core developmental competencies. A variety of studies have shown that the symptom severity of bipolar disorder, depression, ADHD, separation anxiety, somatoform disorder and substance abuse is correlated with the presence, severity and chronicity of childhood abuse and neglect in patients diagnosed with these disorders. The comorbidity literature in trauma is vast (over 1800 published studies to date, 400 of which specifically focus on the sequelae of childhood trauma) [36,39–45].

## Disruption of biological systems by childhood trauma

Interpersonal trauma during childhood has a profoundly negative effect upon key regulatory biological systems. The central nervous system and hormonal regulation appear to be deleteriously impacted by childhood interpersonal trauma. The interpersonal trauma-related disruptions evident in biological systems are consistent with the symptom presentation associated with DTD. It is important to note that the biological systems affected by childhood trauma may, in turn, impact multiple behavioral outcomes, and this may account for the broad range of inter-related outcomes associated with interpersonal trauma. Associations have been documented between interpersonal trauma and structural and functional abnormalities in the prefrontal cortex [22,46,47], corpus callosum [48], amygdala [49], hippocampus [49,50], temporal lobe [22] and cerebellum [51]. Taken together, these areas of the brain represent key pathways for the regulation of consciousness, affect, impulse, sense of self and physical awareness. Numerous additional studies have documented abnormalities in stress hormone reactivity [37,52,53], which may, in turn, exacerbate susceptibility to the physiological manifestations of emotional distress.

## The effect of a diagnosis of developmental trauma disorder on treatment outcome

The treatment outcome literature lends additional credence to both the specificity and the necessity of a complex trauma diagnosis. Numerous studies have documented that the balance between treatment resistance and success in diagnoses such as conduct disorder, bipolar disorder and ADHD can be attributed to occurrence of childhood interpersonal trauma. Therapies which focus on addressing the core disturbances in DTD of affect dysregulation, attention and consciousness, physiological regulation, interpersonal skills and identity show significant treatment gains in trauma survivors [54,55]. These findings suggest that other diagnoses may be serving as "stand-ins" for DTD, to the detriment of traumatized children to whom such diagnoses are applied.

## Implications for clinical assessment and treatment

Since the early 1990s, there have been significant advances in the assessment and treatment of people who have experienced complex trauma. Many of these advances have their foundation in the improved understanding of how trauma affects the developing brain and self-perception. Contemporary neuroscience research suggests that effective treatment needs to involve (a) learning to modulate arousal, (b) learning to tolerate feelings and sensations by increasing the capacity for interoception and (c) learning that, after confrontation with physical helplessness, it is essential to engage in taking effective action.

## Modulating arousal

Describing traumatic experiences in conventional verbal therapy runs the risk of activating implicit memory systems: trauma-related physical sensations and physiological hyper- or hypoarousal. The very act of talking about one's traumatic experiences can make trauma victims feel hyperaroused, afraid and unsafe. These reactions only aggravate post-traumatic helplessness, fear, shame and rage. In order to avoid this, chronically traumatized individuals are prone to seek a supportive therapeutic relationship in which the therapist becomes a refuge from a life of anxiety and ineffectiveness, rather than someone to help them to process the imprints of their traumatic experiences. Learning to modulate one's arousal level autonomously is essential for overcoming the passivity and dependency associated with a fear of reliving the trauma.

## Increasing capacity for interoception

Most clinicians agree that being able to regulate affective arousal is critical to being able to tolerate effective trauma-processing therapy. In recent years, there has been an increasing awareness that people have built-in ways of regulating themselves. Interestingly, there is little in the Western tradition that cultivates this inborn capacity – there has been a tendency to believe that one can lead "a better life through chemistry." In Western cultures, alcohol traditionally has served as the primary way of dealing with excessive arousal and fear. During the past century, alcohol was gradually condemned as a way of coping, and psychopharmacological agents were increasingly substituted to help disturbed people to modulate their emotions. However, in other, largely non-Western, cultures, there are long traditions of cultivating the capacity to regulating one's physiological system. Examples are chi qong and tai chi in China, yoga in India and drumming in parts of Africa. All of these self-regulatory practices involve the activation of the tenth cranial nerve, the vagus nerve, which, as Darwin already pointed out in *The emotional expression of animals and men* [56], is the principal avenue between brain and body.

Contemporary research is beginning to support the notion that breathing, moving, chanting, tapping acupressure points and engaging in rhythmical activities with other human beings can have a profound effect on physiological arousal systems. Clinicians are gradually learning how activating bodily sensations that have become dulled by avoidance of painful stimuli can help clients to regain a sense of pleasure and engagement. Our initial studies of utilizing yoga in the treatment of complex trauma have been very promising [57] and hopefully this will be just the beginning of the exploration of effective body-based self-regulatory practices.

## Taking effective action

Interoceptive, body-oriented therapies can directly deal with a core clinical issue in PTSD: traumatized individuals are prone to experience the present with physical sensations and emotions that are associated with their traumatic past, and to act accordingly. For therapy to be effective, it is useful to focus in on the patient's physical self-experience and increase their self-awareness, rather than focusing exclusively on the meaning that people make of their experience – their narrative of the past. If past experience is embodied in current physiological states and action tendencies, and the trauma is reenacted in breath, gestures, sensory perceptions, movement, emotion and thought, then therapy may be most effective if it facilitates self-awareness and self-regulation. Once patients become aware of their sensations and action tendencies, they can set about discovering new ways of orienting themselves to their surroundings and exploring novel ways of engaging with potential sources of mastery and pleasure.

## Lessons learned

Perhaps one of the most profound lessons from trauma research over the last 50 years has been that the trauma that once was outside, and played itself out in a social setting, has become lodged within people's internal experiences, in the very sinew and muscles of their organism. The greatest task of therapy is enabling a traumatized individual to learn how to tolerate, approach, befriend and nurture their deepest sensations and emotions. Clinical experience shows that traumatized individuals, as a rule, have great difficulty attending to their inner sensations and perceptions – when asked to focus on internal sensations, they often feel overwhelmed or deny having an inner sense of self. When they try to meditate, they often report becoming overwhelmed by residues of trauma-related perceptions, sensations and emotions. Instead, they report feeling disgusted with themselves, helpless or panicked, or they may experience trauma-related images and physical sensations. Trauma victims tend to have a negative body image – they wish to pay as little attention to their bodies and, thereby, to their internal sensations as possible. Yet learning to take care of oneself requires being in touch with the demands and requirements of one's physical self. In order to keep old trauma from intruding into current experience, patients need to deal with the internal residues of the past. Neurobiologically speaking, they need to activate their medial prefrontal cortex, insula and anterior cingulate by learning to tolerate orienting and focusing their attention on their internal experience, while interweaving and conjoining cognitive, emotional and sensorimotor elements of their traumatic experience.

Traumatized individuals need to be effectively taught that it is safe and useful to have feelings and sensations. If they learn to attend to inner experience, they will become aware that bodily experience never remains static. Unlike at the moment of a trauma, when everything seems to freeze in time, physical sensations and emotions are in a constant state of flux. They need to learn to tell the difference between a sensation and an emotion (How do you know you are angry/afraid? Where do you feel that in your body? Do you notice any impulses in your body to move in some way right now?). Once they realize that their internal sensations continuously shift and change, they discover that remembering the past does not inevitably result in overwhelming emotions, particularly as they are able to develop a degree of control over their physiological states by breathing and movement.

Trauma is not primarily remembered as a story but is stored in mind and brain as images, sounds, smells, physical sensations and enactments [58]. Our research showed that talking about traumatic events does not necessarily allow mind and brain to integrate the dissociated images and sensations into a coherent whole. Techniques other than figuring out, talking and understanding can be helpful in the integration of these fragments of the traumatic past.

## Conclusions

The incorporation of DTD into the diagnostic system would represent a significant advance in child psychiatry. The availability of DTD as a diagnosis would improve treatment for children suffering from the consequences of interpersonal trauma. A diagnosis based upon exposure to developmentally adverse interpersonal trauma, maltreatment and neglect during childhood, and which includes the coherent set of DTD symptoms, has the potential to alert clinicians to the influential role of childhood trauma in psychopathology.

As long as the various symptoms suffered by traumatized individuals are relegated to seemingly disconnected diagnoses such as PTSD, ADHD, bipolar illness, attachment disturbances, borderline personality disorder and depression, it will be very difficult to study systematically and scientifically the full range of possible interventions to help those with histories of complex trauma gain control over their lives.

It is ironic that people with complex trauma histories probably make up the bulk of patients seen in mental health centers, yet they remain nameless and diagnostically homeless. In an age of the genome project and highly evolved epidemiological methods and neuroimaging techniques, the treatment of chronically traumatized individuals fundamentally continues to play itself out on a village level of oral traditions and anecdotes. The clinical wisdom that results from intimate exposure to chronically traumatized people continues to be largely anecdotal and transmitted in supervision sessions, small conferences and informal discussions among colleagues. Because dissociation is of little interest to mainstream psychology and psychiatry, it is not being systematically studied. Because affect regulation and its vicissitudes are not central to our scientific work, it is relegated to yoga studios, martial arts classes and meditation centers. As long as self-hatred and disgust are not understood as developmental inevitabilities after abuse and neglect, they will be relegated to the realm of religion rather than the realm of science.

## References

1. American Psychiatric Association (1980). *Diagnostic and statistical manual of mental disorders*, 3rd edn. Washington, DC: American Psychiatric Press.
2. van der Kolk, B. A., Roth, S., Pelcovitz, D., Sunday, S. and Spinazzola, J. (2005). Disorders of extreme stress: The empirical foundation of a complex adaptation to trauma. *Journal of Traumatic Stress*, **18**, 389–399.
3. Toth, S. L., Maughan, A., Manly, J. T., Spagnola, M. and Cicchetti, D. (2002). The relative efficacy of two interventions in altering maltreated preschool children's representational models: Implications for

attachment theory. *Development and Psychopathology*, **14**, 877–908.

4. Putnam, F. and Trickett, P. K. (1997). The psychobiological effects of sexual abuse, a longitudinal study. *Annals of the New York Academy of Science*, **821**, 150–159.

5. Beers, S. R. and De Bellis, M. D. (2002). Neuropsychological function in children with maltreatment-related posttraumatic stress disorder. *Journal of Psychiatry*, **159**, 483–486.

6. Cohen, J., Perel, J., De Bellis, M. D. *et al.* (2002). Treating traumatized children: Clinical implications of the psychobiology of posttraumatic stress disorder. *Trauma Violence and Abuse*, **3**, 91–108.

7. Teicher, M. H., Andersen, S. L., Polcari, A. *et al.* (2003). The neurobiological consequences of early stress and childhood maltreatment. *Neuroscience and Biobehavioral Review*, **27**, 33–44.

8. Lipschitz, D. S., Rasmusson, A. M., Anyan, W. *et al.* (2003). Posttraumatic stress disorder and substance use in inner-city adolescent girls. *Journal of Nervous and Mental Disorders*, **191**, 714–721.

9. Wilson, S. N., van der Kolk, B. A., Burbridge, J. A., Fisler, R. E. and Kradin, R. (1999). Phenotype of blood lymphocytes in PTSD suggests chronic immune activation. *Psychosomatics*, **40**, 222–225.

10. Ackerman, P. T., Newton, J. E. O., McPherson, W. B., Jones, J. G. and Dykman, R. A. (1998). Prevalence of post traumatic stress disorder and other psychiatric diagnoses in three groups of abused children (sexual, physical, and both). *Child Abuse and Neglect*, **22**, 759–774.

11. Freedman, A. M. and Kaplan, H. I. (eds.) (1974). *Comprehensive textbook of psychiatry*, 2nd edn. Baltimore, MD: Williams & Wilkins.

12. Henderson, D. J. (1974). Incest. In A. M. Freedman and H. I. Kaplan (eds.), *Comprehensive textbook of psychiatry*, 2nd edn (p. 1536). Baltimore, MD: Williams & Wilkins.

13. Teicher, M. H., Tomoda, A. and Andersen, S. L. (2006). Neurobiological consequences of early stress and childhood maltreatment: Are results from human and animal studies comparable? *Annals of the New York Academy of Sciences*, **1071**, 313–323.

14. Ito, Y., Teicher, M. H., Glod, C. A. and Ackerman, E. (1998). Preliminary evidence for aberrant cortical development in abused children: A quantitative EEG study. *Journal of Neuropsychiatry and Clinical Neurosciences*, **10**, 298–307.

15. Perry, B. D. (2001). The neurodevelopmental impact of violence in childhood. In Schetky, D. and Benedek, E. (eds.), *Textbook of child and adolescent forensic psychiatry* (pp. 221–238). Washington, DC: American Psychiatric Press, Inc.

16. Felitti, V. J., Anda, R. F., Nordenberg, D. *et al.* (1998). The relationship of adult health status to childhood abuse and household dysfunction. *American Journal of Preventive Medicine*, **14**, 245–258.

17. van der Kolk, B. A., Crozier, J. and Hopper, J. (2001). Child abuse in America: Prevalence, costs, consequences and intervention. *Journal of Aggression, Maltreatment and Trauma*, **4**, 9–31.

18. Anda, R. F., Felitti, V. J., Walker, J. *et al.* (2006). The enduring effects of abuse and related adverse experiences in childhood: A convergence of evidence from neurobiology and epidemiology. *European Archives of Psychiatry and Clinical Neurosciences*, **256**, 174–186.

19. Pynoos, R., Fairbank, J., Steinberg, A. *et al.* (2008). The National Child Traumatic Stress Network: Collaborating to improve standard of care. *Professional Psychology, Research and Practice*, **39**, 389–395.

20. Spinazzola, J., Ford, J., Zucker, M. *et al.* (2005). Survey evaluates complex trauma exposure, outcome, and intervention among children and adolescents. *Psychiatric Annals*, **35**, 433–444.

21. Lanius, R. A., Williamson, M. and Densmore, D. (2001). Neural correlates of traumatic memories in posttraumatic stress disorder: A functional MRI investigation. *American Journal of Psychiatry*, **158**, 1920–1922.

22. Hopper, J. H., Frewen, P., van der Kolk, B. A. and Lanius, R. A. (2007). Neural correlates of reexperiencing, avoidance, and dissociation in PTSD: Symptom dimensions and emotion dysregulation in responses to script-driven trauma imagery. *Journal of Traumatic Stress*, **20**, 713–725.

23. Damasio, A. R. (1999). *The feeling of what happens: Body and emotion in the making on consciousness*. New York: Harcourt Brace.

24. Crittenden, P. M. (1998). The developmental consequences of childhod sexual abuse. In P. Trickett and C. Schellenback (eds.), *Violence against children in the family and the community* (pp. 11–38). Washington, DC: American Psychological Association.

25. Fosha, D. (2003). Dyadic regulation and experiential work with emotion and relatedness in trauma and disorganized attachment. In M. Solomon and D. Siegel, (eds.), *Healing trauma: Attachment, mind, body, and brain* (pp. 221–281). NewYork: Norton.

26. American Psychiatric Association (1994) *Diagnostic and statistical manual of mental disorders*, 4th edn. Washington, DC: American Psychiatric Press.

27. van der Kolk, B. A. (2005). Developmental trauma disorder: Toward a rational diagnosis for children with complex trauma histories. *Psychiatric Annals*, **35**, 401–408.

28. Pynoos, R., Fairbank, J., Steinberg, A. *et al.* (2009). DSM-V PTSD diagnostic criteria for children and adolescents: A developmental perspective and

recommendations. *Journal of Traumatic Stress*, **22**, 391–398.

29. Teisl, M. and Cicchetti, D. (2008). Physical abuse, cognitive and emotional processes, and aggressive/disruptive behavior problems. *Social Development*, **17**, 1–23.

30. Kaplow, J., Hall, E., Koenen, K., Dodge, K. and Amaya-Jackson, L. (2008). Dissociation predicts later attention problems in sexually abused children. *Child Abuse and Neglect*, **32**, 261–275.

31. Neumann, D. A., Houskamp, B. M., Pollock, V. E. and Briere, J. (1996). The long-term sequelae of childhood sexual abuse in women: A meta-analytic review. *Child Maltreatment*, **1**, 6–16.

32. Sachs-Ericsson, N., Verona, E., Joiner, T. and Preacher, K. J. (2006). Parental verbal abuse and mediating role of self-criticism is adult internalizing disorders. *Journal of Affective Disorders*, **93**, 71–8.

33. Weaver, T. L. and Clum, G. A. (1996). Interpersonal violence: Expanding the search for long-term sequelae within a sample of battered women. *Journal of Traumatic Stress*, **9**, 783–803.

34. Briere, J. and Rickards, S. (2007). Self-awareness, affect regulation, and relatedness: Differential sequels of childhood versus adult victimization experiences. *Journal of Nervous and Mental Disorders*, **195**, 497–503.

35. Kim, J. and Cicchetti, D. (2004). A longitudinal study of child maltreatment, mother–child relationship quality and maladjustment: The role of self-esteem and social competence. *Journal of Abnormal Child Psychology*, **32**, 341–354.

36. Ehlert, U., Heim, C. and Hellhammer, D. H. (1999). Chronic pelvic pain as somatoform disorder. *Psychotherapy and Psychosomatics*, **68**, 87–94.

37. Bevans, K., Cerbone, A. and Overstreet, S. (2008). Relations between recurrent trauma exposure and recent life stress and salivary cortisol among children. *Developmental Psychopathology*, **20**, 257–272.

38. Mullett-Hume, E., Anshel, D., Guevara, V. and Cloitre, M. (2008). Cumulative trauma and posttraumatic stress disorder among children exposed to the 9/11 World Trade Center attack. *American Journal of Orthopsychiatry*, **78**, 103–108.

39. Kilpatrick, D. G., Ruggeiro, K. J., Acierno, R. *et al.* (2003). Violence and risk of PTSD, major depression, substance abuse/dependence and comorbidity: Results from the National Survey of Adolescents. *Journal of Consulting and Clinical Psychology*, **71**, 692–700.

40. Rucklidge, J. J. (2006). Impact of ADHD on the neurocognitive functioning of adolescents with bipolar disorder. *Biological Psychiatry*, **60**, 921–928.

41. Weinstein, D., Staffelbach, D. and Biaggio, M. (2000). Attention-deficit hyperactivity disorder and posttraumatic stress disorder; Differential diagnosis in childhood and sexual abuse. *Clinical and Psychological Reviews*, **20**, 359–378.

42. Pelcovitz, D., Kaplan, S. J., DeRosa, R. R., Mandel, F. S. and Salzinger, S. (2000). Psychiatric disorders in adolescents exposed to domestic violence and physical abuse. *American Journal of Orthopsychiatry*, **70**, 360–369.

43. Widom, C. S., DuMont, K. and Czaja, S. J. (2007). A prospective investigation of major depressive disorder and comorbidity in abused and neglected children grown up. *Archives in General Psychiatry*, **64**, 49–56.

44. de Graaf, R., Bijl, R. V., Ravelli, A., Smit, F. and Vollebergh, W. A. (2002). Predictors of first incidence of DSM-III-R psychiatric disorders in the general population: Findings from the Netherlands Mental Health Survey and Incidence Study. *Acta Psychiatrica Scandinavica*, **106**, 303–313.

45. Foote, B., Smolin, Y., Neft, D. I. and Lipschitz, D. (2008). Dissociative disorders and suicidality in psychiatric outpatients. *Journal of Nervous and Mental Disorders*, **196**, 29–36.

46. Lanius, R., Williamson, P., Boksman, K., Densmore, M. *et al.* (2002): Brain activation during script-driven imagery induced dissociative responses in PTSD: A functional magnetic resonance imaging investigation. *Biological Psychiatry*, **52**, 305–311.

47. Schmahl, C. G., Vermetten, E., Elzinga, B. M. and Bremner, J. D. (2004). A positron emission tomography study of memories of childhood abuse in borderline personality disorder. *Biological Psychiatry*, **55**, 759–765.

48. Teicher, M. H., Dumont, N. L., Ito, Y. *et al.* (2004). Childhood neglect is associated with reduced corpus callosum area. *Biological Psychiatry*, **56**, 80–85.

49. Driessen, M., Herrmann, J., Stahl, K. *et al.* (2000). Magnetic resonance imaging volumes of the hippocampus and the amygdala in women with borderline personality disorder and early traumatization. *Archives in General Psychiatry*, **57**, 1115–1122.

50. Lanius, R. A., Williamson, P. C., Bluhm, R. L. *et al.* (2005). Functional connectivity of dissociative responses in posttraumatic stress disorder: A functional magnetic resonance imaging investigation. *Biological Psychiatry*, **57**, 873–884.

51. Anderson, C. M., Teicher, M. H., Polcari, A. and Renshaw, P. F . (2002). Abnormal T2 relaxation time in the cerebellar vermis of adults sexually abused in childhood: Potential role of the vermis in stress-enhanced risk for drug abuse. *Psychoneuroendocrinology,* **27**, 231–244.

52. Cicchetti, D. and Rogosch, F. A. (2001). The impact of child maltreatment and psychopathology on neuroendocrine functioning. *Developmental Psychopathology*, **13**, 783–804.

53. Cicchetti, D. and Rogosch, F. A. (2007). Personality, adrenal steroid hormones, and resilience in maltreated children: A multilevel perspective. *Developmental Psychopathology*, **13**, 787–809.

54. Lanius, R. A. and Tuhan, I. (2003). Stage-oriented trauma treatment using dialectical behavior therapy. *Canadian Journal of Psychiatry*, **48**, 126–127.

55. Sachsse, U., Vogel, C. and Leichsenring, F. (2006). Results of psychodynamically oriented trauma-focused inpatient treatment for women with complex posttraumatic stress disorder (PTSD) and borderline personality disorder (BPD). *Bulletin of the Menninger Clinic*, **70**, 125–144.

56. Darwin, C. (1872). *The expression of the emotions in man and animals*. London: Greenwood Press.

57. van der Kolk, B. A. (2006). Clinical implications of neuroscience research in PTSD. *Annals of the New York Academy of Sciences*, **1071**, 277–293.

58. van der Kolk, B. A. and Fisler, R. (1995). Dissociation and the fragmentary nature of traumatic memories: Background and experimental evidence. *Journal of Traumatic Stress*, **8**, 505–525.

# Complex adult sequelae of early life exposure to psychological trauma

Julian D. Ford

## Introduction

Exposure to psychological trauma may have a profound and lasting impact when it occurs at critical ages or developmental transitions [1], particularly if it also involves disruption in fundamental attachment relationships [2], "betrayal" by caregivers [3], or violation of the self (e.g., sexual or emotional abuse [4]). In epidemiological studies, recalled exposure to interpersonal violence or violation in childhood is associated with high (i.e., 50–75%) risk of post-traumatic stress disorder (PTSD) among adults [5]. Beyond increasing the risk of chronic PTSD, developmentally adverse interpersonal trauma in early life may compromise core psychobiological self-regulatory capacities [6–8]. Although early childhood is a period of resilience [9], psychological trauma places infants and toddlers at risk for anxiety, affective, regulatory and attachment disorders [10]. Early life traumatization is associated with adult vulnerability not only to psychiatric and behavioral morbidity [11,12], but also to chronic stress-related [13] gastrointestinal, metabolic, cardiovascular and immunological illness [14,15].

Although studies have reported substantial psychosocial morbidity following victimization in late childhood or adolescence [16–18] – including higher levels of some types of morbidity or risk than if maltreatment occurred earlier in childhood [12,19] – the more consistent finding is that the earlier the onset of maltreatment the greater the morbidity or risk in late childhood or adolescence [20–23] or in adulthood [12]. Maltreatment in adolescence (rather than earlier in childhood) may be more strongly associated with externalizing behavior problems [12], but traumatic victimization in early childhood (including witnessing domestic violence and experiencing assault or community violence) also increases the risk of externalizing problems later in childhood [24].

Children experience many forms of psychological trauma [5,25], but violent or sexual traumas confer the greatest risk of severe adverse outcomes in pediatric community [26], clinical [24], adult community [5], and healthcare [14] samples. Therefore, this chapter will focus on the sequelae in adulthood of traumatic victimization experienced in early childhood (i.e., infancy, toddlerhood, early school years).

## Adverse outcomes in adulthood following childhood traumatic victimization

Adult survivors of early childhood traumatic victimization are at risk for PTSD [5,12,27,28], and for heightened anxiety [11,28–30], depression and suicidality [11,14,27,28,31,32], addiction [11,14,16,27,29,33], personality disorders [28,34], antisocial or violent behavior [29,35,36], serious mental illness [37,38] and sexual disorders [14]. Abuse survivors also are at risk for medical illness [14,39], overutilization of emergency and specialty medical care and underutilization of routine healthcare [39], impaired work functioning [40] and parenting [41], and traumatic re-victimization in adolescence or adulthood [12,42–46].

The multifaceted sequelae of developmentally adverse interpersonal trauma in early life have been described as complex PTSD [4] or "disorders of extreme stress not otherwise specified" (DESNOS [47,48]). This is defined as a set of persistent adverse alterations in seven aspects of self-regulation and psychosocial functioning: (a) affect and impulse regulation (e.g., unmanageable emotions, risky or self-harming behavior), (b) biological self-regulation (i.e., somatization, such as pain or physical symptoms or impairments that cannot be fully medically explained), (c) attention or consciousness (i.e., dissociation), (d) perception of perpetrator(s) (e.g., idealization, preoccupation with revenge); (e) self-perception (e.g., self as damaged or ineffective; profound shame or guilt), (f) relationships (e.g., inability to trust, re-victimization, avoidance of sexuality), and (g) systems of meaning or sustaining beliefs (e.g., hopelessness, loss of faith).

Whereas PTSD is an anxiety disorder, DESNOS involves a broader set of biopsychosocial self-regulatory impairments consistent with findings that DESNOS is most likely to occur following (a) trauma in *early childhood*, when many self-capacities are formed or malformed, or (b) *interpersonal violence or violation*, rather than non-interpersonal traumas. These findings have been replicated with civilian clinical samples [34,46,47,49,50] as well as with military clinical samples [6,51]. The occurrence of DESNOS has been assessed by structured interview [52] in mid-life and older adult community samples [46,47], in inpatient psychiatric [34] and PTSD [6] treatment and in outpatient mental health [46,47,49] and addiction treatment [50,53] samples have included healthy young adults [54], combat veterans [51] and incarcerated adults [53].

Empirical evaluation of DESNOS was carried out in the American Psychiatric Association's PTSD Field Trial in preparation for the 4th revision of the *Diagnostic and Statistical Manual* [55]. Ultimately, however, DESNOS was not designated as a formal psychiatric diagnosis. Instead, several DESNOS features were included in the DSM-IVR as associated features of the PTSD diagnosis. The utility of DESNOS has been questioned on several counts [56], especially regarding its incremental clinical or scientific benefit in the assessment and treatment of the sequelae of childhood victimization beyond that of the existing psychiatric disorders. As DESNOS is most often found to occur comorbidly with PTSD (although there are exceptions on the syndromal [6] and symptom cluster [54] levels), it may represent a severe variant of PTSD. The concept of DESNOS was developed [4] as a less stigmatizing approach to describing the features of borderline personality disorder, but because the two syndromes share several symptom features and are likely to be comorbid clinically [57], the added value of DESNOS is debatable. One empirical finding that supports the utility of DESNOS as a separate syndrome is the evidence from two studies that show that DESNOS (as a syndrome [58] and on the level of symptoms [59]) was predictive of therapy outcome in intensive PTSD treatment and substance abuse treatment, respectively. The identification of DESNOS was related to poorer outcomes

independent of the effects of comorbid PTSD and other psychiatric disorders [58] or psychiatric and substance abuse symptomatology [59]. At present, DESNOS provides a potentially useful template for concisely summarizing the affective, behavioral, cognitive, sociovocational and spiritual sequelae experienced by many adults who have experienced traumatic victimization in early childhood and now suffer from persistent stress-related psychobiological dysregulation that may not be fully accounted for by PTSD and other diagnoses.

## Limitations of the current knowledge base and future directions

Several methodological limitations suggest caution in interpreting the findings from studies on the effects of childhood traumatic victimization on adult functioning and health. With important exceptions [12,60], trauma history usually is assessed retrospectively without external confirmation. Psychological trauma often is delimited to specific subtypes (e.g., maltreatment, violence, assault). Thorough, behaviorally specific trauma history questionnaires or structured interviews show evidence of reliability and validity [32,61,62], with less risk of underreporting than with archival records [68].

The Structured Interview for Disorders of Extreme Stress (SIDES; the self-report interview measure used to assess DESNOS) has shown evidence of reliability, but the criterion and construct validity of the SIDES subscales are uncertain. Ford and colleagues [54] reported that the SIDES subscales were interrelated but largely distinct among college women, providing additional support for SIDES subscale and syndromal validity [6,47]. However, when exploratory and confirmatory factor analyses of the SIDES were conducted with similar but distinct samples (a convenience sample of substance abusing adults with post-traumatic morbidity, and a representative sample of incarcerated adults), only a somatization factor was robust [53]. Four other factors represented a dismantling of some subscales and combination of others: anger dysregulation, risk/self harm, demoralization and altered sexuality. Dissociation items did not constitute a factor, apparently because there were insufficiently articulated items for that construct. Consequently, the DESNOS construct and its operationalization remain in need of theoretical and methodological refinement.

Most studies on the effects of childhood traumatic victimization do not examine the exact timing of psychological trauma exposure in childhood or adolescence. Given evidence that the timing of trauma in infancy [10] and throughout childhood and adolescence [19] may affect critical outcomes, future studies should examine the effects of the occurrence of psychological trauma at clearly specified developmental epochs or transitions (e.g., in preverbal infants versus toddlers engaged in the separation–individuation transition versus preschoolers versus early elementary age children). A cumulatively increasing risk of morbidity has been reported when victimization in childhood is followed by further traumatization in adolescence and adulthood [26,43,54]. However, only one study explicitly utilized a developmental (i.e., ages 0–2, 3–5, 6–8, 9–11 years) or dichotomous early–late childhood (i.e., 0–5 or 6–11 years) definition of maltreatment onset [12]. In that study, onset of maltreatment was established using child welfare records, and absolute age of onset was *not* predictive of adult outcomes three decades later; however, early childhood onset maltreatment (i.e., 0–2, 3–5 years of age) predicted internalizing problems, while later childhood onset maltreatment (i.e., 6–8, 9–11 years of age) predicted externalizing problems. Although this methodology is an important advance, the findings are still limited because psychological traumas other than maltreatment were not assessed, the exact onset and duration of maltreatment were not assessed, only survivors of childhood maltreatment were included and the court records used to verify maltreatment may substantially underreport its incidence [63].

Although adult sequelae of early life psychological trauma have been investigated in diverse populations, with some exceptions [6,14,29,36,39,53], men are often underrepresented or not included [9,30,34,43,48]. The impact of psychological trauma and the etiology and course of post-traumatic disorders differ for males and females in several respects (e.g., susceptibility to internalizing versus externalizing disorders, risk of exposure to sexual versus physical abuse, and family versus community violence [29]), such that gender may moderate the adverse effects of early life psychological trauma [64]. Race and ethnicity have been found to have differing effects as moderators of the relationship between childhood psychological trauma and adolescent or adult outcomes, with white abuse survivors reporting more severe adverse outcomes in some cases (e.g., depression, substance abuse, conduct problems [65]), and African American or Hispanic abuse survivors reporting worse outcomes in other studies

[66]. Minority ethno-racial background is consistently associated with increased risk of childhood psychological trauma, including loss [67], domestic violence [68] and sexual abuse [69]. However, ethno-racial differences in early childhood trauma exposure and its long-term effects tend to be moderated or attenuated when factors such as family structure (e.g., two biological parents present throughout childhood [69]), immigration history [70], socioeconomic status [33] and biological vulnerability [71] are accounted for.

The role of contextual factors, such as socioeconomic status, which are related to risk of early psychological trauma, have rarely been systematically investigated in order to identify risk factors for trauma exposure [25] and to develop theory-driven data-based longitudinal models of psychological trauma as a mediator, moderator or mechanism in adult psychobiological outcomes [26]. A longitudinal epidemiological study in New Zealand tested the relationships among several contextual factors – socioeconomic status, family history of psychopathology, childhood intelligence and health risk behaviors and child maltreatment – with depressive or anxiety disorders, tobacco dependence, alcohol/drug dependence and cardiovascular illness risk [33]. The study concluded that maltreatment was associated with all adverse adult outcomes studied [33,72], but that socioeconomic status accounted for much of the relationship between child maltreatment and adult alcohol/drug dependence and cardiovascular risks. The authors noted that childhood maltreatment and other contextual factors may mediate the link between low socioeconomic status and poor health outcomes. Another study found that prior childhood abuse was associated with increased adolescent levels of, and vulnerability to, depression after subtraumatic life stressors ("chronic difficulties") [73]. Childhood victimization and other childhood adversities are, therefore, not only highly interrelated [74], but also have separate and combined effects on adolescent and adult illness and functioning.

The precise impact on psychobiological functioning and development of different forms, durations and intensities of early life exposure to psychological trauma remains unknown. In children, "poly-victimization" (i.e., multiple different types of victimization) appears to confer greater risk of internalizing and externalizing problems than the extent of any single type of victimization [75], but with young adults, the severity of specific abuse experiences was also more predictive of poor outcomes than was the number of types of abuse [76].

Different types of traumatic childhood victimization have been investigated, with mixed findings, suggesting both unique and shared effects of sexual and physical abuse, neglect, domestic and community violence [77], and emotional maltreatment [78].

Furthermore, none of the psychobiological mediator pathways or moderator mechanisms that have been hypothesized to account for poor outcomes (e.g., impaired self-regulation, disrupted development, altered attachment working models) has yet been rigorously investigated. Potential psychological mediators such as PTSD [44], negative beliefs about the self and the world [44,79] and shame [80] have been identified, as have potential biological moderators such as genetic alleles related to the monoamine oxidase/serotonin neurotransmitter systems [35,36,71,72] and altered brain size, structure or functioning [81,82]. Prospective studies beginning in early childhood with high- and low-risk samples are needed to assess at repeated intervals beginning in early childhood and continuing through adulthood, using psychometrically sound measures of developmental attainment and psychosocial functioning, and repeated multilevel and multisource measures of trauma exposure and psychobiological outcomes [25,33,60,83,84]. Early results suggest that psychobiological moderator variables (e.g., gene alleles [35,60,71,72]) are important, but temporal trajectories of risk and resilience must be mapped in order to move beyond static formulations of the relationships among traumatic victimization, psychobiological mediators and moderators, and adult outcomes. Population-based epidemiological studies including genetic and molecular-level data [85] are needed to inform traumatic victimization research, consistent with the US National Institutes of Health translational research agenda (http://nihroadmap.nih.gov/) to develop "studies of unique populations, determinants of large variations in [outcomes] among populations and over time, and the long incubation period for many [outcomes]" ([86], p. 1109).

A major question that has received little empirical attention is the nature and predictors of resilience among survivors of childhood psychological trauma. Three longitudinal studies, one with high-risk mothers and children in London [87], one in the USA [88] with child welfare-identified maltreated children and one with an epidemiological community sample in New Zealand [89], have specifically examined predictors of positive functioning in early/mid adulthood by traumatized children. Protective factors included intelligence, female gender, secure attachment with primary caregiver, stable residence and prosocial parents, peers and neighborhood in childhood, as well as subtraumatic life stressors and a primary partner in adulthood. Risk factors included parents with substance use problems, poor school functioning, living in neighborhoods with high crime rates and low cohesion, and informal social control. Risk and protective factors differed based on the subsequent adolescent/adult developmental period and often had direct as well as indirect (moderated) effects on subsequent adjustment and functioning [88].

## Conclusions

A robust clinical research literature indicates that traumatic victimization in early childhood places survivors at risk in adolescence and adulthood not only for PTSD but also for psychiatric, medical and psychosocial morbidity and impairment. The hypothesized links between (a) early life victimization and adversely altered psychobiological development (i.e., biological, affective, cognitive and attachment/relational dysregulation [2,42,81,90]), and (b) impaired self-regulation and compromised functioning and health in adolescence and adulthood remain to be definitively confirmed and elucidated. Whether existing psychiatric syndromes and psychosocial models are necessary and sufficient to clinically and scientifically describe and operationalize the complex sequelae of early childhood victimization remains controversial [91]. However, whether or not DESNOS or developmental trauma disorder become formally recognized diagnoses, it is clear that psychiatric and psychosocial interventions must be designed or adapted to address the potentially wide-ranging and refractory adverse impacts that early childhood traumatic victimization may have on adult and adolescent survivors [92].

## Acknowledgements

The writing of this chapter was supported in part by National Institute of Mental Health grant K23-MH01889–01A, Julian D. Ford, Principal Investigator.

## References

1. Cicchetti, D. and Rogosch, F. (2001). The impact of child maltreatment and psychopathology on neuroendocrine function. *Development and Psychopathology*, **13**, 783–804.

2. Schore, A. (2001). The effects of early relational trauma on right brain development, affect regulation, and

infant mental health. *Infant Mental Health Journal,* **22**, 201–269.

3. Freyd, J. (1994). Betrayal trauma. *Ethics and Behavior,* **4**, 307–329.

4. Herman, J. L. (1992). Complex PTSD. *Journal of Traumatic Stress,* **5**, 377–391.

5. Kessler, R. C., Sonnega, A., Bromet, E., Hughes, M. and Nelson, C. B. (1995). Posttraumatic stress disorder in the national comorbidity survey. *Archives of General Psychiatry,* **52**, 1048–1060.

6. Ford, J. D. (1999). Disorders of extreme stress following war-zone military trauma. *Journal of Consulting and Clinical Psychology,* **67**, 3–12.

7. Manly, J., Kim, J., Rogosch, F. and Cicchetti, D. (2001). Dimensions of child maltreatment and children's adjustment. *Development and Psychopathology,* **13**, 759–782.

8. Miltenburg, R. and Singer, E. (1999). Culturally mediated learning and the development of self-regulation by survivors of child abuse. *Human Development,* **42**, 1–17.

9. McGloin, J. and Widom, C. (2001). Resilience among abused and neglected children grown up. *Development and Psychopathology,* **13**, 1021–1038.

10. Scheeringa, M. and Zeanah, C. (2001). A relational perspective on PTSD in early childhood. *Journal of Traumatic Stress,* **14**, 799–816.

11. McCauley, J., Kern, D., Kolodner, K. *et al.* (1997). Clinical characteristics of women with a history of childhood abuse: Unhealed wounds. *Journal of the American Medical Association,* **277**, 1362–1368.

12. Kaplow, J. B. and Widom, C. S. (2007). Age of onset of child maltreatment predicts long-term mental health outcomes. *Journal of Abnormal Psychology,* **116**, 176–187.

13. Cromer, K. and Sachs-Ericsson, N. (2006). The association between childhood abuse, PTSD, and the occurrence of adult health problems. *Journal of Traumatic Stress,* **19**, 967–971.

14. Felitti, V., Anda, R., Nordenberg, D. *et al.* (1998). Relationship of childhood abuse and household dysfunction to many of the leading causes of death in adults. *American Journal of Preventive Medicine,* **14**, 245–258.

15. Heim, C. and Nemeroff, C. (2001). The role of childhood trauma in the neurobiology of mood and anxiety disorders. *Biological Psychiatry,* **49**, 1023–1039.

16. Gordon, H. (2002). Early environmental stress and biological vulnerability to drug abuse. *Psychoneuroendocrinology,* **27**, 115–126.

17. Mazza, J. and Reynolds, W. (1999). Exposure to violence in young inner-city adolescents. *Journal of Abnormal Child Psychology,* **27**, 203–213.

18. Pelcovitz, D., Kaplan, S., Goldenberg, B. *et al.* (1994). Post-traumatic stress disorder in physically abused adolescents. *Journal of the American Academy of Child and Adolescent Psychiatry,* **33**, 305–312.

19. Thornberry, T., Ireland, T. and Smith, C. (2001). The importance of timing. *Development and Psychopathology,* **13**, 957–979.

20. Bolger, K. E., Patterson, C. J. and Kupersmidt, J. B. (1999). Peer relationships and self-esteem among children who have been maltreated. *Child Development,* **69**, 1171–1197.

21. English, D. J., Graham, J. C., Litrownik, A. J., Everson, M. and Bangdiwala, S. I. (2005). Defining maltreatment chronicity. *Child Abuse & Neglect*, **29**, 575–595.

22. Kaplow, J. B., Dodge, K. A., Amaya-Jackson, L. and Saxe, G. N. (2005). Pathways to PTSD. Part II: Sexually abused children. *American Journal of Psychiatry,* **162**, 1305–1310.

23. Keiley, M., Howe, T., Dodge, K., Bates, J. and Petit, G. (2001). The importance of timing: The varying impact of child hood and adolescent maltreatment on multiple problem outcomes. *Development and Psychopathology,* **13**, 891–912.

24. Ford, J. D., Racusin, R., Ellis, C. *et al.* (2000). Child maltreatment, other trauma exposure, and posttraumatic symptomatology among children with oppositional defiant and attention deficit hyperactivity disorders. *Child Maltreatment,* **5**, 205–217.

25. Costello, E. J., Erklani, A. Fairbank, J. and Angold, A. (2002). The prevalence of potentially traumatic events in childhood and adolescence. *Journal of Traumatic Stress,* **15**, 99–112.

26. Copeland, W., Keeler, G., Angold, A. and Costello, E. J. (2007). Traumatic events and posttraumatic stress in childhood. *Archives of General Psychiatry,* **64**, 577–584.

27. Duncan, R. D., Saunders, B. E., Kilpatrick, D. G., Hanson, R. F. and Resnick, H. S. (1996). Childhood physical assault as a risk factor for PTSD, depression, and substance abuse. *American Journal of Orthopsychiatry,* **66**, 437–448.

28. Krupnick, J. L., Green, B. L., Stockton, P. *et al.* (2004). Mental health effects of adolescent trauma exposure in a female college sample. *Psychiatry,* **67**, 264–279.

29. MacMillan, H., Fleming, J., Streiner, D. *et al.* (2001). Childhood abuse and lifetime psychopathology in a community sample. *American Journal of Psychiatry,* **158**, 1878–1883.

30. Stein, M. B., Walker, J., Anderson, G. *et al.* (1996). Childhood physical and sexual abuse in patients with anxiety disorders and in a community sample. *American Journal of Psychiatry,* **153**, 275–277.

31. Dube, S., Anda, R., Felitti, V. *et al.* (2001). Childhood abuse, household dysfunction, and the risk of attempted suicide throughout the life span. *Journal of the American Medical Association,* **286**, 3089–3096.

32. Widom, C. S., Dumont, K. and Czaja, S. (2006). A prospective investigation of major depressive disorder and comorbidity in abused and neglected children grown up. *Archives of General Psychiatry,* **64**, 49–56.

33. Melchior, M., Moffitt, T., Milne, B., Poulton, R. and Caspi, A. (2007). Why do children from socioeconomically disadvantaged families suffer from poor health when they reach adulthood? *American Journal of Epidemiology,* **166**, 966–974.

34. Zlotnick, C., Mattia, J. and Zimmerman, M. (2001). Clinical features of survivors of sexual abuse with major depression. *Child Abuse & Neglect,* **25**, 3, 357–367.

35. Caspi, A., McClay, J., Moffitt, T. *et al.* (2002). Role of genotype in the cycle of violence in maltreated children. *Science,* **297**, 851–854.

36. Reif, A., Rosler, M., Freitag, C. *et al.* (2007). Nature and nurture predispose to violent behavior. *Neuropsychopharmacology,* **32**, 2375–2383.

37. Lysaker, P., Meyer, P., Evans J., Clements, C. and Marks, K. (2001). Childhood sexual trauma and psychosocial functioning in adults with schizophrenia. *Psychiatric Services,* **52**, 1485–1488.

38. Leverich, G., McElroy, S., Suppes, T. *et al.* (2002). Early physical and sexual abuse associated with an adverse course of bipolar illness. *Biological Psychiatry,* **51**, 288–297.

39. Chartier, J., Walker, M. and Naimark, B. (2007). Childhood abuse, adult health, and healthcare utilization. *American Journal of Epidemiology,* **165**, 1031–1038.

40. Lee, S. and Tolman, R. (2006). Childhood sexual abuse and adult work outcomes. *Social Work Research,* **30**, 83–92.

41. DiLillo, D. and Damashek, A. (2003). Parenting characteristics of women reporting a history of childhood sexual abuse. *Child Maltreatment,* **8**, 319–333.

42. Cloitre, M., Scarvalone, P. and Difede, J. (1997). Posttraumatic stress disorder, self- and interpersonal dysfunction among sexually retraumatized women. *Journal of Traumatic Stress,* **10**, 437–452.

43. Follette, V., Polusny, M., Bechtle, A. and Naugle, A. (1996). Cumulative trauma. *Journal of Traumatic Stress,* **9**, 25–36.

44. Messman-Moore, T., Brown, A. and Koelsch, C. (2005). Posttraumatic symptoms and self-dysfunction as consequences and predictors of sexual revictimization. *Journal of Traumatic Stress,* **18**, 253–261.

45. Risser, H., Hetzel-Riggin, M., Thomsen, C. and McCanne, T. (2006). PTSD as a mediator of sexual revictimization: The role of reexperiencing, avoidance, and arousal symptoms. *Journal of Traumatic Stress,* **19**, 687–698.

46. Whitfield, C., Anda, R., Dube, S. and Felitti, V. (2003). Violent childhood experiences and the risk of intimate partner violence in adults. *Journal of Interpersonal Violence,* **18**, 166–186.

47. Roth, S., Newman, E., Pelcovitz, D., van der Kolk, B. and Mandel, F. (1997). Complex PTSD in victims exposed to sexual and physical abuse. *Journal of Traumatic Stress,* **10**, 539–555.

48. van der Kolk, B., Pelcovitz, D., Roth, S. *et al.* (1996). Dissociation, somatization, and affect dysregulation: Complexity of adaptation to trauma. *American Journal of Psychiatry,* **153** (7 Festschrift Supplement), 83–93.

49. Ford, J. D. and Fournier, D. (2007). Psychological trauma, post-traumatic stress disorder, among women in mental healthcare aftercare following psychiatric intensive care. *Journal of Psychiatric Intensive Care,* **3**, 27–34.

50. Ford, J. D. and Smith, S. F. (2008). Complex post-traumatic stress disorder (PTSD) in trauma-exposed adults receiving public sector outpatient substance abuse disorder treatment. *Addiction Research and Theory,* **16**, 193–203.

51. Newman, E., Orsillo, S., Herman, D., Niles, B. and Litz, B. (1995). Clinical presentation of disorders of extreme stress in combat veterans. *Journal of Nervous and Mental Disease,* **183**, 628–632.

52. Pelcovitz, D., van der Kolk, B., Roth, S. *et al.* (1997). Development of a criteria set and a structured interview for disorders of extreme stress (DESNOS). *Journal of Traumatic Stress,* **10**, 3–16.

53. Scoboria, A., Ford, J. D., Lin, H. and Frisman, L. (2008). Exploratory and confirmatory factor analyses of the structured interview for disorders of extreme stress. *Assessment,* **15**, 404–425.

54. Ford, J. D., Stockton, P., Kaltman, S. and Green, B. L. (2006). Disorders of extreme stress (DESNOS) symptoms are associated with interpersonal trauma exposure in a sample of healthy young women. *Journal of Interpersonal Violence,* **21**, 1399–1416.

55. van der Kolk, B., Roth, S., Pelcovitz, D., Sunday, S. and Spinazzola, J. (2005). Disorders of extreme stress. *Journal of Traumatic Stress,* **18**, 389–399.

56. Kilpatrick, D. (2005). A special section on complex trauma and a few thoughts about the need for more rigorous research on treatment efficacy, effectiveness, and safety. *Journal of Traumatic Stress,* **18**, 379–384.

57. McLean, L. and Gallop, R. (2003). Implications of childhood sexual abuse for adult borderline personality disorder and complex posttraumatic stress disorder. *American Journal of Psychiatry,* **160**, 369–371.

58. Ford, J. D. and Kidd, P. (1998). Early childhood trauma and disorders of extreme stress as predictors of treatment outcome with chronic PTSD. *Journal of Traumatic Stress,* **11**, 743–761.

59. Ford, J. D., Hawke, J., Alessi, S., Ledgerwood, D. and Petry, N. (2007). Psychological trauma and PTSD symptoms as predictors of substance dependence treatment outcomes. *Behaviour Research and Therapy, 45*, 2417–2431.

60. Lyons-Ruth, K., Dutra, L., Schuder, M. and Bianchi, I. (2006). From infant attachment disorganization to adult dissociation: Relational adaptations or traumatic experiences? *Psychiatric Clinics of North America, 29*, 63–86.

61. Green, B. L., Goodman, L. A., Krupnick, J. L. *et al.* (2000). Outcomes of single versus multiple trauma exposure in a screening sample. *Journal of Traumatic Stress, 13*, 271–286.

62. Goodman, L. A., Corcoran, C., Turner, K., Yuan, N. and Green, B. L. (1998). Assessing traumatic event exposure: The Stressful Life Events screening questionnaire. *Journal of Traumatic Stress, 11*, 521–542.

63. Swahn, M., Whitaker, D., Pippin, C. *et al.* (2006). Court records of abuse or neglect among high risk youths. *American Journal of Public Health, 96*, 1849–1853.

64. Tolin, D. and Foa, E. B. (2006). Sex differences in trauma and posttraumatic stress disorder: A quantitative review of 25 years of research. *Psychological Bulletin, 132*, 959–992.

65. Schilling, E., Aseltine, R. and Gore, S. (2007). Adverse childhood experiences and mental health in young adults: A longitudinal survey. *BMC Public Health,* 7, 30.

66. Lau, A., Huang, M., Garland, A. *et al.* (2006). Racial variation in self-labeled child abuse and associated internalizing symptoms among adolescents who are high risk. *Child Maltreatment, 11*, 168–181.

67. Rheingold, A., Smith, D., Ruggiero, K. *et al.* (2004). Loss, trauma exposure, and mental health in a representative sample of 12–17-year-old youth: Data from the National Survey of Adolescents. *Journal of Loss and Trauma, 9*, 1–19.

68. Graham-Bermann, S., DeVoe, E., Mattis, J., Lynch, S. and Thomas, S. (2006). Ecological predictors of traumatic stress symptoms in Caucasian and ethnic minority children exposed to intimate partner violence. *Violence Against Women, 12*, 662–692.

69. Amodeo, A., Griffin, Fassler, Clay, A. and Ellis, (2006). Childhood sexual abuse among black women and white women from two-parent families. *Child Maltreatment, 11*, 237–246.

70. Jaycox, L., Stein, B., Kataoka, S. *et al.* (2002). Violence exposure, posttraumatic stress disorder, and depressive symptoms among recent immigrant schoolchildren. *Journal of the American Academy of Child and Adolescent Psychiatry, 41*, 1104–1110.

71. Widom, C. S. and Brzustowicz, L. (2006). MAOA and the "cycle of violence:" Childhood abuse and neglect, MAOA genotype, and risk for violent and antisocial behavior. *Biological Psychiatry*, 60, 684–689.

72. Caspi, A., Sugden, K., Moffitt, T. *et al.* (2003). Influence of life stress on depression: Moderation by polymorphism in the 5-HTT gene. *Science,* 301, 386–389.

73. Harkness, K., Bruce, A. and Lumley, M. (2007). The role of childhood abuse and neglect in the sensitization to stressful life events in adolescent depression. *Journal of Abnormal Psychology,* 115, 730–741.

74. Dong, M., Anda, R., Felitti, V. *et al.* (2004). The interrelatedness of multiple forms of childhood abuse, neglect, and household dysfunction. *Child Abuse & Neglect, 28*, 771–784.

75. Finkelhor, D., Ormrod, R. and Turner, H. (2007). Poly-victimization: A neglected component in child victimization. *Child Abuse & Neglect, 31*, 7–26.

76. Clemmons, R., Walsh, K., DiLillo, D. and Messman-Moore, T. (2007). Unique and combined contributions of multiple child abuse types and abuse severity to adult trauma symptomatology. *Child Maltreatment, 12*, 172–181.

77. Ford, J. D., Hartman, J. K., Hawke, J. and Chapman, J. (2008). Traumatic victimization, posttraumatic stress disorder, suicidal ideation, and substance abuse risk among juvenile justice-involved youths. *Journal of Child and Adolescent Trauma, 1*, 75–92.

78. Teicher, M., Samson, J., Polcari, A. and McGreenery, C. (2006). Sticks, stones, and hurtful words: Relative effects of various forms of childhood maltreatment. *American Journal of Psychiatry,* 163, 993–1000.

79. Browne, C. and Winkelman, C. (2007). The effect of childhood trauma on later psychological adjustment. *Journal of Interpersonal Violence, 22*, 684–697.

80. Feiring, C. and Traska, L. (2005). The persistence of shame following sexual abuse. *Child Maltreatment, 10*, 337–349.

81. De Bellis, M. (2001). Developmental traumatology. *Psychoneuroendocrinology, 27*, 155–170.

82. Kaufman, J., Plotsky, P., Nemeroff, C. and Charney, D. (2000). Effects of early adverse experiences on brain structure and function: Clinical implications. *Biological Psychiatry,* 48, 778–790.

83. Briggs-Gowan, M. J., Carter, A. S., Bosson-Heenan, J., Guyer, A. E. and Horwitz, S. M. (2006). Are infant–toddler social–emotional and behavioral problems transient? *Journal of the American Academy of Child and Adolescent Psychiatry, 45*, 849–858.

84. Widom, C. S., Dutton, M. A., Czaja, S. and Dumont, K. (2005). Development and validation of a new instrument to assess lifetime trauma and victimization history. *Journal of Traumatic Stress, 18*, 519–531.

85. Thomas, D. C. (2005). The need for a systematic approach to complex pathways in molecular

epidemiology. *Cancer Epidemiology, Biomarkers & Prevention, 14,* 537–539.

86. Kuller, L. (2007). Is phenomenology the best approach to health research? *American Journal of Epidemiology,* **166**, 1109–1115.

87. Bifulco, A. (2008). Risk and resilience in young Londoners. In D. Brom , R. Pat-Horenczyk and J. Ford (eds.), Treating traumatized children: Risk, resilience and recovery (pp. 117–128). London: Routledge.

88. Dumont, K., Widom, C. S. and Czaja, S. (2007). Predictors of resilience in abused and neglected children grown-up. *Child Abuse & Neglect, 31,* 255–274.

89. Jaffee, S., Caspi, A., Moffitt, T., Polo-Tomas, M. and Taylor, A. (2005). Individual, family, and neighborhood factors distinguish resilient from non-resilient maltreated children: A cumultive stressors model. *Child Abuse & Neglect, 31,* 231–253.

90. Ford, J. D. (2005). Treatment implications of altered neurobiology, affect regulation and information processing following child maltreatment. *Psychiatric Annals,* **35**, 410–419.

91. van der Kolk, B. (2005). Developmental trauma disorder. *Psychiatric Annals,* **35**, 439–448.

92. Ford, J. D., Courtois, C., van der Hart, O., Nijenhuis, E. and Steele, K. (2005). Treatment of complex post-traumatic self-dysregulation. *Journal of Traumatic Stress,* **18**, 437–447.

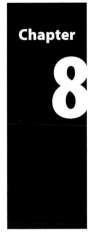

# Chapter 8

# The relationship of adverse childhood experiences to adult medical disease, psychiatric disorders and sexual behavior: implications for healthcare

Vincent J. Felitti and Robert F. Anda

*In my beginning is my end.*

T. S. Eliot, *Four Quartets* [1]

## Introduction

Biomedical researchers increasingly recognize that childhood events, specifically abuse and emotional trauma, have profound and enduring effects on the neuroregulatory systems mediating medical illness as well as on behavior from childhood into adult life. Our understanding of the connection between emotional trauma in childhood and the pathways to pathology in adulthood is still being formed as neuroscientists begin to describe the changes that take place on the molecular level as a result of events that occurred decades earlier.

The turning point in modern understanding of the role of trauma in medical and psychiatric pathology is commonly credited to Freud, who studied patients of the French neurologist Charcot and attributed their unusual behavior to histories of trauma rather than to underlying biomedical pathology [2]. The writings of Freud and Breuer as well as Janet represented a departure from the traditional view that mental illness and unexplained medical disease were the result of divine retribution or demonic possession, instead revealing that they were strongly associated with a history of childhood abuse [2].

The focus of this chapter will be an examination of the relationship between traumatic stress in childhood and the leading causes of morbidity, mortality and disability in the USA: cardiovascular disease, chronic lung disease, chronic liver disease, depression and other forms of mental illness, obesity, smoking and alcohol and drug abuse. To do this, we will draw on our

experience with the Adverse Childhood Experiences (ACE) Study, a major American epidemiological study providing retrospective and prospective analysis in over 17 000 individuals of the effect of traumatic experiences during the first 18 years of life on adolescent and adult medical and psychiatric disease, sexual behavior, healthcare costs and life expectancy [3].

The ACE Study is an outgrowth of repeated counter-intuitive observations made while operating a major weight loss program that used the technique of supplemented fasting, which allows non-surgical weight reduction of approximately 300 lb (135 kg) per year. Unexpectedly, the weight program had a high dropout rate, limited almost exclusively to patients successfully losing weight. Exploring the reasons underlying the high prevalence of patients inexplicably fleeing their own success in the program ultimately led us to recognize that weight loss is often sexually or physically threatening and that certain of the more intractable public health problems such as obesity were *also* unconscious, or occasionally conscious, compensatory behaviors that were put in place as solutions to problems dating back to the earliest years, but hidden by time, by shame, by secrecy and by social taboos against exploring certain areas of life experience. It became evident that traumatic life experiences during childhood and adolescence were far more common than generally recognized, were complexly inter-related and were associated decades later in a strong and proportionate manner with outcomes important to medical practice, public health, and the social fabric of a nation. In the context of everyday medical practice, we came to recognize that the earliest years of infancy and childhood are not lost but, like a child's footprints in wet cement, are often lifelong.

*The Impact of Early Life Trauma on Health and Disease: The Hidden Epidemic*, ed. Ruth A. Lanius, Eric Vermetten and Clare Pain. Published by Cambridge University Press. Copyright © Cambridge University Press 2010.

The findings from the ACE Study provide a remarkable insight into how we become what we are as individuals and as a nation. They are important medically, socially and economically. Indeed, they have given us reason to reconsider the very structure of medical, public health and social services practices in America and other countries.

## The Adverse Childhood Experiences (ACE) Study: outline and setting

The ACE Study was carried out in Kaiser Permanente's Department of Preventive Medicine in San Diego, in collaboration with the US Centers for Disease Control and Prevention (CDC). This particular department provided an ideal setting for such collaboration because detailed biomedical, psychological and social (biopsychosocial) evaluations had been carried out over many years for the adult Kaiser Health Plan members (50 000 a year). The CDC contributed the essential skill sets for study design and the massive data management required for meaningful interpretation of clinical observations.

Kaiser Health Plan patients are middle-class Americans; all have high-quality health insurance. In any 4 year period, 81% of adult members in San Diego choose to come in for comprehensive medical evaluation. A group of 26 000 consecutive adults coming through the department was asked if they would help us to understand how childhood events might affect adult health status. The majority agreed and, after certain exclusions for incomplete data and duplicate participation, the ACE Study cohort had over 17 000 individuals. The study was carried out in two waves, to allow midpoint correction.

The participants were 80% white including Hispanic, 10% black and 10% Asian; 74% had attended college; their average age was 57 years. Almost exactly half were men, half women. This is a solidly middle-class group from the seventh largest city in the USA; it is not a group that can be dismissed as atypical, aberrant or "not in my practice." Disturbingly, it is us – a point not to be overlooked when considering the problems of translating the ACE Study's findings into action.

Eight categories of adverse childhood experiences (ACEs) were studied in the first wave; two categories of neglect were added in the second wave. These categories were selected empirically because of their discovered high prevalence in the weight program. Their prevalence in a general, middle-class population was also unexpectedly high. An ACE Score was created for each individual, a count of the number of *categories* of adverse experience that had occurred during the first 18 years of life. The ACE Score does not tally incidents within a category. The scoring system is simple: the occurrence during childhood or adolescence of any one category of adverse experience is scored as 1 point. There is no further scoring for multiple incidents within a category; thus, an alcoholic and a drug user within a household score the same as one alcoholic; multiple sexual molestations by multiple individuals are totaled as 1 point. If anything, this would tend to understate our findings. The ACE Score, therefore, can range from 0 to 8 or 10, depending on the data being from wave 1 or wave 2. Specifics of the questions underlying each category are detailed in the original article [3].

Only one-third of this middle-class population had an ACE Score of 0. If any one category was experienced, there was 87% likelihood that at least one additional category was present. One in six individuals had an ACE Score of 4 or more, and one in nine had an ACE Score of 5 or more. Consequently, every physician will see several patients with high ACE Scores each day. Typically, they are the most difficult patients of the day. Women were 50% more likely than men to have experienced five or more categories of adverse childhood experiences. We believe that here is a key to what in mainstream epidemiology appears as women's natural proneness to ill-defined health problems such as fibromyalgia, chronic fatigue syndrome, obesity, irritable bowel syndrome and chronic non-malignant pain syndromes. In the light of these findings, we now see these as medical constructs, artifacts resulting from medical blindness to social realities and ignorance of the impact of gender.

Somewhat surprisingly, the ACE categories turned out to be approximately equal to each other in impact; an ACE Score of 4 consists of *any* four of the categories. The categories do not occur randomly; the number of individuals with high ACE Scores is distinctly higher than if the categories exist independently of each other [4]. The 10 reference categories experienced during childhood or adolescence are as below, with their prevalence in parentheses:

- abuse
  - emotional: recurrent threats, humiliation (11%)
  - physical: beating not spanking (28%)
  - contact sexual abuse (28% women, 16% men; 22% overall)

- household dysfunction
  - mother treated violently (13%)
  - household member was alcoholic or drug user (27%)
  - household member was imprisoned (6%)
  - household member was chronically depressed, suicidal, mentally ill or in psychiatric hospital (17%)
  - not raised by both biological parents (23%)
- neglect
  - physical (10%)
  - emotional (15%).

The essence of the ACE Study has been to match retrospectively, approximately a half century after the fact, an individual's current state of health and well-being against adverse events in childhood (the ACE Score), and then to follow the cohort forward to match ACE Score prospectively against doctor office visits, emergency room visits, hospitalization, pharmacy costs and death. The study has recently passed the 14 year mark in the prospective arm.

# Findings

This section illustrates with a sampling from the findings in the ACE Study, the long-lasting, strongly proportionate and often profound relationship between adverse childhood experiences and important categories of emotional state, health risks, disease burden, sexual behavior, disability, and healthcare costs – decades later.

## Psychiatric disorders

The relationship between ACE Score and self-acknowledged chronic depression is illustrated in Fig. 8.1a [5]. Should one doubt the reliability of self-acknowledged chronic depression, there is a similar but stronger relationship between ACE Score and later suicide attempts, as shown in the exponential progression of Fig. 8.1b [6]. The *p* value of all graphic depictions herein is 0.001 or lower.

One continues to see a proportionate relationship between ACE Score and depression by analysis of prescription rates for antidepressant medications after a 10-year prospective follow-up, now approximately 50 to 60 years after the ACEs occurred (Fig. 8.1c) [7]. It would appear that depression, often unrecognized in medical practice, is in fact common and has deep roots, commonly going back to the developmental years of life.

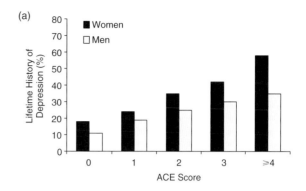

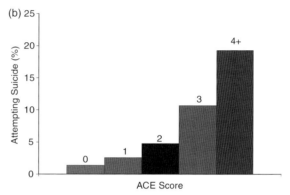

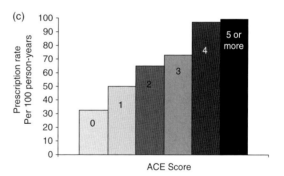

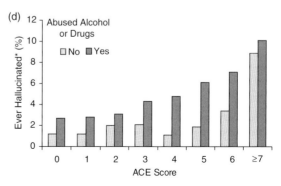

**Fig. 8.1.** Psychiatric disorders. The relationship between ACE Score and chronic depression (a), suicide attempts (b), rates of antidepressant prescriptions approximately 50 years later (c), hallucinations (*adjusted for age, sex, race and education) (d), and impaired memory of childhood (e).

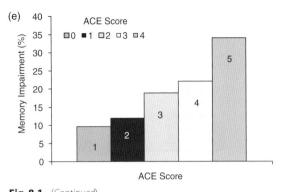

**Fig. 8.1.** (Continued)

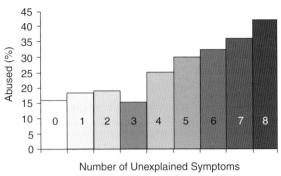

**Fig. 8.2.** The relationship between the likelihood of childhood sexual abuse and the number of unexplained symptoms in adulthood.

An analysis of population attributable risk (that portion of a problem in the overall population whose prevalence can be attributed to specific risk factors) shows that 54% of current depression and 58% of suicide attempts in women can be attributed to adverse childhood experiences. Whatever later factors might trigger suicide, childhood experiences cannot be left out of the equation. Seeman *et al.* [8] have described this general concept of background burden as allostatic load.

A similar relationship exists between ACE Score and later hallucinations, shown in Fig. 8.1d. As it might be suspected that, at ACE Score 7 or higher, people will likely be using street drugs or alcohol to modulate their feelings, and that *these* might be the cause of hallucinations, the results are corrected for alcohol and drug use and the same relationship exists [9].

Clinicians treating somatization or disorders with no clear medical etiology, as well as those dreading such patients, will find Fig. 8.2 of special interest. Indeed, this figure exemplifies the observation in the weight program that what one sees, the presenting problem, is often only the marker for the real problem, which lies buried in time, concealed by patient shame, secrecy and sometimes amnesia – and frequent clinician discomfort. Amnesia, usually considered a theatrical device of Hollywood movies of the 1940s, is in fact alive and well, although unrecognized, in everyday medical practice. In the weight program, 12% of the participants were partially or sometimes totally amnestic for a period of their lives, typically the few years before weight gain began. In the ACE Study, there was a distinct relationship of ACE Score and impaired memory of childhood, and we understand this phenomenon to be reflective of dissociative responses to emotional trauma (Fig. 8.1e) [10].

All told, it is clear that adverse childhood experiences have a profound, proportionate and long-lasting effect on emotional state, whether measured by depression or suicide attempts, by protective unconscious devices such as somatization and dissociation, or by self-help attempts that are misguidedly addressed solely as long-term health risks – perhaps because we physicians are less than comfortable acknowledging the manifest short-term benefits these "health risks" offer to the patient dealing with hidden trauma.

## Health risks

The most common contemporary health risks are smoking, alcoholism, illicit drug use, obesity and high-level promiscuity. Although widely understood to be harmful to health, each is notably difficult to give up. Conventional logic is not particularly useful in understanding this apparent paradox. As opposing forces are not known to exist commonly in biological systems, little consideration is given to the possibility that many long-term health risks might *also* be personally beneficial in the short term. For instance, American Indians understood the psychoactive benefits of nicotine for centuries with their peace pipe, before its risks were recognized. We repeatedly hear from patients of the benefits of these "health risks." Indeed, relevant insights are even built into our language: "Have a smoke, relax." "Sit down and have something to eat. You'll feel better." Or, need "a fix," referring to intravenous drug use. Conversely, the common reference to "drug abuse" serves to conceal the short-term functionality of such behavior. It is perhaps noteworthy that the demonized street drug crystal meth is the very compound that was introduced in pure form and reliable dosage in 1940 as one of the first prescription antidepressants in the USA: methamphetamine.

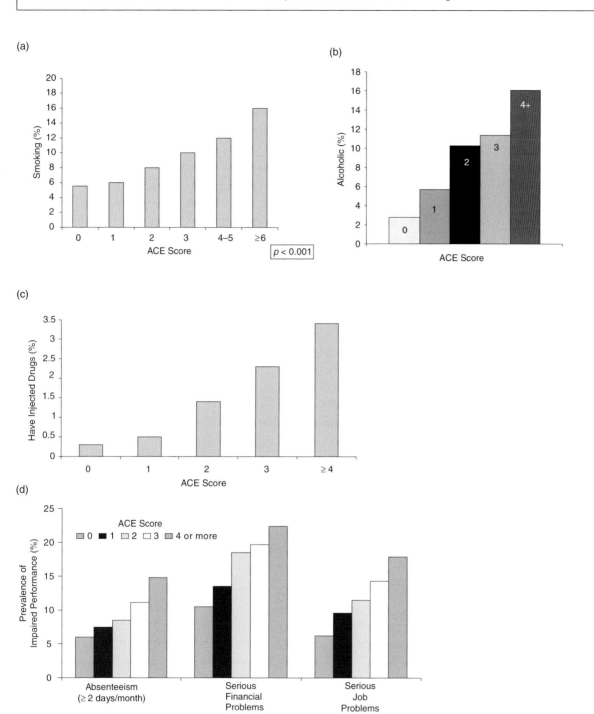

**Fig. 8.3.** Health risks. The relationship between ACE Score and adult smoking (a), adult alcoholism (b), intravenous drug use (c), and indicators of impaired worker performance (d).

In the ACE Study, there were strong, proportionate relationships between ACE Score and the use of various psychoactive materials or behaviors. The saying, "It's hard to get enough of something that *almost* works" provides insight. Three common categories of

what are usually termed addictions (the unconscious compulsive use of psychoactive agents) are illustrated in this section. Self-acknowledged current smoking (Fig. 8.3a) [11,12], self-defined alcoholism (Fig. 8.3b) [3,5,13] and self-acknowledged injection drug use

(Fig. 8.3c) [14] are strongly related in a proportionate manner to the several specific categories of adverse experiences during childhood. Additionally, poor self-rated job performance correlated with ACE Score (Fig 8.3d) [15].

The relationship of intravenous drug use with ACE Score is particularly striking, given that male children with ACE Score 6 or more have a 46-fold increased likelihood of later becoming an injection drug user compared with a male child with an ACE Score 0; this moves the probability from an arithmetic to an exponential progression. Relationships of this magnitude are rare in epidemiology. This, coupled with related information, suggests that the basic cause of addiction is predominantly experience dependent during childhood and not substance dependent. This challenge to the usual concept of the cause of addictions

has significant implications for medical practice and for treatment programs[16].

## Sexual behavior

Using teenage pregnancy and promiscuity as measures of sexual behavior, the ACE Score has a proportionate relationship to these outcomes (Fig. 8.4). So too does miscarriage of pregnancy, indicating the complexity of the relationship of early life psychosocial experience to what are usually considered purely biomedical outcomes [17].

## Medical disease

Biomedical disease in adults had a significant relationship to adverse life experiences in childhood in the ACE Study. The implication of this observation that life experience can transmute into organic disease over time is a profound change from an earlier era when infectious diseases such as rheumatic fever or polio, or nutritional deficiency such as pellagra, would come to mind as the main medical links between childhood events and

(a)

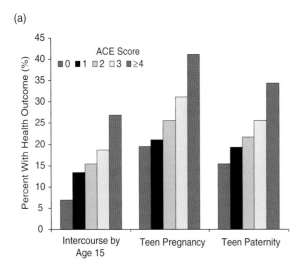

(b)

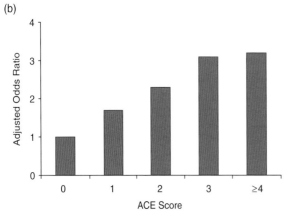

**Fig. 8.4.** Sexual behavior. The relationship between ACE Score and teenage sexual behavior (a) and promiscuity (likelihood of > 50 sexual partners) (b).

(a)

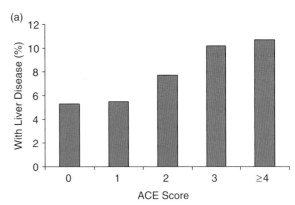

(b)

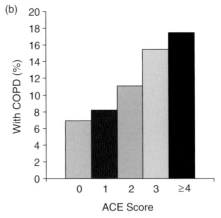

**Fig. 8.5.** Medical disease. The relationship between ACE Score and prevalence of liver disease (hepatitis/jaundice) (a) and chronic obstructive pulmonary disease (COPD) (b).

adult disease. In spite of this change in our understanding of the etiology of biomedical outcomes, we find no evidence that there has been a change in the frequency of overall adverse childhood experiences in various age cohorts spanning the twentieth century [18].

Four examples of the links between childhood experience and adult biomedical disease are the relationship of ACE Score to liver disease (Fig. 8.5a) [19], chronic obstructive pulmonary disease (Fig. 8.5b) [20], coronary artery disease [21] and autoimmune disease [22]. Our data for coronary artery disease show the effect of ACE Score after correcting for, or in the absence of, the conventional risk factors for coronary disease, such as hyperlipidemia, smoking, the likelihood of heart disease was increased in all categories of ACE Score:

- emotional abuse 1.7×
- physical abuse 1.5×
- sexual abuse 1.4×
- domestic violence 1.4×
- substance abuse 1.3×
- mental illness 1.4×
- household criminal 1.7×
- emotional neglect 1.3×
- physical neglect 1.4×.

Certain of these relationships of childhood experience to later biomedical disease might initially be thought to be straightforward, for instance assuming that chronic obstructive pulmonary disease and coronary artery disease are merely the obvious outcomes of cigarette smoking. In this case, one might reasonably assume that the total relationship of adverse childhood experience to later biomedical disease lies in the observation that stressful early life experience leads to a coping behavior like smoking, which becomes the mechanism of biomedical damage. While this hypothesis is true, it is incomplete; the actual situation is more complex. For instance, in our analysis published in *Circulation* [21], we found that there was a strong relationship of ACE Score with coronary disease, *after* correcting for all the conventional risk factors such as smoking, cholesterol and so on. This illustrates that adverse experiences in childhood are related to adult disease by two basic etiologic mechanisms:

- conventional risk factors that actually are attempts at self-help through the use of agents like nicotine, with its documented, multiple psychoactive benefits, in addition to its now well-recognized cardiovascular risks
- the effects of chronic stress as mediated through the mechanisms of chronic hypercortisolemia,

pro-inflammatory cytokines and other stress responses on the developing brain and body systems, dysregulation of the stress response and pathophysiological mechanisms yet to be discovered.

A public health paradox is implicit in these observations. One sees that certain common public health problems, while being often also unconscious attempted solutions to major life problems, harken back to the developmental years. The idea of the problem being a solution, while understandably disturbing to many, is certainly in keeping with the fact that opposing forces routinely coexist in biological systems. Understanding that it is hard to give up something that almost works, particularly at the behest of well-intentioned people who have little understanding of what has gone on, provides us a new way of understanding treatment failure in addiction programs, where typically the attempted solution rather than the core problem is being addressed.

## Healthcare costs

At the 14 year point in the prospective arm of the ACE Study, we have only begun to analyze pharmacy data. Given the average age of the cohort, we are now looking at prescription drug use 50 to 60 years after the fact. Prescription costs are an increasingly significant portion of rapidly rising national healthcare expenditures in the USA. The relationship of ACE Score to antidepressant prescription rates has already been shown in Fig. 8.1c. Figure 8.6 shows the relationship of adverse childhood experiences to the decades-later use of antipsychotic and anxiolytic medications [5]. Analyses of the relationships of ACE Score to doctor office visits, emergency department visits, hospitalization and death are in progress. The economic effect of the results shown in Fig. 8.2 will be intuitively obvious to practitioners who have observed that patients with multiple visits to the doctor commonly do not have a unifying diagnosis underlying all the medical attention. Rather, they have a multiplicity of symptoms: illness, but not disease. Kirkengen has more fully discussed the nature, origins and often-unwitting medical creation of this complex phenomenon in her book *Inscribed Bodies* [23]. The 2000 Nobelist in Economics, James Heckman, has grasped the enormity of the economic and social consequences of the long-term effects of adverse childhood experiences and has written perceptively on the subject [24].

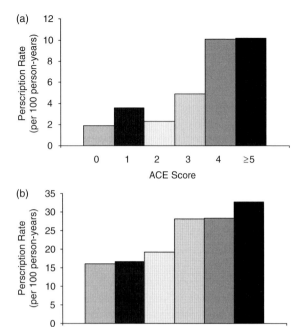

**Fig. 8.6.** Healthcare costs. Rates of issuing prescriptions for antipsychotic drugs (a) and anxiolytic drugs (b).

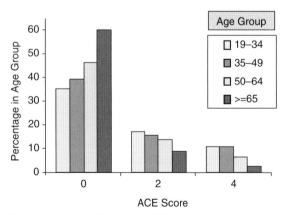

**Fig. 8.7.** Older individuals in the ACE Study are more likely to have low ACE Scores (null hypothesis).

## Life expectancy

Given that the ACE Score has been shown to be strongly related first to health risks and then to disease, it is reasonable to expect that the relationship will continue to the major outcome of disease, premature death. Figure 8.7 shows that the older individuals in the ACE Study are more likely to have a low ACE Scores (ACE Score 0) and are substantially less likely to have higher ACE Scores (ACE Score 2 or 4). One explanation for

this finding is that persons with higher ACE Scores do indeed die younger; thus older people would tend to have lower ACE Scores because others in their birth cohort were less likely to survive to be included in the study.

Reasonably, this interpretation of selective attrition could be challenged by hypothesizing that our patients were progressively so humiliated by exposure of their increasing ACE Scores that they are subsequently avoiding necessary medical care. Such an hypothesis is not supported by the findings. Some years ago we had on site for 6 months a psychoanalytically trained psychiatrist who saw selected patients with high ACE Scores immediately after their comprehensive medical evaluation, rather than after referral to psychiatry. An anonymous questionnaire, returned by 81% of the patients he saw, showed that his hour-long interview was overwhelmingly interpreted by patients as highly desirable and appreciated. Talking about the worst secret of one's life with an experienced person, being understood and coming away feeling still accepted as a human being seems to be remarkably important and beneficial, perhaps not unlike the role of confession in the Roman Catholic Church, a technique whose persistence over nearly two millennia suggests it has functional benefit for those involved in its use.

At the 14 year mark, an analysis of adult death rates has been initiated as they may be related to adverse childhood experiences. Carrying the above approach further, analysis of findings from the prospective phase of the study has confirmed the expectation outlined above with the discovery that individuals with ACE Score 6 and higher had a lifespan almost two decades shorter than seen in those with an ACE Score 0 but otherwise similar characteristics [25]. This finding supports the hypothesis that decreases in ACE Scores with age may be explained by the effects of ACEs on premature mortality.

## Implications for healthcare

We have made a limited but instructive attempt to integrate the ACE Study findings into clinical practice. At Kaiser Permanente's high-volume Department of Preventive Medicine in San Diego, we have used what we learned to expand radically the nature of our Review of Systems (ROS) and Past History questionnaire. We have now asked routinely of over 440 000 adult individuals undergoing comprehensive medical evaluation a number of questions of newly discovered relevance; the following are a sample:

- Have you ever been a combat soldier?
- Have you ever lived in a war zone?
- Have you been physically abused as a child?
- Have you been sexually molested as a child or adolescent?
- Have you ever been raped?
- Who in your family has been murdered?
- Who in your family has had a nervous breakdown?
- Who in your family has been a suicide?
- Who in your family has been alcoholic or a drug user?

Such questions have been accepted by patients in the context of a well-devised medical questionnaire that is filled out at home. Examiners have learned that the most productive response to a "Yes" answer is, "I see that you have …. Tell me how that has affected you later in your life." While not a simple transition for staff, and one requiring an organized training effort, the transition has been effective and with measured benefits. An independent organization carried out a neural network analysis – an artificial intelligence approach to mathematical modeling and data mining – of the data from over 100 000 patient evaluations (2 years' work) using this new approach: a truly biopsychosocial approach to comprehensive medical evaluation. Surprisingly, a 35% reduction in doctor office visits was found in the year subsequent to evaluation, compared with the year before. Additionally, analysis showed an 11% reduction in emergency department visits and a 3% reduction in hospitalizations. This change was dramatically and unexpectedly different from a much smaller, 700-patient evaluation carried out 20 years earlier when we worked in the more usual biomedical mode. That earlier approach provided a net 11% reduction in doctor office visits compared to the antecedent year, in spite of a 14% referral rate. No evaluation was made then of emergency department visits or hospitalization. Finally, we found that the unexpectedly notable reductions in doctor office visits and emergency department visits totally disappeared in the second year after comprehensive evaluation, when there was a reversion to prior baseline. While the underlying biopsychosocial information was present in charts with laser-printed clarity, it was almost never integrated into subsequent medical visits. Interpreting the basis of this major reduction in doctor office visits was not within the purview of the ACE Study design, but the impression of the clinicians initially evaluating these patients is that the reduction represents

the benefit of having, through a comprehensive medical history, the worst secrets of one's life understood by another, and still being accepted as a human being. The Swiss psychologist Alice Miller describes this as the role of "the enlightened witness" [26].

If these first year results are replicable, and we believe they should be, the implications for primary medical care are those of a paradigm shift. While offering tremendous opportunity, paradigm shifts are resisted. The philosopher Eric Hoffer has discussed this problem in his book *The Ordeal of Change* [27]. Jeffrey Masson, in *Assault on Truth* [28], describes the enormous social pressures on Freud to recant his interpretation of his findings of traumatic sexual experiences in childhood as being valid. Louise De Salvo points out in *Virginia Woolf* [29] how literary commentators almost uniformly avoid discussing the themes of incest in Woolf's work in favor of erudite discussions of her style and literary techniques.

If the treatment implications of what we have found in the ACE Study are far reaching, the problems of integrating this information into clinical practice are absolutely daunting. Simply put, it is easier for all of us to deal with the presenting symptom of the moment than to attempt to understand it in the full context of the patient, particularly when that full context involves thematic material of child abuse and household dysfunction that is usually protected by social taboos against exploring these areas of human experience. Although the proposed approach demonstrably would save time and money in the long run, most of us operate in the short term and respond to valid forces that are both external and internal.

The very nature of the material in the ACE Study is such as to make most of us uncomfortable. Why would a physician or leader of any major health agency want to leave the familiarity of traditional biomedical disease and enter this area of threatening uncertainty for which none of us have been trained? As physicians, we typically focus our attention on tertiary consequences, far downstream, while the primary causes are well protected by time, social convention and taboo. We have often limited ourselves to the smallest part of the problem, that part in which we are erudite and comfortable as mere prescribers of medication or users of impressive technologies. Consequently, although the ACE Study and its 50-some publications have generated significant intellectual interest in North America and Europe during the past dozen years, its findings are only beginning to be translated into significant clinical or social action. The reasons for this are important to consider if this information is to be converted into meaningful social and medical opportunity.

## Conclusions

The influence of childhood experience, including often-unrecognized traumatic events, is as powerful as Freud and his colleagues originally described. These influences are long lasting, and neuroscientists are now describing the intermediary mechanisms that develop as a result of these stressors. Unfortunately, and in spite of these findings, the biopsychosocial model and the biomedical model of psychiatry remain at odds rather than taking advantage of the new discoveries to reinforce each other.

Many of our most intractable public health problems are the result of compensatory behaviors such as smoking, overeating, and alcohol and drug use, which provide immediate partial relief from the emotional problems caused by traumatic childhood experiences. The chronic life stress of these developmental experiences is generally unrecognized and hence unappreciated as a second etiologic mechanism. These experiences are lost in time and concealed by shame, secrecy and social taboo against the exploration of certain topics of human experience.

The findings of the ACE Study provide a credible basis for a new paradigm of medical, public health and social service practice that would start with comprehensive biopsychosocial evaluation of all patients at the outset of ongoing medical care. We have demonstrated in our practice that this approach is acceptable to patients, affordable and beneficial in multiple ways. The potential gain is huge. So too is the likelihood of clinician and institutional resistance to this change. Actualizing the benefits of this paradigm shift will depend on first identifying and resolving the various bases for resistance to it. In reality, this will require far more planning than would be needed to introduce a purely intellectual or technical advance. However, our experience suggests that it can be done.

## References

1. Eliot, T. S. (1943). Four Quartets. New York: Harcourt, Brace, and World.
2. Breuer, J. and Freud, S. (1893–95). Studies on hysteria. In J. Strachey (ed.), *The standard edition of the complete psychological works of Sigmund Freud*, Vol. 2. London: Hogarth Press, 1955.
3. Felitti, V. J., Anda, R. F., Nordenberg, D. *et al.* (1998). The relationship of adult health status to childhood abuse and household dysfunction. *American Journal of Preventive Medicine, 14,* 245–258.
4. Dong, M., Anda, R. F., Felitti, V.J. *et al.* (2004). The interrelatedness of multiple forms of childhood abuse, neglect, and household dysfunction. *Child Abuse & Neglect, 28,* 771–784.
5. Anda, R. F., Whitfield, C. L., Felitti, V. J. *et al.* (2002). Alcohol-impaired parents and adverse childhood experiences: The risk of depression and alcoholism during adulthood. *Psychiatric Services, 53,* 1001–1009.
6. Dube, S. R., Anda, R. F., Felitti, V. J. *et al.* (2001). Childhood abuse, household dysfunction and the risk of attempted suicide throughout the life span: Findings from the Adverse Childhood Experiences Study. *Journal of the American Medical Association, 286,* 3089–3096.
7. Anda, R. F., Brown, D. W., Felitti, V. J. *et al.* (2007). The relationship of adverse childhood experiences to rates of prescribed psychotropic medications in adulthood. *American Journal of Preventive Medicine, 32,* 389–394.
8. Seeman, T., McEwen, B., Rowe, J. and Singer, B. (2001). Allostatic load as a marker of cumulative biological risk. *Proceedings of the National Academy of Sciences USA, 98,* 4770–4775.
9. Whitfield, C. L., Dube, S. R., Felitti, V. J. and Anda, R. F. (2005). Adverse childhood experiences and subsequent hallucinations. *Child Abuse and Neglect, 29,* 797–810.
10. Anda, R. F., Felitti, V. J., Walker, J. *et al.* (2006). The enduring effects of abuse and related adverse experiences in childhood: A convergence of evidence from neurobiology and epidemiology. *European Archives of Psychiatry and Clinical Neurosciences, 256,* 174–186.
11. Anda, R. F., Croft, J. B., Felitti, V. J. *et al.* (1999). Adverse childhood experiences and smoking during adolescence and adulthood. *Journal of the American Medical Association, 282,* 1652–1658.
12. Edwards, V. J., Anda, R. F., Gu, D., Dube, S. R. and Felitti, V. J . (2007). Adverse childhood experiences and smoking persistence in adults with smoking-related symptoms and illness. *Permanente Journal, 11,* 5–13.
13. Dube, S. R., Miller, J. W., Brown, D. W. *et al.* (2006). Adverse childhood experiences and the association with ever using alcohol and initiating alcohol use during adolescence. *Journal of Adolescent Health, 38,* 444.
14. Dube, S. R., Anda, R. F., Felitti, V. J., Chapman, D. P. and Giles, W. H. (2003). Childhood abuse, neglect, and household dysfunction and the risk of illicit drug use: The adverse childhood experiences study. *Pediatrics, 111,* 564–572.

15. Anda, R. F., Fleisher, V. I., Felitti, V. J. *et al.* (2004). Childhood abuse, household dysfunction, and indicators of impaired worker performance in adulthood. *Permanente Journal,* **8**, 30–38.

16. Felitti, V. J . (2003). Ursprünge des Suchtverhaltens: Evidenzen aus einer Studie zu belastenden Kindheitserfahrungen. *Praxis der Kinderpsychologie und Kinderpsychiatrie,* **52**, 547–559.

17. Hillis, S. D., Anda, R. F., Dube, S. R. *et al.* (2004). The association between adolescent pregnancy, long-term psychosocial outcomes, and fetal death. *Pediatrics,* **113**, 320–327.

18. Dube, S. R., Felitti, V. J., Dong, M., Giles, W. H . and Anda, R. F . (2003). The impact of adverse childhood experiences on health problems: Evidence from four birth cohorts dating back to 1900. *Preventive Medicine,* **37**, 268–277.

19. Dong, M., Dube, S. R., Felitti, V. J., Giles, W. H. and Anda, R. F . (2003). Adverse childhood experiences and self-reported liver disease: New insights into a causal pathway. *Archives of Internal Medicine,* **163**, 1949–1956.

20. Anda, R. F., Brown, D. W., Dube, S. R. *et al.* (2010). Adverse childhood experiences and chronic obstructive pulmonary disease in adults. *American Journal of Preventive Medicine,* **34**, 396–403.

21. Dong, M., Giles, W. H., Felitti, V. J. *et al.* (2004). Insights into causal pathways for ischemic heart disease: Adverse Childhood Experiences Study. *Circulation,* **110**, 1761–1766.

22. Dube, S., Fairweather, D., Pearson, W. *et al.* (2009). Cumulative childhood stress and autoimmune diseases in adults. *Psychosomatic Medicine,* **71**, 243–250.

23. Kirkengen, A. L. (2001). Inscribed bodies. Dordrecht: Kluwer Academic.

24. Heckman, J., Knudsen, E., Cameron, J. and Shonkoff, J. (2006). Economic, neurobiological, and behavioral perspectives on building America's future workforce. *Proceedings of the National Academy of Sciences USA,* **103**, 10155–10162.

25. Brown, D. W., Anda, R. A., Tiemeier, H. *et al.* (2009). Adverse childhood experiences and the risk of premature mortality. *American Journal of Preventive Medicine,* **37**, 389–396.

26. Miller, A . (2006). *The body never lies.* New York: Norton.

27. Hoffer, E. (1959). *The ordeal of change.* New York: Harper and Row.

28. Masson, J. M . (1984). *Assault on truth.* New York: Farrar, Straus, and Giroux.

29. De Salvo, L . (1989). *Virginia Woolf: The impact of childhood sexual abuse on her life and work.* Boston, MA: Beacon Press.

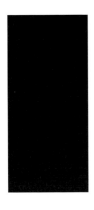

# Part 2 synopsis

Alicia F. Lieberman

## Overview

Part 2 provides a thorough examination of the effects of trauma on physical and mental health, with chapters covering the span from infancy to the adult years.

In Ch. 5, Bureau *et al.* make the thought-provoking proposal that attachment dysregulation may be conceptualized as "hidden trauma" stemming not from physical assault but from maternal failures to regulate the child's affect in the face of fear-evoking events. In their model, early stress may interact with deficits in maternal buffering to result in later psychiatric morbidity through the mechanism of early attachment dysregulation. The authors ground their reasoning in the premises of attachment theory [1–3] to argue that infants cannot evaluate the threat to safety represented by life events (including physical injury) and need the attachment figure to provide protection from external threats and internal distress that trigger emotional dysregulation.

The conceptualization in Ch. 5 of attachment-related dysregulation as a form of trauma represents a departure from the fourth edition of *Diagnosic and Statistical Manual* [4] definition of a traumatic event as involving threat to the person's physical integrity, and resembles instead the definition provided in DC:0-3-R [5] of traumatic events as involving a threat to the *psychological* or physical integrity of the infant or young child. In locating the source of trauma within the child in the form of attachment dysregulation, however, Bureau and colleagues depart from the focus of both nosologies on external threat as the trigger to the traumatic experience, and return to the classic psychoanalytic emphasis on the child's internal processing of interpersonal experience as the locus of psychopathology.

The authors of Ch. 5 review a range of studies that provide evidence for the long-term impact of early

experience on later functioning, including the differential predictive power of maternal depression at different ages in the child's life on the child's depressive symptoms at each of those ages. The inclusion of maternal depression and maternal unresponsiveness in the authors' conceptual framework of "hidden trauma" raises the question of when, in the continuum from stress to trauma, *emotionally costly* experiences become *traumatic* experiences, when trauma is framed in the context of classic definitions that involve unpredictability, horror and helplessness [6,7]. In light of these three markers of trauma, can maternal unresponsiveness in the face of ordinary stress be considered traumatic if it becomes the norm rather than the exception in the infant's emotional life?

The debate about the threshold for "caseness" in a variety of mental health diagnoses is a recurrent feature of efforts to operationalize, predict and classify psychiatric phenomena. Chapter 5 offers a novel angle from which to ponder these issues.

Chapter 6 explores the extreme of the stress–trauma continuum, focusing much-needed attention on the broad array of severe symptoms presented by children victimized by repeated, chronic, co-occurring and cumulative traumatic experiences from a variety of sources, including sexual and physical abuse.

The authors of Ch. 6 review the evidence linking chronic trauma to deviations of functioning in multiple domains, including affect and impulse dysregulation; disturbances of attention, cognition and consciousness; distortions in self perception and systems of meaning; interpersonal difficulties; somatization and biological dysregulation; and co-occurring symptoms. These symptom domains supersede the more circumscribed symptom clusters that characterize post-traumatic stress disorder (PTSD), with the consequence that in clinical practice children exposed to multiple traumas routinely receive multiple psychiatric diagnoses. In effect, there is a clinical expectation of comorbidity as the rule rather than the exception in public health service populations.

Van der Kolk and d'Andrea in Ch. 6 highlight the fact that this routine clinical finding of comorbidity in multiply traumatized children masks the compelling but unrecognized phenomenon of caregiver abuse as a pervasive source of traumatization in large sectors of the pediatric population and it poses an obstacle to the clinician's appreciation of the enormity of the trauma and the crucial importance of appropriately comprehensive treatment. Repeated interpersonal abuse represents a shattering organismic experience that results in multifaceted manifestations of developmental disturbance in biological, emotional, social and emotional functioning. The authors point out that the use of a comorbidity approach to the diagnosis of multiply traumatized children lacks parsimony and etiological clarity and may interfere with a case formulation leading to a comprehensive treatment approach by focusing attention on discrete aspects of the child's symptomatology rather than on the impact of trauma as the organizing substrate for the child's seemingly unrelated symptoms.

In advocating for the adoption and empirical investigation of developmental trauma disorder as a comprehensive, developmentally sensitive interpersonal trauma diagnosis, the authors of Ch. 6 call for a long-overdue recognition that the disparate symptoms presented by multiply traumatized children tend to co-occur and represent a single, coherent diagnostic construct. It is important to note as well that Ch. 6 represents much more than a persuasive appeal to investigate the scientific and clinical value of developmental trauma disorder as an alternative to current diagnostic approaches. The authors are, in effect, issuing an urgent call to action by highlighting the discrepancy between the staggering prevalence of cumulative interpersonal trauma in children and adolescents and the abysmal insufficiency of research funds, clinical services and public policy initiatives designed to prevent and alleviate this public health emergency [8,9].

Chapter 7 provides a comprehensive critical analysis of the literature linking early exposure to psychological trauma with complex psychiatric sequelae in adulthood. Ford's review provides converging evidence from numerous studies showing that the child's age at the onset of maltreatment and the type of trauma are key predictive variables, with earlier ages at onset of violence or sexual abuse associated with increased morbidity in later childhood and adolescence. The literature review also makes clear the multifinality of early victimization: adults who were abused as children show a heterogeneity of disorders that include PTSD, anxiety, depression, suicidality, addiction, personality disorders, antisocial or violent behavior and sexual disorders, as well as risk for a range of physical illnesses and impaired role functioning. Ford links this wide array of outcomes with early and ongoing efforts to provide empirical support for diagnostic categories that encompass the multifaceted sequelae of early interpersonal trauma, including complex PTSD [10], disorders of extreme stress not otherwise specified (DESNOS [11,12]) and developmental trauma disorder (Ch. 6).

The author of Ch. 7 reviews the conceptual and methodological arguments that have to date prevented the formal recognition and adoption of these diagnostic categories, including the absence of external confirmation for trauma history, which is assessed retrospectively in the majority of studies, and the frequent focus on a specific subtype of trauma (e.g., domestic violence, sexual abuse, physical abuse) instead of comprehensive assessment of the entire range of traumatic events to which a person might have been exposed. This occurs in spite of evidence that there is substantial overlap in exposure to different trauma subtypes, such as physical abuse, domestic violence and community violence. Although these methodological and conceptual problems exist in the literature, there is also evidence that trauma history questionnaires and interviews that are behaviorally specific have evidence of reliability and validity.

Ford concludes his chapter with the argument that interventions should be designed to incorporate the well-established findings that childhood victimization has wide-ranging adverse impacts on adolescent and adult survivors.

This part closes with a detailed description by Felitti and Anda of their landmark Adverse Childhood Experiences (ACE) Study (Ch. 8), a longitudinal investigation that has had a powerful impact on current thinking about the long-term repercussions on both physical and mental health of early trauma and other adversities.

The ACE Study is a model of the fruitful synergy that is created when clinical acumen, in the form of observing individual phenomena and seeking meaning in patterns of clinical findings, is linked with methodological expertise and institutional support to envision, develop and implement a groundbreaking initiative that simultaneously creates new knowledge and uses that knowledge to change clinical practice.

The ACE Study is rooted in self-reports of trauma and adversity exposure, but the potential flaw of this method is mitigated, as the authors of the chapter point out, by the demonstrated psychometric properties of behavior-specific questionnaires as well as by the long-term prospective component and the unusually large sample size of the investigation. In the first wave of the study, eight categories of adverse experience were selected on the basis of their high incidence in a population of obese individuals seeking treatment at Kaiser Permanente; two additional categories were added in the second wave. The categories used were emotional abuse; physical abuse; contact sexual abuse; mother treated violently; household member with alcoholism or drug use; imprisoned household member; household member chronically depressed, suicidal, mentally ill or in psychiatric hospital; not being raised by both biological parents; physical neglect; and emotional neglect.

In analysis after analysis, Felitti and Anda demonstrate the powerful statistical effect of childhood or adolescent exposure to four or more of these categories on a range of adult physical and mental health outcomes charted prospectively over the course of 14 years, including chronic depression, suicide attempts, hallucinations, unexplained symptoms, smoking, alcoholism, intravenous drug use, impaired work performance, likelihood of more than 50 sexual partners, liver disease, heart disease, drug prescriptions (written for antidepressant, antipsychotic and anxiolytic medication), medical costs and life expectancy.

The findings can be discussed from a variety of angles, but some conclusions stand out. In this middle-class population, the prevalence of trauma and adversity is much higher than conventionally assumed, yet systematic assessment of these conditions tends to be the exception rather than the rule in medical and mental health practice. Felitti and Anda provide evidence that questions about risk factors are well accepted by patients when they are administered in the context of a well-devised questionnaire filled out at home, and the approach is linked to reductions in doctor office visits and emergency department

visits when the information becomes incorporated into the patient's medical care. Sadly, but also predictably, the information is not systematically used to inform care: in the second year after the comprehensive evaluation, the reduction in visits all but disappeared, perhaps because the information was now in the charts but not in the medical provider's continued awareness.

Felitti and Anda argue for the need for a profound paradigmatic shift in primary medical care that incorporates attention to the health consequences of trauma and adversity at the forefront of the provider's practice. The same prescription can be applied to the practice of mental health. The avoidance of knowing and remembering traumatic events is not only a clinical phenomenon relegated to patients, it pervades the practice of clinicians as well.

This section of the book provides a powerful antidote to the resistance to incorporate trauma knowledge as an essential clinical tool that must become an expected component of the professional practice of clinicians across disciplines.

## Future directions

The future directions for the field emerge clearly from the issues presented in the chapters comprising this part. The definition of trauma is still subject to debate, as is evident in the range of conditions (such as maternal depression and child affective dysregulation) that are encompassed within the umbrella of trauma in some of the chapters.

Prospective longitudinal research linking the effects of trauma to developmental course, symptom clusters and neuroscience is needed to refine the definition of trauma and create a more cohesive definitional consensus in the field. The issue of equifinality versus multifinality needs to be systematically addressed in efforts to determine the heuristic value of new diagnostic categories. Multiple types of exposure to traumatic events may lead to a common outcome such as PTSD, while a specific event such as sexual abuse can lead to multiple outcomes depending on constitutional and environmental factors and on the specific configuration of risk and protective factors in the child, the family and the community.

Steady progress is being made, but there is a need for empirically validated, objective measures of dose exposure as well as measures of child functioning in social and emotional domains across developmental stages, including measures of child–parent interaction that are culturally informed and developmentally appropriate. These measures will facilitate research on stress diathesis linking genetic, temperamental, relational and environmental domains to elucidate mechanisms linking exposure to outcome.

Research also needs to cut across discrete sources of trauma to study trauma in all its many facets, in recognition of the widely documented overlap between different types of trauma in the lives of children and their families. The systematic inclusion of infants, toddlers and preschoolers in epidemiological studies on the incidence and impact of different forms of trauma, including exposure to domestic violence and child abuse, is essential to elucidate the earliest underpinnings of later dysfunction.

The most urgently needed direction in the field of trauma, however, involves the search for and implementation of effective treatments for multiply traumatized children. The routine experience of violence in the home, the school, the street and the community at large has grown to epidemic proportions for large sectors of the population – precisely those sectors most bereft of protective factors that may moderate both the incidence and the impact of violence, such as adequate housing, education, income and healthcare. Steven Sharfstein [9] stated that "interpersonal violence, especially violence experienced by children, is the largest single preventable cause of mental illness. What cigarette smoking is to the rest of medicine, early childhood violence is to psychiatry." Yet there is a persistent discrepancy between the availability, efficacy and effectiveness of treatment available to multiply traumatized children and the scope of the need. Harris and colleagues [8] coined the term "supraclinical" to describe the nature of the interventions needed to address the sequelae of multiple trauma in the context of poverty and intergenerational transmission of maladaptive patterns of adaptation, including the overlap of different forms of trauma. We need to develop, implement and evaluate multifaceted interventions that address the child's dysfunctions in the context of the family and the environment and provide access to safe and responsive settings that palliate rather than exacerbate the child's vulnerabilities.

At present, treatment outcome research for the sequelae of trauma seems divided between the ideal of scientific rigor on one hand and the urge for action that redresses the mental health disparities for poor and minority children on the other hand.

Scientific rigor is applied to discrete phenomena in tightly controlled experimental settings, but the lessons learned in those circumscribed conditions lose their power and validity, as a rule, when efforts are made to implement them in the chaotic conditions of families and communities with multiple adversities. Reconciling the search for scientific soundness with the urgent need for using science to address the seemingly intractable problems of multiply traumatized children is the most important direction beckoning those working with trauma victims.

# References

1. Bowlby, J. (1969). *Attachment and loss, Vol. 1: Attachment*. New York: Basic Books.
2. Main, M. and Hesse, E. (1990). Parents' unresolved traumatic experiences are related to infant disorganized attachment status: Is frightened and/or frightening parental behaviour the linking mechanism? In M. Greenberg, D. Cicchetti and E. M. Cummings (eds.), *Attachment in the preschool years: Theory, research and intervention* (pp. 161–184). Chicago, IL: University of Chicago Press.
3. Schuder, M. and Lyons-Ruth, K. (2004). "Hidden trauma" in infancy: Attachment, fearful arousal, and early dysfunction of the stress response system. In J. Osofsky (ed.). *Trauma in infancy and early childhood* (pp. 69–104). New York: Guilford.
4. American Psychiatric Association (2000). *Diagnostic and statistical manual of mental disorders,* 4th edn., revised. Washington, DC: Americal Psychiatric Press.
5. Zero to Three: National Center for Infants, Toddlers and Families (2005). *Diagnostic classification of mental health and developmental disorders of infancy and early childhood*, revised edn *(DC:0–3R)*. Washington, DC: Zero to Three.
6. Freud, S. (1926). Inhibitions, symptoms and anxiety. In S. James (ed.), *The standard edition of the complete psychological works of Sigmund Freud*, Vol. 20 (pp. 70–174). London: Hogarth Press and the Institute of Psychoanalysis, 1959.
7. Pynoos, R. S., Steinberg, A. M. and Piacentini, J. C. (1999). A developmental psychopathology model of childhood traumatic stress and intersection with anxiety disorders. *Biological Psychiatry,* **46**, 1542–1554.
8. Harris, W. W., Lieberman, A. F. and Marans, S. (2007). In the best interests of society. *Journal of Child Psychology and Psychiatry,* **48**, 392–411.
9. Sharfstein, S. (2006). New task force will address early childhood violence. *Psychiatric News,* **41**, 3.
10. Herman, J. L. (1992). Complex PTSD. *Journal of Traumatic Stress*, **5**, 377–391.

11. Roth, S., Newman, E., Pelcovitz, D., van der Kolk, B. and Mandel, F. (1997). Complex PTSD in victims exposed to sexual and physical abuse. *Journal of Traumatic Stress*, **10**, 539–555.

12. van der Kolk, B., Pelcovitz, D., Roth, S. *et al.* (1996). Dissociation, somatization, and affect dysregulation: Complexity of adaptation to trauma. *American Journal of Psychiatry*, **153** (7 Festschrift Supplement), 83–93.

# Biological approaches to early life trauma

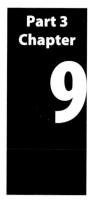

**Part 3
Chapter
9**

# The impact of early life trauma: psychobiological sequelae in children
# Juvenile stress as an animal model of childhood trauma

Gal Richter-Levin and Shlomit Jacobson-Pick

## Introduction

Danger, trauma, fear and anxiety are embedded in the human condition. There is a wide spectrum of appraisal, response and adaptation to danger within the lifecycle of the individual. A developmental psychopathology approach recognizes the intricate matrix of intrinsic factors, developmental maturation, experience and life events that contribute to proximal and distal outcomes.

Traumatic experiences are common in the lives of children and adolescents. Approximately 15% to 20% of juveniles will encounter some form of relatively severe trauma [1]. Trauma exerts approximately two-fold increased risk for various forms of psychopathology, including anxiety [2], major depression [3] and behavior problems [4]. These disorders span the full range of human existence from childhood to old age, although symptoms may vary considerably owing to developmental differences and related factors [5].

## Reaction to stress

One of the key factors of trauma-related states is "stress." Stress may be defined as a real or interpreted threat to the physiological or psychological integrity of an individual that results in physiological and/or behavioral responses [6].

The basic neuroendocrine core of acute stress response, also known as the fight-or-flight response, does not seem to vary substantially between species and/or gender. Humans, monkeys and rodents experience a cascade of hormonal responses to threat that appears to begin with the rapid release of oxytocin, vasopressin, corticotropin-releasing factor (CRF) and possibly other hormones produced in the paraventricular nucleus of the hypothalamus. Direct neural activation of the adrenal medulla triggers release of the catecholamines

norepinephrine and epinephrine, and concomitant sympathetic responses. Hypothalamic release of CRF and other hormones stimulate the release of adreno-corticotropic hormone (ACTH) from the anterior pituitary, which, in turn, stimulates the synthesis and secretion of glucocorticoids, especially cortisol or corticosterone, depending upon the species [7–9].

This hypothalamic–pituitary–adrenal (HPA) axis is involved in the regulation of threats to homeostasis [10,11] and can be activated by a wide variety of stressors. Some of the most potent stressors are psychological or processive stressors (i.e., stressors that involve higher order sensory–cognitive processing, as opposed to physiological or systemic stressors) [12,13].

The HPA response has a close relationship to behavioral traits, such as fear and anxiety [14–17]. Moreover, through the actions of glucocorticoid hormones in the brain, the HPA axis is involved in programming responses to future challenges, thereby potentially rendering the animal more vulnerable or more successful at coping with environmental challenges [18].

However, while an important role of normal HPA response to stressors is to restore physiological balance and prevent overreaction of defense mechanisms to stress [11], prolonged exposure to high levels of glucocorticoids has damaging effects on many systems of the body, including the central nervous system [10].

Abnormal reaction to stress can have a disastrous impact on human lives. The reaction to an extremely stressful event can lead to mood and anxiety disorders [19]. People who are exposed to such events are at increased risk for post-traumatic stress disorder (PTSD) as well as for major depression, panic disorder generalized anxiety disorder, and substance abuse compared with those who have not experienced traumatic events [19–21].

## Effects of exposure to early life stress

Although the blueprint of the mammalian brain is genetically programmed, the interaction between environmental factors and gene expression is required for normal brain development and the formation of the neural circuits which enable normal brain function throughout life. Therefore, the brain is vulnerable to alterations generated by external and internal stimuli during infancy, childhood and adolescence [22].

Stressful life events during childhood have a powerful impact on the neuronal mechanisms that mediate the reaction to stress via systems such as the endocrine and immune systems [23]. Compelling evidence from a variety of studies suggests that an array of early life stressors, constitute a major risk factor for the development and persistence of both mood and anxiety disorders, as they are associated with increased rates of stress-related mental and physical disorders in adulthood [24–27]. This suggested that adverse experience during cerebral development may induce a vulnerability to the effects of stress later in life. Possibly this may occur through induction of a persistent sensitization of stress-responsive neural circuits, which augments the consequences of later experiences, thus predisposing these individuals to the risk of developing a wide array of stress-related mental and physical disorders [25,27,28].

Studies examining the impact of early life experiences in rats usually refer to "early life" as the first 14 postnatal days. Several protocols have been used to examine the effects of stress during this time period: foot shock or isolation [29], hypoxia [30], cold stress [31] and maternal deprivation, which is the most prevalent model [32–35]. At the behavioral level, maternal deprivation for 24 hours results in hyperresponsiveness to stress and increased reaction to fear. At the physiological level, a similar maternal deprivation protocol altered plasma levels of ACTH and corticosterone secretion. These hormonal responses modulate the functioning of the HPA axis in ways that, if continued, may increase the risk of immune disorders and heighten sensitivity to future stress, potentially leading to cognitive deficits and social–emotional problems [36,37].

Accumulating evidence from laboratory animal studies on early life stress suggests persistent changes in the function of brain regions pivotal to the meditation of stress and emotion that are similar to the neurobiological alterations exhibited in patients suffering from depression or anxiety disorders. These include persistent changes in CRF neurotransmission, disregulation of central and peripheral HPA axis responsiveness and alterations in other neurotransmitter systems implicated in the regulation of the stress responses including noradrenergic, serotonergic and GABAergic functions [25,27]. Collectively, animal models of early life stress demonstrated that stressful experiences occurring during critical periods of brain development (perinatal to pre-weaning) persistently and perhaps permanently change the behavior and the response of the HPA axis to stress, thereby increasing the vulnerability to mood and anxiety disorders [27].

## The juvenile stress model

Most studies concerned with the impact of early life stress on development and behavior in rodents have traditionally focused on the postnatal pre-weaning period, involving some form of maternal separation/deprivation [38]. However, Heim *et al.* [26,39] have argued that any form of stress – short term, acute or chronic as long as it occurs prior to sexual maturity onset – may be classified as early life stress; hence, it may constitute a risk factor for the development of depression and other stress-related psychopathologies.

The post-weaning prepuberty period (juvenile stage) is a potentially sensitive time in which adversities may result in enduring stress effects. Relatively little research has been conducted on the post-weaning prepuberty period, a time of significant brain development [40,41] and a time of great importance for mental and physical health. The risk for the development of various psychopathologies, such as schizophrenia, depression and drug abuse, increases during this period (see reviews by Hayward and Sanborn [42], Masten [43] and McGue and Iacono [44]), and stressors have been implicated as predisposing factors in these disorders (see reviews by Goodyer *et al.* [45] and Grant *et al.* [46]).

Juvenile rats resemble children and preteenagers in several behavioral features, such as the need for maternal care, independence and increased play behaviors with peers, that diminish at puberty [47–49]. During this period, substantial remodeling occurs in the hippocampus and amygdala, brain areas sensitive to stress and also involved in emotional and learning processing (for review see Spear [49]). Indeed the brain's development continues well after the pre-weaning period and substantial maturation processes continue well into the pubertal period. Pre-teen humans exhibit enhanced stress perception and responses. Therefore, traumatic life events during this period are associated with later socioemotional maladaptive behaviors [49,50] and constitute a significant risk factor for later development of stress-related psychopathologies [26,51]. Moreover, as in human neural development, although the HPA axis response in rats reaches its developmental asymptote during the juvenile period [52], this response still lasts considerably longer than in adults [52,53]. Romeo et al. [53] suggested that this slower shutoff of the HPA axis during the juvenile period might derive from less central feedback activity by the not fully developed forebrain limbic regions, such as the hippocampus and amygdala-based neurocircuits, which are still undergoing significant maturation processes [49].

## Long-term effects of juvenile stress exposure

Exposing rats to stress during the juvenile period has been reported to produce more pronounced effects than exposure at earlier or later ages. Social isolation at the age of 25–45 days, as opposed to earlier (16–25 days), or later (older than 45 days) ages, resulted in more pronounced and longer lasting effects on object exploration tasks in an open field [54]. More significant effects of social isolation during juvenility were also reported in terms of water intake, with single housing stress increasing fluid intake of juvenile but not adult animals [55]. Preventing juvenile rats from engaging in social play behaviors disrupted adulthood social and non-social behaviors, effects that were found to be associated with alteration of the response to morphine and of the endogenous opioid system in the amygdala [56–59]. Furthermore, similar to patients with PTSD, adult rats exposed to long-term variable stress as juveniles (21–32 days) demonstrated an enhanced acoustic startle response [60].

Tsoory and Richter-Levin [61] acutely exposed juvenile rats to variable stressors (forced swim, elevated platform, foot shock) over days 27–29 or later (toward adolescence) over days 33–35 and tested them in adulthood. Both groups showed reduced exploratory behavior and reduced avoidance learning, but poorer performance was greater in those stressed at the earlier age of adolescence, namely during their juvenile stage [61]. Avital and Richter-Levin [62] have shown that acute juvenile stress may produce increased vulnerability to stressful events in adulthood, resulting in an augmented response to adverse experiences. The combination of exposure to acute stress at juvenility and reexposure in adulthood, at 60 or 90 days of age, was found to increase anxiety levels, as measured in the open field and startle reflex response tests, and affected water maze performance not only in comparison with control rats but also in comparison with rats that were exposed and then reexposed to the stress protocol only in adulthood (i.e., at 60 and 90 days of age) [62].

## Short-term effects of juvenile stress exposure

Epidemiological studies of child and adolescent mood disorders have been carried out for many years; nevertheless, progress in the field of mood disturbances in children has been hindered by two misconceptions: mood disorders are rare before adulthood [63] and mood disturbances are a normative and self-limiting aspect of child and adolescent development [64–66]. Clinical research now makes it clear that neither of these beliefs is true [67]. Since the mid 1990s, early onset of affective illness and the risk of psychiatric disorder among children that are associated with adverse life events have been recognized as major public health problems [68,69].

Kessler et al. [70] have shown that, although treatment of mood and anxiety disorders typically begins in early adulthood, the first onset of mental disorders usually takes place during childhood and adolescence. The median age of onset (i.e., 50th percentile on the age-of-onset distribution) was found to be 11 years of age, during juvenility [70]. It has been hypothesized that traumatized children initially exhibit complex environmentally induced developmental disorders that may without treatment later branch toward more specific and adult-like pathologies, such as depression and anxiety [71].

Although considerable amounts of animal research have dealt with the long-term effects of exposure to stress during juvenility [61,62,72–75], relatively little is known about the short-term effects of exposure to stress during this distinct developmental period.

We have recently assessed whether exposure to stress during juvenility elicits abnormal behavior soon after the stressful experience in comparison with the behavioral consequences of adult rats subjected to stress during juvenility but examined in adulthood. Surprisingly, not only did stress during juvenility have significant short-term effects on animals' behavior, but this reaction also shows an opposite pattern of behavior compared with the long-term behavioral effects of juvenile stress. Therefore, while adult rats exhibited "classic anxious behavior" (i.e., reduced total activity level, spent less time and were less active in the "unsafe regions" of the open field and elevated plus maze apparatuses), juvenile rats exhibited a "reverse" pattern of behavior (increased total activity level, spent more time and were more active in the "unsafe regions" of these apparatuses) soon after the exposure to the juvenile stress.

It is important to note that the stressed rats exhibited both immediate and long-term alterations in anxiety-related behaviors while, the behavior of the age-matched controls remained mostly unchanged between juvenility and adulthood. Hence, the observed age-related behavioral effects were indeed induced by the juvenile stress and could not be attributed to age-related changes in baseline behavior.

The age-related juvenile stress-induced behavioral pattern are of particular interest given that they correspond to clinical studies demonstrating that while children experience anxiety and depression in much the same way as adults they display these symptoms differently [76]. For example, a child with major depression may exhibit irritable mood and anxiety rather than overt depression as the prominent feature, and a child with bipolar disorder can initially demonstrate symptoms of hyperactivity and inattention, although children often do not exhibit the more typical euphoria and grandiosity of adults [77].

Costello *et al.* [65] have argued that usually "early-onset" affective disorders are undiagnosed, since the diagnostic tools for mood and anxiety disorders in children are not yet fully developed [66]. Our findings suggest that the juvenile stress model might serve as an animal model for developmental-stage-specific symptoms of mood and anxiety disorders, which could then promote the search for a valid diagnostic tool of these disorders in children and adolescents. The need of developmental-stage-specific diagnostic criteria is crucial for a number of reasons. First, although the first onset of mental disorders usually takes place during childhood and adolescence, these disorders typically remain undiagnosed and untreated until early adulthood [67]. Second, for many disturbed children, the relationship between disorder and impairment is a reciprocal one, with impairment leading to continued exacerbation of anxiety symptoms, which, in turn, results in worse impairment. It has been suggested that traumatized children initially exhibit complex developmental disorders, which may later branch to more specific and adult-like pathologies such as depression and anxiety [71], as noted above. Third, over time, early-onset mood and anxiety disorders are likely to develop additional comorbid conditions. For example, early-onset

depressives tend to develop conduct disorders, anxiety disorders and substance abuse disorder [5,78,79].

One limitation of the available preclinical literature on behavioral neuroscience is that much of the literature discussing stages of development has utilized a male only population, and yet the demands of development and of the environment differ for males and females. It may be that the consequences of exposure to stressors would differ for females and males, particularly since the HPA axis is regulated by sex hormones [18]. However, emotionally challenging juvenile-stressed female rats demonstrated age-related "reverse" behavior similar to the behavior demonstrated by male rats. Nevertheless, when examined in the open field test, female rats' behavior did differ slightly from that of the males: juvenile stressed female rats showed no difference in total exploratory behavior when tested soon after the exposure to the juvenile stress or in adulthood. Additionally, unlike male rats, no difference was found in the activity level and percentage of time spent in the center of the open field arena at juvenility, again suggesting that differences do exist between the response of male and female rats to juvenile stress.

Research indicates that gender differences exist in the prevalence of both mood and anxiety disorders [80–82]. A large body of evidence from general population surveys confirms that each of the *Diagnostic and Statistical Manual of Mental Disorders* (DSM) IV anxiety disorders [83] is more common in females than in males. For example, during their lifetime females are twice as likely as men to have PTSD (10% compared with 5%) [84]. These differences in prevalence have been attributed to the greater risk for women of adverse experiences such as sexual abuse, in particularly child abuse [27]. In our studies, life circumstances were controlled and male and female rats experienced the same adversities. In addition, the behavioral response of each stressed group, juvenile/adult and male/female, was assessed in comparison with their matching control. This experimental design allowed the relative pattern of behavior within each age group and between the sexes to be assessed. To that end, the results indicate that overall female and male rats are both affected by adverse experiences during juvenility. Nevertheless, some aspects of female rat's behavior differed from males' response to the same adverse experiences. These observations correspond to previous studies showing that, while sex differences characterize certain behavioral aspects, males and females exhibit a similar degree of response to induced stress [80]. For instance, while sex differences were observed in head swinging in the forced swim test, rats' duration of immobility was increased in both male and female rats during the second session of the test [85]. It is, therefore, possible that the differences between males and females are less in the frequency of symptoms than in the pattern of symptoms.

Our data and those from other studies highlight the need for studies comparing male and female behavior utilizing different stress protocols, behavioral paradigms and physiological–biochemical correlates during various developmental stages.

Rats exposed to juvenile stress and challenged in either juvenility or adulthood exhibit similar blood corticosterone levels. Nevertheless, injecting corticosterone to juvenile or adult naive rats elicited an opposite pattern of behavioral effects, similar to the immediate and long-term behavioral effects of juvenile stress exposure. Overall, this pattern of behavior was demonstrated among male and female rats, although it was more pronounced among male rats. Therefore, acute corticosterone application mimics the age-related "reverse" pattern of behavior elicited by exposure to stress during juvenility in male and female rats.

During adolescence, the brain goes through a transitional phase towards final maturation [49,86]. It is plausible that corticosterone applied at two different developmental stages – in juvenility and adulthood – cause different effects on the developing and mature brain.

Obviously, corticosterone and alterations in responses to it cannot by themselves explain the entire spectrum of mood and anxiety. However, understanding its contribution to inducing age-specific anxiety-like behaviors might advance our knowledge of early- versus late-onset of mood and anxiety disorders. The pivotal role of corticosterone in the immediate and long-term behavioral outcomes of juvenile stress exposure may serve to promote our understanding of the differences between mood and anxiety disorder symptoms in children and adults.

## Conclusions

It is imperative that findings from the preclinical studies of reaction to juvenile stress among juvenile and adult rats be translated into increased knowledge of the physiological correlates, associated neural mechanisms and pharmacological agents that can account

for the signs, symptoms and treatment in children and adult patients with mood and anxiety disorders.

Recently, we were able to demonstrate that, while the exposure to juvenile stress has long-term behavioral, endocrinological and biochemical consequences, the exposure of juvenile-stressed animals to enriched environment from juvenility to adulthood could prevent those adverse outcomes [87]. The ability of enriched environment to reverse cognitive impairments resulting from isolation or early life stress has been demonstrated [88]. The ameliorating effects this manipulation may have on emotional consequences of early life stress may be of great therapeutic importance. Yang et al. [89] have already demonstrated that an enriched environment could prevent negative emotional consequences of prenatal stress. Our data extend these findings to demonstrate that enriched environment may also be effective when the stress occurs at a later early life period, juvenility.

Adapting these findings to the human condition, enriched environment treatment might be an important therapeutic intervention to confront at least part of the adverse consequences of early life stress in adulthood.

## References

1. Breslau, N. (2002). Psychiatric morbidity in adult survivors of childhood trauma. *Seminars in Clinical Neuropsychiatry*, 7, 80–88.

2. Yule, W., Bolton, D., Udwin, O. *et al.* (2000). The long-term psychological effects of a disaster experienced in adolescence: I: The incidence and course of PTSD. *Journal Child Psychology and Psychiatry*, **41**, 503–511.

3. Brown, E. S., Rush, A. J. and McEwen, B. S. (1999). Hippocampal remodeling and damage by corticosteroids: Implications for mood disorders. *Neuropsychopharmacology*, **21**, 474–484.

4. Shaw, J. A., Applegate, B., Tanner, S. *et al.* (1995). Psychological effects of Hurricane Andrew on an elementary school population. *Journal of the American Academy of Child and Adolescent Psychiatry*, **34**, 1185–1192.

5. Stein, M. B. and Lang, A. J. (2002). Anxiety and stress disorders: course over the lifetime. In K. L. Davis, D. Charney, J. T. Coyle and C. Nemeroff (eds.), *Neuropsychopharmacology: The fifth generation of progress* (pp. 859–866). Philadelphia, PA: Lippincott, Williams and Wilkins.

6. Kalueff, A. V. and Tuohimaa, P. (2004). Experimental modeling of anxiety and depression. *Acta Neurobiologiae Experimentalis (Wars)*, **64**, 439–448.

7. Arborelius, L., Owens, M. J., Plotsky, P. M. and Nemeroff, C. B. (1999). The role of corticotropin-releasing factor in

depression and anxiety disorders. *Journal of Endocrinology,* **160**, 1–12.

8. Jezova, D., Skultetyova, I., Tokarev, D. I., Bakos, P. and Vigas, M. (1995). Vasopressin and oxytocin in stress. In G. P. Chrousos, R. McCarty, K. Pacak, *et al.* (eds.), *Stress: Basic mechanisms and clinical implications,* Vol. 771 (pp. 192–203). New York: Annals of the New York Academy of Sciences.

9. Sapolsky, R. M. (1999). Glucocorticoids, stress, and their adverse neurological effects: Relevance to aging. *Experimental Gerontology,* **34**, 721–732.

10. McEwen, B. S. (2000). Allostasis, allostatic load, and the aging nervous system: Role of excitatory amino acids and excitotoxicity. *Neurochemistry Research,* **25**, 1219–1231.

11. Munck, A., Guyre, P. M. and Holbrook, N. J. (1984). Physiological functions of glucocorticoids in stress and their relation to pharmacological actions. *Endocrine Reviews,* **5**, 25–44.

12. Anisman, H. and Matheson, K. (2005). Stress, depression, and anhedonia: Caveats concerning animal models. *Neuroscience and Biobehavioral Reviews,* **29**, 525–546.

13. McEwen, B. S. (2000). The neurobiology of stress: From serendipity to clinical relevance. *Brain Research,* **886**, 172–189.

14. Dellu, F., Piazza, P. V., Mayo, W., Le Moal, M. and Simon, H. (1996). Novelty-seeking in rats: Biobehavioral characteristics and possible relationship with the sensation-seeking trait in man. *Neuropsychobiology,* **34**, 136–145.

15. Kabbaj, M., Devine, D. P., Savage, V. R. and Akil, H. (2000). Neurobiological correlates of individual differences in novelty-seeking behavior in the rat: Differential expression of stress-related molecules. *Journal of Neuroscience,* **20**, 6983–6988.

16. Landgraf, R. and Wigger, A. (2003). Born to be anxious: Neuroendocrine and genetic correlates of trait anxiety in HAB rats. *Stress,* **6**, 111–119.

17. Steimer, T. and Driscoll, P. (2003). Divergent stress responses and coping styles in psychogenetically selected Roman high-(RHA) and low-(RLA) avoidance rats: Behavioural, neuroendocrine and developmental aspects. *Stress,* **6**, 87–100.

18. McCormick, C. M. and Mathews, I. Z. (2007). HPA function in adolescence: role of sex hormones in its regulation and the enduring consequences of exposure to stressors. *Pharmacology, Biochemistry and Behavior,* **86**, 220–233.

19. Yehuda, R. (2002). Post-traumatic stress disorder. *New England Journal of Medicine,* **346**, 108–114.

20. Hanson, R. K. (1990). The psychological impact of sexual assault on women and children: A review. *Annual Review of Sex Research,* **3**, 187–232.

21. Epstein, J. N., Saunders, B. E. and Kilpatrick, D. G. (1997). Predicting PTSD in women with a history of childhood rape. *Journal of Trauma and Stress,* **10**, 573–588.

22. Levitt, P., Reinoso, B. and Jones, L. (1998). The critical impact of early cellular environment on neuronal development. *Preventive Medicine,* **27**, 180–183.

23. van der Kolk, B. A. (1994). The body keeps the score: Memory and the evolving psychobiology of posttraumatic stress. *Harvard Review of Psychiatry,* **1**, 253–265.

24. Heim, C. and Nemeroff, C. B. (1999). The impact of early adverse experiences on brain systems involved in the pathophysiology of anxiety and affective disorders. *Biological Psychiatry,* **46**, 1509–1522.

25. Heim, C. and Nemeroff, C. B. (2001). The role of childhood trauma in the neurobiology of mood and anxiety disorders: Preclinical and clinical studies. *Biological Psychiatry,* **49**, 1023–1039.

26. Heim, C., Plotsky, P. M. and Nemeroff, C. B. (2004). Importance of studying the contributions of early adverse experience to neurobiological findings in depression. *Neuropsychopharmacology,* **29**, 641–648.

27. Nemeroff, C. B. (2004). Neurobiological consequences of childhood trauma. *Journal of Clinical Psychiatry* **65**(Suppl. 1), 18–28.

28. Agid, O., Kohn, Y. and Lerer, B. (2000). Environmental stress and psychiatric illness. *Biomedicine and Pharmacotherapy,* **54**, 135–141.

29. Goodwin, G. A., Bliven, T., Kuhn, C., Francis, R. and Spear, L. P. (1997). Immediate early gene expression to examine neuronal activity following acute and chronic stressors in rat pups: Examination of neurophysiological alterations underlying behavioral consequences of prenatal cocaine exposure. *Physiological Behavior,* **61**, 895–902.

30. Hermans, R. H. and Longo, L. D. (1994). Altered catecholaminergic behavioral and hormonal responses in rats following early postnatal hypoxia. *Physiological Behavior,* **55**, 469–475.

31. Gonzalez, A. S., Rodriguez Echandia, E. L., Cabrera, R., Foscolo, M. R. and Fracchia, L. N. (1990). Neonatal chronic stress induces subsensitivity to chronic stress in adult rats. I. Effects on forced swim behavior and endocrine responses. *Physiological Behavior,* **47**, 735–741.

32. Ogawa, T., Mikuni, M., Kuroda, Y. *et al.* (1994). Periodic maternal deprivation alters stress response in adult offspring: Potentiates the negative feedback regulation of restraint stress-induced adrenocortical response and reduces the frequencies of open field-induced behaviors. *Pharmacology, Biochemistry and Behavior,* **49**, 961–967.

33. Levine, S., Huchton, D. M., Wiener, S. G. and Rosenfeld, P. (1991). Time course of the effect of maternal deprivation on the hypothalamic–pituitary–adrenal axis in the infant rat. *Developmental Psychobiology,* **24**, 547–558.

34. Vazquez, D. M., van Oers, H., Levine S. and Akil, H. (1996). Regulation of glucocorticoid and mineralocorticoid receptor mRNAs in the hippocampus of the maternally deprived infant rat. *Brain Research, 731*, 79–90.

35. Rosenfeld, P., Wetmore, J. B. and Levine, S. (1992). Effects of repeated maternal separations on the adrenocortical response to stress of preweanling rats. *Physiological Behavior, 52*, 787–791.

36. Bugental, D. B., Martorell, G. A. and Barraza, V. (2003). The hormonal costs of subtle forms of infant maltreatment. *Hormones and Behavior, 43*, 237–244.

37. Cirulli, F., Santucci, D., Laviola, G., Alleva, E. and Levine, S. (1994). Behavioral and hormonal responses to stress in the newborn mouse: Effects of maternal deprivation and chlordiazepoxide. *Developmental Psychobiology, 27*, 301–316.

38. Levine, S. (1994). The ontogeny of the hypothalamic–pituitary–adrenal axis. The influence of maternal factors. *Annals of the New York Academy of Sciences, 746*, 275–288; discussion 289–293.

39. Heim, C., Newport, D. J., Bonsall, R., Miller A. H. and Nemeroff C. B. (2001). Altered pituitary–adrenal axis responses to provocative challenge tests in adult survivors of childhood abuse. *American Journal of Psychiatry, 158*, 575–581.

40. O'Donnell, S., Noseworthy, M. D., Levine, B. and Dennis, M. (2005). Cortical thickness of the frontopolar area in typically developing children and adolescents. *NeuroImage, 24*, 948–954.

41. Sowell, E. R., Thompson, P. M., Tessner, K. D. and Toga, A. W. (2001). Mapping continued brain growth and gray matter density reduction in dorsal frontal cortex: Inverse relationships during postadolescent brain maturation. *Journal of Neuroscience, 21*, 8819–8829.

42. Hayward, C. and Sanborn, K. (2002). Puberty and the emergence of gender differences in psychopathology. *Journal of Adolescent Health, 30*, 49–58.

43. Masten, A. S. (2004). Regulatory processes, risk, and resilience in adolescent development. *Annals of the New York Academy of Sciences, 1021*, 310–319.

44. McGue, M. and Iacono, W. G. (2005). The association of early adolescent problem behavior with adult psychopathology. *American Journal of Psychiatry, 162*, 1118–1124.

45. Goodyer, I. M., Park, R. J., Netherton, C. M. and Herbert, J. (2001). Possible role of cortisol and dehydroepiandrosterone in human development and psychopathology. *British Journal of Psychiatry, 179*, 243–249.

46. Grant, K. E., Compas, B. E., Stuhlmacher, A.F. *et al.* (2003). Stressors and child and adolescent psychopathology: Moving from markers to mechanisms of risk. *Psychology Bulletin, 129*, 447–466.

47. Pellis, S. M. and Pellis, V. C. (1990). Differential rates of attack, defense, and counterattack during the developmental decrease in play fighting by male and female rats. *Developmental Psychobiology, 23*, 215–231.

48. Pellis, S. M. and Pellis, V. C. (1997). The prejuvenile onset of play fighting in laboratory rats (Rattus norvegicus). *Developmental Psychobiology, 31*, 193–205.

49. Spear, L. P. (2000). The adolescent brain and age-related behavioral manifestations. *Neuroscience and Biobehavioral Reviews, 24*, 417–463.

50. Spear, L. (2000). Modeling adolescent development and alcohol use in animals. *Alcohol Research and Health, 24*, 115–123.

51. Penza, K. M., Heim, C. and Nemeroff, C. B. (2003). Neurobiological effects of childhood abuse: Implications for the pathophysiology of depression and anxiety. *Archives of Women's Mental Health, 6*, 15–22.

52. Vazquez, D. M. (1998). Stress and the developing limbic–hypothalamic–pituitary–adrenal axis. *Psychoneuroendocrinology, 23*, 663–700.

53. Romeo, R. D., Lee, S. J., Chhua, N., McPherson, C. R. and McEwen, B. S. (2004). Testosterone cannot activate an adult-like stress response in prepubertal male rats. *Neuroendocrinology, 79*, 125–132.

54. Einon, D. F. and Morgan, M. J. (1977). A critical period for social isolation in the rat. *Developmental Psychobiology, 10*, 123–132.

55. McGivern, R. F., Henschel, D., Hutcheson, M. and Pangburn, T . (1996). Sex difference in daily water consumption of rats: Effect of housing and hormones. *Physiological Behavior, 59*, 653–658.

56. van den Berg, C. L., van Ree, J. M. and Spruijt, B. M. (1999). Sequential analysis of juvenile isolation-induced decreased social behavior in the adult rat. *Physiological Behavior, 67*, 483–488.

57. van den Berg, C. L., van Ree, J. M., Spruijt, B. M. and Kitchen, I. (1999). Effects of juvenile isolation and morphine treatment on social interactions and opioid receptors in adult rats: Behavioural and autoradiographic studies. *European Journal of Neuroscience, 11*, 3023–3032.

58. van den Berg, C. L., Pijlman, F. T., Koning, H. A. *et al.* (1999). Isolation changes the incentive value of sucrose and social behaviour in juvenile and adult rats. *Behavioral and Brain Research, 106*, 133–142.

59. van den Berg, M. D., Oldehinkel, A. J., Brilman, E. I., Bouhuys, A. L. and Ormel, J. (2000). Correlates of symptomatic, minor and major depression in the elderly. *Journal of Affective Disorders, 60*, 87–95.

60. Maslova, L. N., Bulygina, V. V. and Popova, N. K. (2002). Immediate and long-lasting effects of chronic stress in the prepubertal age on the startle reflex. *Physiological Behavior, 75*, 217–225.

61. Tsoory, M. and Richter-Levin, G. (2006). Learning under stress in the adult rat is differentially affected by "juvenile" or "adolescent" stress. *The International Journal of Neuropsychopharmacology,* **9**, 713–728.

62. Avital, A. and Richter-Levin, G. (2005). Exposure to juvenile stress exacerbates the behavioural consequences of exposure to stress in the adult rat. *The International Journal of Neuropsychopharmacology,* **8**, 163–173.

63. Anthony, J. and Scott, P. (1960). Manic depressive psychosis in childhood. *Journal Child Psychology and Psychiatry,* **1**, 52–72.

64. Douvan, E. A. and Adelson, J. (1966). *The adolecent experience*. New York: Wiley.

65. Costello, E. J., Pine, D. S., Hammen, C. *et al.* (2002). Development and natural history of mood disorders. *Biological Psychiatry,* **52**, 529–542.

66. Lewinsohn, P. M., Solomon, A., Seeley, J. R. and Zeiss, A. (2000). Clinical implications of "subthreshold" depressive symptoms. *Journal of Abnormal Psychology,* **109**, 345–351.

67. Kessler, R. C., Avenevoli, S. and Ries Merikangas, K. (2001). Mood disorders in children and adolescents: An epidemiologic perspective. *Biological Psychiatry,* **49**, 1002–1014.

68. Tiet, Q. Q., Bird, H. R., Davies, M. *et al.* (1998). Adverse life events and resilience. *Journal of the American Academy of Child and Adolescent Psychiatry,* **37**, 1191–1200.

69. Pynoos, R. S., Steinberg, A. M. and Piacentini, J. C. (1999). A developmental psychopathology model of childhood traumatic stress and intersection with anxiety disorders. *Biological Psychiatry,* **46**, 1542–1554.

70. Kessler, R. C., Angermeyer, M., Anthony, J. C. *et al.* (2007). Lifetime prevalence and age-of-onset distributions of mental disorders in the World Health Organization's World Mental Health Survey Initiative. *World Psychiatry,* **6**, 168–176.

71. Cicchetti, D. (1996). Child maltreatment: Implications for developmental theory and research. *Human Development,* **39**, 18–39.

72. Jacobson-Pick, S., Elkobi, A., Vander, S., Rosenblum, K. and Richter-Levin, G. (2008). Juvenile stress-induced alteration of maturation of the GABAA receptor alpha subunit in the rat. *The International Journal of Neuropsychopharmacology,* **1**, 13.

73. Maslova, L. N., Bulygina, V. V. and Markel, A. L. (2002). Chronic stress during prepubertal development: Immediate and long-lasting effects on arterial blood pressure and anxiety-related behavior. *Psycho-neuroendocrinology,* **27**, 549–561.

74. Spear, L. P. (2004). Adolescent brain development and animal models. *Annals of the New York Academy of Sciences,* **1021**, 23–26.

75. Tsoory, M., Cohen, H. and Richter-Levin, G. (2007). Juvenile stress induces a predisposition to either anxiety or depressive-like symptoms following stress in adulthood. *European Neuropsychopharmacology,* **17**, 245–256.

76. Bostic, J. Q., Rubin, D. H., Prince, J. and Schlozman, S. (2005). Treatment of depression in children and adolescents. *Journal of Psychiatric Practice,* **11**, 141–154.

77. Volkmar, F. R. (2002). Changing perspectives on mood disorders in children. *American Journal of Psychiatry,* **159**, 893–894.

78. Kandel, D. B. and Davies, M. (1986). Adult sequelae of adolescent depressive symptoms. *Archives of General Psychiatry,* **43**, 255–262.

79. Kovacs, M., Gatsonis, C., Paulauskas, S. L. and Richards, C. (1989). Depressive disorders in childhood. IV. A longitudinal study of comorbidity with and risk for anxiety disorders. *Archives of General Psychiatry,* **46**, 776–782.

80. Bennett, D. S. Ambrosini, P. J., Kudes, D., Metz, C. and Rabinovich, H. (2005). Gender differences in adolescent depression: do symptoms differ for boys and girls. *Journal of Affective Disorders,* **89**, 35–44.

81. Klose, M. and Jacobi, F . (2004). Can gender differences in the prevalence of mental disorders be explained by sociodemographic factors? *Archives of Women's Mental Health,* **7**, 133–148.

82. Kornstein, S. G., Schatzberg, A. F., Thase, M. E. *et al.* (2000). Gender differences in chronic major and double depression. *Journal of Affective Disorders,* **60**, 1–11.

83. American Psychiatric Association . (1994). *Diagnostic and statistical manual of mental disorders,* 4th edn., Washington, DC: American Psychiatric Press.

84. Kessler, R. C., Sonnega, A., Bromet, E., Hughes, M. and Nelson, C.B. (1995). Posttraumatic stress disorder in the National Comorbidity Survey. *Archives of General Psychiatry,* **52**, 1048–1060.

85. Drossopoulou, G., Antoniou, K., Kitraki, E. *et al.* (2004). Sex differences in behavioral, neurochemical and neuroendocrine effects induced by the forced swim test in rats. *Neuroscience,* **126**, 849–857.

86. Walker, E. F., Sabuwalla, Z. and Huot, R. (2004). Pubertal neuromaturation, stress sensitivity, and psychopathology. *Developmental Psychopathology,* **16**, 807–824.

87. Ilin, Y. and Richter-Levin, G. (2009). Enriched environment experience overcomes learning deficits and depressive-like behavior induced by juvenile stress. *PLoS ONE,* **4**, e4329.

88. Koo, J. W., Park, C. H., Choi, S. H. *et al.* (2003). The postnatal environment can counteract prenatal effects on cognitive ability, cell proliferation, and synaptic protein expression. *FASEB Journal,* **17**, 1556–1558.

89. Yang, J., Li, W., Liu, X. *et al.* (2006). Enriched environment treatment counteracts enhanced addictive and depressive-like behavior induced by prenatal chronic stress. *Brain Research,* **1125**, 132–137.

# Chapter 10

# Lateral asymmetries in infants' regulatory and communicative gestures

Rosario Montirosso, Renato Borgatti and Ed Tronick

## Introduction

Lateralization of function is considered a central characteristic of brain organization [1–3] and is well established in adulthood. However, the nature of the lateralization during early development is controversial and findings are inconsistent. Our primary aim was to examine whether differences in the lateralization of expressive and regulatory gestures may reflect different hemispheric activity. To that end, the differential deployment of infant regulatory and social expressive gestures were examined during the non-stressful and stressful episodes of the Face-to-Face Still-Face paradigm (FFSF). Beyond the general importance of understanding the development of lateralization, examining the lateralization of emotional expressive as well as regulatory processes may have implications for infants' and young children's vulnerability to trauma and its effects such as dissociation.

Although neurophysiological and behavioral studies suggest an early functional brain asymmetry for emotional processing [4–8], the nature and even the presence of the specialization are debatable. According to some authors, the right hemisphere is specialized for the expression of emotion *regardless* of the hedonic valence or motivational significance of emotions [9,10]. In contrast, others argue that the hemispheres are more specialized, with the right hemisphere the seat of negative and avoidance-related emotions and the left hemisphere more specialized for positive emotions [11,12]. Despite the generality of the argument, few studies have looked at a range of emotional behaviors including gestures, postural changes and head movements as a way of examining lateralization, yet these behaviors are a critical feature of emotional expression and regulation and might be expected to be lateralized. Trevarthen [13] has argued that emotional gestures and self-regulatory gestures play an expressive function[1] and are a class of movement distinct from movements (either gratuitous or action-specific) related to posture, locomotion, object grasping and exploration. Gianino and Tronick [14] described infants as having two different kinds of emotional behavior: self-directed regulatory behaviors (e.g., looking away, self-comforting and even self-stimulation) to modulate their levels of arousal and affect and other-directed regulatory behaviors that function to express the infants' communicative or relational intent and solicitation of external regulation. Gianino and Tronick [14] hypothesized that self-directed regulatory behaviors would be expected in negative or possibly highly aroused positive states and stressful conditions, while other-directed behaviors would be expected during emotionally positive states with low levels of stress.

Note that the distinction between self- and other-directed behaviors is not hard and fast. Self-regulatory behaviors (e.g., thumb sucking) are utilized by the infant to regulate their emotional arousal, but they also simultaneously communicate the infant's state of regulatory stability and possible need for regulatory scaffolding from the caregiver, whereas other-directed behaviors may express infants' need for regulatory scaffolding from the caregiver (e.g., pick-me-up gestures). Although difficult to fully justify or document, a possible distinction between other- and self-directed behaviors may be that self-directed behaviors function

---

[1] Besides *emotional gestures* and *self-regulating* gestures, Trevarthen [13] proposed three other types of gestures: (a) *gratuitous gestures*, reflecting the infant's ability to pick up information from the environment such as grasping and manipulating an object; (b) *indicating gestures*, directing attention or action and aimed to show another person an object or place of interest in the environment; and (c) *symbolic gestures (emblems)*, constructing representations of actions, events, objects or situations.

*The Impact of Early Life Trauma on Health and Disease: The Hidden Epidemic*, ed. Ruth A. Lanius, Eric Vermetten and Clare Pain. Published by Cambridge University Press. Copyright © Cambridge University Press 2010.

inadvertently to communicate a need for regulation, the intent or goal associated with them being *self-regulation*, whereas other-directed behaviors are intentional solicitations. Whatever may turn out to be the case, these different functions suggest a differential deployment of self- and other-directed behaviors related to infants' affective state and contextual stress. Consequently, although such behaviors are complicated and not well understood, it is important to keep in mind that other-directed and self-directed regulatory behaviors are concurrent and reciprocal to each other such that each may affect the other [14–16]. Effective self-regulation, for example looking away, likely reduces the need for external regulatory scaffolding conveyed by other-directed gestures (e.g., banging hand on a surface). The regulatory system is highly dynamic over time.

Some research supports the suggestion of a differential deployment of self- and other-directed behaviors related to the stressfulness of the context to the infant. Gaze aversion as a component of the still-face effect can be seen as a form of self-directed regulation by the infant. Gianino and Tronick [14] found higher levels of self-soothing during the still-face. These behaviors are suggestive of self-directed attempts by infants to control high levels of arousal, negative emotions and behavioral dysregulation. These studies and others (for a review see Adamson and Frick [17]) have also found that infants actively engage in what can be seen as other-directed regulatory behaviors that function to express infants' interactive intent (vocalizing, gesturing and communicating distress) and attempts to reengage the mother. But are self- and other-directed behaviors lateralized? Certainly if there is lateralization of emotional expressive functioning one might expect the regulation of emotion to be lateralized as well. This is an important issue because trauma is not only about the emotions experienced but also about how they are regulated, a function that may be even more critical than the emotional experience in and of itself. Most of the lateralization hypotheses about emotions do not deal with the issue of regulation. An exception is that of Schore [18], who has brought together a broad array of research, too extensive to review here, and forcefully argued that the right hemisphere not only controls the expression of *all* emotions but is also the seat of emotion regulation.

Unfortunately, little evidence is available on lateralization of regulation. In a widely cited study Trevarthen [13,19] concluded that expressive and regulatory gestures (i.e., other-directed gestures) are asymmetrically organized to the left side of the brain. Trevarthen coded only active fingering of their cloths or free moving of the body as indicators of self-directed regulatory behaviors. Although he states that he found asymmetries, he also notes – and our examination of his data confirms – that the observed asymmetries were highly labile, varied from visit to visit and were different in different ways for boys and girls. The observed variability and gender differences do not fit the lateralization hypothesis. Using the same sample and set of still photographs, Trevarthen further argued that when the infants were mildly distressed (e.g., when they were confronted with an unresponsive mother), the pattern of gestures changed. The left hand was more active and the infants made more self-touching movements. This finding too suffers the same problems as those of the findings on other-directed behaviors (e.g., variability over sessions). Furthermore, Trevarthen did not find an increase in asymmetries with age, an expected finding based on the general principle that differentiation of function generally characterizes development.

There is other evidence suggestive of an asymmetrical organization of expressive gestures. Fogel and Hannan [20] observed asymmetric hand movements (i.e., other-directed gestures) indicating right-side activation when mothers were asked to "chat" with their 3-month-old infants during a 2 minute spontaneous face-to-face interaction. Murray [21], using a television replay test (i.e., loss of contingency simulated through a videotape replay of the mothers' responses) that disturbed the infants, found that 2-month-old infants increased touching of their clothes with *both* hands and showed increased and longer touching of their faces by their left hand, while expressive (other-directed) right-arm raising decreased. Neither the findings by Fogel and Hannan [20] nor those of Murray [21] support Trevarthen's conclusion [13,19], but they seem to support Schore's argument [18]. Therefore, the question of lateralization of either form of expressive gesture remains open.

Using the FFSF paradigm in the study described in this chapter, we evaluated if there is a differential distribution of self- and other-directed expressive gestures related to the context of the different episodes, and if there are differences in the lateralization of expressive gestures in infants during normal and stressful interactions, which would indicate differential emotional hemispheric activity during the second half of the first year of life. Our first hypothesis was that there would be a differential distribution of self- and other-directed gestures related to stress. Specifically, that there would be a greater use of other-directed gestures during normal interactions and a greater use of self-directed regulatory gestures during the still-face episode. In other words, we were expecting a *normal interaction gestures effect*, with more other-directed behaviors and a decrease in self-directed behaviors during the normal interaction compared with the still-face, and a reciprocal *still-face gestures effect*, with a reduction in other-directed gestures and an increase in self-directed gestures when the mother was unresponsive. Given Schore's hypothesis [18,22] of the role of the right hemisphere in the regulation of emotions, our second hypothesis was that there would be a prevalence of self-directed regulatory gestures performed with the left side of the body (right hemisphere) during the stressful condition. However, although Schore would predict lateralization of other-directed gestures, given the inconclusiveness of the literature on early functional left brain asymmetry for expressive emotional behaviour, we did not expect a lateralization of other-directed gestures during any episode.

## Research study

We studied 30 healthy full-term infants (14 females, 16 males). Infants were tested between 6 to 12 months of age (mean age, 8.3 ± 1.6). The infants were clinically normal and had uncomplicated prenatal, perinatal and neonatal courses. Left-handed mothers were excluded from the study because we found one study [23] that presented evidence for a maternal effect on infant hand-use preferences, as well as the more well-established finding of the genetics of hand preferences [24]. Mothers and infants were videotaped during the FFSF procedure based on the original paradigm developed by Tronick (see Tronick *et al.* [25] for details). Infants' gestures were coded using the Infant Self-directed Regulatory and Other-directed Gestures Coding System (ISOG; R. Montirosso, S. Marseglia and C. Pupino, unpublished data 2005). The ISOG was specifically designed for scoring the gestures that infants can make during the face-to-face interaction (R. Montirosso, R. Borgatti and T. Tronick unpublished data). The ISOG cover two areas: other-directed gestures and self-regulatory gestures. The other-directed gestures cover hand movements that express emotions and are usually associated with making interpersonal contact. These movements are accompanied by facial expressions, eye movements and vocalizations that further convey the subject's expressive intent to communicate (e.g., extending one or more fingers, arm moving upwards, banging hand on table, reaching out for mother, touching mother with hand). The self-directed regulatory gestures include hand movements aimed at facilitating, protecting or stimulating the body and at regulating the infant's inner state (e.g., touching a close surface, touching clothes, touching head or face, touching arm or hand, touching mouth or sucking one or more fingers). Only unilateral gestures were considered as these single-handed gestures are mutually exclusive. The ISOG coding used software developed by the Bioengineering Laboratory of Scientific Institute "E. Medea" (Picture Analyzer and Behavior Coder – PACO). This software allows coders to indicate the time unit to 1 second for each observed behavior. To evaluate reliability, one-third of the videotaped data was separately coded with each of two coding systems by independent coders blind to the study purposes and hypotheses. Different coders were used for the Infant and Caregiver Engagement Phases System [26] and the ISOG systems. Reliability was evaluated in two ways. The mean proportion of agreement ranged from 0.82 to 0.91% and Cohen's kappa values ranged from 0.71, caregiver engagement to 0.75.

The ISOG codes were grouped into four configurations: right-sided other-directed gestures; left-sided other-directed gestures; right-sided self-directed regulatory gestures; left-sided self-directed regulatory gestures. The proportion of time for the four ISOG configurations of gestures was calculated. To examine if there was a global lateral bias affecting the gestures, two combined variables were obtained by separately totaling the proportions of two kinds of expressive gestures produced by each infant with the left side of the body (left-sided gestures combined left-sided other-directed and self-directed gestures) and the right side (right-sided gestures combined right-sided other-directed and self-directed gestures). These measures reflect the proportions of gestures for each side of the body during each episode of the FFSF, regardless of type. To examine if there was an expressive gestures effect related to episode, two combined variables were obtained by summing the proportions of self-directed regulatory gestures (combining right-sided and left-sided self-directed gestures) and other-directed gestures (combining right-sided and left-sided other-directed gestures). These measures reflect the overall amount of self-directed regulatory gestures and other-directed

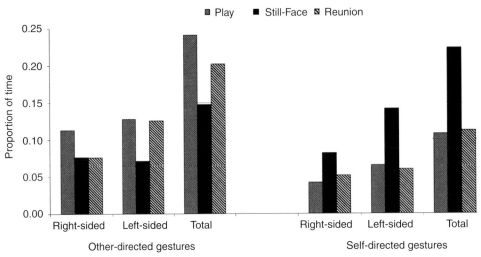

**Fig. 10.1.** Mean proportion time of infant's gestures performed with the right or left hemibody across the Face-to-Face Still-Face paradigm.

gestures produced by each infant during each episode of the FFSF, regardless of body side. The following questions were pursued using the generated data.

*Was there an overall left-side or right-side gestures bias and a gender effect?* The findings suggested that infants showed no significant overall lateral bias of gestures, that is, no tendency to have more movements on one side compared to the other; there were no findings for gender.

*Were there increases in other-directed behaviors and decreases in self-directed gestures during the normal interaction and reductions in other-directed gestures and increases in self-directed gestures during the still-face?* The findings supported the hypothesis of a self-other-directed gestures effect by episode (Fig. 10.1). Self-directed gestures significantly increased from play episode to still-face and decreased from still-face to the reunion episode, returning to the levels of the play episode. Other-directed gestures significantly decreased from play to still-face and significantly increased from still-face to reunion, but did not return to the level in the play episode. These findings highlight a *still-face gestures effect* and a *reunion gestures effect*, supporting the interpretation that the reunion episode is a challenging task for the infant (Fig. 10.1).

*Was there a prevalence of self-directed regulatory gestures performed with the left-side of the body (right hemisphere activation) during the stressful condition?* Self-directed regulatory gestures performed with the left side were significantly more common during the still-face than during the play and reunion episodes, supporting the hypothesis that there would be an asymmetry of left-sided self-directed regulatory gestures.

*Was there a lateralization of other-directed gestures?* Analysis revealed a significant overall main effect of episode for left-sided other-directed gestures as well (Fig. 10.1). Other-directed regulatory gestures performed with the left side were significantly more common during the play and reunion than during the still-face. There were no significant main effects for other-directed gestures and self-directed gestures performed with the right side.

## Discussion

This study evaluated the differential utilization and lateralization by infants of socioemotional expressive gestures and self-directed coping (self-directed regulatory gestures versus other-directed gestures). The findings support the hypothesis that there is a differential distribution of self-directed and other-directed gestures related to the stress experienced by the infant. Other-directed gestures were more common during the play and reunion and self-directed behaviors were more common during the still-face phases of the FFSF. Self-directed as well as other-directed gestures were lateralized to the left side. These findings suggest that during the FFSF infants showed greater right hemisphere activation and that the activation is associated with different kind of gestures related to episode.

The findings confirm our first hypothesis. The findings on the preferential distribution of self-directed gestures related to stress are consistent with studies reporting an increase of self-touching behaviors for infants during several stressful situations, such as being left alone by the mother, the entrance of a stranger, a television replay test or maternal still-face [21,27–30]. They are also consistent with the findings of increased infant self-clasping and oral self-comfort behaviors in infants of depressed mothers. Thus infants make a greater use of gestures to self-regulate the negative states experienced during the still-face. One might well expect that infants and children who experience trauma will show much more extreme, perhaps chronic, differential distributions of self- versus other-directed behaviors, with self-directed gestures in greater prominence. The occurrence of such extremes may be possible signs of trauma (see below).

The findings suggest that gestures are an essential component of the mix of modalities that are assembled for self-regulatory purposes and that they should be given more consideration in future studies. The results also confirm that infant self-regulation increases in various distress situations. Furthermore, the findings in the reunion episode support that there also is a differential deployment of self- and other-directed regulatory behaviors and make clear just how complex the interplay is between forms of regulation and affect. Although the levels of negative affect in the reunion episode remain at the levels seen with still-face, the level of positive affect returns to play episode levels. Self-directed gestures reduce from still-face levels and return to the play episode levels, while other-directed gestures are still below the level seen in the play but higher than during the still-face. The finding on the high level of negative affect supports the argument advanced by Weinberg and Tronick [31] that the reunion episode actually is stressful because of the carryover of negative affect from the recent experience of the still-face and because the dyad also has to renegotiate and repair the stress of mismatches inherent to normal interactions [15].

This explanation however, does not seem complete because it would also be reasonable to expect a very high level of self-directed gesturing to regulate the stress of the reunion, something not seen. Perhaps the findings suggest that self-directed regulation even in the face of high levels of negative affect can be modulated or offset by high levels of positive affect, as seen in the reunion episode. A further speculation is that because of the immediate past negative experience of the still-face episode, infants are still hesitant to use other-directed gestures with the mother for fear that she will not respond. In a sense it may be that following the still-face, infants are unable to make sense out of the mothers' intent during the reunion – she simultaneously is saying "hello" and "goodbye" [25] – and as a consequence the infants do not yet trust that she will respond to their other-directed gestures. Consequently, their intention to communicate remains diminished and other-directed behaviors remain relatively low. Such confusion may well characterize children who have experienced trauma and may lead to their hesitancy to interact even with individuals who were not part of their traumatic experience.

Overall differential distribution of self- and other-directed behaviors in relation to the different social contexts suggests that the regulatory capacities of the infant are highly tuned and quite sophisticated. The infants experience the different contexts differently, appear to quickly make sense of them, and to organize a different regulatory strategy in each. This degree of regulatory sophistication is greater than one might expect from many existing brain models of regulatory control, which suggest that cortical development of executive centers is requisite for effective self-regulation [32]; however, a different view is put forward by Wager et al. [33]. Rather, the findings suggest that regulatory control is found in the limbic or other lower structures that control emotions and their expression and the regulation of emotions, and that the mechanisms controlling them change with development. Thus, it might be more reasonable to suggest that regulation and activation are always coupled regardless of the mechanisms involved. Brazelton [34], for example, has shown that even newborns are capable of self-regulating their levels of arousal using gestures (e.g., thumb sucking) or the deployment of attention (e.g., looking at objects, attending to sounds) long before cortical or possibly even limbic mechanisms are developed. One might picture a functional organization of the brain in which action capacities generated at one level of the brain at one developmental stage are part of a larger organization that is capable of regulating those same capacities. In a sense, there are functional arcs in which capacities – for example, for action and inhibition – develop together to be replaced in development by more advanced action and inhibitory capacities [35]. Therefore, during the episodes of the FFSF paradigm, infants can engage in other- and self-directed behaviors that involve both these action-oriented behaviors and simultaneously regulate them, and the control is found in limbic and other brain areas without any great involvement of cortical mechanisms.

Another of the findings on gestures during the reunion episode is noteworthy. Prior work has shown that facial and vocal communication during the reunion episode return to the levels seen in the first play episode. Here we found that other-directed gestures did not. These findings indicate that the different expressive systems – facial expressions, vocalization and gestures – are not as tightly linked as was previously thought [30]. The less-tight coupling among the different modalities suggests the speculation that infants can make blended configurations or assemblages of expressive gestures in which one modality enhances or diminishes the meaning or intensity of another modality. For example, blended intermodality configurations might convey different messages at the same time – smiles communicating an intention for social engagement while simultaneous self-touching communicates the intention to disengage. Blended communicative configurations might also convey differences in the intensity of the message (e.g., smiling while self-touching conveys that the infant intends to play, but that the play should be low-key, whereas a smile coupled with a big other-directed gesture conveys the intention to play intensely). Certainly, consideration of gestures in relation to other expressive modalities suggests that infants' communicative repertoires are not only complexly organized but also nuanced and subtle. The existence of this blending would contradict the view held by those examining facial expressions that blended emotions are a later development [36]. The findings suggest that we should look more carefully at the interplay of expressive systems and the subtleties of facial expression that have typically been seen as disorganized. Such an examination might reveal an orderliness in the relations of the subtle facial changes and gestural expressions.

As expected, we found that left-sided regulatory gestures were more frequent during the still-face than during the play and reunion episodes, indicative of a greater activation of the right hemisphere. We also found that during normal interactions infants performed other-directed gestures with the left side. These findings suggest that right hemisphere activation is associated with behaviors related to normal and stressful interactive conditions. The finding is consistent with the work of Bazhenova and colleagues [37] and with electrophysiological investigations performed during separation from the mother and withdrawal

as a result of negative emotional conditions. During these conditions, a selective activation of the right frontotemporal anterior regions has been documented [38,39]. These findings support a growing body of evidence showing that the neural circuitry of the stress system is located in the right brain [22,40–43]. Consequently, it seems plausible that infants cope with the emotional distress caused by unresponsive mothers through self-regulation behaviors associated with a greater activation of the right hemisphere. In sum, this finding supports the view that during a stressful condition there is a state-dependent activation of the right hemisphere [22,39]. Our finding of increased left-sided other-directed behaviors during normal interaction associated with making interpersonal contact (e.g., touching mother with hand) is inconsistent with previous experimental findings and with theoretical views suggesting that it is the left side of the brain that controls the approach behaviors [44]. Therefore, it is possible to suggest that the right hemisphere is involved in both positive interpersonal contact and its regulation. More generally, these findings suggest that the right hemisphere is more involved in the social and biological functions involved in infant–caregiver emotional bonding [22,45]. Alternatively, our findings on the lateralization of self- and other-directed behaviors to the right hemisphere could be explained in the light of the well-established observation that the right side of the brain matures more quickly than the left side [46–48]. Such a left–right gradient could be evaluated by looking at asymmetries of other-directed behaviors in *younger* infants and following them longitudinally. We think Schore would predict strong lateralization of other-directed behaviors in younger infants that continues with development or, perhaps, with the development of increasing complex and explicit social behavior, the control shifting to the left side of the brain with a concomitant a reduction in asymmetry. This suggestion would integrate Schore's and Davidson's views with a developmental perspective.

## Conclusions

Our study shows self- and other-directed behaviors to be differentially deployed in relation to the stressfulness of the context, a finding which suggests that infants are sensitive to what is going on in an interaction and adjust their behaviors in highly specific ways. Support for a lateralization of self- and other-directed behaviors to the right hemisphere was found, lending support to views of the specialization of the right

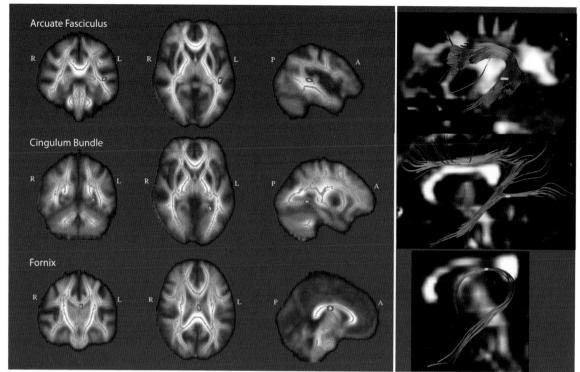

**Fig. 11.2.** Three white matter tract regions (shown in red) differed significantly in fractional anisotropy (FA) between subjects with history of exposure to high levels of parental verbal aggression and healthy controls. Region 1 contained fibers from arcuate fasciculus. Region 2 contained fibers from the cingulum bundle near the tail of the hippocampus. Region 3 is part of the left fornix. Green shows the mean FA skeleton and background image is in MNI 152. Tractography (far right panel) from representative subjects show tracts passing through the region of reduced FA identified by tract-based spatial statistics. (Modified from Choi *et al.* [47] with permission.)

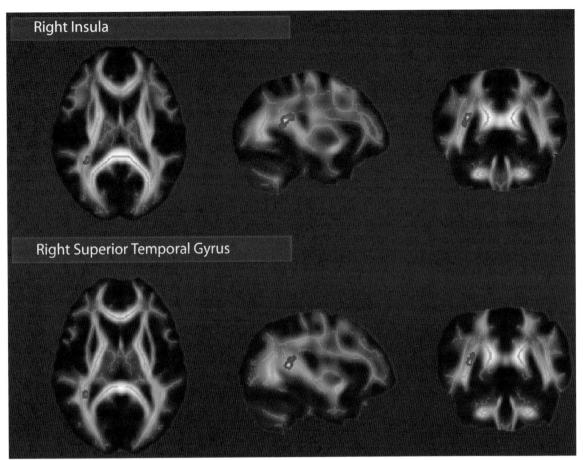

**Fig. 11.3.** Regions identified by tract-based spatial statistics (shown in red) in which there was an inverse correlation between degree of exposure to peer verbal bullying and fractional anisotropy in white matter tracts. Regions identified were in the right insula (Brodmann's area 13; MNI coordinates: 31, −39, 18; 33 voxels; $p = 0.024$), and right superior temporal gyrus (MNI coordinates: 34, −44, 10; 11 voxels; $p = 0.018$).

hemisphere for both regulatory and communicative emotional processing. The findings suggest the need to study the use of different gestures with simultaneous measurement of brain function over a wider age span. Such studies would also be useful with samples of high-risk infants whose behavior and brain organization may be compromised (e.g., preterm infants, infants with lateralized white matter disorder). This hypothesis about preterm infants is currently under investigation at our laboratory.

One final point. Infant gestures are a lifelong form of human communication that is used to convey meaning even earlier than the onset of language. However, it remains controversial as to whether gestures should be considered part of the linguistic system or a separate system for conveying meaning. It is well established that the left hemisphere is specialized for language. Even infant babbling is lateralized to the left hemisphere [49]. In contrast, the neural sites for the expression of social–emotional communication are generally viewed as lateralized to the right hemisphere. Had we found other-directed gestures lateralized to the right side of the body it would suggest that, like babbling, they are linguistic in nature. However, we found that these were preferentially distributed to the left side of the body, suggesting that the neural basis of gestures develops independently from the development of the linguistic system and that the gestural system for conveying meaning is an independent meaning-making system.

In conclusion, the present research demonstrates the need to consider gestures when evaluating regulatory and interactive behavior and the usefulness of these behaviors for exploring the development of lateralization and the subtlety of expressive behavior in infants. Micro-analytic study of gestures and other expressive modalities over time in different contexts with samples of low- and high-risk infants and dyads is needed to further explore these issues.

## Acknowledgements

This research was supported by funds of the Italian Health Minister (Ricerca Corrente 2004), partially supported by an unrestricted educational grant from Chiesi Farmaceutici, and NICHD grants (Ed Tronick, PI). We wish to thank Patrizia Cozzi for her help in the video recording of the mother-child interactions. Also, we are grateful to Sara Marseglia and Chiara Pupino for their help in data coding. Finally, our special thanks go to all the infants and their mothers participating in this study.

## References

1. Vallortigara, G. (2006). The evolutionary psychology of left and right: Costs and benefits of lateralization. *Developmental Psychobiology,* **48**, 418–427.

2. Corballis, M. C. (2009). Review. The evolution and genetics of cerebral asymmetry. *Philososphical Transactions of The Royal Society of London, Series B, Biological Sciences,* **364**, 867–879.

3. Schaafsma, S. M., Riedstra, B. J., Pfannkuche, K. A., Bouma, A. and Groothuis, T. G. (2009). Epigenesis of behavioural lateralization in humans and other animals. *Philososphical Transactions of The Royal Society of London, Series B, Biological Sciences,* **364**, 915–927.

4. Vargha-Khadem, F. and Corballis, M. C. (1979). Cerebral asymmetry in infants, *Brain and Language,* **8**, 1–9.

5. Davidson, R. J. and Tomarken, A. J. (1989). Laterality and emotion: An electrophysiological approach. In: F. Boller and J. Grafman (eds.), *Handbook of neuropsychology,* Vol. 3 (pp. 419–441). Amsterdam: Elsevier.

6. Fox, N. A. (1991). If it's not left, it's right: Electroencephalograph asymmetry and the development of emotion. *American Psychologist,* **46**, 863–872.

7. Davidson, J. R. (1992). Emotion and affective style: Hemispheric substrates. *Psychological Science,* **3**, 39–43.

8. Olko, C. and Turkewitz, G. (2001). Cerebral asymmetry of emotion and its relationship to olfactory in infancy. *Laterality: Asymmetries of Body, Brain and Cognition,* **6**, 29–37.

9. Campbell, R. (1978). Asymmetries in interpreting and expressing a posed facial expression. *Cortex,* **14**, 327–342.

10. Sackeim, H. A. and Gur, R. C. (1978). Lateral asymmetry in intensity of emotional expression. *Neuropsychologia,* **16**, 473–481.

11. Buss, K. A., Malmstadt Schumacher, J. R., Dolski, I. *et al.* (2003). Right frontal brain activity, cortisol, and withdrawal behavior in 6-month-old infants. *Behavioral Neuroscience,* **117**, 11–20.

12. Davidson, R. J. (1984). Affect, cognition and hemispheric specialization. In C. E. Izard, J. Kagan and R. Zajonc (eds.), *Emotion, cognition and behavior* (pp. 320–365). New York: Cambridge University Press.

13. Trevarthen, C. (1986). Form, significance and psychological potential of hand gestures of infants. In: J. L. Nespoulos, P. Peron and A. R. Lecours (eds.), *The biological foundation of gestures: Motor and semiotic aspects* (pp. 149–202). Hillsdale, NJ: Lawrence Erlbaum.

14. Gianino, A. and Tronick, E. Z. (1988). The mutual regulation model: The infant's self and interactive regulation and coping and defensive capacities. In T. Field, P. McCabe and N. Schneiderman (eds.), *Stress and coping* (pp. 47–68). Hillsdale, NJ: Lawrence Erlbaum.

15. Tronick, E. Z. (1989). Emotions and emotional communication in infants. *American Psychologist,* **44,** 112–119.

16. Beebe, B. and Lachmann, F. M. (2002). *Infant research and adult treatment: Co-constructing interactions.* Hillsdale, NY: Analytic Press.

17. Adamson, L. B. and Frick, J. E. (2003). The still-face: A history of a shared experimental paradigm. *Infancy,* **4,** 451–473.

18. Schore, A. N. (2003). *Affect dysregulation and disorders of the self.* New York: Norton.

19. Trevarthen, C. (1996). Lateral asymmetries in infancy: Implications for the development of the hemispheres, *Neuroscience and Biobehavioral Reviews,* **20,** 571–586.

20. Fogel, A. and Hannan, T. E. (1985). Manual actions of nine- to fifteen-week-old human infants during face-to-face interaction with their mothers. *Child Development,* **56,** 1271–1279.

21. Murray, L. (1980). *The sensitivities and expressive capacities of young infants in communication with their mothers.* PhD Thesis. University of Edinburgh.

22. Schore, A. N. (2005). Back to basics: Attachment, affect regulation, and the developing right brain – linking developmental neuroscience to pediatrics. *Pediatrics in Review,* **26,** 204–217.

23. Harkins, D. A. and Michel, G. F. (1988). Evidence for a maternal effect on infant hand-use preferences. *Developmental Psychobiology,* **21,** 535–541.

24. Annet, M. (1985). *Left, right, hand and brain: The right shift in theory.* Hillsdale, NJ: Lawrence Erlbaum.

25. Tronick, E. Z., Als, H., Adamson, L., Wise, S. and Brazelton, T. B. (1978). The infant's response to entrapment between contradictory messages in face-to-face interaction. *Journal of the American Academy of Child Psychiatry,* **17,** 1–13.

26. Weinberg, M. K. and Tronick, E. Z. (1999). *Infant and caregivers engagement phases (ICEP).* Boston, MA: Harvard Medical School.

27. Trevarthen, C. (1977). Descriptive analyses of infant communicative behavior. In R. Schaffer (ed.), *Studies in mother–infant interaction* (pp. 227–270). London: Academic Press.

28. Trevarthen, C. (1979). Communication and cooperation in early infancy: A description of primary intersubjectivity. In M. Bullowa (ed.), *Before speech: The beginnings of human communication* (pp. 321–347). London: Cambridge University Press.

29. Murray, L. and Trevarthen, C. (1985). Emotional regulation of interactions between two-months-olds and their mothers. In: T. M. Field and N. A. Fox (eds.), *Social perception in infants* (pp. 177–198). Norwood, NJ: Ablex.

30. Weinberg, M. K. and Tronick, E. Z. (1994). Beyond the face: An empirical study of infant affective configurations of facial, vocal, gestural and regulatory behaviors. *Child Development,* **65,** 1503–1515.

31. Weinberg, M. K. and Tronick, E. Z. (1996). Infant affective reactions to the resumption of maternal interaction after the still-face. *Child Development,* **67,** 905–914.

32. Quirk, G. J. and Beer, J. S. (2006). Prefrontal involvement in the regulation of emotion: Convergence of rat and human studies. *Current Opinion in Neurobiology,* **16,** 723–727.

33. Wager, T. D., Davidson, M. L., Hughes, B. L., Lindquist, M. A. and Ochsner, K. N. (2008). Prefrontal–subcortical pathways mediating successful emotion regulation. *Neuron,* **59,** 1037–1050.

34. Brazelton, T. B. (1972). Implications of infant development among the Mayan Indians of Mexico. *Human Development,* **15,** 90–111.

35. Anokhin P. K. (1974). *Biology and neurophysiology of the conditioned reflex and its role in adaptive behaviour.* Oxford: Pergamon Press.

36. Ekman, P. and Friesen, W. V. (1975). *Unmasking the face: A guide to recognizing emotions from facial clues.* Englewood Cliffs, NJ: Prentice-Hall.

37. Bazhenova, O. V., Stroganova, T. A., Doussard-Roosevelt, J. A., Posikera, I. A. and Porges, S. W. (2007). Physiological responses of 5-month-old infants to smiling and blank faces. *International Journal of Psychophysiology,* **63,** 64–76.

38. Davidson, R. J. and Fox, N. A. (1989). Frontal brain asymmetry predicts infants' response to maternal separation. *Journal of Abnormal Psychology,* **98,** 127–131.

39. Davidson, R. J. (2004). What does the prefrontal cortex "do" in affect: Perspectives on frontal EEG asymmetry research. *Biological Psychology,* **67,** 219–233.

40. Sullivan, R. M. and Gratton, A. (1999). Lateralized effects of medial prefrontal cortex lesions on neuroendocrine and autonomic stress responses in rats. *Journal of Neuroscience,* **19,** 2834–2840.

41. Sullivan, R. M. (2004). Hemispheric asymmetry in stress processing in rat prefrontal cortex and the role of mesocortical dopamine. *Stress,* **7,** 131–143.

42. Spence, S., Shapiro, D. and Zaidel, E. (1996). The role of the right hemisphere in the physiological and cognitive components of emotional processing. *Psychophysiology,* **33,** 112–122.

43. Wittling, W. (1997). The right hemisphere and the human stress response. *Acta Physiologica Scandinavica Supplementum,* **640,** 55–59.

44. Davidson, R. J., Ekman, P., Saron, C. D., Senulis, J. A. and Friesen, W. V. (1990). Approach-withdrawal and cerebral asymmetry. *Journal of Personality and Social Psychology,* **58,** 330–341.

45. Siegel, D. (1999). *The developing mind.* New York: Guilford Press.

46. Joseph, R. (1982). The neuropsychology of development hemispheric laterality, limbic language, and the origin of thought. *Journal of Clinical Psychology*, **38**, 4–33.

47. Saugstad, L. F. (1998). Cerebral lateralisation and rate of maturation. *International Journal of Psychophysiology*, **28**, 37–62.

48. Best, C. T. and Queen, H. F. (1989). Baby, it's in your smile: Right hemiface bias in infant emotional expressions. *Developmental Psychology,* **25**, 264–276.

49. Holowka, S. and Petitto, L. A. (2002). Left hemisphere cerebral specialization for babies while babbling. *Science*, **297**, 1515.

# Neurobiology of childhood trauma and adversity

Martin H. Teicher, Keren Rabi, Yi-Shin Sheu, Sally B. Seraphin, Susan L. Andersen, Carl M. Anderson, Jeewook Choi and Akemi Tomoda

## Introduction

Exposure to childhood adversity leads to the early initiation of drug, alcohol and nicotine use and risky sexual behaviors [1] and accounts for 50–75% of the population attributable risk for alcoholism, drug abuse, depression and suicide [2,3]. It also substantially increases risk for ischemic heart disease, chronic obstructive pulmonary disease, liver disease and obesity [4]. This powerful adverse relationship is best understood as a cascade. Exposure to early adversity alters trajectories of brain development, which, in turn, leads to social emotional and cognitive impairment, followed by the adoption of health-risk behaviors [1].

Childhood adversity is the result of exposure to traumatic events, as well as exposure to dysregulation in the quality of parent–child interactions (e.g., Lyons-Ruth et al. [5]). Hence, the Adverse Childhood Experience study (Ch. 8) quantified adversity based on occurrence of specific types of abuse (physical abuse [PA], sexual abuse [SA], witnessing domestic violence [WDV], verbal abuse–threats), and on the presence of risk factors associated with disruption in parent–child interactions. These include having a family member mentally ill, abusing substances, or incarcerated, along with parental loss through death, divorce or separation [1,4].

Research efforts since the mid 1990s have identified a host of structural and functional neurobiological abnormalities associated with exposure to early life trauma, most specifically PA, SA or neglect. This chapter will review the major findings stemming from this research and present new data suggesting that there are sensitive periods when particular brain regions may be most susceptible to the effects of abuse. Finally, new findings looking at the neurobiological correlates of exposure to other forms of adversity will be considered including parental verbal abuse (PVA), peer verbal bullying (VB) and WDV.

## Neurobiological effects of physical abuse, sexual abuse or neglect

The following section will first summarize preclinical studies that delineate the effects of early stress on specific brain regions found to be vulnerable. It will then discuss clinical studies reviewing the effects of childhood abuse on the development of these regions in humans. We should emphasize from the outset that research on the "effects of childhood trauma on brain development" is correlational. Children are not randomly assigned to abused or non-abused conditions. The studies conducted to date provide evidence for associations between abuse history and neurobiological differences; they do not prove causality. Alternative explanations are possible. For instance, the abused subjects may have had a preexisting neurobiological abnormality that increased their risk of being abused. It is also possible that the abused subjects had an inherited abnormality that increases the risk of abusive behavior by family members or relatives. (Evidence that neurobiological differences occur in subjects abused by unrelated individuals tends to rule out this possibility.) Preclinical studies demonstrating that early stress exerts comparable CNS effects helps to support a causal link [6]. The literature reviewed here is consistent with the hypothesis that early abuse alters brain development, and we present it from this perspective. Nevertheless, it is important to emphasize that these studies demonstrate significant associations and not a direct cause–effect relationship.

## Corpus callosum and hemispheric integration

Myelinated regions such as the corpus callosum are potentially vulnerable to the impact of early exposure to excessive levels of stress hormones, which suppress

*The Impact of Early Life Trauma on Health and Disease: The Hidden Epidemic*, ed. Ruth A. Lanius, Eric Vermetten and Clare Pain. Published by Cambridge University Press. Copyright © Cambridge University Press 2010.

glial cell division critical for myelination. Pioneering studies by Victor Denenberg and colleagues showed that corpus callosum size was markedly affected by early experience, and that the effects were gender dependent [7]. Sanchez *et al.* [8] found that rearing male monkeys in an isolating environment attenuated the development of the corpus callosum, and that diminished size was associated with defects in learning tasks. The first hint that the corpus callosum may be adversely affected by childhood trauma was provided by Teicher *et al.* in 1997 [9]. This observation was extended by De Bellis [10], who showed that reduced corpus callosum size was the most prominent anatomical finding in children with a history of abuse and post-traumatic stress disorder (PTSD). Males were more affected than females. More recently, the corpus callosum of boys has been shown to be particularly vulnerable to the effects of neglect [11]. The corpus callosum of girls appears to be more vulnerable to SA [11]. Reduced size of the corpus callosum has been associated with diminished communication between the hemispheres. Schiffer *et al.* [12] used probe auditory evoked potentials to study laterality and hemispheric integration of memory in adults with a history of childhood maltreatment. Maltreatment was associated with increased hemispheric laterality and decreased hemispheric integration.

## Hippocampus

Preclinical studies have demonstrated the vulnerability of the hippocampus to the ravages of stress. This region has a protracted ontogeny, persistent postnatal neurogenesis [13] and a high density of glucocorticoid receptors. Exposure to corticosteroids can markedly alter pyramidal cell morphology and can even produce pyramidal cell death [14]. Stress also suppresses production of new granule cells [13], and early stress prevents the normal peripubertal overproduction of synapses in the hippocampus of rats but does not prevent pruning, thus leading to an enduring deficit in synaptic density [15].

Bremner *et al.* [16] and Stein [17] first reported a reduction in left hippocampal volume in adults with a history of childhood trauma and a current diagnosis of PTSD or dissociative identity disorder. Driessen and colleagues [18] reported a 16% reduction in hippocampal volume bilaterally in women with borderline personality disorder (BPD) and a history of childhood abuse. More recently, Vythilingam *et al.*, [19] reported a 15–18% reduction in left hippocampal volume in

women with prepubertal PA and/or SA and depression relative to healthy control or depressed women who had not been exposed to childhood abuse. Vermetten and colleagues [20] reported a 19.2% hippocampal reduction bilaterally in women with childhood abuse and dissociative identity disorder. However, De Bellis *et al.* [10] conducted detailed volumetric analysis of the hippocampus in 44 maltreated children with PTSD and in 61 controls. They failed to observe a significant difference in hippocampal volume. Carrion *et al.*, [21] also failed to find a significant reduction in hippocampal volume in abused children with PTSD, as did De Bellis [22] in a separate sociodemographically matched sample. We conducted a complete volumetric analysis of the hippocampus in 17 healthy female young adult controls (18–22 years of age) and 26 young women with repeated childhood SA [23]. Unlike previous studies, these were not patients, but a non-clinical community sample. Only 6 of the 26 abused subjects met current criteria for PTSD and no subjects had a history of drug or alcohol use. Hippocampal volume was reduced bilaterally (6.8%), and loss of hippocampal volume was most apparent in young adults who indicated that SA occurred between 3 and 5 or 11 and 13 years of age (see below) [23].

Why might six studies consistently report reduced hippocampal volume in adults with a history of childhood abuse while three studies consistently failed to find any differences in children? As we have discussed [6,15], there are several possibilities. One possibility is that PTSD and depression exert a very gradual degenerative effect so that the adverse consequences are not discernable in children. Another possibility is that reduced hippocampal size may be an artifact of the high levels of alcohol abuse that often occur in adults with PTSD, BPD or depression. Still another possibility is that reduced hippocampal size is not a consequence of exposure to stress but a risk factor for development of chronic PTSD, as Gilbertson *et al.* [24] proposed based on their study of twins discordant for combat exposure. We proposed that stress exerts a delayed effect on hippocampal morphometry that becomes manifest in early adulthood, as we have observed in rats exposed to maternal isolation stress [15]. This may occur through stress-induced programming of neurotropic factors regulating overproduction and pruning.

## Amygdala

The amygdaloid nuclei are some of the most sensitive structures in the brain for the emergence of kindling, an important phenomenon in which repeated inter-mittent stimulation produces greater and greater alteration in neuronal excitability, which may even-tually result in seizures [25]. However, the emergence of seizure activity is not critical; kindling results in long-term alterations in neuronal excitability that can have major impact on behavioral control [25]. Early stress alters development and subunit structure of the GABA$_A$ receptor supramolecular complex in the amygdala, reducing the density of both the central benzodiazepine-binding sites and the high affinity GABA-binding sites on the receptors [26]. Gamma-aminobutyric acid (GABA) is a crucial inhibitory neurotransmitter that attenuates electrical excitabil-ity. Polymorphisms in GABA subunits may be asso-ciated with anxiety, neuronal irritability and seizure susceptibility [27].

Abnormalities in amygdala or hippocampal devel-opment and a diminished density of benzodiazepine-binding sites and high-affinity GABA-binding sites receptors may lead to the emergence of temporal lobe or limbic seizure-like activity. In our initial studies on the impact of childhood abuse, we reasoned that early stress could affect the development of the amygdala or hippocampus and produce seizure-like psychomotor phenomenon in the absence of seizures. We created the Limbic System Checklist-33 (LSCL-33) to rate the occurrence of the symptoms that often emerge dur-ing temporal lobe seizures (e.g., perceptual distor-tions, brief hallucinatory events, motor automatisms, dissociative phenomenon) to ascertain whether such symptoms, which we refer to as "limbic irritability," were associated with exposure to early abuse [28]. Adult outpatients with self-reported history of PA or SA had increased LSCL-33 scores, and these scores were dra-matically elevated in patients with a history of com-bined abuse [28]. Subsequently, it was demonstrated that psychiatrically hospitalized children with a history of abuse had a twofold increased incidence of clinically significant electroencephalograph (EEG) abnormalities [29]. The abnormalities were frontotemporal in origin and consisted of spikes, sharp waves or paroxysmal slowing. There was also a strong association between EEG abnormalities and history of self-destructive or violent behaviors. Children with a Massachusetts Department of Social Services confirmed diagnosis of depressive signs and symptoms and a history of severe PA or SA (without head trauma) had a 72% incidence of EEG abnormalities. Interestingly, Davies [30] found the same high rate of EEG abnormalities in a sample of incest survivors. However, he did not believe that this was a consequence of the SA, but a risk factor for being molested [30].

## Cerebral cortex

The neocortex as a whole matures slowly through cyclic processes of reorganization [31]. Delayed myelination of the cerebral cortex enables the two hemispheres to develop relatively independently. Language and motor lateralization is largely established before 5 years of age. Right hemisphere specialization for perception of human faces emerges between 8 and 13 years. Early experience can exert marked effects on lateralization in laboratory animals [6].

The prefrontal cortex has the most delayed func-tional ontogeny of any brain region. Major projections to the prefrontal cortex scarcely begin to myelinate until adolescence, and this process continues into the third decade of life. We have theorized that early stress activates the prefrontal cortex and alters its develop-ment. This may produce precocious maturation of the prefrontal cortex, leading to signs of early maturation ("parentified child"), but may arrest the development of this region, preventing it from reaching full adult capacity [32].

The effects of childhood trauma on the devel-opment of the left versus right hemisphere was investigated using EEG coherence, which provides information regarding the nature of the brain's wiring and circuitry [33]. Coherence measures indicated that left hemisphere development of abused subjects lagged substantially behind healthy controls [9,34].

De Bellis et al. [35] used single-voxel proton mag-netic resonance spectroscopy to measure the relative concentration of N-acetylaspartate and creatine in the anterior cingulate cortex of 11 abused children and adolescents with PTSD and 11 healthy matched com-parison subjects. They found a significant reduction in the ratio of N-acetylacetate to creatine in the abused subjects. N-acetylacetate to creatine is located prima-rily within neurons, and reduction of N-acetylacetate to creatine is a marker of neuronal loss or dysfunction.

Carrion and colleagues [21] quantified cortical volumes in 24 children exposed to trauma (50% with PTSD) versus 24 matched archived controls. They found a significant reductions in total brain and cer-ebral gray matter volume (GMV), and most strikingly a loss of normal left–right asymmetry in the frontal lobes of children exposed to trauma [21]. More refined analysis showed that children with PTSD symptoms had a significantly larger GMV in the delineated middle-inferior and ventral regions of the prefrontal cortex than did controls [36]. Decreased GMV in the dorsal prefrontal cortex correlated with increased impairment scores [36].

## Voxel-based morphometry

Most recently, the most significant effect of exposure to repeated episodes of SA seen with voxel-based morphometry was a reduction in GMV of the visual cortex. Screenings were conducted on 723 volunteers to recruit 30 subjects with SA and 30 controls for magnetic resonance imaging (MRI). (Sexual abuse was defined as at least three episodes of forced sexual contact accompanied by threats of harm to self or others, and feelings of fear or terror, which occurred before age 18 and at least 2 years prior to enrolment.) A disproportionate number of subjects with SA were female. Hence, the study was limited to 23 females with SA (mean age 19.1 ± 1.1 years) and to 14 female controls (20.1 ± 1.3 years). Abused and control subjects were predominantly middle class or higher (96%); both groups had similar measures of cognitive abilities and parental socioeconomic status. All but two subjects experienced childhood SA outside the family. Voxel-based morphometry is a fully automated, unbiased, whole-brain morphometric technique that detects regional differences in GMV between groups on a voxel-by-voxel basis.

The most prominent finding was a highly significant reduction in GMV in the left primary visual (V-1) and visual association cortices (V-2) (Brodmann's area [BA] 17 to 18; $p < 0.0001$, corrected cluster level). There was 18.1% lower average GMV in these regions in the abused subjects. The degree of reduction in GMV of left V-1 was closely related to the duration of the abuse that occurred prior to 12 years of age ($r = -0.559$; $p = 0.0003$), but was not related to the duration of abuse that occurred from 12 years of age onwards ($r = 0.088$; $p > 0.5$).

There was a significant correlation between visual memory and GMV of BA 17 among all subjects ($r = 0.45$; $P = 0.005$), and a significant positive correlation between GMV of left V-1 and the subject's capacity ($d'$) to discriminate targets versus other stimuli on a Go/No-Go/Stop cognitive control task ($r = 0.58$).

Although voxel-based morphometry is a potentially powerful technique for identifying morphometric differences between groups, it hinges on a number of assumptions, particularly the accuracy of image coregistration. Hence, these findings were reevaluated using an independent technique that does not rely on image coregistration. Cortical surface-based analysis was performed using FreeSurfer [37]. Parcellation regions selected for analysis were those that were located in and around the areas of greatest difference identified by voxel-based morphometry, and included the lingual, fusiform, middle occipital and inferior occipital gyri, plus the cuneus and occipital pole.

FreeSurfer revealed a reduction in GMV of the entire left visual cortex of 8.0% ($p = 0.007$). There was an 18.0% reduction in the left fusiform gyrus ($p = 0.004$) and a 9.5% reduction in the left middle occipital gyrus ($p = 0.041$). Cortical surface-based analysis also indicated that there was a 5% reduction in GMV for the entire right visual cortex ($p = 0.038$). The most specific association was an 8.9% reduction in the right lingual gyrus ($p = 0.002$).

The fusiform gyrus is also known as the occipito-temporal gyrus, and it plays a very important role in the recognition of faces, words, objects and colors. Activity in the fusiform gyrus tends to be right lateralized for unfamiliar faces, bilateral for objects and left lateralized for printed words. The right fusiform gyrus appears to be specialized for processing a face as a whole, and the left fusiform specialized for processing based on facial features [38]. The left fusiform was found to be specifically activated when viewing one's own face [39] and remembered faces [40]. Patients with BPD, who often have histories of exposure to SA and other forms of trauma, appear to have heightened sensitivity to facial emotional expression, and may be more prone to interpret ambiguous facial expressions as angry [41]. It is conceivable that a reduction in GMV of left but not right fusiform gyrus may bias perception in this way.

The right lingual gyrus appears to be involved in the global aspects of figure recognition and object naming. It may also be a critical substrate for dreaming [42]. This brain region consistently shows reduced blood flow after sleep deprivation or disruption [43]. Nightmares and sleep disruption are frequently reported sequelae of SA. Sleep disruption as a result of SA may diminish activity and blood flow to this region, and consequently alter its developmental trajectory.

Reduced GMV in V-1 and V-2 are commensurate with a recent report from Fennema-Notestine et al. [44], who conducted a volumetric region-of-interest analysis of victims of intimate-partner violence. These

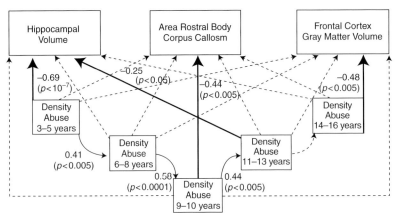

**Fig. 11.1.** Path analysis indicating relationships between density of abuse during different stages of development and measures of brain size derived from structural equation modeling (Amos Graphics). Path analysis examined two main components. The first was that child sexual abuse (CSA) (or absence of CSA) during one period would predict CSA (or absence of CSA) during the subsequent period. The second component examined the association between density of CSA during each stage and all morphometric measures. Numerical values represent standardized beta weights and their associated p values. The dotted lines were evaluated in the model but were not significantly predictive of any relationship between the variables. (From Andersen et al. [23] with permission.)

individuals had significantly reduced occipital GMV. However, it appeared that loss of GMV was a consequence of exposure to childhood abuse and not a result of intimate-partner violence or development of PTSD [44].

## Sensitive periods

Based on differential rates of maturation, we have hypothesized that specific brain regions should have differing periods of sensitivity to the effects of abuse [23]. We recruited 26 right-handed women, 18–22 years of age, with three or more episodes of forced contact SA accompanied by fear or terror. Controls were 17 healthy women (18–22 years) with no history of SA or axis I disorders, raised in families with comparable socioeconomic status. Hippocampal and amygdala volume, frontal cortex GMV and midsagittal area of the corpus callosum were selected as a-priori regions of interest and were measured from volumetric MRI scans. Data were analyzed using multiple regression and path analysis to assess the effect of SA occurring during different developmental stages (3–5, 6–8, 9–10, 11–13 and 14–16 years of age). Hippocampal volume was reduced in association with SA at 3–5 and 11–13 years (Fig. 11.1). The corpus callosum was reduced with SA at 9–10 years, and frontal cortex GMV was attenuated in subjects with SA at ages 14–16 years.

These findings provide the first preliminary evidence in humans that brain regions have different windows of vulnerability to the effects of exposure to childhood maltreatment.

## Neurobiological effects of other forms of childhood adversity

### Neuropsychiatric effects of exposure to parental verbal abuse and peer verbal bullying

Childhood maltreatment research has focused primarily on the effects of PA, SA or WDV. By comparison, PVA has received little attention as a specific form of abuse. We have compared the impact of exposure to PVA versus WDV, PA and SA on psychiatric symptoms [6]. Symptoms and exposure ratings were collected from 554 subjects 18–22 years of age (68% female) who responded to advertisements. Exposure to PVA was assessed using the Verbal Abuse Scale (VAS). Outcome measures included dissociation and symptoms of limbic irritability, (see above), depression, anxiety and anger-hostility.

Parental verbal abuse was associated with moderate to large statistical effects, comparable to those associated with WDV or non-familial SA, and larger than those associated with PA. Exposure to multiple forms of maltreatment had an effect size that was often greater than the component sum. These findings provide evidence that PVA is a potent form of maltreatment [6].

Subsequently, we hypothesized that exposure to VB would exert similar effects, given that VB has been linked to depression and suicidal ideation [45], along with risk for aggressive retaliation. Ratings scores and

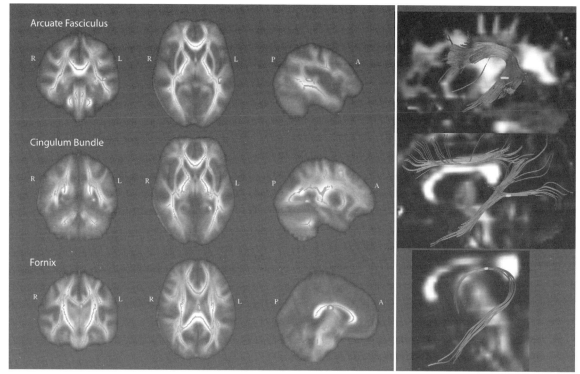

**Fig. 11.2.** Three white matter tract regions (shown in red) differed significantly in fractional anisotropy (FA) between subjects with history of exposure to high levels of parental verbal aggression and healthy controls. Region 1 contained fibers from arcuate fasciculus. Region 2 contained fibers from the cingulum bundle near the tail of the hippocampus. Region 3 is part of the left fornix. Green shows the mean FA skeleton and background image is in MNI 152. Tractography (far right panel) from representative subjects show tracts passing through the region of reduced FA identified by tract-based spatial statistics. (Modified from Choi *et al.* [47] with permission.) Please refer to color plate section.

exposure history were collected on a separate group of 1662 respondents (18–25 years of age) to an advertisement entitled "Memories of Childhood." Subjects rated their degree of exposure to male and female VB using the VAS [46]. Briefly, exposure to VB was fully comparable to the effects of exposure to PVA on all measures. Moreover, twice as many individuals were exposed to VB than PVA.

## White matter tract abnormalities in young adults exposed to parental verbal abuse

Diffusion tensor imaging (DTI) was used to ascertain whether PVA was associated with abnormalities in brain white matter tract integrity [47]. A group of 1271 healthy young adults were screened for exposure to childhood adversity and DTI scans were collected for 16 unmedicated subjects with a history of high-level exposure to PVA but no other form of maltreatment (4 male, 12 female; mean age 21.9 ± 2.4 years), and 16 healthy controls (5 male, 11 female; mean age 21.0 ± 1.6 years). Group differences in fractional anisotropy

(FA), covaried by parental education and income, were evaluated using tract-based spatial statistics, and correlated with symptom ratings and verbal intelligence quotient (IQ) (Fig. 11.2).

Three white matter tracts had significantly reduced FA: region 1, the arcuate fasciculus in the left superior temporal gyrus; region 2, the cingulum bundle in the fusiform gyrus by the posterior tail of the left hippocampus; and region 3, the left body of the fornix. The FA values were strongly associated with the maximal PVA scores ($r_s$ = −0.701, −0.801, −0.524, respectively; all $p \leq 0.002$). The FA value in region 1 correlated with verbal IQ ($r_s$ = 0.411; $p$ = 0.024). In region 2 the FA value was inversely associated with ratings of depression ($r_s$ = −0.504), dissociation ($r_s$ = −0.373) and limbic irritability ($r_s$ = −0.602). The FA value in region 3 was inversely correlated with ratings of somatization ($r_s$ = −0.389) and anxiety ($r_s$ = −0.311). The arcuate fasciculus connects Wernicke's and Broca's area. The cingulum bundle is a major pathway between the limbic system and the neocortex, particularly the cingulate cortex. The fornix interconnects hippocampus with the mammillary bodies and septal nuclei. Interestingly, the hippocampus receives serotonin fibers from the midbrain raphe via two pathways: the cingulum bundle (which predominantly innervates dorsal hippocampus), and the fornix (which innervates all portions) [48].

## White matter tract abnormalities in young adults who witnessed domestic violence

Subjects were right-handed, healthy, unmedicated young adults recruited from the community by advertisements. They were selected based on a complete absence of exposure to any type of abuse (control group), or if they had a history of WDV but no history of PA, SA or exposure to other traumatic events. Controls had no history of axis I psychopathology. Screenings were conducted on 1402 volunteers to recruit 20 carefully selected subjects with a history of WDV (4 male, 16 female; mean age 22.4 ± 2.48 years) and 27 healthy control subjects (8 male, 19 female; mean age 21.9 ± 1.97 years).

The FA in the white matter tract of the left lateral occipital lobe (inferior longitudinal fasciculus) was significantly reduced ($p < 0.05$, corrected) in the WDV group. The FA values in this region were significantly associated with depression, anxiety, somatization, dissociation and limbic irritability. The inferior longitudinal fasciculus connects occipital and temporal cortex and is the main component of the visual–limbic pathway that subserves emotional, learning and memory functions that are modality specific to vision.

## Signals strength abnormalities in $T_2$-weighted signals in young adults exposed to parental verbal abuse

Voxel-based relaxometry [49] was performed on $T_2$-relaxometry scans from 22 unmedicated subjects with PVA (7 male, 15 female) and 22 matched controls of equivalent age and socioeconomic status, with no history of trauma [50]. The technique identified regional clusters of $T_2$ relaxation times that differed between controls and subjects exposed to PVA. Elevated $T_2$ relaxation times are indicative of reduced blood flow[50] but could also be indicative of fibrosis and sclerosis. These $T_2$-signal abnormalities are frequently observed in the hippocampus, amygdala and parahippocampal gyrus of patients with temporal lobe epilepsy and hippocampal sclerosis [49].

Exposure to PVA was associated with increased $T_2$ signal strength in parahippocampal gyrus ($p < 0.017$, corrected), anterior cingulate cortex ($p < 0.01$, corrected) and cerebellar vermis ($p < 0.001$, uncorrected). A previous study found increased $T_2$ relaxation times in cerebellar vermis of subjects exposed to SA [51]. Voxel-based relaxometry of subjects exposed to SA also revealed increased signal in parahippocampal gyrus, which correlated strongly with LSCL-33 limbic irritability scores. Hence, this technique revealed similar effects of early stress exposure in subjects exposed to SA and those exposed to PVA.

## Effects of peer verbal bullying on gray matter volume and fractional anisotropy

Data were analyzed from 47 subjects (17 male, 30 female; mean age 22.1 ± 1.9 years) selected as controls from other studies. These subjects had no history of exposure to domestic violence, SA or PA, and had never experienced any form of trauma (e.g., motor vehicle accidents, natural disasters). They had no history of axis I disorders, and all had very low levels of exposure to PVA. They did, however, differ substantially in their degree of exposure to VB.

Global analyses were conducted to identify voxel clusters in which GMV correlated with VB scores. One cluster was identified with a positive correlation between VB and GMV. This was a relatively large cluster located in the lingual gyrus of the left occipital lobe (BA 18). Functional MRI studies have frequent found that this region is involved in emotional processing of both visually and verbally presented information [52]. There are two major ways to interpret this finding. First, exposure to VB may stimulate this region, resulting in a significant increase in GMV. An equally compelling alternative is that this was a preexisting difference that resulted in an increased capacity to detect emotional slights, and resulted in elevated ratings of VB exposure.

Data were collected on 42 of these subjects and analyzed using tract-based spatial statistics. Two regions emerged in which FA was inversely correlated with degree of exposure to VB. As shown in Fig. 11.3, one region was located in white matter in the right insula, the other in the right superior temporal gyrus.

The insula is a complex structure in which visceral, somatosensory, motor, vestibular and auditory functions converge and generate subjective feelings such as pain and craving. The anterior insula, particularly on the right side, can recast these feelings as social

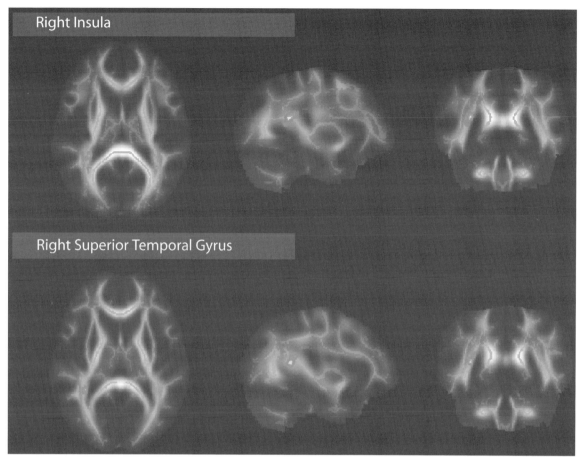

**Fig. 11.3.** Regions identified by tract-based spatial statistics (shown in red) in which there was an inverse correlation between degree of exposure to peer verbal bullying and fractional anisotropy in white matter tracts. Regions identified were in the right insula (Brodmann's area 13; MNI coordinates: 31, −39, 18; 33 voxels; $p = 0.024$), and right superior temporal gyrus (MNI coordinates: 34, −44, 10; 11 voxels; $p = 0.018$). Please refer to color plate section.

emotions [53]. Hence, this part of the brain is activated during expressions of anger/indignation, empathy, love, hate, disgust, joy and contempt (e.g., [54,55]). It seems plausible that exposure to VB could alter the development of pathways interconnecting this region, or that a preexisting anomaly in these pathways could bias the perception of peer interactions. Similarly, the right superior temporal gyrus appears to be involved in interpreting emotional prosody and communicative intention, such as the tone of voice used to convey irony [56].

## Conclusions

Exposure to early life trauma is associated with a host of structural abnormalities. There is consistent evidence for a reduction in the midsagittal area of the corpus callosum [9–11,22,23]. Similarly, there is compelling evidence for reduction in hippocampal volume in adults [16,18–20,23] but not children [10,21,22]. There is also evidence from multiple laboratories for alterations in symmetry, GMV, neuronal integrity, and EEG coherence in portions of the neocortex [10,21–23,34,36]. Our latest findings, using automated unbiased global analytical techniques, have identified new pathways and regions. It is particularly striking that exposure to repeated episodes of SA most significantly attenuated GMV in the occipital cortex and reduced GMV in the left fusiform and right lingual gyri. These regions appear to play an important role in recognition of familiar faces [39,40] and dreaming [42]. Witnessing domestic abuse was associated with reduced FA in the inferior longitudinal fasciculus, which relays visual information to the limbic system. Exposure to VB was associated with reduced FA in the insula, where multi-sensory information is integrated, and with a reduction in the left lingual gyrus, which is involved in processing emotional response to visual or verbal stimuli. There was a substantial reduction in FA in subjects exposed to PVA along a portion of the arcuate fasciculus, which connects regions involved in the perception and expression of language. We also found, but did not discuss here, that exposure to harsh corporal punishment was associated with alteration in FA and mean diffusivity throughout components of the cortical pain pathway. Hence, these findings suggest that exposure to various forms of maltreatment affect sensory systems or pathways through which the aversive stimulus is processed or interpreted. These findings are consistent with the idea that sensory systems are malleable and strongly influenced by early experience [57].

Another important observation was our finding that different brain regions may have unique windows of vulnerability during which they are maximally sensitive to the effects of exposure to childhood stress. One implication of this finding is that different neuropsychiatric sequelae of maltreatment may arise based on ages of exposure. We are continuing to pursue this observation in larger samples and are exploring the inter-relationship between stages of exposure and psychiatric manifestations.

The final point to emphasize is that the developing brain appears to be affected by exposure to multiple forms of adversity including neglect, PVA, VB and harsh corporal punishment, and not just those that meet the A(1) and A(2) criteria for trauma of the *Diagnostic and Statistical Manual*, fourth edition [58]. Hence, we need to bear in mind that exposure to childhood adversity is a complex psychosocial stressor that can lead to a host of adverse outcomes. The occurrence of PTSD is a relatively rare consequence of early abuse. All of the adverse neurobiological correlates that we have observed are unrelated to and independent of the presence of PTSD. As we mentioned at the outset of this chapter, childhood adversity is a developmental stressor that accounts for 50–75% of the population attributable risk for alcoholism, depression, suicidal behavior and drug abuse [2,3]. It is our hope that by delineating the neurobiological consequences of exposure to different forms of adversity across different developmental stages, we will shed new light on this pathological relationship, which affects millions of people and results directly or indirectly in many of the major causes of death, disability and human suffering.

## Acknowledgements
This work was supported, in part, by National Institute of Mental Health RO1 grants MH53636 and MH-66222, and National Institute of Drug Abuse RO1 grants DA-016934 and DA-017846 to MHT, and by the Joanne B. Simches Research Endowment. This work would not have been possible without the diligent efforts of Drs. Ann Polcari, Carryl Navalta and Katherine Flagg and Ms. Cynthia McGreenery and Elizabeth Bolger for recruitment, assessment and evaluation of subjects.

## References
1. Anda, R. F., Felitti, V. J., Bremner, J. D. *et al.* (2006). The enduring effects of abuse and related adverse experiences in childhood: A convergence of evidence from neurobiology and epidemiology. *European Archives of Psychiatry and Clinical Neuroscience,* **256**, 174–186.
2. Anda, R. F., Whitfield, C. L., Felitti, V. J. *et al.* (2002). Adverse childhood experiences, alcoholic parents, and later risk of alcoholism and depression. *Psychiatric Services,* **53**, 1001–1009.
3. Dube, S. R., Felitti, V. J., Dong, M. *et al.* (2003). Childhood abuse, neglect, and household dysfunction and the risk of illicit drug use: The adverse childhood experiences study. *Pediatrics,* **111**, 564–572.
4. Felitti, V. J., Anda, R. F., Nordenberg, D. *et al.* (1998). Relationship of childhood abuse and household dysfunction to many of the leading causes of death in adults. The Adverse Childhood Experiences (ACE) Study. *American Journal of Preventive Medicine,* **14**, 245–258.
5. Lyons-Ruth, K., Bronfman, E. and Parsons, E. (1999). Atypical attachment in infancy and early childhood among children at developmental risk. IV. Maternal frightened, frightening, or atypical behavior and disorganized infant attachment patterns. *Monographs of the Society for Research in Child Development,* **64**, 67–96; discussion 213–220.
6. Teicher, M. H., Tomoda, A. and Andersen, S. L. (2006). Neurobiological consequences of early stress and childhood maltreatment: Are results from human and animal studies comparable? *Annals of the New York Academy of Sciences,* **1071**, 313–323.
7. Berrebi, A. S., Fitch, R. H., Ralphe, D. L. *et al.* (1988). Corpus callosum: Region-specific effects of sex, early experience and age. *Brain Research,* **438**, 216–224.
8. Sanchez, M. M., Hearn, E. F., Do D., Rilling, J. K. and Herndon, J. G. (1998). Differential rearing affects corpus callosum size and cognitive function of rhesus monkeys. *Brain Research,* **812**, 38–49.
9. Teicher, M. H., Ito, Y., Glod, C. A. *et al.* (1997). Preliminary evidence for abnormal cortical development in physically and sexually abused children

using EEG coherence and MRI. *Annals of the New York Academy of Sciences,* **821**, 160–175.

10. De Bellis, M. D., Keshavan, M. S., Clark, D. B. *et al.* (1999). Developmental traumatology. Part II: Brain development. *Biological Psychiatry,* **45**, 1271–1284.

11. Teicher, M. H., Dumont, N. L., Ito, Y. *et al.* (2004). Childhood neglect is associated with reduced corpus callosum area. *Biological Psychiatry,* **56**, 80–85.

12. Schiffer, F., Teicher, M. H. and Papanicolaou, A. C. (1995). Evoked potential evidence for right brain activity during the recall of traumatic memories. *Journal of Neuropsychiatry and Clinical Neurosciences,* **7**, 169–175.

13. Gould, E. and Tanapat, P. (1999). Stress and hippocampal neurogenesis. *Biological Psychiatry,* **46**, 1472–1479.

14. Sapolsky, R. M., Uno, H., Rebert, C. S. and Finch, C. E. (1990). Hippocampal damage associated with prolonged glucocorticoid exposure in primates. *Journal of Neuroscience,* **10**, 2897–2902.

15. Andersen, S. L. and Teicher, M. H. (2004). Delayed effects of early stress on hippocampal development. *Neuropsychopharmacology,* **29**, 1988–1993.

16. Bremner, J. D., Randall, P., Vermetten, E. *et al.* (1997). Magnetic resonance imaging-based measurement of hippocampal volume in posttraumatic stress disorder related to childhood physical and sexual abuse: A preliminary report. *Biological Psychiatry,* **41**, 23–32.

17. Stein, M. B. (1997). Hippocampal volume in women victimized by childhood sexual abuse. *Psychological Medicine,* **27**, 951–959.

18. Driessen, M., Herrmann, J., Stahl, K. *et al.* (2000). Magnetic resonance imaging volumes of the hippocampus and the amygdala in women with borderline personality disorder and early traumatization. *Archives of General Psychiatry,* **57**, 1115–1122.

19. Vythilingam, M., Heim, C., Newport, J. *et al.* (2002). Childhood trauma associated with smaller hippocampal volume in women with major depression. *American Journal of Psychiatry,* **159**, 2072–2080.

20. Vermetten, E., Schmahl, C., Lindner, S., Loewenstein, R. J. and Bremner, J. D. (2006). Hippocampal and amygdalar volumes in dissociative identity disorder. *American Journal of Psychiatry,* **163**, 630–636.

21. Carrion, V. G., Weems, C. F., Eliez, S. *et al.* (2001). Attenuation of frontal asymmetry in pediatric post-traumatic stress disorder. *Biological Psychiatry,* **50**, 943–951.

22. De Bellis, M. D., Keshavan, M. S., Shifflett, H. *et al.* (2002). Brain structures in pediatric maltreatment-related posttraumatic stress disorder: A sociodemographically matched study. *Biological Psychiatry,* **52**, 1066–1078.

23. Andersen, S. L., Tomada, A., Vincow, E. S. *et al.* (2008). Preliminary evidence for sensitive periods in the effect of childhood sexual abuse on regional brain development.

*Journal of Neuropsychiatry and Clinical Neuroscience,* **20**, 292–301.

24. Gilbertson, M. W., Shenton, M. E., Ciszewski, A. *et al.* (2002). Smaller hippocampal volume predicts pathologic vulnerability to psychological trauma. *Nature Neuroscience,* **5**, 1242–1247.

25. Post, R. M., Rubinow, D. R. and Ballenger, J. C. (1984). Conditioning, sensitization and kindling: Implications for the course of affective illness. In R. M. Post and J. C. Ballenger (eds.), *Neurobiology of mood disorders* (pp. 432–466). Baltimore, MD: Williams & Wilkins.

26. Caldji, C., Diorio, J. and Meaney, M. J. (2003). Variations in maternal care alter GABA(A) receptor subunit expression in brain regions associated with fear. *Neuropsychopharmacology,* **28**, 1950–1959.

27. Mizielinska, S., Greenwood, S. and Connolly, C. N. (2006). The role of GABAA receptor biogenesis, structure and function in epilepsy. *Biochemical Society Transactions,* **34**, 863–867.

28. Teicher, M. H., Glod, C. A., Surrey, J. and Swett, C. Jr. (1993). Early childhood abuse and limbic system ratings in adult psychiatric outpatients. *Journal of Neuropsychiatry and Clinical Neurosciences,* **5**, 301–306.

29. Ito, Y., Teicher, M. H., Glod, C. A. *et al.* (1993). Increased prevalence of electrophysiological abnormalities in children with psychological, physical, and sexual abuse. *Journal of Neuropsychiatry and Clinical Neurosciences,* **5**, 401–408.

30. Davies, R. K. (1979). Incest: Some neuropsychiatric findings. *International Journal of Psychiatry and Medicine,* **9**, 117–121.

31. Thatcher, R. W. (1992). Cyclic cortical reorganization during early childhood. *Brain and Cognition,* **20**, 24–50.

32. Teicher, M. H., Ito, Y., Glod, C. A., Schiffer, F. and Gelbard, H. A. (1996). Neurophysiological mechanisms of stress response in children. In C. Pfeffer (ed.), *Severe stress and mental disturbance in children* (pp. 59–84). Washington, DC: American Psychiatric Association Press.

33. Thatcher, R. W., Walker, R. A. and Giudice, S. (1987). Human cerebral hemispheric development at different rates and ages. *Science,* **236**, 1110–1113.

34. Ito, Y., Teicher, M. H., Glod, C. A. and Ackerman, E. (1998). Preliminary evidence for aberrant cortical development in abused children: A quantitative EEG study. *Journal of Neuropsychiatry and Clinical Neurosciences,* **10**, 298–307.

35. De Bellis, M. D., Keshavan, M. S., Spencer, S. and Hall, J. (2000). N-Acetylaspartate concentration in the anterior cingulate of maltreated children and adolescents with PTSD. *American Journal of Psychiatry,* **157**, 1175–1177.

36. Richert, K. A., Carrion, V. G., Karchemskiy, A. and Reiss, A. L. (2006). Regional differences of the prefrontal cortex in pediatric PTSD: An MRI study. *Depression Anxiety,* **23**, 17–25.

37. Fischl, B., Salat, D. H., Busa, E. *et al.* (2002). Whole brain segmentation: Automated labeling of neuroanatomical structures in the human brain. *Neuron,* **33**, 341–355.

38. Rossion, B., Dricot, L., Devolder, A. *et al.* (2000). Hemispheric asymmetries for whole-based and part-based face processing in the human fusiform gyrus. *Journal of Cognitive Neuroscience,* **12**, 793–802.

39. Sugiura, M., Kawashima, R., Nakamura, K. *et al.* (2000). Passive and active recognition of one's own face. *NeuroImage,* **11**, 36–48.

40. Druzgal, T. J. and D'Esposito, M. (2001). A neural network reflecting decisions about human faces. *Neuron,* **32**, 947–955.

41. Domes, G., Czieschnek, D., Weidler, F. *et al.* (2008). Recognition of facial affect in borderline personality disorder. *Journal of Personality Disorders,* **22**, 135–147.

42. Bischof, M. and Bassetti, C. L. (2004). Total dream loss: A distinct neuropsychological dysfunction after bilateral PCA stroke. *Annals of Neurology,* **56**, 583–586.

43. Joo, E. Y., Tae, W. S., Han, S. J., Cho, J. W. and Hong, S. B. (2007). Reduced cerebral blood flow during wakefulness in obstructive sleep apnea–hypopnea syndrome. *Sleep,* **30**, 1515–1520.

44. Fennema-Notestine, C., Stein, M. B., Kennedy, C. M., Archibald, S. L. and Jernigan, T. L. (2002). Brain morphometry in female victims of intimate partner violence with and without posttraumatic stress disorder. *Biological Psychiatry,* **52**, 1089–1101.

45. van der Wal, M. F., de Wit, C. A. and Hirasing, R. A. (2003). Psychosocial health among young victims and offenders of direct and indirect bullying. *Pediatrics,* **111**, 1312–1317.

46. Teicher, M. H., Samson, J. A., Polcari, A. and McGreenery, C. E. (2006). Sticks, stones, and hurtful words: Relative effects of various forms of childhood maltreatment. *American Journal of Psychiatry,* **163**, 993–1000.

47. Choi, J., Jeong, B., Rohan, M. L., Polcari, A. M. and Teicher, M. H. (2008). Preliminary evidence for white matter tract abnormalities in young adults exposed to parental verbal abuse. *Biological Psychiatry,* **65**, 227–234.

48. Patel, T. D., Azmitia, E. C. and Zhou, F. C. (1996). Increased 5-HT1A receptor immunoreactivity in the rat hippocampus following 5,7-dihydroxytryptamine lesions in the cingulum bundle and fimbria-fornix. *Behavioral and Brain Research,* **73**, 319–323.

49. Pell, G. S., Briellmann, R. S., Waites, A. B., Abbott, D. F. and Jackson, G. D. (2004). Voxel-based relaxometry: A new approach for analysis of T2 relaxometry changes in epilepsy. *NeuroImage,* **21**, 707–713.

50. Anderson, C. M., Kaufman, M. J., Lowen, S. B. *et al.* (2005). Brain T2 relaxation times correlate with regional cerebral blood volume. *Magma,* **18**, 3–6.

51. Anderson, C. M., Teicher, M. H., Polcari, A. and Renshaw, P. F. (2002). Abnormal T2 relaxation time in the cerebellar vermis of adults sexually abused in childhood: Potential role of the vermis in stress-enhanced risk for drug abuse. *Psychoneuroendocrinology,* **27**, 231–244.

52. Rama, P., Martinkauppi, S., Linnankoski, I. *et al.* (2001). Working memory of identification of emotional vocal expressions: An fMRI study. *NeuroImage,* **13**, 1090–1101.

53. Craig, A. D. (2004). Human feelings: Why are some more aware than others? *Trends in Cognitive Science,* **8**, 239–241.

54. Zahn, R., Moll, J., Paiva, M. *et al.* (2008). The neural basis of human social values: Evidence from functional MRI. *Cerebral Cortex,* **2**, 336–352.

55. Sambataro, F., Dimalta, S., Di Giorgio, A. *et al.* (2006). Preferential responses in amygdala and insula during presentation of facial contempt and disgust. *European Journal of Neuroscience,* **24**, 2355–2362.

56. Wang, A. T., Lee, S. S., Sigman, M. and Dapretto, M. (2007). Reading affect in the face and voice: Neural correlates of interpreting communicative intent in children and adolescents with autism spectrum disorders. *Archives of General Psychiatry,* **64**, 698–708.

57. Hubel, D. H. and Wiesel, T. N. (1998). Early exploration of the visual cortex. *Neuron,* **20**, 401–412.

58. American Psychiatric Association. (1994). *Diagnostic and statistical manual of mental disorders,* 4th edn, Washington, DC: American Psychiatric Press.

# The neurobiology of child neglect

Michael D. De Bellis

## Introduction

Child neglect is the most chronic and prevalent form of child maltreatment. There are few standardized measures that examine the absence of culturally expected caregiver behaviors. This chapter will discuss definitions, preclinical studies of maternal deprivation, the field of developmental traumatology, studies of neglected children and future directions.

## Definitions

Child protective services (CPS) defines child neglect by law as a significant omission in care by a caregiver, which causes (the Harm Standard) or creates an imminent risk of (the Endangerment Standard) serious physical or mental harm to a child. Child neglect is defined as physical, medical educational and emotional neglect (US child Abuse Prevention and Treatment Act 42 U.S.C.A. §5106g). Physical neglect is abandonment, lack of supervision and failure to provide for a child's basic needs of nutrition, clothing, hygiene and safety. Medical neglect is the failure to provide necessary medical or mental health treatment. Emotional neglect is defined as refusals or delays in psychological care, inadequate attentions to a child's needs for affection, emotional support, attention or competence, *exposure of the child to extreme domestic violence* and permitting a child's maladaptive behaviors. Educational neglect is permitted chronic truancy, failure to enroll a child in mandatory schooling and inattention to a child's special needs. Various forms of child neglect and abuse commonly coexist in CPS-referred children [1].

## Review of preclinical studies of maternal deprivation

The social attachment between mother and infant is an essential experience-dependent interaction for normal development. Frequent touching by the maternal caregiver is a biologic necessity for physical and psychological growth [2]. Maternal deprivation causes persistent problems in the social, behavioral and cognitive development of offspring in studies of infant rats as well as primates.

The seminal studies of Harlow and colleagues [3] suggested that the nature, age of onset, duration of neglect and the availability of an enriched environment during primate infancy are important contributors to normal adult function. Rhesus monkey infants who were reared in "total social isolation" (i.e., separated from their mothers, peers and social group) for their first 6 months of life were adversely affected as adults. These "isolates" spent their time primarily engrossed in autistic-like behaviors (e.g., stereotyped movements, compulsive non-nutritional sucking and self-mutilatory behaviors when they reached puberty), showed a lack of recognition of social cues, an inability to develop normal social relationships and increased anxiety and aggression. These behaviors were more severe when rhesus monkey infants were raised in total social isolation for their first year of life. For these 12-month old "isolates," play and exploration were non-existent and all social interactions resulted in extremely anxious behaviors. They froze in reactions to aggression from other animals and sustained serious injuries. However, rhesus monkey infants who were reared in "total social isolation" for their first 3 months of life and then allowed to interact with age-mates appeared normal as adults.

## Historical review of child neglect

In the early 1900s, the US pediatrician Henry Dwight Chapin noted that, despite the improvements in food and hygiene, institutionalized infants suffered death rates of 31.7% to 75% from infections or failure to

*The Impact of Early Life Trauma on Health and Disease: The Hidden Epidemic*, ed. Ruth A. Lanius, Eric Vermetten and Clare Pain. Published by Cambridge University Press. Copyright © Cambridge University Press 2010.

thrive [4]. In 1902, Chapin began the foster care movement by forming the Speedwell Society and boarding out orphaned infants to willing foster parents. He reported only a 2% death rate in the 266 infants his Speedwell Society fostered compared with the institution infant death rate [5]. Although improvements were made in hygienic and nutritional standards in the 1940s and the institutionalized (Foundling Home) infant mortality rate was under 10% (similar to the national rates at the time), studies continued to show that institutionalized infants suffered from an increased susceptibility to infections [6]. Spitz [7] showed that, as institutionalized children began to live past infancy, severe deficits in social, behavioral, and emotional development were noted. These institutionalized children suffered from progressive developmental deterioration in cognitive functioning that was felt to be irremediable if institutionalization occurred in the first 3 years of life [8]. Spitz reported maturational delays and evidence of symptoms in these Foundling Home infants that would now be described as a reactive attachment disorder under the criteria of the Diagnosis and Statistical Manual, Fourth edition [9] when comparing them with infants raised in poverty or raised by their natural young mothers, with staff assistance, in a penal institution [7]. Spitz concluded that fostering an adequate and satisfactory mother–child relationship in infancy would decrease the unavoidable and irreparable psychiatric consequences to children deriving from early emotional neglect. Bowlby [10] stated that a selective, non-interchangeable relationship with a single adult primary "attachment figure was required" for an infant's development to proceed normally, and this relationship could not be provided in an institution.

## Developmental traumatology

Developmental traumatology is the systemic investigation of the neurobiological and psychological impact of early life adversity on the developing child [11]. It is a relatively new field of study that synthesizes knowledge from developmental psychopathology, developmental neuroscience and stress and trauma research. The development of the brain is regulated by genes, which interact with life experiences. In this research, CPS-defined abuse and neglect are seen as extreme forms of early life stress. Other early life stressors commonly seen in neglected children are poverty and parental substance use disorders. These may additionally contribute to and confound the relationship between child neglect and children's brain development. An important aim for the field of developmental traumatology is to unravel the complex interactions between an individual's genetic constitution, their unique psychosocial environment and the proposed critical periods of vulnerability for and resilience to maltreatment experiences, and to determine how such factors may influence changes in biological stress systems and brain development, thus leading to the known serious consequences of early life stress.

It can be effectively argued that childhood neglect may be experienced by the human child, a member of a social species, as traumatic, causing anxiety and distress. The degree of the traumatic experience perceived by the child may depend on the age of the child at the time of neglect and the duration of neglect. The high rates of infection and early death seen in institutionized infants may be associated with stress-induced suppression of the immune system (reviewed by De Bellis [12]). Infants have been known to aspirate and die from the stress of severe and continued unanswered crying. A toddler who is not fed does not develop a "secure base" and is in a chronic state of severe anxiety [13]. An unsupervised non-abused young child may be more likely to witness interpersonal traumas, experience traumatic accidents or suffer from abuse outside of the home.

In developmental traumatology research, it is hypothesized that there are an infinite number of stressors that can cause anxiety and distress in a child but there are finite ways in which the brain and the body (i.e., biological stress response systems) can respond to those stressors. For the neglected child, the nature of the stressor is the dysfunctional parent–child interpersonal relationship. This type of stressor is the failure to attain the experience-dependent trust in a parent or an authority figure and the socially expected behaviors that follow from knowing such trust. Child neglect may be more detrimental to the child's developing biological stress systems and brain than adversity experienced in adulthood, secondary to interactions between this lack of experience of expected environmental stimulation and brain maturation. Neglect, without social intervention, is a chronic stressor that may negatively influence the development of biological stress system responses and may lead to adverse brain, cognitive and psychological development. This is seen as delays in or deficits of multisystem developmental achievements in behavioral and emotional regulation, cognitive and psychosocial function, antisocial behaviors, poor academic achievement, and serious psychopathology in adulthood [14,15].

# Biological stress response systems

Multiple neurotransmitter systems and neuroendocrine axes are activated during stress [12]. Stress exposure affects the neurotransmitter systems, the neuroendocrine system and the immune system. These systems are interconnected to modulate response to acute and chronic stressors. The sympathetic nervous system or catecholamine system, the hypothalamic–pituitary–adrenal (HPA) axis and the serotonin system are the three major neurobiological stress response systems implicated in mood, anxiety and impulse control disorders (reviewed by Vermetten and Bremner [16]). Arousal, stress response, behavior, emotional regulation and neurodevelopment are all dependent on these systems.

# The "fight or flight or freeze" reaction

Traumatic experiences impact neurodevelopment through activation of the body's biological stress systems. Stress responses are activated when external stimuli perceived via the senses are processed through the brain's thalamus, activating the amygdala fear detection circuit; projections from the amygdala then transmit fear signals to connections in the prefrontal cortex, paraventricular nucleus of the hypothalamus, and locus ceruleus in the brainstem [12]. Intense anxiety activates the locus ceruleus, an ancient structure, and the sympathetic nervous system, leading to the biological changes of the "fight or flight or freeze" reaction. The locus ceruleus is the major norepinephrine containing nucleus in the brain. Norepinephrine, serotonin and dopamine are major catecholamine brain neurotransmitters. Direct and indirect effects of this activation include increases in catecholamine turnover in the brain, the sympathetic nervous system and the adrenal medulla. The adrenals, endocrine glands located above the kidneys, secrete the stress hormones cortisol and epinephrine. This "fight or flight or freeze" reaction is directly caused by elevated levels of epinephrine and sympathetic nervous system activity and is manifested by increases in heart rate, blood pressure, metabolic rate and alertness. This reaction prepares the body to fight, run or in some other way protect itself from ancient enemies (e.g., snakes, lions).

During the stress response, the amygdala, a brain structure involved in the regulation of fear, anxiety and novelty, is in turn stimulated by the locus ceruleus. The amygdala then stimulates the hypothalamus, which results in release of corticotropin-releasing hormone or factor. This causes the pituitary to secrete adrenocorticotropic hormone (ACTH) and also stimulates brain regions of the cortex. Release of ACTH then results in release of cortisol from the adrenal gland, with feedback to the sympathetic nervous system, causing further activation [17]. Cortisol acts to attenuate the stress response via negative feedback inhibition on the hypothalamus, pituitary, the hippocampus, and the medial PFC, suppressing the HPA axis and leading to restoration of basal cortisol levels so that the stress response and its effects on immune suppression are contained (homeostasis). The amygdala has the opposite effect, promoting the stress response [18].

Through complex mechanisms, the amygdala also stimulates dopaminergic inputs to the medial PFC. These dopaminergic inputs to PFC appear to be particularly sensitive to stress. Enhanced dopamine PFC function in response to stress may reflect the heightened attention or cognitive processes needed to cope with the stressor [19]. However, chronic stress may result in more PFC dopamine than is functionally necessary and may impair PFC function, causing a host of problems in developing children, including inattention and difficulties in problem solving [20], hypervigilance, problems in learning new material, psychotic symptoms and paranoia.

The serotonin system is a stress response system that activates both anxiogenic and anxiolytic pathways and serotonin is regarded as a master control neurotransmitter of complex neuronal communication [21]. Serotonin plays important roles in the regulation of mood and behaviors (e.g., aggression, impulsivity). Serotonin is dysregulated in major depression, impulsivity and suicidal behaviors. Low serotonin function is associated with suicidal and aggressive behaviors in adults, children and adolescents [12]. In primate studies of chronic stress, serotonin levels decrease in the PFC [22]. In animal studies of unpredictable and uncontrollable stress (e.g., inescapable shock, restraint stress), serotonin levels decrease in the amygdala, medial PFC, nucleus accumbens and lateral hypothalamus. These processes of serotonin depletion result in behaviors of "learned helplessness" and severe behavioral dysregulation [23].

# Neglect and the development of neurotransmitter and neuroendocrine systems

Primates subjected to maternal and social deprivation have altered catecholamine [24], cortisol [25] and immune [26] function. Similarly, maltreated children show alterations in cortisol and catecholamine levels. Levels of 24-hour urinary norepinephrine were elevated in severely neglected male children who suffered from clinical depression [27]. Abused and neglected children with post-traumatic stress disorder (PTSD), who had experienced abuse and witnessed domestic violence, had greater levels of urinary norepinephrine and dopamine and free cortisol than non-maltreated controls [28]. Measures of epinephrine, norepinephrine and dopamine showed positive correlations with duration of the maltreatment trauma and PTSD symptoms. An increase in baseline functioning of the catecholamine system in childhood PTSD is further suggested by two separate, open-label treatment trials of the medications clonidine (a central $\alpha_2$-adrenergic partial agonist) and propranolol (a $\beta$-adrenergic antagonist); both of these drugs dampen catecholamine transmission. Clonidine treatment was associated with general clinical improvement and decreases in the arousal cluster of PTSD symptoms and basal heart rate [29]. Propranolol treatment was associated with decreases in aggressive behaviors and insomnia [30]. Elevated catecholamines can lead to health problem such as high blood pressure and cardiovascular disease. However, the evidenced-based treatment of choice for PTSD is trauma-focused cognitive behavioral therapy rather than medications [31]. This therapy likely lessens amygdala activity through strengthening the inhibitory connections of the medial PFC to the amygdala.

Maltreated children also show alterations of the development of the HPA axis. In pediatric studies of abused and neglected children, dysregulation of the HPA axis, with increased cortisol secretion, is supported. Increased cortisol levels are found in most studies of maltreated young and latency age children, while most studies have shown that the opposite is evidenced in adolescents and adults (reviewed by De Bellis [11]). Elevated salivary cortisol levels were found in children aged 6–12 years who had been raised in Romanian orphanages for more than 8 months of their lives, compared with levels in early-adopted and Canadian-born children 6.5 years after adoption [32]. Elevated salivary cortisol has been described in maltreated children with depression [33] and in maltreated children with PTSD who experienced or witnessed interpersonal violence [34]. In addition, elevated 24-hour urine levels of free cortisol [28] and greater increases in pituitary volume with age [35] were observed in prepubertal abused children with PTSD, many of whom witnessed domestic violence, compared with non-maltreated children.

Neglected children are at higher risk for externalizing behavioral problems and adult antisocial behavior [15]. These problems are hypothesized to be the result of stress-induced serotonin dysregulation and may be related to witnessing family violence.

# Child neglect and the immune system

During chronic stress, biological stress response systems signal to the immune system via the HPA axis and the sympathetic nervous sytem. As early as 1936, Selye [36] showed that restraining rats produced involution of the thymus and stress-induced lymphopenia. An extensive review of the literature on the effects of stress on cellular immune response in animals concluded that a variety of stressors are associated with suppression of immune responses [37]. Stressed animals are at significantly greater risk for development of infections, tumors and death after experimentally induced immune (antigenic) challenge. As discussed above, institutionalized infants suffer from increased rates of infection and early death. There are no child studies to date published in this area, an important area for investigation, as stress-induced immune dysregulation is likely seen in neglected children.

# Brain development

## Healthy childhood brain development

The time from birth to adulthood is marked by the development of skills consecutively in physical, behavioral, cognitive and emotional domains. Progressive maturational processes, such as myelination of newly formed neuronal networks, parallel these stages. Myelin, a fatty white substance produced by supportive glial cells, is a vital component of the brain. Myelin encases the axons of neurons, forming an insulator, the myelin sheath. It is responsible for the color of white matter. Human brain development takes place by an overproduction of neurons in utero, increases in synaptic neuropil (neuron size and synapses) during childhood and then selective elimination of some neurons (apoptosis), with corresponding increases in myelination, during adolescence and young adulthood. Synapses, dendrites, cell bodies and unmyelinated axons, which form the brain's gray matter, decrease during development [38].

Magnetic resonance imaging (MRI) provides a safe method of measuring brain maturation in healthy children. Cross-sectional and longitudinal MRI studies of high-functioning healthy children and adolescents have greatly advanced our knowledge of human brain development [39]. Cortical myelination (the growth of white matter) can easily be examined through MRI-based morphometry of cerebral white matter volume and the midsagittal corpus callosum area, a white matter structure made up of axons that connect major subdivisions of the cerebral cortex. There are regionally specific non-linear preadolescent increases in cortical gray matter followed by postadolescent decreases [40,41]. The most dramatic increase in myelination is reflected by the corpus callosum, which peaks in early childhood but continues linearly into the third decade [41–43]. The PFC, which subserves executive cognitive functions and regulates the stress responses, continues its development into young adulthood [44].

In the developing brain, stress and elevated levels of stress chemicals may lead to adverse brain development through the mechanisms of accelerated loss (or metabolism) of neurons [45–48], delays in myelination [49], abnormalities in developmentally appropriate pruning [50,51], the inhibition of neurogenesis [52–54], or a stress-induced decrease in brain growth factors (e.g., brain-derived neurotropic factor) [55]. It is hypothesized that dysregulation of a neglected child's major stress systems contributes to adverse brain development and leads to psychopathology and an increased risk for medical problems [56].

Sex steroids influence neurodevelopment throughout the lifespan [57]. In one pediatric neuroimaging study, boys showed significantly greater loss of gray matter volume and an increase in both white matter volume and corpus callosum area compared with girls over a similar age range, suggesting sex differences in both cerebral gray and white matter maturational processes in childhood [58]. This is of interest because males seem to be more vulnerable to the adverse psychosocial [59] and neurobiological [60] consequences of neglect.

## Preclinical and human brain maturation investigations of early life neglect

The medial PFC and myelinated areas of the brain appear particularly susceptible to the effects of early life stress. Medial PFC inhibits activation of the parts of the limbic system involved in anxiety (i.e., the amygdala and related neurocircuitry) [61]. The PFC subserves executive cognitive functions [62]. However, severe stress can "turn off" this frontal inhibition of the

limbic system [20]. This "turning off" of frontal inhibition to the amygdala is seen in distressed adults who were maltreated as children [63,64]. Maternal deprivation of infant primates is associated with deficits in PFC functions of attention and motivation [65–67]. Sanchez and colleagues [68] studied brain differences in one group of infant rhesus monkeys who were separated from their mothers at 2 months of age, and another group who were not separated. The separated monkeys demonstrated a reduction in the midsagittal size of the corpus callosum. This decrease occurred in parallel to a decrease in white (but not gray) matter volume in the PFC and parietal cortices, and impairment in cognitive function. Therefore, primates who suffer maternal deprivation have deficits in PFC functions and in normal age-related myelination.

Child neglect likely interferes with the effective development of PFC and executive functions, leading to inattention, inability to focus and poor academic achievement. Most studies of neglected children have focused on intellectual ability and academic function. In prospective studies, child neglect is associated with significantly delayed cognitive development and head growth in young children [69], and lower intelligence quotient (IQ) and academic achievement in adulthood [14]. Chugani and colleagues [70] reported that previously institutionalized Romanian adoptees exhibited deficits on tasks dependent on PFC function (i.e., social and attention deficits). These children showed significantly decreased metabolism in the orbital frontal gyrus, temporal cortex, PFC, amygdala and brainstem (brain structures involved in cognitive function, social intelligence and anxiety) compared with children with chronic epilepsy and healthy adults.

The corpus callosum appears particularly susceptible to the effects of early life stress. A lack of experience-dependent stimulation may lead to delays in myelination in neglected children [71,72]. To date, only a handful of studies involving maltreated children have been reported. The results of these studies suggest that pediatric maltreatment-related PTSD is associated with adverse brain development [73]. In one study, a reduction in the middle portion of the corpus callosum in maltreated pediatric psychiatric patients was seen compared with control psychiatric patients. This negative effect appeared to be more significant in males [74].

In a study of 44 children and adolescents with PTSD secondary to maltreatment and 61 matched controls, decreased total midsagittal area of the corpus callosum and decreased brain volume were seen in children with PTSD compared with controls [75]. Most of the children with PTSD had witnessed domestic violence. Earlier onset of abuse and longer duration of abuse correlated with smaller intracranial volume. The PTSD symptoms of intrusion, avoidance, hyperarousal and dissociation correlated with decreased intracranial volume and smaller total corpus callosum area. These findings suggest that adverse effects may be greater with exposure to trauma in early childhood. The correlation of lower intracranial volume with longer duration of abuse also suggests that chronic abuse may have a cumulative, harmful effect on brain development.

Another study from different investigators reported that children with PTSD or subthreshold PTSD showed smaller total brain and cerebral volumes when compared with healthy age- and gender-matched archival controls [76]. In addition, attenuation of frontal lobe asymmetry in children with maltreatment-related PTSD was observed.

In an imaging study that controlled for socioeconomic status, 28 psychotropic drug-naive children and adolescents with maltreatment-related PTSD showed smaller intracranial, cerebral cortex, PFC, PFC cortical white matter and right temporal lobe volumes in comparison with 66 sociodemographically matched healthy controls [73]. Again, total brain volume positively correlated with age of onset of trauma-causing PTSD (i.e., smaller volumes with earlier onset of trauma), and negatively correlated with duration of abuse (i.e., longer duration of abuse with smaller volumes). Most of these subjects with PTSD had experienced abuse and witnessed domestic violence.

Findings from a secondary analysis of sex differences in the published data of DeBellis *et al.* [28,75] suggest that there are sex differences in the brain structures of maltreated children with PTSD [60]. Findings of larger prefrontal lobe cerebrospinal fluid volumes and smaller midsagittal area of the corpus callosum sub region 7 (splenium) were seen in both boys and girls with maltreatment-related PTSD compared with their gender-matched comparison subjects [60]. Additionally, subjects with PTSD did not show the normal age-related increases in the area of the total corpus callosum and its subregion 7 compared with non-maltreated subjects, indicating deficits in age-appropriate myelination in these traumatized children. This latter white matter finding is similar to the work in non-human primates and extends the earlier work. Interestingly, the failure to achieve normal age-related increases in the area of the corpus callosum was more prominent in males with

PTSD. Greater lateral ventricular volumes were seen in maltreated males with PTSD than in control males and were not seen in maltreated females with PTSD, suggesting sex differences leading to more adverse brain maturation in boys compared with girls with maltreatment-related PTSD [60]. These sex differences persisted despite similar ages of onset, duration, length of time since disclosure and similar types of abuse between the boys and girls with PTSD.

The smaller hippocampal volumes seen in adult PTSD secondary to child abuse [77] were not seen in these cross-sectional studies of pediatric PTSD [73,75,76] or in a longitudinal study of pediatric maltreatment-related PTSD [78], although there was some indication that hippocampal volumes may be larger in pediatric maltreatment-related PTSD [79]. Stress-induced hippocampal damage may not be evident until postpubertal development or it may be an inherent vulnerability for chronic PTSD that persists into adulthood [80]. Teenage drinking problems may negatively influence the hippocampus and PFC [81,82]. Neglected children are at higher risk for adolescent alcohol and substance use disorders (reviewed by De Bellis [83]). These double insults (neglect and adolescent onset substance use disorders) may further damage the developing adolescent brain.

In summary, smaller intracranial, cerebral and cerebellar volumes and total midsagittal area of corpus callosum and its posterior subregion, a lack of the normal age-related growth of myelination and larger prefrontal cerebrospinal fluid volumes were seen in maltreated boys and girls with PTSD compared with non-maltreated comparison subjects [60,84]. However, gender effects reveal a more complex developmental picture. The tendency for males to show evidence for more adverse brain development than females while showing similar levels of childhood psychopathology may be a marker for future antisocial behavior. Since child neglect is associated with adolescent and adult antisocial behavior, this is another area of neurobiological study that warrants examination.

## Genetics and child neglect

Recently, researchers have examined genetic variables and early life stress to understand the contribution of each variable to child outcomes. In a large-scale twin study of 1116 monozygotic and dizygotic 5-year-old twin pairs, domestic violence, a form of neglect, was associated with a negative effect on IQ in a dose-dependent fashion [85]. Children exposed to high levels of domestic violence had IQ scores eight points lower than children who were not exposed. This effect did not differ by gender and persisted after controlling for other maltreatment.

Researchers have examined the interaction of genetic variables with early life stress to understand why some children experience conduct problems associated with neglect while others are more resilient. The gene for monoamine oxidase A (*MAOA*), which is located on the X chromosome, has two variants of different transcriptional efficiencies. It has a short, less active allele and a long, more active allele. It is the focus of research examining gene-by-environment interactions with respect to antisocial behavior. Monoamine oxidase A selectively degrades the biogenic amines dopamine, serotonin and norepinephrine after their reuptake from the synaptic cleft, and through this mechanism influences behavioral regulation [86]. Child neglect and antisocial behavior was significantly stronger in boys with the short version of *MAOA*, suggesting that this variant of the *MAOA* genotype confers greater vulnerability [87]. Additionally, adolescent boys with the short *MAOA* allele who were exposed to maltreatment or poor-quality family relations were found to exhibit more alcohol-related problems than maltreated boys with the longer *MAOA* allele [88]. Early prevention and interventions for at-risk children with these genetic vulnerabilities are important ethical issues in the field of developmental traumatology and in public health policy.

## Conclusions

Neglected children have adverse outcomes. However, neglected children may suffer from various types of neglect and other early life stressors and have different genetic vulnerabilities, which contribute to adverse brain development and compromised psychosocial outcomes. Novel non-invasive neuroimaging methods, valid measures of social support, and genetic studies will allow for pioneering studies in developmental traumatology. The study of the effects of child neglect and childhood brain development is only in its infancy. Longitudinal investigations are a promising strategy to further our understanding of the neurobiology of neglect and to help to identify the best predictors for the permanence and the therapeutic reversibility of the adverse effects associated with child neglect. There is a vast literature examining risks for child abuse and neglect. Consequently, we know which children will be at greater risk of neglect. Longitudinal investigations

using effective interventions to prevent child abuse and neglect, such as the Nurse Family Partnership Model [89], in combination with these novel brain imaging methods, will further our understanding of child health.

## Acknowledgements

This work was supported by NIMH grants K24 MH071434 and RO1-MH61744 (Principal Investigator for both, M. D. De Bellis).

## References

1. Levy, H. B., Markovic, J., Chaudry, U. *et al.* (1995). Reabuse rates in a sample of children followed for 5 years after discharge from a child abuse inpatient assessment program. *Child Abuse and Neglect*, **11**, 1363–1377.

2. Hofer, M. A. (1996). On the nature and consequences of early loss. *Psychosomatic Medicine*, **58**, 570–581.

3. Harlow, H. F., Harlow, M. K. and Suomi, S. J. (1971). From thought to therapy: Lessons from a primate laboratory. *American Scientist*, **59**, 538–549.

4. Chapin, H. D. (1995). Are institutions for infants necessary? *Journal of the American Medical Association*, **XIV**, 1–3.

5. Chapin, H. D. (1917). Systematized boarding out vs. institutional care for infants and young children. *New York Medical Journal*, **CV**, 1009–1011.

6. Bakwin, H. (1942). Loneliness in infants. *American Journal of Diseases of Children*, **63**, 30–40.

7. Spitz, R. A. (1945). Hospitalism: An inquiry into the genesis of psychiatric conditions in early childhood Part I. *Psychoanalytic Study of the Child*, **I**, 53–74.

8. Bender, L. and Yarnell, H. (1941). An observation nursery: A study of 250 children in the psychiatric division of Bellevue hospital. *American Journal of Psychiatry*, **97**, 1158–1174.

9. American Psychiatric Association. (1994). *Diagnostic and statistical manual of mental disorders*, 4th edn, Washington, DC: American Psychiatric Press.

10. Bowlby, J. (1982). *Attachment: Attachment and loss*, 2nd edn. New York: Basic Books.

11. De Bellis, M. D. (2001). Developmental traumatology: The psychobiological development of maltreated children and its implications for research, treatment, and policy. *Development and Psychopathology*, **13**, 537–561.

12. De Bellis, M. D. (2003). The neurobiology of posttraumatic stress disorder across the life cycle. In: J. C. Soares and S. Gershon (eds.), *The handbook of medical psychiatry* (pp. 449–466). New York: Marcel Dekker.

13. Rutter, M. (1981). *Maternal deprivation reassessed*. New York: Penguin.

14. Perez, C. and Widom, C. S. (1994). Childhood victimization and long-term intellectual and academic outcomes. *Child Abuse and Neglect,* **18**, 617–633.

15. Widom, C. S., DuMont, K. and Czaja, S. J. (2007). A prospective investigation of major depressive disorder and comorbidity in abused and neglected children grown up. *Archives of General Psychiatry,* **64**, 49–56.

16. Vermetten, E. and Bremner, J. D. (2002). Circuits and systems in stress II. Applications to neurobiology and treatment in posttraumatic stress disorder. *Depression and Anxiety,* **16**, 14–38.

17. Chrousos, G. P. and Gold, P. W. (1992). The concepts of stress and stress system disorders: Overview of physical and behavioral homeostasis. *Journal of the American Medical Association,* **267**, 1244–1252.

18. Herman, J. P., Ostrander, M. M., Mueller, N. K. *et al.* (2005). Limbic system mechanisms of stress regulation: Hypothalamic–pituitary–adrenocortical axis. *Progress in Neuropsychopharmacology and Biological Psychiatry,* **29**, 1201–1213.

19. Bertolucchi-D'Angio, M., Serrano, A. and Scatton, B. (1990). Involvement of mesocorticolimbic dopaminergic systems in emotional states. *Progress in Brain Research,* **85**, 405–416.

20. Arnsten, A. F. T. (1998). The biology of being frazzled. *Science,* **280**, 1711–1712.

21. Lesch, K. P. and Moessner, R. (1998). Genetically driven variation in serotonin update: Is there a link to affective spectrum, neurodevelopmental and neurodegenerative disorders? *Biological Psychiatry,* **44**, 179–192.

22. Fontenot, M. B., Kaplan, J. R., Manuck, S. B. *et al.* (1995). Long-term effects of chronic social stress on serotonergic indices in the prefrontal cortex of adult male cyanomolgus macaques. *Brain Research,* **705**, 105–108.

23. Petty, F., Kramer, G. L. and Wu, J. (1997). Serotonergic modulation of learned helplessness. *Annuals of the New York Academy of Sciences,* **821**, 538–541.

24. Martin, L. J., Sackett, G. P., Gunderson, V. M. *et al.* (1988). Auditory evoked heart rate responses in pigtailed macaques raised in isolation. *Developmental Psychobiology,* **22**, 251–260.

25. Lyons, D. M., Yang, C., Mobley, B. W. *et al.* (2000). Early environment regulation of glucocorticoid feedback sensitivity in young adult monkeys. *Journal of Neuroendocrinology,* **12**, 723–728.

26. Lubach, G. R., Coe, C. L. and Erhler, W. B. (1995). Effects of early rearing environment on immune responses of infant rhesus monkeys. *Brain, Behavior and Immunity,* **9**, 31–46.

27. Queiroz, E. A., Lombardi, A. B., Santos Furtado, C. R.H. *et al.* (1991). Biochemical correlate of depression in children. *Arquiros de neuro-psiquiatria,* **49**, 418–425.

28. De Bellis, M. D., Baum, A., Birmaher, B. *et al.* (1999). A. E. Bennett Research Award. Developmental traumatology: Part I: biological stress systems. *Biological Psychiatry,* **45**, 1259–1270.

29. Perry, B. D. (1994). Neurobiological sequelae of childhood trauma: PTSD in children. In M. M. Murburg (ed.), *Catecholamine function in posttraumatic stress disorder: Emerging concepts* (pp. 233–255). Washington, DC: American Psychiatric Press.

30. Famularo, R., Kinsherff, R. and Fenton, T. (1988). Propranolol treatment for childhood posttraumatic stress disorder, acute type. *American Journal of the Diseases of Children,* **142**, 1244–1247.

31. Cohen, J. A., Mannarino, A. P., Perel, J. M. *et al.* (2007). A pilot randomized controlled trial of combined trauma-focused CBT and sertraline for childhood PTSD symptoms *Journal of the American Academy of Child and Adolescent Psychiatry,* **46**, 811–819.

32. Gunnar, M. R., Morison, S. J., Chisholm, K. *et al.* (2001). Salivary cortisol levels in children adopted from Romanian orphanages. *Development and Psychopathology,* **13**, 611–628.

33. Hart, J., Gunnar, M. and Cicchetti, D. (1996). Altered neuroendocrine activity in maltreated children related to symptoms of depression. *Development and Psychopathology,* **8**, 201–214.

34. Carrion, V. G., Weems, C. F., Ray, R. D. *et al.* (2002). Diurnal salivary cortisol in pediatric posttraumatic stress disorder. *Biological Psychiatry,* **51**, 575–582.

35. Thomas, L. A. and De Bellis, M. D. (2004). Pituitary volumes in pediatric maltreatment related PTSD. *Biological Psychiatry,* **55**, 752–758.

36. Selye, H. (1936). A syndrome produced by diverse nocuous agents. *Nature,* **138**, 32.

37. Weiss, J. M. and Sundar, S. (1992). Effects of stress on cellular immune responses in animals. In A. Tasman and M. B. Riba (eds.), *Review of psychiatry* (pp. 145–168). Washington, DC: American Psychiatric Press.

38. Jernigan, T. L. and Sowell, E. R. (1997). Magnetic resonance imaging studies of the developing brain. In M. S. Keshavan and R. M. Murray (eds.), *Neurodevelopment and adult psychopathology* (pp. 63–70). Cambridge, UK: Cambridge University Press.

39. Durston, S., Hulshoff Pol, H. E., Casey, B. J. *et al.* (2001). Anatomical MRI of the developing human brain: What have we learned? *Journal of the American Academy of Child and Adolescent Psychiatry,* **40**, 1012–1020.

40. Giedd, J. N., Blumenthal, J., Jeffries, N. O. *et al.* (1999). Brain development during childhood and adolescence: A longitudinal MRI study. *Nature Neuroscience,* **2**, 861–863.

41. Thompson, P. M., Giedd, J. N., Woods, R. P. *et al.* (2000). Growth patterns in the developing brain detected by using continuum mechanical tensor maps. *Nature,* **404**, 190–193.

42. Paus, T., Collins, D. L., Evans, A. C. *et al.* (2001). Maturation of white matter in the human brain: A

review of magnetic resonance studies. *Brain Research Bulletin,* **54**, 255–266.

43. Giedd, J. N., Blumenthal, J., Jeffries, N. O. *et al.* (1999). Development of the human corpus callosum during childhood and adolescence: A longitudinal MRI study. *Progress in Neuropsychopharmacology and Biological Psychiatry,* **23**, 571–588.

44. Alexander, G. E. and Goldman, P. S. (1978). Functional development of the dorsolateral prefrontal cortex: An analysis utilizing reversible cryogenic depression. *Brain Research,* **143**, 233–249.

45. Smythies, J. R. (1997). Oxidative reactions and schizophrenia: A review-discussion. *Schizophrenia Research,* **24**, 357–364.

46. Sapolsky, R. M. (2000). Glucocorticoids and hippocampal atrophy in neuropsychiatric disorders. *Archives of General Psychiatry,* **57**, 925–935.

47. Simantov, R., Blinder, E., Ratovitski, T. *et al.* (1996). Dopamine induced apoptosis in human neuronal cells: Inhibition by nucleic acids antisense to the dopamine transporter. *Neuroscience,* **74**, 39–50.

48. Edwards, E., Harkins, K., Wright, G. *et al.* (1990). Effects of bilateral adrenalectomy on the induction of learned helplessness. *Behavioral Neuropsychopharmacology,* **3**, 109–114.

49. Dunlop, S. A., Archer, M. A., Quinlivan, J. A. *et al.* (1997). Repeated prenatal corticosteroids delay myelination in the ovine central nervous system. *Journal of Maternal–Fetal Medicine,* **6**, 309–313.

50. Lauder, J. M. (1988). Neurotransmitters as morphogens. *Progress in Brain Research,* **73**, 365–388.

51. Todd, R. D. (1992). Neural development is regulated by classical neuro-transmitters: Dopamine D2 receptor stimulation enhances neurite outgrowth. *Biological Psychiatry,* **31**, 794–807.

52. Tanapat, P., Galea, L. A. and Gould, E. (1998). Stress inhibits the proliferation of granule cell precursors in the developing dentate gyrus. *Journal of Developmental Neuroscience,* **16**, 235–239.

53. Gould, E., Tanapat, P. and Cameron, H. A. (1997). Adrenal steroids suppress granule cell death in the developing dentate gyrus through an NMDA receptor-dependent mechanism. *Developmental Brain Research,* **103**, 91–93.

54. Gould, E., Tanapat, P., McEwen, B. S. *et al.* (1998). Proliferation of granule cell precursors in the dentate gyrus of adult monkeys is diminished by stress. *Proceedings of the National Academy of Sciences USA,* **95**, 3168–3171.

55. Smith, M. A., Makino, S., Kvetnansky, R. *et al.* (1995). Effects of stress on neurotrophic factor expression in the rat brain. *Annals of the New York Academy of Sciences,* **771**, 234–239.

56. Felitti, V. J., Anda, R. F., Nordenberg, D. *et al.* (1998). Relationship of childhood abuse and household dys-

function to many of the leading causes if death in adults. *American Journal of Preventive Medicine,* **14**, 245–258.

57. McEwen, B. S. (1981). Neural gonadal steroid actions. *Science,* **211**, 1303–1311.

58. De Bellis, M. D., Keshavan, M. S., Beers, S. R. *et al.* (2001). Sex differences in brain maturation during childhood and adolescence. *Cerebral Cortex,* **11**, 552–557.

59. McGloin, J. M. and Widom, C. S. (2001). Resilience among abused and neglected children grown up. *Development and Psychopathology,* **13**, 1021–1038.

60. De Bellis, M. D. and Keshavan, M. S. (2003). Sex differences in brain maturation in maltreatment-related pediatric posttraumatic stress disorder. *Neurosciences and Biobehavioral Reviews,* **27**, 103–117.

61. LeDoux, J. (1998). Fear and the brain: Where have we been, and where are we going? *Biological Psychiatry,* **44**, 1229–1238.

62. Posner, M. I. and Petersen, S. E. (1990). The attention system of the human brain. *Annual Review of Neuroscience,* **13**, 25–42.

63. Bremner, J. D., Narayan, M., Staib, L. *et al.* (1999). Neural correlates of memories of childhood sexual abuse in women with and without posttraumatic stress disorder. *American Journal of Psychiatry,* **156**, 1787–1795.

64. Shin, L. M., McNally, R. J., Kosslyn, S. M. *et al.* (1999). Regional cerebral blood flow during script-imagery in childhood sexual abuse-related PTSD: A PET investigation. *American Journal of Psychiatry,* **156**, 575–584.

65. Gluck, J. P. and Sachiltz, K. A. (1976). Extinction deficits in socially isolated rhesus monkeys (Macaca mulatta). *Developmental Psychology,* **12**, 173–174.

66. Beauchamp, A. J. and Gluck, J. P. (1988). Associative processes in differentially reared monkeys (Macaca mulatta): Sensory preconditioning. *Developmental Psychobiology,* **21**, 355–364.

67. Beauchamp, A. J., Gluck, J. P. and Lewis, M. H. (1991). Associative processes in differentially reared rhesus monkeys (Macaca mulatta): Blocking. *Developmental Psychobiology,* **24**, 175–189.

68. Sanchez, M. M., Hearn, E. F., Do, D. *et al.* (1998). Differential rearing affects corpus callosum size and cognitive function of rhesus monkeys. *Brain Research,* **812**, 38–49.

69. Strathearn, L., Gray, P. H., O'Callaghan, F. *et al.* (2001). Childhood neglect and cognitive development in extremely low birth weight infants: A prospective study. *Pediatrics,* **108**, 142–151.

70. Chugani, H. T., Behan, M. E., Muzik, O. *et al.* (2001). Local brain functional activity following early deprivation: A study of post-institutionalized Romanian orphans. *NeuroImage,* **14**, 1290–1301.

71. Diamond, M. C., Krech, D. and Rosenzweig, M. R. (1964). The effects of an enriched environment on

the histology of the rat cerebral cortex. *Journal of Comparative Neurology,* **123**, 111–120.

72. Juraska, J. M. and Kopcik, J. R. (1988). Sex and environmental influences on the size and ultrastructure of the rat corpus callosum. *Brain Research,* **450**, 1–8.

73. De Bellis, M. D., Keshavan, M., Shifflett, H. *et al.* (2002). Brain structures in pediatric maltreatment-related PTSD: A sociodemographically matched study. *Biological Psychiatry,* **52**, 1066–1078.

74. Teicher, M. H., Ito, Y., Glod, C. A. *et al.* (1997). Preliminary evidence for abnormal cortical development in physically and sexually abused children using EEG coherence and MRI. *Annals of the New York Academy of Sciences,* **821**, 160–175.

75. De Bellis, M. D., Keshavan, M., Clark, D. B. *et al.* (1999). A. E. Bennett Research Award. Developmental traumatology, Part II: Brain development. *Biological Psychiatry,* **45**, 1271–1284.

76. Carrion, V. G., Weems, C. F., Eliez, S. *et al.* (2001). Attenuation of frontal asymmetry in pediatric post-traumatic stress disorder. *Biological Psychiatry,* **50**, 943–951.

77. Bremner, J. D., Randall, P., Vermetten, E. *et al.* (1997). Magnetic resonance imaging-based measurement of hippocampal volume in posttraumatic stress disorder related to childhood physical and sexual abuse: A preliminary report. *Biological Psychiatry,* **41**, 23–32.

78. De Bellis, M. D., Hall, J., Boring, A. M. *et al.* (2001). A pilot longitudinal study of hippocampal volumes in pediatric maltreatment-related posttraumatic stress disorder. *Biological Psychiatry,* **50**, 305–309.

79. Tupler, L. A. and De Bellis, M. D. (2006). Segmented hippocampal volume in children and adolescents with posttraumatic stress disorder. *Biological Psychiatry,* **59**, 523–529.

80. Gilbertson, M. W., Shenton, M. E., Ciszewski, A. *et al.* (2002). Smaller hippocampal volume predicts pathologic vulnerability to psychological trauma. *Nature Neuroscience,* **5**, 1242–1247.

81. De Bellis, M. D., Clark, D. B., Beers, S. R. *et al.* (2000). Hippocampal volume in adolescent onset alcohol use disorders. *American Journal of Psychiatry,* **157**, 737–744.

82. De Bellis, M. D., Narasimhan, A., Thatcher, D. L. *et al.* (2005). Prefrontal cortex, thalamus and cerebellar volumes in adolescents and young adults with adolescent onset alcohol use disorders and co-morbid mental disorders. *Alcoholism: Clinical and Experimental Research,* **29**, 1590–1600.

83. De Bellis, M. D. (2002). Developmental traumatology: A contributory mechanism for alcohol and substance use disorders. *Psychoneuroendocrinology,* **27**, 155–170.

84. De Bellis, M. D. and Kuchibhatla, M. (2006). Cerebellar volumes in pediatric maltreatment-related posttraumatic stress disorder. *Biological Psychiatry,* **60**, 697–703.

85. Koenen, K. C., Moffitt, T. E., Caspi, A. *et al.* (2003). Domestic violence is associated with environmental suppression of IQ in young children. *Development and Psychopathology,* **15**, 297–311.

86. Shih, J. C., Chen, K. and Ridd, M. J. (1999). Monoamine oxidase: from genes to behavior *Annual Review of Neuroscience,* **22**, 197–217.

87. Caspi, A., McClay, J., Moffitt, T. *et al.* (2002). Role of genotype in the cycle of violence in maltreated children. *Science,* **297**, 851–854.

88. Nilsson, K. W. Sjoberg, R. L. Wargelius, H. L. *et al.* (2007). The monoamine oxidase A (MAO-A) gene, family function and maltreatment as predictors of destructive behaviour during male adolescent alcohol consumption. *Addiction,* **102**, 389–398.

89. Olds, D. L. (2002). Prenatal and infancy home visiting by nurses: From randomized trials to community replication. *Prevention Science,* **3**, 153–172.

# Chapter 13

# Early life stress as a risk factor for disease in adulthood

Philip A. Fisher and Megan Gunnar

## Introduction

Early life stress (ELS) and trauma are often thought to virtually guarantee negative outcomes over the course of development. Although there is little doubt that stressful and traumatic experiences early in life often play a deterministic role in the emergence of later pathology and disease, studies employing animal models and those focusing on high-risk human populations are revealing an increasingly complex, interdependent and multidetermined set of processes that influence outcomes. These include individual-specific factors such as genetics and temperament, a variety of dimensions of the ELS (e.g., type, duration, age at onset) and, perhaps most importantly, what occurs in the environment of the individual following the traumatic experiences. In this chapter, we draw on this emerging research, and particularly on our past and ongoing studies of children in foster care, to provide a framework for understanding the interplay of these multiple factors influencing positive versus negative outcomes.

Children enter foster care because they have been maltreated – via acts of commission (physical, sexual or psychological abuse) or omission (neglect of physical and social needs). To result in an out-of-home placement, such maltreatment needs to pose an imminent and ongoing risk to the child. Consequently, foster children have rarely experienced only a single episode of maltreatment; rather, multiple instances of maltreatment over prolonged periods of time are common by the time children enter foster care [1].

The experience of a single form of maltreatment also appears to be fairly unusual among foster children. Pears et al. [2] employed retrospective methods for coding maltreatment from official case records. They found that, although neglect and emotional maltreatment occurred more frequently than other types of maltreatment among foster children (i.e., in over

80% of cases), the co-occurrence of neglect and emotional maltreatment was most common, occurring in 62% of the cases. The co-occurrence of multiple types of abuse in combination with neglect was common to a lesser degree.

Maltreatment experiences have a strong impact on a foster child's well-being. In epidemiological studies of foster children in comparison with their non-maltreated counter-parts, researchers have documented widespread disparities among numerous indicators of psychological adjustment [3,4]. In addition, delays in cognitive and emotional development are common, elevated substance abuse rates in adolescence have been reported and physical health appears to be compromised in many instances [5–9].

Although maltreatment has long been considered a root cause of foster children's poor outcomes, placement in foster care might further exacerbate existing risks. In a recent report, Kessler et al. [10] found that adults who had spent time in foster care as children had disproportionately high rates of anxiety, depression, substance use disorders and physical health disorders. In a similar retrospective study of foster care alumni, Juon et al. [11] found higher rates of psychiatric disorders and mortality. Although these results do not provide causal evidence of the link between foster care and poor outcomes, several studies have documented poorer outcomes for foster children who spend more time in care and who experienced more placement transitions [12,13].

A number of explanations have been offered for the potentially pathogenic nature of foster care. By definition, foster care involves the disruption of a child's primary caregiver relationship. At best, most foster children experience two disruptions, one at placement into foster care and another when they return home or are adopted. However, in many instances, there are additional disruptions – sometimes numerous, as a result of failed foster placements, failed reunifications and failed adoptions. From the perspective of attachment theory, each disruption represents a significant challenge to healthy development [14,15]. In addition to the stress of these relationship disruptions, foster homes might not be well suited to meet the needs of the child for several reasons: a lack of parental experience/skills in dealing with difficult behaviors exhibited by traumatized children; an absence of training, support and consultation; and/or a lack of resources in the system that results in placements of multiple children with substantial emotional and behavioral problems in the same foster home [16].

The limitations of conventional foster care in providing an environment that can help to mitigate the effects of early maltreatment are acknowledged public health concerns and have led to efforts to develop effective intervention strategies to improve foster children's outcomes [10,17–19]. As we have noted in several prior publications, however, not all children in foster care fare poorly [2,20]. Indeed, some foster children's outcomes are positive despite the adversity they have faced. This might result from a combination of factors, including constitutional factors on the part of the children associated with resilience (e.g., intelligence and easy temperament), aspects of the children's early environments that support healthy development in spite of the presence of maltreatment (e.g., a supportive relationship with at least one adult), particularly skilled foster parents and/or caseworkers and the availability of high-quality services to address problems.

# A translational neurobiological model to describe pathways towards risk and resiliency following early life stress

The scientific literature contains few empirically grounded conceptual models that help to explicate differential trajectories towards positive and negative outcomes among foster children. Such models are of critical importance because they have the potential to advance knowledge beyond existing "hydraulic" conceptualizations of risk and protection, in which negative influences are summed and subtracted from positive influences to predict outcomes. As such, more precise and specific models might guide theory, policy and practice.

In several prior publications, we have described a translational conceptual model developed in the context of our research on children reared under adverse conditions to explain differential pathways between risk and resilience [20,21]. This model was developed drawing from the vast literature on the neurobiological effects of ELS on development, much of it using animal models. Our work has focused specifically on the neurobiological systems involved in the reaction and the regulation of physiological responses to stressors.

One area of emphasis in our research involves patterns of activity of the hypothalamic–pituitary–adrenal (HPA) system, which produces cortisol, a steroid hormone. The HPA system activates in response to stressors, including psychosocial stressors, which then activates a number of neural systems involved in the appraisals and responses to threats, with the central nucleus of the amygdala and bed nucleus of the stria terminalis as the final common pathways to the HPA system. The regulation of responses to psychosocial threats also involves forebrain systems, predominantly the hippocampus and regions of the prefrontal cortex involved in executive functioning (i.e., anterior cingulate cortex and medial prefrontal cortex). These forebrain regions are also critical to emotion and behavior regulation.

Alterations in HPA system regulation and problems with emotion and behavior regulation have been widely associated with later psychopathology [22]. Moreover, there is clear evidence that the development of these systems is strongly tied to the quality of early care [23]. However, only recently has knowledge from basic cognitive and developmental neuroscience begun to be applied to such populations as foster children. This work has considerable potential significance because it might provide more precise explanatory models than achieved with purely psychosocial formulations for high-risk populations (e.g., characterizing why many foster children fail to respond to improved environmental conditions even when the psychosocial variables posited to be the cause of their problems are no longer present) and might provide specific targets for interventions (e.g., addressing deficits in inhibitory control and working memory).

In our original formulation of this model, we emphasized specific dimensions of ELS suggested by prior research to be strongly deterministic of positive versus negative outcomes. In particular, we focused on the *timing* of ELS. Animal studies have shown that the impact of inadequate or inappropriate care experiences on the development of the HPA system is greatest when it occurs early in life, during periods roughly comparable to the first 5 years in humans [24]. The long-term effects of stressors during this period might reflect epigenetic effects (i.e., effects that permanently alter gene expression in neural systems regulating reactivity to stressors) [25]. They might also result from the impact of stress hormones (e.g., cortisol) and associated neuroactive peptides (e.g., corticotropin-releasing hormone) on the maturation of key neural systems (e.g., amygdala, hippocampus and prefrontal cortex) involved in emotion and behavior regulation through mechanisms such as apoptosis (programmed cell death), neurogenesis in the hippocampus and processes impacting neural plasticity [26–28].

Interestingly, the period during which ELS has the most impact in animal models is the period during which appropriate parental care is associated with maintenance of the HPA system in a nearly quiescent state. That is, during this period, in the context of supportive parental care, stressors that in an older animal would provoke large activations of this neuroendocrine system provoke little or no increases in activity. It has been argued that the sensitivity of the developing stress and emotion regulatory system to variations in parental care during this period functions to aid later survival. Meaney and Szyf [25] postulated that such sensitivity prepares individuals to face a hostile, threatening world that requires rapid and frequent shifts to a defensive posture focused on immediate survival or a more supportive, benign world that allows the individual to place more physical and mental resources towards preparation for the future.

These findings from animal studies have been extended to children through evidence that, during infancy and early childhood, sensitive, responsive and supportive care (of the type necessary for the development of secure infant–caregiver attachment) provides a powerful buffer or regulator of the human HPA system [29,30]. This type of care appears to prevent or vastly ameliorate elevations in cortisol in response to events that nonetheless provoke distress and apprehensive behavioral reactions from young children. In the absence of responsive caregiving (e.g., children living in institutions in Romania), young children show marked aberrations in HPA system activity [31]. These aberrations are particularly salient when cortisol samples are taken across the day. Under conditions of low stress, the HPA system follows a diurnal pattern of basal cortisol production, with peak levels around the time of morning awakening and near zero levels

around the onset of nighttime sleep. Under conditions of chronic stress, however, the diurnal pattern is attenuated or absent because of the system's failure to inhibit production later in the day or to generate the early morning surge in hormone production [32].

In examining the chronic stress signature in foster children, similar atypical diurnal HPA system patterns are found among foster children when compared with non-maltreated community children [33]. The patterns in foster children are consistent with those obtained from institutionally reared children. Attenuated morning cortisol levels were observed in approximately 33% of the foster children; in contrast, this pattern was observed in only 10% of the community children. Parallel results were obtained in a similar study of young foster children conducted by Dozier and colleagues [34]. Therefore, alterations in diurnal cortisol production appear to be a hallmark of ELS in many (although certainly not all) foster children.

Although this model is useful as a descriptive tool, a number of recent scientific developments suggest that it warrants elaboration. For the remainder of this chapter, we concentrate on three areas of model development that are the focus of our ongoing investigations. First, we present data showing how differential impacts to specific neural regulatory systems are associated with variations by the *type* of ELS experienced. Second, we describe how studies of the *severity* of ELS are providing a new basis for understanding trajectories towards risk versus resilience among foster children and other populations who experience ELS. Third, we describe a growing body of evidence documenting the *plasticity* of these neural systems in response to psychosocial, family-based therapeutic interventions. After describing these model extensions, we discuss the implications of these developments for future intervention research, practice and public policy.

## Recent extensions of the translational model

### Variations in the type of early life stress

As is described above, there is growing evidence that ELS affects the development of stress regulatory neural systems in foster children (and similar populations of post-institutional adoptees). However, not all children in these populations exhibit characteristic patterns of neural dysregulation. This led us to explore whether there are specific dimensions of ELS that are more strongly associated with alterations in the neural systems that form our model.

The first investigations in this area focused on the HPA system. Associations were examined between different types of maltreatment (coded retrospectively from child welfare case records), foster placement history variables (e.g., age at first placement and number of placements) and alterations in preschool-aged foster children's diurnal HPA system function [35]. Among the maltreatment variables, only neglect was significantly associated with atypical cortisol levels. Neither physical nor sexual abuse was predictive of atypical diurnal cortisol. In addition, none of the foster placement history variables was associated with atypical diurnal cortisol. Notably, neglect was associated specifically with attenuated morning cortisol levels, similar to that observed among post-institutional adoptees, whose early care is strongly characterized by neglect [36]. These results suggest that ELS effects might arise from the presence of traumatic events and the absence of responsive caregiving.

As our conceptual model has expanded beyond the HPA system to include the structurally and functionally connected forebrain regions involved in executive cognitive functions, we have looked at how different dimensions of ELS affect the development of these systems. Interestingly, neither prior abuse nor prior neglect appears to be significantly associated with deficits in this area. Rather, this domain of functioning appears to be more strongly affected by foster placement history variables. In particular, Pears et al. [2] found that the number of unique caregivers young foster children lived with was positively associated with poorer performance on a composite measure of executive functioning neuropsychological tasks. Similarly, Lewis et al. [13] reported that foster children's performance on a day/night Stroop task was negatively affected by prior placement instability.

It is important to acknowledge that the current evidence regarding how the type of ELS differentially affects specific neural systems is correlational in nature. Consequently, it would be premature to conclude at this point that different types of ELS cause alterations in different neural systems. Nevertheless, some conclusions of this work are highly promising: (a) low early morning cortisol levels and the resulting attenuated diurnal cortisol pattern might be most associated with neglect rather than other ELS variables, and (b) the

development of neural systems involved in executive functioning is more adversely affected by placement instability than by other ELS variables. These finding might help to explain why certain domains of functioning appear to be remarkably intact in some children, despite their having experienced considerable adversity. For example, for children whose maltreatment might not have included severe neglect and who have spent relatively little time in one foster home before achieving a permanent placement, their experiences might leave psychological scars but not significantly impact the neurobiological systems in question. Our research in this area is ongoing.

## Variations in the severity of early life stress

At this point, it might seem that the best conditions for foster children's later adaptive functioning would involve the elimination of all ELS or the provision of adequate caregiving to prevent atypical stress regulatory neural system activity. However, emerging evidence suggests this view is inaccurate. Recent studies with non-human primates (with ages equivalent to toddler- or preschool-aged children) have shown that a repeated stressor (e.g., maternal separation) provokes large increases in HPA system activity but results in better self-regulatory skills, improved executive functioning and better modulated stress hormone activation in adulthood [37]. The authors of this work argue that experiencing stressors that are significant but manageable early in life provides a form of "stress inoculation." In a recent study with children adopted from overseas, Gunnar et al. [38] observed that children adopted following several months of foster care had lower cortisol levels and smaller cortisol activations to a standardized laboratory stressor task when they were 10–11 years of age than children reared in their birth families in the USA. This was not the case for children adopted following prolonged periods of institutional care overseas. Although children adopted internationally from foster care have experienced disruptions in early care, other work has shown that, if adopted early, these children do not show problems with various measures of executive functioning, memory or learning [39]. Therefore, similar to the non-human primates studied by Parker et al. [37,40], mild ELS might ultimately stimulate the development of a better-regulated stress system. This hypothesis, which requires additional confirmation, would be consistent with arguments by Boyce and Ellis [41] that too few opportunities to develop stress-coping capacities or too many (or overwhelming) challenges can contribute to hypersensitivity to stressors later in life.

### Individual differences and stress inoculation

Arguments about moderate versus severe ELS and resilience pose the problem of defining, a priori, what constitutes ELS that produces stress inoculation versus stress vulnerability. This problem is exacerbated by mounting evidence indicating that the dividing line varies at the individual level. Research on resilience has shown that, to some degree, environmental factors (e.g., the presence of at least one supportive adult) differentiate individuals who are resilient or vulnerable to ELS [42]. However, other work has strongly suggested that heritable factors play a critical role in the sequelae of, for example, childhood maltreatment [43]. Studies of stress reactivity among adults with significant ELS exposure previously emphasized hyper-responsivity of the HPA system that was comparable to the sequelae observed in many animal models [44]. However, recent studies examining psychologically health adults with ELS histories have shown that these individuals exhibit increased regulation (reduced responding) of the HPA system in response to acute laboratory stressors, with regulation increasing with more ELS exposures [45]. It is not that these individuals have experienced less ELS than those who later show hyper-reactions to stress, as those with the same criteria for ELS exposures have hyperreactive or hyperregulated patterns depending on whether the adult is clinically depressed or is free from psychiatric illness [46]. Consequently, it is possible that some experiences typically viewed as stressors (potentially capable of undermining the development of emotion, behavior and stress regulation) might, in fact, inoculate some foster children against the effects of future stress, assuming that the experiences are not overwhelming.

There is also evidence that genetic variation underlies individual differences in stress response. For example, Binder and colleagues [47] studied depression associated with polymorphisms in the gene *FKBP5*, which is involved in cortisol receptor activity and thus HPA system regulation. They found that, for individuals who had experienced childhood abuse, only those with a particular version of *FKBP5* developed depression. Those with similar abuse histories but without this specific gene variant did not exhibit higher incidence of depressive episodes. Interestingly, Oulette-Morin and colleagues [48] conducted a twin study examining the effects of early adversity on the development of HPA system functioning and found that genetic

effects (i.e., similar responses by twins to stressors) occurred under conditions of low but not high family adversity. Here, again, under ELS circumstances that an individual experiences as overwhelming, the long-term effects might have little potential to be anything other than pathogenic. In less stressful contexts, however, there might be considerable variation in the potential outcomes. Variation in outcomes in these less stressful contexts might have strong genetic determinants and might range from enhanced resilience to increased psychopathology and maladjustment. Our ongoing research emphasizes clearer characterizations of individual perceptions of ELS experience along the continuum of low to high adversity as well as efforts to identify specific polymorphisms that exhibit deterministic qualities regarding risk versus resilience trajectories.

## Plasticity of stress regulatory neural systems

Although the above extensions of our translational model of ELS have been helpful in postulating differential effects and trajectories from the vast heterogeneity of experiences among foster children, there is a potentially negatively deterministic quality in these studies. The future for children whose experiential profiles and genetic predispositions are associated with resilience and positive outcomes might be somewhat protected. Conversely, the futures for children whose experiential profiles and genetic predispositions are associated with elevated risk for poor outcomes are less hopeful.

However, one of the major emphases of our work has been to examine how therapeutic interventions, situated in caregiving/family contexts (which animal and human studies have shown to be basic to the successful development of these neural systems), mitigate the effects of ELS and optimize the plasticity of these systems. Put simply, systematic interventions could help caregivers to facilitate functional development in these systems despite the accumulation of risk factors. In the context of prevention science, preventive interventions aim to alter individuals' life course trajectories away from poor outcomes and towards positive outcomes. The application of this conceptualization to our translation model is that caregiver-based interventions have the potential to impact individuals whose neurobiology and behavior has been adversely affected by ELS and to improve the functioning of their neural systems and later psychosocial adjustment. Randomized trials of caregiver-based therapeutic interventions are providing evidence of the plasticity of stress regulatory neural systems following exposure to ELS.

In a series of papers, we have shown that a therapeutic foster care intervention called Multidimensional Treatment Foster Care for Preschoolers (MTFC-P) impacts a variety of neurobiological and psychosocial domains. In the context of a randomized clinical trial comparing MTFC-P with regular foster care, the intervention was associated with increased stabilization of diurnal HPA system activity [49]. More recently, Fisher and Stoolmiller [50] have shown that the effects of the MTFC-P intervention on HPA system activity are inversely associated over time with caregiver-reported stress in managing problem behavior. That is, more stable diurnal HPA system activity was associated with lower caregiver stress in managing problem behavior in the intervention group. In addition, the MTFC-P intervention has been found to be effective at increasing secure and decreasing insecure attachment-related behaviors and at increasing permanent placement stability [19,20,51].

In addition to our findings with the MTFC-P program, there is emerging evidence from other scientifically robust studies that caregiver-based interventions have the potential to yield effects on stress regulatory neural systems. For example, Dozier *et al.* [52] reported similar normalization of cortisol levels in response to a laboratory stressor among young foster children randomized into their intervention condition. Moreover, in a randomized trial of a psychosocial intervention with inner-city, socially disadvantaged youth (not in foster care), Brotman *et al.* [53] reported normalization of cortisol levels in response to social stressors.

Evidence of neural plasticity in humans following ELS, long anticipated in seminal animal research involving the effects of enriched environments on brain and behavioral development, is beginning to extend beyond the HPA system to other neural systems that make up our translational model [54]. For example, Bruce *et al.* [55] conducted a pilot study of the effects of the MTFC-P intervention on foster children's event-related potentials measured by electroencephalography in response to a computer flanker task, which is known to activate areas of the prefrontal cortex associated with inhibitory control, a domain of executive function. Children were provided with visual feedback on the computer screen, based on whether they made correct or incorrect responses. Results indicated that foster children in the MTFC-P intervention condition showed significantly more activation of prefrontal regions following incorrect responses. Such increased sensitivity to error-related feedback provides highly promising, albeit preliminary, evidence that we are approaching an era in which existing deterministic models of the effects of ELS on outcomes are tempered by emerging studies regarding the plasticity of key neural systems in response to interventions.

# Conclusions

The period since the mid 1990s has seen the emergence of translational developmental science, which involves synergistic, cross-disciplinary collaborations among preclinical scientists, molecular and behavioral geneticists, human developmental psychologists and neuropsychologists, clinical and prevention researchers, physicians, clinicians, policy makers and others. This new discipline has the potential to rapidly advance our knowledge and understanding of social afflictions and their amelioration. Only time will tell if this potential will be realized.

A core goal for this new discipline is to emphasize the cross-fertilization of selective knowledge across multiple levels of analysis (e.g., molecular, genetic, neurobiological, behavioral, individual, familial, racial, cultural and societal) to lead to increasingly precise prediction models for differentiating individuals in any risk group who, when faced with adversity, are likely to fail or prevail. As is discussed in this chapter, an equally important goal is to employ translational developmental science in designing and evaluating systematic interventions to positively impact the life course trajectories and the related underlying neural systems of individuals who have experienced ELS. The research described here may serve as a model for how basic research on the neurobiology of ELS can be used to inform interventions for high-risk children in general. Much work remains to be done across the spectrum of risk and resilience following ELS in order to improve the identification of individuals in need of services and to specify the techniques most likely to improve outcomes.

# Acknowledgements

Support for this research was provided by the following grants: MH059780 (NIMH, US PHS) MH065046 (NIMH, US PHS) and MH052135 (NIMH, US PHS).

# References

1. Manly, J. T., Kim, J. E., Rogosch, F. A. *et al.* (2001). Dimensions of child maltreatment and children's adjustment: Contributions of developmental timing and subtype. *Developmental Psychopathology,* **13**, 759–782.

2. Pears, K. C., Kim, H. K. and Fisher, P. A. (2008). Psychosocial and cognitive functioning of children with specific profiles of maltreatment. *Child Abuse & Neglect,* **32**, 958–971.

3. Burns, B. J., Phillips, S., Wagner, R. *et al.* (2004). Mental health need and access to mental health services by youth involved with child welfare: A national survey. *Journal of the American Academy of Child and Adolescent Psychiatry,* **43**, 960–970.

4. Landsverk, J. A., Garland, A. F. and Leslie, L. K. (2001). Mental health services for children reported to child protective services. In J. E. B. Myers, C. T. Hendrix, L. Berliner, *et al.* (eds.), *APSAC handbook on child maltreatment,* 2nd edn (pp. 487–507). Thousand Oaks, CA: Sage.

5. Pears, K. C. and Fisher, P. A. (2005). Developmental, cognitive, and neuropsychological functioning in preschool-aged foster children: Associations with prior maltreatment and placement history. *Journal of Developmental and Behavioral Pediatrics,* **26**, 112–122.

6. Pears, K. C. and Fisher, P. A. (2005). Emotion understanding and theory of mind among maltreated children in foster care: Evidence of deficits. *Developmental Psychopathology,* **17**, 47–65.

7. Aarons, G. A., Brown, S. A., Hough, R. L., Garland, A. F. and Wood, P. A. (2001). Prevalence of adolescent substance use disorders across five sectors of care. *Journal of the American Academy of Child and Adolescent Psychiatry,* **40**, 419–426.

8. Simms, M. D., Dubowitz, H. and Szilagyi, M. A. (2000). Health care needs of children in the foster care system. *Pediatrics,* **106**, 909–918.

9. Simms, M. D. and Halfon, N. (1994). The Health Care Needs of Children in Foster Care: A Research Agenda. *Child Welfare,* **73**, 505–524.

10. Kessler, R. C., Pecora, P. J., Williams, J. *et al.* (2008). Effects of enhanced foster care on the long-term physical and mental health of foster care alumni. *Archives of General Psychiatry,* **65**, 625–633.

11. Juon, H.-S., Ensminger, M. E. and Feehan, M. (2004). Childhood adversity and later mortality in an urban African American cohort. *American Journal of Public Health,* **93**, 2044–2046.

12. Newton, R. R., Litrownik, A. J. and Landsverk, J. A. (2000). Children and youth in foster care: Disentangling the relationship between problem behaviors and number of placements. *Child Abuse & Neglect,* **24**, 1363–1374.

13. Lewis, E., Dozier, M., Ackerman, J. and Sepulveda-Kozakowski, S. (2007). The effect of placement instability on adopted children's inhibitory control abilities and oppositional behavior. *Developmental Psychobiology,* **43**, 1415–1427.

14. Harden, B. J. (2004). Safety and stability for foster children: A developmental perspective. *The Future of Children,* **14**, 30–47.

15. Smith, D. K., Stormshak, E., Chamberlain, P. and Bridges Whaley, R. (2001). Placement disruption in treatment foster care. *Journal of Emotional and Behavioral Disorders,* **9**, 200–205.

16. Reddy, L. A. and Pfeiffer, S. I. (1997). Effectiveness of treatment foster care with children and adolescents: A review of outcome studies. *Journal of the American Academy of Child and Adolescent Psychiatry,* **36**, 581–588.

17. Nemeroff, C. B. (2008). Fostering foster care outcomes: Quality of intervention matters in overcoming early adversity. *Archives of General Psychiatry,* **65**, 623–624.

18. Chamberlain, P., Price, J., Leve, L. D. *et al.* (2008). Prevention of behavior problems for children in foster care: Outcomes and mediation effects. *Prevention Science,* **9**, 17–27.

19. Fisher, P. A., Burraston, B. and Pears, K. (2005). The Early Intervention Foster Care Program: Permanent placement outcomes from a randomized trial. *Child Maltreatment,* **10**, 61–71.

20. Fisher, P. A., Gunnar, M. R., Dozier, M., Bruce, J. and Pears, K. C. (2006). Effects of a therapeutic intervention for foster children on behavior problems, caregiver attachment, and stress regulatory neural systems. *Annals of the New York Academy of Sciences,* **1094**, 215–225.

21. Gunnar, M. R. and Fisher, P. A. (2006). For the Early Experience, Stress, and Prevention Network. Bringing basic research on early experience and stress neurobiology to bear on preventive intervention research on neglected and maltreated children. *Developmental Psychopathology,* **18**, 651–677.

22. Pine, D. S. and Charney, D. S. (2002). Children, stress, and sensitization: An integration of basic and clinical research on emotion? *Biological Psychiatry,* **52**, 773–775.

23. Levine, S. (1994). The ontogeny of the hypothalamic–pituitary–adrenal axis. The influence of maternal factors. *Annals of the New York Academy of Sciences,* **746**, 275–288.

24. Sapolsky, R. M. and Meaney, M. J. (1986). Maturation of the adrenocortical stress response: Neuroendocrine control mechanisms and the stress hyporesponsive period. *Brain Research Reviews,* **11**, 65–76.

25. Meaney, M. and Szyf, M. (2005). Environmental programming of stress responses through DNA methylation: Life at the interface between a dynamic environment and a fixed genome. *Dialogues in Clinical Neuroscience,* **7**, 103–123.

26. Zhang, L. X., Levine, S., Dent, G. *et al.* (2002). Maternal deprivation increases cell death in the infant rat brain. *Developmental Brain Research, 133,* 1–11.

27. Gould, E. and Tanapat, P. (1999). Stress and hippocampal neurogenesis. *Biological Psychiatry,* **46,** 1472–1479.

28. McEwen, B. S., Coirini, H., Westlind-Danielson, M. *et al.* (1991). Steroid hormones as mediators of neural plasticity. *Journal of Steroid Biochemistry and Molecular Biology,* **39,** 223–232.

29. Gunnar, M. R. (1998). Quality of early care and buffering of neuroendocrine stress reactions: Potential effects on the developing human brain. *Preventive Medicine, 27,* 208–211.

30. Gunnar, M. and Donzella, B. (2002). Social regulation of the cortisol levels in early human development. *Psychoneuroendocrinology, 27,* 199–220.

31. Carlson, M. and Earls, F. (1997). Psychological and neuroendocrinological sequelae of early social deprivation in institutionalized children in Romania. *Annals of the New York Academy of Sciences,* **807,** 419–428.

32. Miller, G. E., Chen, E. and Zhou, E. S. (2007). If it goes up, must it come down? Chronic stress and the hypothalamic–pituitary–adrenocortical axis in humans. *Psychology Bulletin,* **133,** 25–45.

33. Bruce, J., Fisher, P. A., Pears, K. C. and Levine, S. (2009). Morning cortisol levels in preschool-aged foster children: Differential effects of maltreatment type. *Developmental Psychobiology,* **51,** 14–23.

34. Dozier, M., Manni, M., Peloso, E. *et al.* (2007). Foster children's diurnal production of cortisol: An exploratory study. *Child Maltreatment, 11,* 189–197.

35. Bruce, J., Fisher, P. A., Pears, K. C. and Levine, S. (2009). Morning cortisol levels in preschool-aged foster children: Differential effects of maltreatment type. *Developmental Psychobiology,* **51,** 14–23.

36. Gunnar, M. R. and Vazquez, D. M. (2001). Low cortisol and a flattening of expected diurnal rhythm: Potential indices of risk in human development. *Developmental Psychopathology,* **13,** 515–538.

37. Parker, K. J., Buckmaster, C. L., Sundlass, K., Schatzberg, A. F. and Lyons, D. M. (2006). Maternal mediation, stress inoculation, and the development of neuroendocrine stress resistance in primates. *Proceedings of the National Academy of Sciences,* **103,** 3000–3005.

38. Gunnar, M. R., Frenn, K., Wewerka, S. and Van Ryzin, M. J. (2009). Moderate versus severe early life stress: Associations with stress reactivity and regulation in 10- to 12-year old children. *Psychoneuroendocrinology,* **34,** 62–74.

39. Pollak, S. D., Nelson, C. A., Schlaak, M. *et al.* (2010). Neurodevelopmental effects of early deprivation in post-institutionalized children. *Child Development,* **81,** 224–236.

40. Lyons, D. M. and Parker, K. J. (2007). Stress inoculation-induced indications of resilience in monkeys. *Journal of Trauma and Stress,* **20,** 423–433.

41. Boyce, W. T. and Ellis, B. J. (2005). Biological sensitivity to context: I. An evolutionary–developmental theory of the origins and functions of stress reactivity. *Developmental Psychopathology,* **17,** 271–301.

42. Masten, A. S. and Reed, M.-G. (2002). Resilience in development. In: C. R. Snyder and S. J. Lopez (eds.), *The handbook of positive psychology.* Oxford: Oxford University Press.

43. Caspi, A., McClay, J., Moffitt, T. E. *et al.* (2002). Role of genotype in the cycle of violence in maltreated children. *Science, 297,* 851–854.

44. Heim, C. and Nemeroff, C. B. (2001). The role of childhood trauma in the neurobiology of mood and anxiety disorders: Preclinical and clinical studies. *Biological Psychiatry,* **49,** 1023–1039.

45. Elzinga, B. M., Roelofs, K., Tollenaar, M. S. *et al.* (2008). Diminished cortisol responses to psychosocial stress associated with lifetime adverse events. A study among healthy young subjects. *Psychoneuroendocrinology,* **33,** 227–237.

46. Heim, C., Plotsky, P. and Nemeroff, C. B. (2004). The importance of studying the contributions of early adverse experiences to the neurobiological findings in depression. *Neuropsychopharmacology,* **29,** 641–648.

47. Binder, E. B., Bradley, R. G., Wei, L. *et al.* (2008). Association of FKBP5 polymorphisms and childhood abuse with risk of posttraumatic stress disorder symptoms in adults. *Journal of the American Medical Association,* **299,** 1291–1305.

48. Oulette-Morin, I., Boivin, M., Dionne, G. *et al.* (2008). Variations in heritability of cortisol reactivity to stress as a function of early familial adversity among 19-month-old twins. *Archives of General Psychiatry,* **65,** 211–218.

49. Fisher, P. A., Stoolmiller, M., Gunnar, M. R. and Burraston, B. (2007). Effects of a therapeutic intervention for foster preschoolers on diurnal cortisol activity. *Psychoneuroendocrinology,* **32,** 892–905.

50. Fisher, P. A. and Stoolmiller, M. (2008). Intervention effects on foster parent stress: Associations with child cortisol levels. *Developmental Psychopathology,* **20,** 1003–1021.

51. Fisher, P. A. and Kim, H. K. (2007). Intervention effects on foster preschoolers' attachment-related behaviors from a randomized trial. *Prevention Science,* **8,** 161–170.

52. Dozier, M., Peloso, E., Lewis, E., Laurenceau, J.-P. and Levine, S. (2008). Effects of an attachment-based intervention on the cortisol production of infants and toddlers in foster care. *Developmental Psychopathology,* **20,** 845–859.

53. Brotman, L. M., Gouley, K. K., Huang, K.-Y. *et al.* (2007). Effects of a psychosocial family-based preventive

intervention on cortisol response to a social challenge in preschoolers at high risk for antisocial behavior. *Archives of General Psychiatry,* **64**, 1172–1179.

54. Greenough, W. T., Black, J. E. and Wallace, C. S. (1987). Experience and brain development. *Child Development,* **58**, 539–559.

55. Bruce, J., Martin McDermott, J. N., Fisher, P. A. and Fox, N. A. (2009). Using behavioral and electrophysiological measures to assess the effects of a preventive intervention: a preliminary study with preschool-aged foster children. *Prevention Science,* **10**, 129–140.

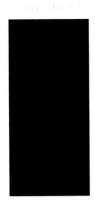

# Part 3 synopsis

Allan N. Schore

## Overview

Although the authors in this part have offered important individual contributions to a deeper understanding of the essential role of early life trauma on brain organization and later psychobiological functioning, they also present a remarkable overlap and a common interdisciplinary perspective. In the following overview, I will emphasize what I see as the major themes that are clearly emerging from a large body of developmental, neurobiological and psychiatric studies on early life trauma. I will then offer comments on directions for future research and clinical applications of this rapidly expanding body of knowledge.

In Ch. 11, Teicher and his colleagues document the well-established principle that exposure to early life trauma alters trajectories of brain development, which, in turn, leads to enduring social, emotional and cognitive impairments. They review the enduring untoward effects of early physical abuse, sexual abuse and neglect (which is now finally being researched) on brain systems. Towards that end, they cite a number of studies showing decreased myelination of the corpus callosum and reduced interhemispheric communication; some although not all reports indicate reduced (especially left) hippocampal volume, abnormalities of amygdala gamma-aminobutyric acid (GABA) activity and "limbic irritability," and altered maturation and asymmetry of cerebral cortical areas, including the anterior cingulate and frontal lobes.

Teicher et al., in their most recent work, have demonstrated that repeated exposures to sexual abuse in adolescence, a period of intense brain reorganization, is associated with reduction of gray matter volume in left visual association cortex and fusiform gyrus, and right lingual gyrus. The authors contend that specific brain regions have differing periods of sensitivity to the effects of sexual abuse, beginning at 3–5 years. They then discuss other forms of adolescent adversity, including parental verbal abuse, peer verbal bullying and witnessing of domestic violence in late adolescent subjects. They conclude that different forms of maltreatment specifically affects sensory systems that process and interpret aversive stimuli, and they allude to lateralization effects in their observation that the two hemispheres develop relatively independently. A major tenet of their work is that different brain regions have unique windows of vulnerability during which they are maximally sensitive to the exposure to various forms of childhood trauma. It should be noted that this group is studying late and not early childhood trauma.

Richter-Levin and Jacobson-Pick in Ch. 9 also concentrate on trauma in later childhood, examining juvenile stress. Although they describe the brain as being vulnerable to alterations generated by stressful stimuli during infancy, childhood and adolescence, their animal studies focus not on pre- and postnatal periods but on the prepuberty stage of development. Importantly, they refute two common misconceptions in the clinical literature: that mood disorders are rare before adulthood and that they are normative and self-limited during childhood and adolescence. In reality, these disorders are now well documented in the juvenile period (and before). Their important contribution here is to show that stress during the juvenile period is apparent immediately, and not only later in adulthood. These authors assert that the anxiety and depression that ensues from juvenile stress clinically presents with a different symptomatology to that occurring in adulthood, and that this developmental psychopathological perspective is clinically relevant to early diagnosis and treatment. This perspective clearly implies that early intervention will be more successful in reestablishing a more normal developmental trajectory if we can more deeply understand the developmental stage-dependent expressions of various emotional disorders.

*The Impact of Early Life Trauma on Health and Disease: The Hidden Epidemic*, ed. Ruth A. Lanius, Eric Vermetten and Clare Pain. Published by Cambridge University Press. Copyright © Cambridge University Press 2010.

In Ch. 12, De Bellis focuses on perhaps the least studied and yet most detrimental form of early life trauma, neglect. Indeed he concludes that child neglect is the most chronic and prevalent form of child maltreatment. As opposed to the authors of Chs. 9 and 11, he brings the concept of attachment directly into the conceptualization of early life trauma. Reviewing Harlow's classic studies of maternal deprivation and citing John Bowlby's seminal work, De Bellis notes, "the social attachment between mother and infant is an essential experience-dependent interaction of normal development." Thus, along with a large number of other current researchers, he moves the timeline of early trauma back to infancy. Citing studies of institutionalized infants, De Bellis asserts the principle that the degree of the traumatic experience perceived by the child may depend on the age of the child at the time of neglect. Therefore, neglect, which represents a chronic stressor, is more detrimental to the child's early developing biological stress systems and brain maturation than adversity at other developmental stages. He also articulates the essential concept of not just early life trauma but relational trauma: for the neglected child, the nature of the stressor is the dysfunctional parent–child interpersonal relationship.

De Bellis outlines the detrimental effects of neglect on the development of the child's neurotransmitter, neuroendocrine and immune systems. He then briefly discusses an important theme frequently omitted in discussions of early trauma, healthy childhood brain development (although he focuses on early childhood rather than infancy). In agreement with Chs. 9 and 11, he suggests that neglect interferes with prefrontal development, including particularly the orbitofrontal areas, but also temporal, amygdala and brainstem, citing among others his 2002 study showing smaller right temporal lobe volumes in children with post-traumatic stress disorder after maltreatment. He ends by calling for longitudinal studies on the neurobiology of neglect and investigations of therapeutic interventions.

Chapter 13 on early life stress focuses on data from foster care and covers the themes of the essential role of the social environment in trauma, attachment, emotional maltreatment and neglect. Fisher and Gunnar note that, in addition to the ruptured attachment bond with the primary caregiver, the child is also exposed to the potentially pathogenic nature of foster care. Citing their substantial work on children reared under adverse conditions such as institutional care, they offer data that show that poor quality early care is associated with alterations in the HPA system and dysregulation of cortisol production. In accord with earlier chapters, they suggest that adverse care has its greatest negative impact on the HPA axis in the first years of life. They then present recent updates of their model, focusing on variations in the types, severity and plasticity of the neural systems involved in early life trauma.

Interestingly these authors are now also observing the negative impact of neglect in generating attenuated morning cortisol levels. In recent modeling they are moving up the neuroaxis to implicate impairment of forebrain regions that are connected with the HPA axis (amygdala, hippocampus), as well as prefrontal systems involved in executive functions and inhibitory control. In discussing individual differences, they speculate on the differential routes to pathology and resilience, but in the end assert that under early life stress conditions which are overwhelming to the child the long-term effects are ultimately pathogenic. That being the case they argue for preventive caregiver-based therapeutic interventions that might optimize the plasticity of the implicated neural systems in order to alter an individual's life trajectory towards more positive outcomes. They report an intervention that leads to stabilized diurnal HPA activity, and indeed to decreases in insecure attachments and increases in secure attachments. They conclude that treatment-induced neural plasticity extends beyond a more regulated HPA axis and includes more adaptive and efficient prefrontal cortical systems.

Chapter 10 discusses an area of developmental neuroscience and stress psychology that is gaining increasing attention, lateral asymmetries in brain organization. Montirosso et al. ask whether differences in the lateralization of expressive and regulatory gestures reflect different hemispheric activity. Focusing on relational trauma in infancy, they use the Face-to-Face Still-Face (FFSF) paradigm to show that the neural circuitry of the infant's developing stress system that responds to early life trauma is located in the early developing right brain. As opposed to other chapters in this part, which use a retrospective approach, this work directly observes and details the detrimental effects of interpersonal trauma on the developing brain of infants aged 6 to 12 months and offers a model of a neurobiological imprint of early life trauma that endures over later life stages.

These researchers report a number of interesting results, including the observation that under the stress of the FFSF infants showed more left-sided self-directed regulatory emotional expressive gestures and greater right hemisphere activation. They speculate that relational trauma in the first year of life activates limbic structures that regulate emotion, and cite a growing body of studies which indicate that the neural circuitry of the stress system is located in the right brain. With direct relevance to the problem of neglect, they conclude that infants cope with emotional stress caused by unresponsive mothers through right lateralized self-regulation behaviors. In addition, their results support the proposal that the right hemisphere, which matures more quickly than the left, is involved in both negative and positive affect regulation, and in attachment bonding. These data provide further evidence for the mechanism by which early life attachment trauma alters the developmental trajectory of stress and affect regulating mechanisms over the course of the lifespan. This work is also relevant to the fundamental problem of the intergenerational transmission of relational trauma and the early pathogenesis of later-forming psychiatric disorders.

## Future directions

In this section I attempt to tie together the common themes of these chapters, as well as to offer ideas about what I see as the progression of a complex interdisciplinary model of early life trauma, one which integrates current developmental psychological, neurobiological and psychiatric data. Two basic trends are emerging from this rapidly expanding area that are impacting the methodologies of experimental studies as well as on the incorporation of recent data on early life trauma into updated models of diagnosis and treatment.

The first emergent trend is within the psychological disciplines of developmental traumatology and attachment theory. Both researchers and clinicians are now moving towards forms of early life trauma that occur in the earliest stages of development. This is expressed in a shift down from models of sexual abuse in later childhood to relational attachment trauma in infancy as the major factor in altered development and psychopathogenesis [1]. Associated with this is a move away from the effects of early trauma in the physical environment to trauma in the social environment, that is relational trauma, including stressors that result from a dysfunctional parent–child interpersonal socioemotional attachment relationship [2,3].

This trend reflects the current paradigm shift across all disciplines from cognition into emotion. Recent models of early life trauma have altered their focus from deficits in later-maturing conscious, verbal, explicit and voluntary behavior to impairments of early maturing non-conscious, non-verbal, implicit and automatic adaptive social emotional functions. Thus attachment trauma in early infancy leads to enduring deficits in the unconscious reception, expression and regulation of stressful bodily based affects, a central psychopathogenic mechanism of all personality and psychiatric disorders [4,5].

In parallel with these psychological shifts, a second trend is seen in neuroscience. Developmental neuroscience is now moving from studies of later-maturing left brain conscious verbal cognitive processes into the early preverbal development of adaptive emotion-processing right brain systems in pre- and postnatal periods ("very early life"). This is accompanied by an increase in affective neuroscience research exploring the enduring effects of early life trauma on the early developing right brain, "the emotional brain." An essential principle of developmental psychopathology is that we need to understand the psychology and neurobiology of both normal development and resilience, as well as abnormal socioemotional development and psychopathogenesis. Ultimately we need a theoretical model that can integrate the psychological and biological realms: an interdisciplinary perspective that can both interpret the scientific research data and generate more complex clinical models of healthy development, psychopathogenesis and treatment. My work on regulation theory and the interpersonal neurobiology of attachment directly addresses this matter.

A growing body of studies now supports the proposal that the long-enduring effects of attachment in mammalian species result from their impact on brain development [2,6]. Because the emotion-processing human limbic system myelinates in the first 18 months and the early-maturing right hemisphere – which is deeply connected into the limbic system – is undergoing a growth spurt at this time, maternal–infant right brain to right brain visual–facial, auditory–prosodic and tactile–gestural socioemotional attachment communications specifically impact critical periods of growth of subcortical limbic–autonomic circuits and cortical areas of the developing right brain [2]. Attachment transactions in the first year are occurring during the brain growth spurt, when total brain volume is increasing by 101%, and the volume of the subcortical areas by 130% [7]. The highest centers of the early developing right hemisphere, especially the orbitofrontal (ventromedial) cortex, the locus of

Bowlby's attachment system, act as the brain's most complex affect and stress regulatory system [2,3,8].

Confirming this right brain model of attachment, Howard and Reggia [9] concluded, "Earlier maturation of the right hemisphere is supported by both anatomical and imaging evidence" (p. 112). Schuetze and Reid [10] asserted, "Although the infant brain was historically reported to be undifferentiated in terms of cerebral lateralisation until 2 years of age, evidence has accumulated indicating that lateralised functions are present much earlier in development" (p. 207). Studies now show that the development of the capacity to efficiently process information from faces requires visual input to the right (and not left) hemisphere during infancy [11], that, specifically, the 5-month-old child's right hemisphere responds to images of adult female faces [12], and that prosodic processing in 3-month-old infants activates the right temporoparietal region [13]. Furthermore, a functional magnetic resonance imaging (fMRI) study of mother–infant emotional communication offers data "supporting the theory that the right hemisphere is more involved than the left hemisphere in emotional processing and thus, mothering" [14]. A near-infrared spectroscopy study of infant–mother attachment at 12 months [15] concluded, "our results are in agreement with that of Schore (2000) who addressed the importance of the right hemisphere in the attachment system" (p. 289).

It is important to stress that a growth-facilitating emotional environment is required for a child to develop an internal system that can adaptively regulate arousal and an array of psychobiological states (and thereby affect, cognition and behavior). In contrast to caregivers who foster secure attachment, an abusive or neglectful caregiver not only plays less but also induces enduring negative affect in the child. There is now extensive evidence which indicates that stress is a critical factor that affects social interactions, especially the mother–child interaction. Disorganized–disoriented insecure attachment, a pattern common to infants abused and/or neglected in the first 2 years of life, is psychologically manifest as an inability to generate a coherent strategy for coping with relational stress [4,5]. During these episodes of hyperarousal and dissociation–hypoarousal, the infant is matching the rhythmic structures of the mother's dysregulated states, and this synchronization is registered in the firing patterns of the stress-sensitive cortical and limbic regions of the infant's brain, especially in the right brain which is in a critical period of growth (see Schore

[3] for attachment as an evolutionary mechanism of the apoptotic sculpting of brain circuits).

I have suggested that a critical period of amygdala development occurs from the last trimester of pregnancy though the second postnatal month, followed by a critical period of limbic anterior cingulate development from 3 to 10 months, and lastly an orbitofrontal developmental period at 10 to 18 months [3]. Depending upon the nature, severity and timing of relational trauma in these critical periods, traumatic attachments are imprinted into the developing limbic (amygdala, then anterior cingulate, then orbitofrontal) and autonomic (insula) nervous systems of the early maturing right brain. Thus the overwhelming stress of very early life attachment trauma (abuse and neglect) alters the developmental trajectory of the right brain, which is dominant for coping with negative affects [16] and for "regulating stress – and emotion-related processes" [17]. This developmental model asserts that sexual abuse in later stages of development impacts later-maturing left hemispheric hippocampal and dorsolateral prefrontal verbal systems, as well as the callosal system that integrates the two hemispheres. These later forms of life trauma will overlie earlier attachment right brain non-verbal imprints.

These two accelerating trends of early life trauma research into relational attachment trauma and impairments of socioemotional development and into critical periods of right brain cortical–subcortical limbic–autonomic circuits are reflected in very recent studies. This representative current research portends the direction of future studies, and it now supports not only the fundamental principle of the asymmetry of the cerebral hemispheres but also the laterality of even subcortical systems, especially those of the right "emotional brain." A very large body of data now indicates that "The right and left human brain hemispheres differ in macrostructure, ultrastructure, physiology, chemistry, and control of behavior" [18, p. 97].

In a major review of the right brain, now described as "the human social brain," Brancucci and his colleagues [19] concluded that "the neural substrates of the perception of voices, faces, gestures, smells, and pheromones, as evidenced by modern neuroimaging techniques, are characterized by a general right-hemispheric functional asymmetry" (p. 895). In describing "the importance of the right hemisphere in complex social functioning" Fournier et al. [20] offered an important observation that bears on future methodologies for studying early life trauma (p. 466).

Neuropsychological examination of social functioning has traditionally involved the presentation of static displays of posed emotional expressions (e.g., faces in a photograph) or the reading of short paragraphs that illustrate specific aspects of social-related behavior… Although they have the advantage of being easy to administer, these tests often bear little resemblance to the types of interactions and complex problems faced in normal everyday life.

Basic research in traumatology and affective neuroscience also provides clues to future studies. Experimental investigations of right lateralized limbic–autonomic circuits of the amygdala, anterior cingulate and orbitofrontal (ventromedial) cortex now document that the right brain, more so than the left regulates the HPA axis [17]. Root et al. [21], in an fMRI study of cortisol response to emotional stimuli (World Trade Center Attack images), showed right frontolimbic activity and a positive correlation between activation of the right amygdala and cortisol changes. In accord with these data, Polli et al. [22] reported from their fMRI research (p. 401) as follows.

> Given the theoretical role of the rostral anterior cingulate cortex in appraising the affective or motivational significance of errors, these findings suggest that the right amygdala and right rostral anterior cingulate cortex work together to modulate affective responses to errors and to learn to prevent their occurrence. They are consistent with animal and human studies that suggest a right amygdala dominance for aversive conditioning.

Representative of a very large body of current research on the right frontal lobe, the electroencephalography study by Balconi and Pozzoli [23] of emotional face comprehension described "a general right hemisphere dominance of gamma and theta" and the authors suggested that this "clear localized right frontal response by the two frequency bands" is involved in "emotion-related evaluation" (p. 461). Perez-Cruz et al. [24] reported that chronic stress reduced the length of dendrites in only the right (and not the left) medial prefrontal cortex (p. 738).

> [T]he reaction of mPFC [medial prefrontal cortex] to stress is lateralized, in that responses to minor challenges stimulate the left hemisphere whereas severe stress activates the right mPFC. Our recent investigations indicated that hemispheric structural lateralization might exist at the cellular level in the mPFC … These findings highlight the importance of analyzing the two hemispheres separately and suggest that pooling data from the two hemispheres may confound reliable effects of a treatment.

Returning to the problem of early life stress and its enduring impact on brain development, a recent study of adolescent adoptees in the UK with histories of early severe institutional deprivation show altered (greater) amygdala volumes, especially on the right, but no differences in hippocampal or corpus callosum volumes [25]. The authors suggest that "the effects of very early negative or stressful experiences on brain structure and function will be qualitatively different from negative experiences later in childhood or adulthood" (p. 948). A parallel study of preadolescent adoptees in the USA separated at birth and institutionally reared for the first 32 months of life showed white matter abnormalities in the right uncinate fasciculus (UNF), including the region adjacent to the right amygdala [26]. This area is a fiber tract that connects right orbitofrontal areas with the right amygdala in the medial temporal lobe, allowing these limbic structures to be involved in socioemotional, memory and executive functions; therefore, this structural impairment could underlie maladaptive interpersonal functions. Indeed, the amount of early severe socioemotional deprivation-induced white matter disorganization was significantly correlated with duration of the stay in the orphanage as well as with neuropsychological and behavioral outcomes. These researchers call for further studies of early severe socioemotional deprivation and limbic changes (i.e., orbital frontal and anterior temporal cortices).

In summary, this large body of interdisciplinary research on early life trauma, brain organization and later psychobiological functioning clearly has direct implications for clinical models of the intergenerational transmission of a predisposition for psychiatric disorders, prevention in pre- and postnatal periods and therapeutic intervention in later periods of life.

# References

1. Cirulli, F., Berry, A. and Alleva, E. (2002). Early disruption of the mother–infant relationship: Effects on brain plasticity and implications for psychopathology. *Neuroscience and Biobehavioral Reviews*, **272**, 73–82.

2. Schore, A. N. (1994). *Affect regulation and the origin of the self*. Mahweh, NJ: Lawrence Erlbaum.

3. Schore, A. N. (2003). *Affect dysregulation and disorders of the self*. New York: Norton.

4. Schore, A. N. (2002). Dysregulation of the right brain: A fundamental mechanism of traumatic attachment and the psychopathogenesis of posttraumatic stress disorder. *Australian and New Zealand Journal of Psychiatry*, **36**, 9–30.

5. Schore, A. N. (2009). Relational trauma and the developing right brain: An interface of psychoanalytic

self psychology and neuroscience. *Annals of the New York Academy of Sciences*, **1159**, 189–203.

6. Schore, A. N. (2005). Attachment, affect regulation, and the developing right brain: Linking developmental neuroscience to pediatrics. *Pediatrics in Review*, **26**, 204–211.

7. Knickmeyer, R. C., Gouttard, S., Kang, C. *et al.* (2008). A structural MRI study of human brain development from birth to 2 years. *Journal of Neuroscience*, **28**, 12176–12182.

8. Sullivan, R. M. and Gratton, A. (2002). Prefrontal cortical regulation of hypothalamic–pituitary–adrenal function in the rat and implications for psychopathology: Side matters. *Psychoneuroendocrinology*, **27**, 99–114.

9. Howard, M. F. and Reggia, J. A. (2007), A theory of the visual system biology underlying development of spatial frequency lateralization. *Brain and Cognition*, **64**, 111–123.

10. Schuetze, P. and Reid, H. M. (2005). Emotional lateralization in the second year of life: Evidence from oral asymmetries. *Laterality*, **10**, 207–217.

11. Le Grand, R., Mondloch, C. J., Maurer, D. and Brent, H. P. (2003). Expert face processing requires visual input to the right hemisphere during infancy. *Nature Neuroscience*, **6**, 1108–1112.

12. Nakato, E., Otsuka, Y., Kanazawa, S. *et al.* (2009). When do infants differentiate profile face from frontal face? A near-infrared spectroscopic study. *Human Brain Mapping*, **30**, 462–472.

13. Homae, F., Watanabe, H., Nakano, T., Asakawa, K. and Taga, G. (2006). The right hemisphere of sleeping infants perceives sentential prosody. *Neuroscience Research*, **54**, 276–280.

14. Lenzi, D., Trentini, C., Pantano, P. *et al.* (2009). Neural basis of maternal communication and emotional expression processing during infant preverbal stage. *Cerebral Cortex*, **19**, 1124–1133.

15. Minagawa-Kawai, Y., Matsuoka, S., Dan, I. *et al.* (2009). Prefrontal activation associated with social attachment: Facial–emotion recognition in mothers and infants. *Cerebral Cortex*, **19**, 284–292.

16. Davidson, R. J., Ekman, P., Saron, C., Senulis, J. and Friesen, W. V. (1990). Approach/withdrawal and cerebral asymmetry: 1. Emotional expression and brain physiology. *Journal of Personality and Social Psychology*, **58**, 330–341.

17. Sullivan, R. M. and Dufresne, M. M. (2006). Mesocortical dopamine and HPA axis regulation: Role of laterality and early environment. *Brain Research*, **1076**, 49–59.

18. Braun, C. M. J., Boulanger, Y., Labelle, M. *et al.* (2002). Brain metabolic differences as a function of hemisphere, writing hand preference, and gender. *Laterality*, **7**, 97–113.

19. Brancucci, A., Lucci, G., Mazzatenta, A. and Tommasi, L. (2009). Asymmetries of the human social brain in the visual, auditory and chemical modalities. *Philosophical Transactions of the Royal Society, Series B, Biological Sciences*, **364**, 895–914.

20. Fournier, N. M., Calverly, K. L., Wagner, J. P., Poock, J. L. and Crossley, M. (2008). Impaired social cognition 30 years after hemispherectomy for intractable epilepsy: The importance of the right hemisphere in complex social functioning. *Epilepsy and Behavior*, **12**, 460–471.

21. Root, J. C., Tuescher, O., Cunningham-Bussel, A. *et al.* (2009). Frontolimbic function and cortisol reactivity in response to emotional stimuli. *Neuroreport*, **20**, 429–434.

22. Polli, F. E., Wright, C. I., Milad, M. R. *et al.* (2009). Hemispheric differences in amygdala contributions to response monitoring. *Neuroreport*, **20**, 398–402.

23. Balconi, M. and Pozzoli, U. (2009). Arousal effect on emotional face comprehension. Frequency band changes in different time intervals. *Physiology and Behavior*, **97**, 455–462.

24. Perez-Cruz, C., Simon, M., Czeh, B., Flugge, G. and Fuchs, E. (2009). Hemispheric differences in basilar dendrites and spines of pyramidal neurons in the rat prelimbic cortex: Activity- and stress-induced changes. *European Journal of Neuroscience*, **29**, 738–747.

25. Mehta, M. A., Golembo, N. I., Nosarti, C. *et al.* (2009). Amygdala, hippocampal and corpus callosum size following severe early institutional deprivation: The English and Romanian adoptees study pilot. *Journal of Child Psychology and Psychiatry*, **50**, 943–951.

26. Govindan, R. M., Behen, M. E., Helder, E., Makki, M. I. and Chugani, H. T. (2009). Altered water diffusivity in cortical association tracts in children with early deprivation identified with tract-based spatial statistics (TBSS). *Cerebral Cortex*, in press; doi: 10.1093/cercor/bhp122.

# The impact of childhood trauma: psychobiological sequelae in adults

## Early life stress and psychiatric risk/resilience: the importance of a developmental neurobiological model in understanding gene by environment interactions

Kelly Skelton, Tamara Weiss and Bekh Bradley

## Introduction

Exposure to early life adverse events, including physical and sexual abuse, significantly increases the risk for a number of physical and psychiatric disorders in adulthood. Several factors are proposed to account for the variable impact of exposure to early life adverse events on risk/resilience to psychopathology. Evidence supports the importance of heredity and environment, as well as their interplay, in determining risk and resilience for psychopathology [1,2]. Despite consensus about the role of biological interactions between genes and environment (G×E), there is disagreement about the usefulness of research examining G×E because of concerns related to methodology and statistical analysis for studying these interactions [3,4]. One criticism is that the number of potential environmental variables will prompt researchers to examine multiple subgroups of subjects until a spurious G×E effect becomes statistically significant, leading to unreliable and non-replicable positive findings of interaction [5]. Among the suggestions for countering this concern is selecting candidate genes and environments based on relevant theory and research [6,7]. Such research requires investigators to focus their work on gene–environment relationships relevant to the putative biological pathways underlying psychiatric illnesses [6,7].

Early life stress (ELS) and abuse are the most commonly assessed environmental exposures in psychiatric G×E interaction studies, partly because of the strength of evidence that ELS plays a role in risk for multiple psychiatric disorders. Other environmental factors that have been examined include those thought to affect risk for psychiatric illness by altering neurodevelopment at key stages during infancy and childhood. The most robust area of research focuses on the impact of early experiences on the development of biological systems responsible for stress reactivity and regulation. Early rearing environments, in particular maternal care, influence gene-controlled patterns of stress responsivity, promoting a more or less resilient neural architecture of stress-response pathways that persists across the lifespan. Moreover, the relationship between genetic makeup, brain structure/function and behavior varies across the course of developmental stages such that some periods of development allow for increased plasticity of neural organization in response to environmental factors [8,9].

A number of reviews have examined specific G×E interactions as they relate to particular psychiatric illnesses or specific genes (e.g., [10–12]). However, these reviews have often come to disparate conclusions on reliability and generalizability of findings on G×E interactions [10,11]. For example, two recently published reviews on G×E interactions involving the serotonin transporter linked polymorphic region (*5-HTTLPR*) in depression came to different conclusions, with one suggesting that positive findings of G×E are likely attributable to chance and the other concluding that the findings are reliable when based on clearly defined outcomes (e.g., recent onset versus chronic depression) and environments (e.g., childhood maltreatment versus recent life stressors).

Disagreement about interpretation of the existing literature stems in part from the approach that investigators have taken in studying the role of G×E interactions in risk and resilience following ELS. First, there is a tendency to organize data based primarily on specific candidate genes rather than key neural systems and related developmental neurobiology. In contrast, environmental exposures have been defined with greater breadth (e.g., "life stress" and "adverse early life events"), rather than specifically delineated based on extant knowledge of environmental factors associated with risk/resilience. These would include factors such as the developmental timing of the stressor and the context in which the stressor occurs (e.g., interpersonal domestic violence versus natural disaster). Last, a growing body of research suggests the benefits of defining outcomes according to constitutive psychological processes and states (e.g., emotion regulation, impulsivity, attention, negative affectivity) that may cut across specific psychiatric diagnoses. With these factors in mind, this review of research on G×E interactions is organized by the presumed underlying neurobiological systems and by the broader classification of psychiatric outcomes (mood/anxiety disorders and externalizing disorders). Following this, we discuss the importance of clearly defining and measuring both the proposed environmental risk/resilience factors as well as the predicted diagnostic and behavioral outcomes. This will allow investigators to conduct G×E studies that will better inform our understanding of the role of ELS in predicting psychiatric risk/resilience.

## Risk/resilience for mood and anxiety disorders

### The serotonin transporter linked polymorphic region

Initial evidence for G×E interactions in depressive disorders was established in twin studies, including a notable study that identified an increased risk of new onset depressive disorder following a negative life event in twins with a higher genetic liability for depression [13]. Given the role of serotonergic neurotransmission in the treatment of depressive disorders, this system was a logical starting point for finding candidate genes that might mediate G×E interactions in mood disorders. In 1996, Lesch and colleagues [14] reported that the short allele version of a functional polymorphism in 5-HTTLPR was associated with an increased risk for depression. However, after other investigators were unable to replicate this finding, Caspi and colleagues [15] hypothesized that this lack of replication was because the genetic risk was dependent on the concomitant presence of an adverse environment. This hypothesis was supported by animal research in rhesus monkeys demonstrating that the presence of the short allele variant of 5-HTTLPR was associated with negative psychiatric outcomes, including increased aggression in monkeys exposed to the adverse environment of peer-rearing versus maternal rearing [16]. The study by Caspi et al. [15] found no significant main effect for serotonin transporter genotype on risk for the onset of depression but did find that the short allele variant was associated with an increased risk for depression in those individuals exposed to childhood maltreatment between the ages of 3 and 11 years or stressful life events between the ages of 21 and 26 years. Since then, the research on this topic has been inconsistent, with replications in some samples [17,18] but not others [19,20], and some suggestion that this G×E effect is strongest for young adults, particularly females, with a history of ELS [21,22]. As anxiety disorders are highly comorbid with depressive disorders, it is not surprising that the short allele variant of 5-HTTLPR has also been implicated in anxiety sensitivity in individuals with a history of childhood abuse [23] and with anxiety related to daily life stressors in young adults [24]. While most of the above studies have examined the interaction of 5-HTTLPR with adverse environments alone, two studies have demonstrated that the protective environmental factor of positive social support can mitigate the risk for depression associated with the interaction of the short allele variant and childhood maltreatment [25,26].

### The hypothalamic–pituitary–adrenal axis

Although the interaction between serotonin transporter genotype and adverse environment in the development of depressive disorders is well established, this association does not elucidate the mechanism that underlies the interaction. Based on what is known about the underlying pathophysiology of depression, one plausible mechanism accounting for a G×E interaction in this case involves the reactivity of the hypothalamic–pituitary–adrenal (HPA) axis to environmental stressors. Beginning with the release of hypothalamic corticotropin-releasing factor (or hormone CRF) and ending with the release of cortisol from the adrenal glands, the HPA axis mediates the primary hormonal response to stress, and activation of the HPA axis is a key indicator of biological reactivity to stress. Hyperactivation of CRF neurotransmission has long been hypothesized to play a principal role in the pathophysiology of depressive and anxiety disorders, and hypercortisolemia is a well-replicated finding in a significant subset of individuals with depressive disorders [27]. Furthermore, hyper-reactivity of the HPA axis in response to physiological and psychological stressors has been demonstrated in both preclinical animal models based on adverse early life experience [28] and humans with a history of childhood maltreatment [29].

The potential role of HPA axis reactivity in mediating or moderating an interaction between serotonin transporter promoter polymorphism and stressful life events in depressive disorders has been examined in two recent studies. Adult females homozygous for the short allele variant of 5-HTTLPR exhibited increased cortisol release in response to a psychological stressor task compared with those females possessing the long allele variant [30]. Interestingly, this heightened cortisol release was not demonstrated in males possessing the short allele genotype, mirroring and perhaps providing a biological basis for the gender discrepancy reported in prior studies showing that serotonin promoter polymorphism was more strongly associated with depressive disorders in females exposed to stressors. Similarly, in a study of adolescent females, those individuals possessing the short allele variant of 5-HTTLPR demonstrated increased cortisol response to a psychological stressor task, while those possessing either one or two copies of the long allele variant demonstrated only a minimal increase in cortisol, potentially indicating a protective effect of the long allele in reducing biological sensitivity to stress [31].

Promising research points to epigenetic processes as a mechanism by which environmental cues may alter gene expression involved in control of the HPA axis, via DNA methylation or histone acetylation. Methylation of DNA is an active process during early development that is typically associated with the inactivation of genes. In a rat model, Weaver et al. [32] have demonstrated that the promoter region of gene for the glucocorticoid receptor (GR) in the hippocampus is regulated through early experience, including the quality of maternal behavior towards her pups, and produces lifelong alterations in endocrine responsivity to stress. These genetic changes in response to environment developed over the first week of life – a critical

period for epigenetic alterations that persist into adulthood. Further studies suggest that the mechanism by which early maternal behavior alters expression of the gene for GR in the offspring is via changes in serotonin activity.

Variations in HPA axis sensitivity to stress may provide a common biological pathway through which other genetic polymorphisms mediate their association with onset of depressive/anxiety disorders in response to stress. Multiple single nucleotide polymorphisms (SNPs) within the gene for the CRF type 1 (CRF-1) receptor are associated with increased depressive symptoms in those individuals exposed to childhood abuse [33]. As increased CRF-1 receptor binding density in limbic brain regions is associated with persistent hyperactivity of the HPA axis in preclinical studies of ELS [28,34], it is very possible that the causal mechanism by which these SNPs in the gene for CRF-1 convey their risk for increased depressive symptoms in those with a history of childhood abuse is at least partially moderated by altered stress responsivity of the HPA axis.

Another recent G×E finding potentially mediated by altered HPA axis reactivity is the interaction of four SNPs in FKBP5 with severity of childhood abuse as a prediction of the level of post-traumatic stress disorder (PTSD) symptoms in adults [35]. The expression of FKBP5 is induced by glucorticoids and is part of a GR-mediated negative feedback loop impacting HPA axis activity. Some of the SNPs associated with PTSD severity in those with a history of childhood abuse in this study had previously been linked with increased FKBP5 expression [36]. Increased FKBP5 expression would theoretically predict decreased sensitivity to glucocorticoid-mediated negative feedback. However, in our study, these SNPs actually correlated with enhanced suppression of cortisol response to the synthetic glucocorticoid dexamethasone. This enhanced dexamethasone suppression thus represents an environment-dependent reversal of the expected functional association with these FKBP5 SNPs, and it correlates with the controversial but often-reported finding of hypocortisolemia in individuals with PTSD as opposed to the hypercortisolemia often reported in depression. Therefore, this alteration of HPA axis sensitivity to negative feedback regulation by glucocorticoids may represent a mechanism by which genetic polymorphisms in FKBP5 mediate the risk for worsened symptomatic severity of PTSD.

Beyond the HPA axis, another neurobiological mechanism that may be involved in mediating the increased risk for depressive disorders in those individuals with both the short variant of *5-HTTLPR* and exposure to stressful environments involves alteration in the functional activity of the amygdala, a limbic region whose activation has been consistently associated with states of increased fear and anxiety. Functional imaging studies report that individuals possessing a short copy of *5-HTTLPR* exhibited greater amygdala neural activity to fearful visual stimuli than did individuals who were homozygous for the longer allele. In addition, it has been demonstrated that in those with the short allele variant, there is a relative uncoupling of the feedback circuit between the amygdala and the perigenual cingulate cortex (a region within the prefrontal cortex [PFC]). As the PFC exerts inhibitory influence on the amygdala and is necessary for extinction of fear conditioning, this finding suggests that decreased PFC inhibition of the amygdala in individuals possessing the short allele genotype may be a plausible biological mechanism for findings of increased negative affect and anxiety in these individuals [37].

# Risk/resilience for externalizing disorders

## Monoamine oxidase A

In contrast to internalizing disorders, such as depression, which are manifested by negative internal thoughts and feelings, externalizing disorders are characterized by problematic, often disruptive, external behaviors. Examples of externalizing disorders include attention-deficit hyperactivity disorder (ADHD) and conduct disorder. Deficits in the activity of monoamine oxidase A (MAO-A), the enzyme responsible for intraneuronal breakdown of catecholamines, have been associated with a risk for violence in animal models and humans. Further, a history of childhood maltreatment has long been established as a risk factor for antisocial behavior, albeit with significant individual variability in this response. A functional polymorphism in the promoter region of the gene (*MAOA*) associated with low production of the enzyme has been demonstrated to predict the outcomes of increased risk for conduct disorder, adult antisocial personality disorder and adult violence in response to childhood maltreatment in preadolescent males [38]. Since publication of this finding, several other studies including a meta-analysis have replicated the association between the low expression *MAOA* genotype and conduct disorder,

antisocial behavior and impulsivity in response to childhood maltreatment in males [39–41], although negative studies have also been published [42].

In a neuroimaging study designed to examine the underlying biological substrate mediating this G×E interaction, the low expression variant of *MAOA* was found to be structurally associated with decreased volume of both the bilateral amygdalae and the anterior cingulate cortex. However, it was functionally associated with increased amygdala activation but decreased activation in PFC regions in response to a task of perceptual matching of angry and fearful faces [43], suggesting lack of "top-down" cortical inhibition of aggressive actions. Thus, similar environment exposures (childhood maltreatment) have been demonstrated to produce different phenotypic outcomes (depressive disorders versus externalizing behaviors, such as violence/sociopathy) based on the effect of underlying genotype of intervening biological substrates.

## Dopamine

Another central catecholeamine, dopamine, plays a key role in motivation, reward seeking and executive function. Mesocortical dopamine pathways in the PFC are particularly important in coordinating executive functions, such as attention, organization, planning, time management, impulse control and judgment. Many studies have focused on G×E interactions in the dopamine system as predictive of impulsivity, violence and ADHD symptomology. In a cohort of children followed from 6 months to 5 years of age, those homozygous for the 480 base pair (bp) allele for the dopamine transporter who were exposed to the environment of prenatal maternal smoking exhibited increased hyperactivity and impulsivity [44]. A different set of polymorphisms of this allele (40 bp variable number of tandem repeats [VNTRs] and/or the 6-repeat allele of the 30 bp VNTR) predicted increased inattentiveness and hyperactivity/impulsivity for those adolescents who grew up in adverse conditions [45].

Another relevant G×E interaction in this system involves the dopamine $D_4$ receptor. The 7-repeat allele of its gene, *DRD4*, has been associated with increased sensitivity to environmental influences in children. The possession of this allele by children exposed to poorer parenting quality was associated with increased sensation seeking in the children [46]. As would be expected for children with a high degree of novelty seeking, this 7-repeat *DRD4* allele has also been associated with increased externalizing traits in children exposed to insensitive parenting. Conversely, children possessing this same long *DRD4* allele demonstrated lower externalizing traits than children without this allele when raised in the presence of sensitive parenting behaviors, suggesting that genetic variation in dopamine neurotransmission modulates attachment and responsivity to parenting style [47].

A plausible explanation for the biological mechanism by which altered gene expression in the dopamine system modulates risk for externalizing behavior in response to particular environmental exposures during development is through impact on the process of attachment. Dopamine has the potential to modulate attachment security in several ways. At the level of the mother, impaired executive function as a result of altered PFC dopamine neurotransmission could interfere with secure attachment by promoting an inconsistent pattern of maternal responsivity to infants' cues. Parental sensitivity has been acknowledged to play a crucial role in the development of a child's capacity to establish attachments to protective adults and to regulate stress. Mothers who are heterogenous in the gene for catechol O-methyltransferase (Val/Val and Val/Met forms) plus carrying the 7-repeat *DRD4* allele have exhibited either decreased parenting sensitivity in the face of increased daily hassles or increased parenting sensitivity in the face of decreased daily hassles [48]. This suggests a pattern of enhanced environmental sensitivity in which individuals are very responsive to a cue-rich environment but can easily become derailed when the environment is chaotic.

At the level of the child, altered dopamine neurotransmission may influence the child's sensitivity to his or her mother's pattern of response. Evidence suggests that children vary with respect to susceptibility to environmental influence [49] and that decreased levels of dopaminergic efficiency correlate with increased vulnerability to parental stress [47]. In a relevant G×E finding, the 7-repeat *DRD4* polymorphism has been associated with an increased risk for disorganized attachment, but only in the presence of maternal unresolved loss or trauma [47]. An intriguing recent study [50] of a parenting intervention targeted at improving maternal sensitivity and attachment quality reported that children with the 7-repeat *DRD4* allele demonstrated a reduction in daily cortisol production, suggesting that children with this polymorphism are more biologically sensitive to this parenting intervention. As this same group has reported an inverse relationship between basal cortisol levels and externalizing behaviors [50], it is plausible to extrapolate that these children may also demonstrate a greater reduction in externalizing behavior as a consequence of this parenting intervention.

## Implications and directions

The above reviewed literature provides evidence grounded in neurobiological models supporting the hypothesis that a variety of adverse early life events interact with genetic variations to influence levels of depression and anxiety, as well externalizing behaviors, across the lifespan. However, the findings also vary widely in terms of replicability, with many findings supported by a single or only a few studies.

## Defining the environment

As has been noted, G×E research is complicated by the wide range of candidate environmental factors. However, the sheer quantity of potential environments does not imply that all environments should be considered equally suitable candidates for G×E studies. Rather, a subset of strong candidate environments emerges from developmental psychopathology research on the neurobiology of psychiatric risk/resilience. These include prenatal maternal factors and exposure to childhood maltreatment, as well as adult exposure to traumatic events. In addition, these environmental factors are complemented by a growing body of research on many other adverse early life events [51].

Even within these categories of environmental stressors, a number of factors related to both assessment and definition of relevant variables need to be taken into account. To examine this issue more closely, we will focus on childhood physical, sexual and emotional abuse, which are currently among the most well-researched environmental risk variables in human psychopathology research. First, the method by which data on childhood abuse is gathered needs to be considered. The majority of G×E studies to date are cross-sectional and rely on adult self-reported history of childhood abuse. These data come with a number of limitations, including recall biases. However, despite these limitations, instruments assessing adult self-reported childhood abuse are valid and in many cases related predictably and reliably to multiple measures of adult physical and mental health. A smaller number of studies, including both cross-sectional and longitudinal study designs, evaluate children. As with adult self-report, these methods have limitations, including bias with respect to types and levels of abuse reported to child protection agencies and fears/motivations of both children and parents. Across these studies, the types of question used to assess child abuse range from those requiring self-identification of abuse to those asking about the occurrences of specific experiences. Given that both genetic and childhood environmental factors impact on cognitive capacities such as memory and verbal expression, it is reasonable to expect that memories of abuse may be influenced by these same G×E risk factors.

In addition to assessing the presence or absence of childhood abuse, a number of other abuse-related factors can be evaluated, including identity of perpetrator(s), age at onset, duration and frequency of abuse and severity of abuse. Assessment of these characteristics may be crucial to our ability to identify and understand G×E risk factors as they relate to child abuse. Distinct abuse characteristics may differentially impact a range of biological processes that could be relevant to potential G×E interplay, even when candidate genetic polymorphisms are held constant. Other abuse-related factors, including child gender, type of abuse and developmental timing of abuse, may also combine and lead to different patterns of neurobiological response. As an example, recent preliminary research finds that sexual abuse which occurs between either 3 and 5 years of age or 12 and 13 years of age is associated with reduced hippocamal volume, while sexual abuse with onset at age 9 or 10 is associated with reduced size of the corpus callosum, and sexual abuse with onset between ages 14 and 16 is associated with reduced frontal cortex gray matter volume [52]. In a similar vein, several studies are now suggesting that childhood emotional abuse may be as predictive of risk for adult psychopathology as sexual and physical abuse [53]. Lastly, childhood abuse and other early adverse life events demonstrate a dose–response effect with respect to risk and resilience. Exposure to abuse and other adverse early life events is not distributed at random in the population, meaning that exposure to one type of childhood abuse increases risk for exposure to other types of childhood abuse. Moreover, exposure to childhood abuse and other early adverse life events is associated with an increased risk of exposure to adult interpersonal violence. Therefore, in a population reporting a history of childhood abuse, there is likely to be a subgroup of people who are multiply traumatized across the lifespan, and another subset

who experienced only limited childhood abuse and exposure to adult trauma.

## Defining the outcome

Likewise, research on G×E risk factors needs to take into account the definition and method of assessment for the outcome variable being predicted. In their recent review of studies on interactions of *5-HTTLPR* with stressful life experiences, Brown and Harris [11] pointed out that childhood abuse appears to be specifically predictive of chronic depression in adulthood. It is reasonable to expect that the childhood risk factors and associated developmental processes may not be the same for chronic depression as for a single major depressive episode in reaction to recent stressful life events. This same phenomenon is likely true across varying subtypes of many psychiatric disorders, given that these subtypes may be associated with different levels and types of early life risk factor and later impairment. Another rational approach to G×E research would involve examining broader psychological traits (e.g., anxiety sensitivity, negative affect and emotional dysregulation) that are common across multiple psychiatric diagnoses. Thus, evaluating the reliability of G×E research by comparing studies that assess "stressful life events" as the common environmental stressor is problematic given that within this broad category are stressful experiences for which the underlying neurobiological processes contributing to risk/resilience are likely to be different. This becomes even more problematic when these variations in environment are combined with outcome variables that are determined by differing underlying processes.

## Conclusions

The challenges described above, however, do not preclude the possibility of conducting meaningful and replicable G×E research on risk/resilience for psychiatric disorders. Drawing from the research on developmental neurobiology, scientists will be able to design studies with environmental factors selected based on extant research and theory, and to measure aspects of these environmental stressors that are relevant to the underlying model of risk and resilience. In comparing across studies, we can also use empirically driven models when deciding which risk factors to define as "common." For example, developmental timing/duration of adverse early life events may be more important than the specific type of adverse event, which would allow for comparisons across studies measuring different types of early adverse event when controlling for temporal factors. One drawback of this approach is that it is driven only by current knowledge and has less potential for the identification of unknown G×E risk factors. This limitation can be addressed by the developing area of genome-wide association studies, but this type of research raises the potential for chance findings and necessitates utilizing appropriate methods for controlling for this risk and for conducting and evaluating replication studies. As in other areas of scientific enquiry, there is an inherent trade-off in controlling for false positives versus avoiding false negatives. Despite these challenges, this research holds potential for increasing our understanding of the developmental neurobiology of risk and resilience. For example, even given the uncertainty and variability in current research on *5-HTTLPR* × ELS, the process of following the scientific lead created by initial findings has led to increased knowledge about the mechanism by which ELS alters developmental processes and has potential impact on understanding risk and resilience across the lifespan.

This knowledge lays the foundation for research addressing the best approaches towards the prevention and treatment of psychopathology. The hope is that such research will inform the development of psychopharmacological and psychotherapeutic interventions that target specific paths associated with risk/resilience. As scientific knowledge increases about the differential neurobiological impact created by varying developmental timing and duration of abuse, as well as gender differences, this may allow for the development of targeted psychotherapeutic and psychopharmacologic interventions that would be expected to have increased efficacy in specific populations. Likewise, knowledge about the developmental periods in which environmental enrichment has mitigated the negative impact associated with developmental risk factors will allow for better timed interventions. While we recognize that the creation of such focal interventions as these, based on the current state of developmental neurobiology and G×E research, is limited, examples of such interventions have been proposed and lay the groundwork for future treatment.

## Acknowledgements

This work was supported by National Institutes of Mental Health (MH071537) and by support provided to Dr. Bradley from an American Suicide Foundation Prevention (AFSP) young investigator grant.

## References

1. Thapar, A., Harold, G., Rice, F., Langley, K. and O'Donovan, M. (2007). The contribution of gene–environment interaction to psychopathology. *Development and Psychopathology*, **19**, 989–1004.

2. Reiss, D. and Leve, L. D. (2007). Genetic expression outside the skin: Clues to mechanisms of genotype × environment interaction. *Development and Psychopathology*, **19**, 1005–1027.

3. Zammit, S . (2008). Commentary on "The case for gene–environment interactions in psychiatry." *Current Opinion in Psychiatry*, **21**, 326–327.

4. McClellan, J. M., Susser, E., King, M. C. *et al.* (2008). Forum: The interplay of genes and environment in psychiatric disorders. *Current Opinion in Psychiatry*, **21**, 322–323.

5. Flint, J. and Munafò, M. R .(2008). Forum: Interactions between gene and environment. *Current Opinion in Psychiatry*, **21**, 315–317.

6. Rutter, M . (2008). Biological Implications of gene–environment Interaction. *Journal of Abnormal Child Psychology,* **36**, 969–975.

7. Moffitt, T. E., Caspi, A. and Rutter, M. (2006). Measured gene–environment interactions in psychopathology. *Perspectives on Psychological Science,* **1**, 5–27.

8. Gunnar, M. and Quevedo, K. (2007). The Neurobiology of Stress and Development. *Annual Reviews in Psychology,* **58**, 145–173.

9. Fox, N. A., Hane, A. A. and Pine, D. S . (2007). Plasticity for affective neurocircuitry: How the environment affects gene expression. *Current Directions in Psychological Science,* **16**, 1–5.

10. Munafò, M. R., Durrant, C., Lewis, G. and Flint, J. (2008). Gene × environment interactions at the serotonin transporter locus. *Biological Psychiatry,* **13**, 131–146.

11. Brown, G. W. and Harris, T. O. (2008). Depression and the serotonin transporter 5-HTTLPR polymorphism: A review and a hypothesis concerning gene–environment interaction. *Journal of Affective Disorders,* **111**, 1–12.

12. Taylor, A. and Kim-Cohen, J. (2007). Meta-analysis of gene–environment interactions in developmental psychopathology. *Development and Psychopathology,* **19**, 1029–1037.

13. Kendler, K. S., Kessler, R. C., Walters, E. E. *et al.* (1995). Stressful life events, genetic liability, and onset of an episode of major depression in women. *American Journal of Psychiatry,* **152**, 833–842.

14. Lesch, K. P., Bengel, D., Heils, A. *et al.* (1996). Association of anxiety-related traits with a polymorphism in the serotonin transporter gene regulatory region. *Science,* **274**, 1527–1531.

15. Caspi, A., Sugden, K., Moffitt, T. E. *et al.* (2003). Influence of life stress on depression: Moderation by a

polymorphism in the 5-HTT gene. *Science*, **301**, 386–389.

16. Suomi, S. J. (2006). Risk, resilience, and gene × environment Interactions in Rhesus monkeys. *Annals of the New York Academy of Sciences*, **1094**, 52–62.

17. Taylor, S. E., Way, B. M., Welch, W. T. *et al.* (2006). Early family environment, current adversity, the serotonin transporter promoter polymorphism, and depressive symptomatology. *Biological Psychiatry*, **60**, 671–676.

18. Kendler, K. S., Kuhn, J. W., Vittum, J., Prescott, C. A. and Riley, B. (2005). The interaction of stressful life events and a serotonin transporter polymorphism in the prediction of episodes of major depression: A replication. *Archives of General Psychiatry*, **62**, 529–535.

19. Gillespie, N. A., Whitfield, J. B., Williams, B., Heath, A. C. and Martin, N. G. (2005). The relationship between stressful life events, the serotonin transporter (5-HTTLPR) genotype, and major depression. *Psychological Medicine*, **35**, 101–111.

20. Surtees, P. G., Wainwright, N. W., Willis-Owen, S. A. *et al.* (2006). Social adversity, the serotonin transporter (5-HTTLPR) polymorphism and major depressive disorder. *Biological Psychiatry*, **59**, 224–229.

21. Eley, T. C., Sugden, K., Corsico, A. *et al.* (2004). Gene–environment interaction analysis of serotonin system markers with adolescent depression. *Molecular Psychiatry*, **9**, 908–915.

22. Grabe, H. J., Lange, M., Wolff, B. *et al.* (2005). Mental and physical distress is modulated by a polymorphism in the 5-HT transporter gene interacting with social stressors and chronic disease burden. *Molecular Psychiatry*, **10**, 220–224.

23. Stein, M. B., Schork, N. J. and Gelernter, J. (2007). Gene-by-environment (serotonin transporter and childhood maltreatment) interaction for anxiety sensitivity, an intermediate phenotype for anxiety disorders. *Neuropsychopharmacology*, **33**, 312–319.

24. Gunthert, K. C., Conner, T. S., Armeli, S. *et al.* (2007). Serotonin transporter gene polymorphism (5-HTTLPR) and anxiety reactivity in daily life: A daily process approach to gene–environment interaction. *Psychosomatic Medicine*, **69**, 762–768.

25. Kaufman, J., Yang, B. Z., Douglas-Palumberi, H. *et al.* (2006). Brain-derived neurotrophic factor-5-HTTLPR gene interactions and environmental modifiers of depression in children. *Biological Psychiatry*, **59**, 673–680.

26. Kaufman, J., Yang, B. Z., Douglas-Palumberi, H. *et al.* (2004). Social supports and serotonin transporter gene moderate depression in maltreated children. *Proceedings of the National Academy of Sciences of the United States of America*, **101**, 17316–17321.

27. Nemeroff, C. B. and Vale, W. W. (2005). The neuro-biology of depression: Inroads to treatment and new drug discovery. *Journal of Clinical Psychiatry, Supplement*, **66**, 5–13.

28. Plotsky, P. M., Thrivikraman, K. V., Nemeroff, C. B. *et al.* (2005). Long-term consequences of neonatal rearing on central corticotropin-releasing factor systems in adult male rat offspring. *Neuropsychopharmacology*, **30**, 2192–2204.

29. Heim, C., Newport, D. J., Heit, S. *et al.* (2000). Pituitary–adrenal and autonomic responses to stress in women after sexual and physical abuse in childhood. *Journal of the American Medical Association*, **284**, 592–597.

30. Jabbi, M., Korf, J., Kema, I. P. *et al.* (2007). Convergent genetic modulation of the endocrine stress response involves polymorphic variations of 5-HTT, COMT and MAOA. *Molecular Psychiatry*, **12**, 483–490.

31. Gotlib, I. H., Joormann, J., Minor, K. L. and Hallmayer, J. (2007). HPA axis reactivity: A mechanism underlying the associations among 5-HTTLPR, stress, and depression. *Biological Psychiatry*, **9**, 847–851.

32. Weaver, I. C. G., Cervoni, N., Champagne, F. A. *et al.* (2004). Epigenetic programming by maternal behavior. *Nature Neuroscience*, **7**, 847–854.

33. Bradley, R. G., Binder, E. B., Epstein, M. P. *et al.* (2008). Influence of child abuse on adult depression: Moderation by the corticotropin-releasing hormone gene. *Archives of General Psychiatry*, **65**, 190–200.

34. Ladd, C. O., Huot, R. L., Thrivikraman, K. V. *et al.* (2000). Long-term behavioral and neuroendocrine adaptations to adverse early experience. *Progress in Brain Research*, **122**, 81–103.

35. Binder, E., Bradley, R., Liu, W. *et al.* (2008). Association of FKBP5 polymorphisms and childhood abuse with risk of posttraumatic stress disorder symptoms in adults. *Journal of the American Medical Association*, **299**, 1291–1305.

36. Binder, E. B., Salyakina, D., Lichtner, P. *et al.* (2004). Polymorphisms in FKBP5 are associated with increased recurrence of depressive episodes and rapid response to antidepressant treatment. *Nature Genetics*, **36**, 1319–1325.

37. Pezawas, L., Meyer-Lindenberg, A., Drabant, E. M. *et al.* (2005). 5-HTTLPR polymorphism impacts human cingulate–amygdala interactions: A genetic susceptibility mechanism for depression. *Nature Neuroscience*, **8**, 828–834.

38. Caspi, A., McClay, J., Moffitt, T. E. *et al.* (2002). Role of genotype in the cycle of violence in maltreated children. *Science*, **297**, 851–854.

39. Kim-Cohen, J., Caspi, A., Taylor, A. *et al.* (2006). MAOA, maltreatment, and gene–environment interaction predicting children's mental health: New evidence and a meta-analysis. *Molecular Psychiatry*, **11**, 903–913.

40. Foley, D. L., Eaves, L. J., Wormley, B. *et al.* (2004). Childhood adversity, monoamine oxidase a genotype,

and risk for conduct disorder. *Archives of General Psychiatry,* **61**, 738–744.

41. Huang, Y. Y., Cate, S. P., Battistuzzi, C. *et al.* (2004). An association between a functional polymorphism in the monoamine oxidase A gene promoter, impulsive traits and early abuse experiences. *Neuropsychopharmacology,***29**, 1498–1505.

42. Huizinga, D., Haberstick, B. C., Smolen, A. *et al.* (2006). Childhood maltreatment, subsequent antisocial behavior, and the role of monoamine oxidase a genotype. *Biological Psychiatry*, **60**, 677–683.

43. Meyer-Lindenberg, A., Buckholtz, J. W., Kolachana, B. *et al.* (2006). Neural mechanisms of genetic risk for impulsivity and violence in humans. *Proceedings of the National Academy of Sciences United States of America,* **103**, 6269–6274.

44. Kahn, R. S., Khoury, J., Nichols, W. C. and Lanphear, B.P. (2003). Role of dopamine transporter genotype and maternal prenatal smoking in childhood hyperactive–impulsive, inattentive, and oppositional behaviors. *Journal of Pediatrics,* **143**, 104–110.

45. Laucht, M., Skowronek, M. H., Becker, K. *et al.* (2007). Interacting effects of the dopamine transporter gene and psychosocial adversity on attention-deficit/ hyperactivity disorder symptoms among 15-year-olds from a high-risk community sample. *Archives of General Psychiatry,* **64**, 585–590.

46. Sheese, B. E., Voelker, P. M., Rothbart, M. K. and Posner, M. I. (2007). Parenting quality interacts with genetic variation in dopamine receptor D4 to influence temperament in early childhood. *Development and Psychopathology,* **19**, 1039–1046.

47. Bakermans-Kranenburg, M. J. and van Ijzendoorn, M. H. (2006). Gene–environment interaction of the dopamine D4 receptor (DRD4) and observed maternal insensitivity predicting externalizing behavior in preschoolers. *Developmental Psychobiology,* **48**, 406–409.

48. van Ijzendoorn, M. H., Bakermans-Kranenburg, M. J. and Mesman, J. (2008). Dopamine system genes associated with parenting in the context of daily hassles. *Genes, Brain, and Behavior,* 7, 403–410.

49. Belsky, J., Bakermans-Kranenburg, M. J. and van Ijzendoorn, M. H. (2007). For better and for worse: Differential susceptibility to environmental influences. *Current Directions in Psychological Science,* **16**, 300–304.

50. Bakermans-Kranenburg, M. J., van Ijzendoorn, M. H., Mesman, J., Alink, L. R. A. and Juffer, F. (2008). Effects of an attachment-based intervention on daily cortisol moderated by dopamine receptor D4: A randomized control trial on 1- to 3-year-olds screened for externalizing behavior. *Development and Psychopathology,* **20**, 805–820.

51. Anda, R. F., Felitti, V. J. and Bremner, J. D. *et al.* (2006). The enduring effects of abuse and related adverse experiences in childhood. A convergence of evidence from neurobiology and epidemiology. *European Archives of Psychiatry and Clinical Neuroscience,* **256**, 174–186.

52. Andersen, S. L. and Teicher, M. H. (2008). Stress, sensitive periods and maturational events in adolescent depression. *Trends in Neurosciences,* **31**, 183–191.

53. Yates, T. M. (2007). The developmental consequences of child emotional abuse: A neurodevelopmental perspective. *Journal of Emotional Abuse,* 7, 9–34.

# Chapter 15

# The neuroendocrine effects of early life trauma

Jamie L. LaPrairie, Christine M. Heim and Charles B. Nemeroff

## Introduction

Over the last several decades, the relative contribution of both genetic and environmental influences in the pathogenesis of psychiatric illness has been explored extensively. A predisposing genetic contribution to the development of many mental disorders has now been demonstrated. In addition, compelling evidence exists for a critical role of early life adverse experiences in the increased vulnerability to several psychiatric disorders, including mood and anxiety disorders and schizophrenia. Given the high incidence of childhood maltreatment and neglect, many studies have focused on the neurobiological and neuroendocrine mechanisms underlying this relationship between early life stress (ELS) and adult psychopathology. The present chapter summarizes available findings on the neuroendocrine effects of exposure to trauma during early development, with a focus on a role for such alterations in the increased risk of mood and anxiety disorders in adulthood.

## Early life stress

### Definition

Stress is defined as a physically, mentally or emotionally disruptive or threatening condition occurring in response to adverse intrinsic or extrinsic influences, for which adequate coping resources are unavailable [1]. Individual perception and behavioral adaptations are vital to the experience of stress. A disruption in homeostasis and the subsequent behavioral and physiological adaptive responses can occur throughout the lifespan, including during prenatal development. In humans, ELS has been defined as any such incident occurring within the defined development period from gestation through to either the onset of puberty

or 18 years of age. Developmental trauma is characterized by stress associated with extreme fear and great emotional charge. The most widespread forms of ELS in humans are sexual, physical and emotional maltreatment and neglect. Sexual abuse can be defined as exposure of a child to sexually explicit situations, the use of children as sexual stimuli, and sexual contact between children and adults. Physical abuse involves any non-accidental physical injury to the child's body. Emotional abuse involves injury to the psychological capacity or emotional stability of the child by a parent or caregiver. Neglect is defined as parental deprivation of adequate food, clothing, shelter, medical care, supervision or support [2]. Other forms of early life trauma include parental loss, natural disasters, war, accidents, physical illness, poverty, inadequate parental care as a result of mental or physical illness, and maternal stress during pregnancy.

## Prevalence

Child maltreatment occurs at alarmingly high rates worldwide. According to the US Department of Health and Human Services Children's Bureau, 3.6 million cases of child abuse and neglect are reported annually in the USA. According to *Child Maltreatment 2006* [3], over 900 000 of these reported allegations are determined to be severe in nature, with an estimated 1500 child fatalities resulting from extreme maltreatment each year. Indeed, neglect is the most frequent form of maltreatment, as 62.8% of child victims experience this type of abuse. Because of cultural and various other factors, most abused and neglected children never come to the attention of proper authorities. Therefore, the national rates are most likely a gross underestimate of the actual prevalence of childhood abuse in society. There is also a considerable overlap between physical, emotional and sexual abuse, and children who are subject to one form of abuse are significantly more likely to suffer other forms of abuse. Prevalence estimates of sexual abuse in females range from 7 to 62 in the USA. According to the United Nations, worldwide estimates of female sexual child abuse exceed 150 million and 47.3% of child sexual abuse victims are male, with one in every six boys having endured sexual abuse prior to the age of 16 years [14]. The prevalence of physical abuse ranges from 10 to 30% in females and is generally higher in males. According to the US Department of Health and Human Services, emotional and psychological maltreatment is reported in 7% of children [3]. In addition, a vast number of children experience inadequate parental care through parental mental illness, with up to 50% of mothers suffering from depressive episodes [5]. Variation in rates of maltreatment across studies may be due in part to differences in sample populations, definitions of abuse and methods of assessment.

## Physiological systems involved in the regulation of the stress response

Three major brain circuits initiate and maintain the stress response. The principal components of the stress system are the hypothalamic–pituitary–adrenal (HPA) axis, the locus ceruleus–norepinephrine (LC-NE) system and the extrahypothalamic corticotropin-releasing factor (CRF) systems. Activation of the stress response leads to behavioral, endocrine, immune and autonomic alterations that improve the ability of an individual to adjust homeostasis, and neutralize or minimize the potential impact of a threat. Activation of the stress system in response to acute stress is meant to be salutary, whereas chronic stress system activation may lead to maladaptation and dysfunction.

### The hypothalamic–pituitary–adrenal axis

In response to acute stress, CRF is released into hypothalamo-hypophyseal portal circulation from nerve terminals of the paraventricular nucleus (PVN) of the hypothalamus, and subsequently stimulates the synthesis and secretion of adrenocorticotropic hormone (ACTH) from the anterior pituitary. The release of ACTH, in turn, elicits the secretion of glucocorticoid hormones from the adrenal cortex. Arginine-vasopressin acts synergistically with CRF in increasing the secretion of ACTH but alone has very little ACTH secretagogue activity. Glucocorticoids are the final effectors of the HPA axis and are key regulators in

maintaining the basal activity of the HPA axis and terminating the neuroendocrine response to stress. Glucocorticoids exert their effects via two types of cytoplasmic receptors, mineralocorticoid receptors (MR), located mainly in the hippocampus, and glucocorticoid receptors (GR), which are widely distributed. The negative glucocorticoid feedback on ACTH secretion acts to limit excessive glucocorticoid exposure, thus minimizing the potentially detrimental antireproductive and immunosuppressive effects of these hormones [6,7].

### The locus ceruleus–norepinephrine system

In concert with endocrine activation via the HPA axis, stress concurrently engages the LC-NE system. The LC is a small compact group of norepinephrine-containing cells located in the pons. The LC sends widespread, branching projections to all areas of the neocortex, thalamus, limbic system, hypothalamus and the spinal cord. Within these regions, axons of LC cells extensively branch, resulting in widespread NE release. Norepinephrine serves globally as an alarm system, which contributes to increases in autonomic and neuroendocrine responses to stress including HPA axis activation. It also activates the amygdala, the principal brain region involved in fear-related behaviors, and enhances the storage of aversely charged emotional memories in the hippocampus and striatum. The main role of the LC-NE system is in the integration and orchestration of the adaptive central nervous system (CNS) response to various stressors, resulting in increased vigilance, attention and arousal during a state of stress [7].

### The corticotropin-releasing factor systems

Stress is a potent activator of CRF release from the hypothalamus, as well as at extrahypothalamic sites including the neocortex, limbic system, LC and spinal cord. Moreover, CRF receptor-binding sites are also found in various peripheral tissues. Whereas CRF in the PVN of the hypothalamus is primarily involved in the regulation of pituitary ACTH secretion, extrahypothalamic CRF systems are critical for the assessment of threatening stimuli and for the implementation of appropriate motor responses to threatening stimuli. The CRF neurons found in abundance in the neocortex are likely involved in cognitive function and behavioral responses to stress. High densities of CRF neurons are also found in the central nucleus of the amygdala, a principal site in the regulation of emotion, and have been implicated in the affective response to stress [8]. These CRF neurons influence the endocrine stress response via projections from the central nucleus of the amygdala to the PVN. Moreover, CRF neurons project to the brainstem, which contains the majority of noradrenergic and serotonergic projections to the forebrain. Two distinct subtypes of CRF receptor designated CRFR-1 and CRFR-2 are widely and differentially expressed throughout the brain and periphery. Microinjection of CRF directly into the CNS produces many symptoms of anxiety and depression. Therefore, CRF pathways and CRF receptors are uniquely situated to participate in a number of the different neuronal pathways that are involved in the acute and chronic responses to stress [6,7].

## Neurobiology of disorders related to early life stress

The impact of childhood physical, sexual and emotional abuse on long-term mental and physiological well-being is profound. Acutely, more than half of all abused children display symptoms of anxiety, fear, irritability, low self-esteem, withdrawal, aggression, anger and depression. In addition, increased rates of major depression, post-traumatic stress disorder (PTSD) and attention-deficit hyperactivity disorder (ADHD) have been reported in maltreated children. There is also evidence that victims of child sexual abuse are at greater risk during adolescence of sexually transmitted diseases, teenage pregnancy, multiple sexual partnerships, sexual re-victimization and cardiovascular disease [9]. Similarly, children who have experienced inadequate care through parental loss or mental illness display more psychiatric symptoms than children of intact families [10].

Compelling evidence from numerous studies has shown that ELS results in a substantially increased risk for the development of major depressive disorder. Indeed, women with a history of childhood abuse are four times as likely to develop syndromal depression compared with non-abused females, and the magnitude of the abuse is correlated with the severity of depressive symptoms [11]. Childhood abuse also results in greater propensity for the development of adulthood anxiety disorders, including generalized anxiety disorder, panic disorders, social anxiety disorder and PTSD. Similarly, other forms of ELS, such as inadequate parental care and prenatal stress, also predispose individuals to the development of depression, anxiety disorders, bipolar disorder and schizophrenia in adulthood.

## Depression

A substantial body of evidence suggests that the stress response system is chronically dysfunctional in depressive disorders. To this end, approximately half of all individuals with major depressive disorder demonstrate excessive HPA axis activity, as measured by chronically elevated plasma cortisol concentrations. Administration of the synthetic glucocorticoid dexamethasone does not suppress HPA axis activity in many depressed patients, indicative of diminished feedback inhibition [12]. Moreover, depressed patients display a reduced ACTH response following intravenous CRF administration, suggesting a down-regulation of pituitary CRFR-1 density as a result of chronic hypersecretion of CRF [13]. These findings parallel the reduction in pituitary CRF receptors in maternally deprived rodents and the blunted ACTH response to CRF stimulation in depressed females with a history of childhood abuse. Together, these data are indicative of a hyperactive HPA axis, resulting from excessive CRF drive and overstimulation of pituitary CRFR-1 in depression. Another key clinical finding in patients with untreated major depression is the elevation of CRF-like immunoreactivity in cerebrospinal fluid (CSF), which also provides evidence for hyperactivity of central, extrahypothalamic CRF pathways.

Further support for CRF dysfunction is provided by postmortem analyses of brains of depressed suicide victims, which have revealed increased CRF mRNA expression and CRF concentrations in multiple brain areas associated with emotion and attentional processes, as well as concomitant decreased CRFR-1 mRNA in the frontal cortex [14]. Hippocampal atrophy is a key feature in many depressed patients, perhaps a direct result of persistent hypercortisolism. Hippocampal atrophy may be associated with impaired inhibition of CRF secretion and further increases in glucocorticoid secretion. Depressed patients, as noted above, exhibit impaired cortisol suppression following dexamethasone administration and decreased glucocorticoid receptor expression. These findings are consistent with observations in maternally separated rats.

Postmortem studies have also demonstrated increases in CRF concentrations in brainstem monoaminergic nuclei, including noradrenergic cells of the LC and serotonergic cells of the dorsal raphe [15]. Stress-modulating serotonergic pathways are altered in depression, and administration of a tryptophan-depleting diet to reduce serotonin availability in the CNS results in increased CRF concentrations in CSF as well as depressive symptoms in healthy volunteers [16]. Altered noradrenergic activity has been reported in patients with melancholic depression. These findings are interesting in light of the many reports of noradrenergic and serotonergic dysfunction in animal models of early life stress.

## Anxiety disorders

Considerable evidence suggests that CRF pathways and CRF-R1 in the stress response system are dysfunctional in anxiety disorders, particularly in PTSD and obsessive–compulsive disorder. As in depression, CRF pathways are persistently activated in PTSD, as indicated by increased CRF-like immunoreactivity in CSF. Dysregulation of the HPA axis is also a prominent feature of PTSD, where CRF stimulation results in blunted ACTH responses similar to those observed in depressed patients [5]. In contrast, an increased ACTH response has been observed in response to CRF in patients with panic disorder [17]. Women with PTSD and a history of childhood abuse display low plasma cortisol levels but mount an exaggerated cortisol response to acute stressors [18]. This implies that the HPA axis is in a state of hypoactivity in patients with PTSD but is hyper-responsive to stress. This HPA axis dysfunction is similar to that observed in depressed patients with a past history of ELS. These findings suggest that exposure to a prior stressor may sensitize the HPA axis to subsequent stressors. Structural brain imaging studies have demonstrated alterations in patients with PTSD. Decreased hippocampal volume and hippocampal memory-associated deficits have been reported [19]. These findings are of interest in light of reports suggesting chronic hypocortisolism and increased glucocorticoid feedback inhibition as features of PTSD. One proposed mechanism is that patients with PTSD display markedly increased cortisol responses to everyday stress, resulting in sustained neurotoxic effects in the hippocampus.

Almost 30% of patients with major depression have a comorbid syndromal anxiety disorder. This subpopulation is characterized by a greater severity of depressive illness, including increased rates of suicide, as well as increased treatment resistance. Compared with individuals with only one disorder, patients with comorbid depression and anxiety displayed increased HPA axis activation in response to social stress [20]. Measurement of CRF concentrations in CSF have not been conducted in patients with mixed depression and anxiety; however, neuroendocrine evidence

for a highly sensitized HPA axis is consistent with the hypothesis that psychiatric patients who are more severely affected would display greater CRF system hyperactivity.

Hypersensitive noradrenergic pathways in the brain have been implicated in several anxiety disorders. Previous studies have reported an exaggerated behavioral response to the $\alpha_2$-adrenergic antagonist yohimbine in patients with PTSD and panic disorder [21]. This parallels evidence in non-human primates reared in a variable foraging demand environment. Together, these data suggest a possible interaction between CRF and NE neurons, whereby increased CRF availability may sensitize noradrenergic systems and increase reactivity in patients with anxiety disorders. Serotonergic dysfunction has also been implicated in the expression of PTSD and panic disorder, likely forming the basis for the efficacy of selective serotonin release inhibitors in the treatment of several anxiety disorders. Taken together, these findings support the concept that anxiety-related disorders involve alterations in multiple neurotransmitter systems.

# Neurobiological and neuroendocrine effects of early life stress

Over the past several decades, considerable evidence from both clinical and non-human animal studies suggests a preeminent role for psychological stress and untoward life events in the pathogenesis of psychiatric illness. The relationship between early adverse experiences and the development of adult psychopathology is likely mediated by alterations in neurobiological systems involved in the regulation of stress.

## Studies of early life stress in rodents

The use of various rodent models of early life adversity has revealed that prenatal and early postnatal stressful experiences have profound and permanent consequences on the behavioral and neuroendocrine response to stress stimuli in adulthood. The most common models of postnatal ELS in rodents involve experimental disruption of normal mother–infant interactions, namely a model of maternal neglect. In response to early life manipulations, infant rats display a characteristic corticosterone surge, despite the stress-hyporesponsive period normally ascribed to postnatal days 4–14. Previous research has shown that, compared with non-separated controls, 180 minutes per day of maternal separation during the first approximately 20 days of life in neonatal rats resulted in higher basal and stress-induced plasma ACTH and corticosterone concentrations, increased CRF immunoreactivity in the median eminence, decreased pituitary CRFR-1 binding and increased CRF concentrations and CRF binding to receptors in extrahypothalamic CRF systems in adulthood [22]. Similarly, animals that experienced 180 minutes of daily maternal separation from postnatal day 2 to day 14 displayed increased ACTH and corticosterone concentrations in response to stressors, increased median eminence CRF concentrations, increased CRF mRNA expression in the PVN and decreased hippocampal GR binding compared with undisturbed controls [23]. Moreover, maternal deprivation for 24 hours in 12-day-old rats produce heightened basal and stress-induced ACTH and altered CRFR expression in brain regions involved in the pathophysiology of depression and anxiety [22]. This maternal deprivation on postnatal days 3 or 8 resulted in enhanced ACTH and corticosterone responses to stress, whereas the same manipulation at postnatal day 13 had no effect on stress responsiveness in adulthood [24]. These results suggest that a critical developmental period exists in which ELS may exert differential effects on neurobiological function. Maternal separation paradigms also result in marked behavioral alterations characteristic of affective disorders. Taken together, these findings indicate that brief perinatal disruptions of maternal care produce CRF hypersecretion in the median eminence with associated CRFR and GR downregulation, as well as diminished HPA axis negative feedback regulation, which persist into maturity.

In contrast to the deleterious effects of maternal separation on the HPA axis, brief bouts of handling during the perinatal period result in a fear and anxiety hyporesponsive phenotype. Interestingly, brief (15 minute) separations of pups from the dam (i.e., handling) results in a significant increase in maternal caregiving behavior in the form of licking/grooming and arched-back nursing. Indeed, naturally occurring variations in maternal care can have a profound impact on behavioral and neuroendocrine stress responsiveness, and anxiety-related neurocircuitry [25]. Grown offspring of high-responding mothers display reduced fearfulness, decreased stress-induced ACTH and corticosterone, increased hippocampal GR mRNA expression, enhanced glucocorticoid negative feedback sensitivity, and reduced CRF mRNA in the hypothalamus compared with offspring whose mothers demonstrated low levels of maternal behavior. Differences in

DNA methylation between the offspring of high- and low-licking/grooming dams are reversed with cross-fostering, persist into adulthood and are associated with altered histone acetylation and transcription factor binding to the GR gene promoter. Furthermore, additional neurotransmitter systems and brain regions implicated in fear and anxiety expression are altered, where recipients of more maternal attention demonstrate increased CRF receptor and $\alpha_2$-adrenergic receptor densities in the LC and increased central benzodiazepine receptor density in the amygdala and LC [25,26].

## Studies of early life stress in non-human primates

Consistent with previous findings in rodents, early adversity in non-human primates profoundly impacts the long-term behavioral and neuroendocrine response to stress. One of the most widely used models to study the consequences of early adverse experiences and the increased vulnerability to later psychopathology in non-human primates is maternal separation. In response to acute separation from their mother, non-human primate infants respond with intense distress vocalizations, defecation and increased HPA function. Maternal and social deprivation for up to 12 months results in profound, long-term behavioral alterations, including increased fearfulness and anxiety, social and sexual dysfunction, and aberrant stereotypic and self-directed behaviors. Moreover, alterations in the sympathetic stress response have been noted. Despite the compelling evidence from rodent studies that maternal separation produces profound alterations in the function of HPA axis, the impact of early deprivation on the neuroendocrine response to stress in non-human primates remains unclear. Basal and stress-induced activation of the HPA axis has been reported to be both increased and reduced. Rhesus macaques that are reared without their mothers but allowed to socialize with conspecifics show enhanced stress-induced ACTH and cortisol secretion as well as increased distress vocalizations in adulthood compared with mother-reared monkeys [27]. Similarly, monkeys exposed to repeated social separations display reduced cortisol responses in response to stress and increased glucocorticoid feedback sensitivity [28].

An unpredictable foraging demand paradigm that aims to disrupt normal social and maternal behavior has also been used as a model of early adversity in bonnet macaques. Interestingly, animals confronted with a variable foraging demand (unpredictable alternation of periods of strenuous foraging with periods of free access to food) display the most profound effects on the mother–infant dyad. The manipulation experimentally reduces the quantity and quality of maternal care toward the infants for the first 3 months of life, thereby resulting in increased fearfulness, exaggerated behavioral and physiological responses to stressful stimuli and decreased social competence in adulthood compared with animals reared with consistent low- or high-foraging demands. The animals also exhibit persistent elevations in CRF concentrations in the CSF, as well as alterations in somatostatin and biogenic amines [29].

The model that most closely resembles human child maltreatment is the spontaneous occurrence of infant physical abuse and neglect in large social groups of rhesus and pigtail macaques. Up to 10% of infants born into these primate social groups are subjected to physical abuse and neglect by their mothers. The types of abusive behaviors that the infants endure are hitting, biting, dragging, throwing and rejection. Highly rejected infants display significantly decreased CSF monoamine metabolites (5-hydroxyindoleacetic acid and homovanillic acid) compared with less-rejected infants, suggesting reduced serotonergic and dopaminergic function following early maternal rejection [30]. Furthermore, abused infants exhibit increased anxiety, distress calls and altered play behavior compared with non-abused controls.

## Clinical studies of early life stress

A number of clinical investigations have examined the impact of ELS on HPA axis dysfunction and the development of subsequent psychopathology in children, adolescents and adults.

Studies in children and adolescents who have endured various types of ELS have demonstrated contradictory results. Increased morning cortisol in former Romanian orphans and elevated diurnal cortisol secretion in institutionalized children have been reported [31]. Similarly, maltreated children with pediatric PTSD symptoms displayed elevated salivary cortisol levels and increased 24 hour urinary cortisol excretion compared with control subjects [32]. However, reduced morning cortisol in socially deprived and sexually abused children has also been shown [31].

In response to CRF stimulation, children who have been sexually abused demonstrate significantly reduced ACTH responses compared with non-abused children [33]. This has been hypothesized to be a result of pituitary CRFR down-regulation subsequent to hypersecretion of CRF from the hypothalamus. Abused children with current depression, however, display enhanced ACTH and normal cortisol responses following CRF stimulation [34]. Consistent with these findings, children reared by mothers diagnosed with a psychiatric illness exhibit exaggerated ACTH activation in response to CRF challenge compared with subjects not exposed to such parenting [35].

Following exposure to a traumatic earthquake, adolescents displayed lower morning salivary cortisol and greater cortisol suppression in response to the dexamethasone suppression test [36]. The same test yields opposite results in children who have experienced parental loss [37]. Accordingly, children who experience trauma early in life, in the form of sexual and physical abuse, social deprivation, parental loss, natural disasters and serious parental illness, display markedly increased risk of depression, anxiety and PTSD-related disorders.

Childhood abuse with and without PTSD also affects NE, epinephrine and dopamine urinary excretion, with all levels being significantly elevated in comparison with controls [38]. Extrapolation of such findings to the CNS remains obscure. Abused children with depression and children who experienced adverse rearing conditions demonstrate an increased prolactin response to L-5-hydroxytryptophan and fenfluramine, respectively [39]. Prolactin secretion is mediated by $5\text{-}HT1_A$ receptors and, therefore, these results suggest serotonergic sensitization of this receptor subtype following early life stress. Taken together, it is evident based on these investigations that abnormalities in neuroendocrine function associated with ELS are highly variable and likely dependent upon the nature of abuse, developmental timing and duration of stress exposure, concomitant stress and psychopathology.

Consistent with preclinical evidence, studies in adult humans have found that exposure to ELS results in neuroendocrine dysregulation and an increased vulnerability to mood and anxiety disorders. Female victims of sexual abuse with PTSD demonstrate increased urinary cortisol excretion and increased glucocorticoid feedback sensitivity [40]. However, reports of plasma and salivary cortisol levels in women with a history of childhood abuse are inconsistent. Similarly, increased basal and psychosocial stress-induced cortisol responses are demonstrated by adults with a history of early parental death and are moderated by the quality of the parent–child relationship [41].

Our group has demonstrated that adult survivors of child abuse with and without major depression display significantly increased cortisol responses to psychological stress compared with healthy control subjects and abused women without depression [42,43]. Childhood abuse victims with current depression suffer more from comorbid PTSD and exposure to recent stressful life events compared with females with a history of abuse without current depressive symptoms; this group also demonstrated increased cortisol and heart rate responses to a standardized stressor. In response to CRF stimulation, childhood abuse victims without depression exhibit enhanced ACTH responses. However, abuse victims with comorbid depression display blunted ACTH responses, possibly as a result of chronic overexposure of the pituitary to CRF [44]. These findings suggest that distinct endophenotypes of depression with differential resultant pathophysiologies exist, dependent upon the presence or absence of ELS. We believe that ELS results in hypersecretion of hypothalamic and extrahypothalamic CRF systems in response to stress. This ultimately leads to downregulation of adenohypophyseal CRFRs and enhanced CRF activity at extrahypothalmic sites, resulting in psychopathological symptoms later in life.

Similar to findings in children, adult victims with a history of abuse and PTSD display elevated urinary NE secretion [40]. Furthermore, blunted prolactin responses to meta-chlorophenylpiperazine have been noted in victims of childhood abuse, suggesting altered serotonergic function [45].

## The genetic contribution

Although numerous studies suggest a robust genetic basis for most psychiatric illnesses, including mood and anxiety disorders, the search for direct genetic influences contributing to the risk for these disorders has been inconclusive. Indeed, recent studies suggest that predisposing genetic variants interact with environmental variables such as ELS to contribute to adult pathology. Several groups have demonstrated that the presence of a short allele in the promoter region of the gene for the serotonin transporter (5-HTTLPR) increases the risk of depression in the presence of substantiative life stress. The 5-HTTLPR allele polymorphism may impact "emotional responsivity" to stress, thereby increasing the risk for the development of anxiety and depression consequent to maltreatment in childhood [46]. Genetic predisposition for depression has also been associated with polymorphisms of the gene for the brain-derived neurotrophic factor (BDNF). The combination of polymorphisms of BDNF and 5-HTTLPR and ELS increase the risk of depression in children and also in the adult population [47]. Moreover, recent evidence suggests that multiple polymorphisms associated with the gene CRFR1 appear to exacerbate or diminish the impact of early life trauma on the vulnerability for major depressive disorder [48]. This provides further support for the hypothesis that dysregulation of the CRF and CRFR-1 system associated with adult psychopathology is a function of early life trauma.

The relationship between genetic, neurobiological and environmental factors, and the relative contributions of each in the expression of adult PTSD, has also been examined. Variation in 5-HTTLPR as well as polymorphisms in the glucocorticoid stress-related gene FKBP5 have been implicated in the development of PTSD symptoms and appear to interact with childhood abuse to predict the risk of PTSD in adulthood. For example, four SNPs in FKBP5 significantly interact with the severity of childhood abuse to predict adult PTSD symptoms [49]. Taken together, heritable differences in stress-associated genes modulate the effects of early adversity on neurobiological system involved in stress, thereby altering the risk for certain disorders upon further exposure to stress in adulthood.

## Conclusions

In summary, it is highly evident based on preclinical and clinical studies that severe stress early in life induces persistent maladaptations in multiple neurotransmitter systems involved in the regulation of stress, specifically characterized by enhanced behavioral, neuroendocrine and autonomic stress responsiveness. Early adverse experiences in combination with predisposing genetic factors combine with additional exposure to acute and chronic life stress to substantially increase the vulnerability for stress-related diseases. Future studies should focus on the nature and developmental timing of early adverse events on the development of psychiatric illness, as well as the novel psychotherapeutic and pharmacological interventions that might mitigate or prevent the deleterious effects of ELS. Findings from this research would have important implications for the development of optimized treatment strategies that directly target different neurobiological pathways involved in depression and anxiety disorders in victims of early child maltreatment.

# References

1. Lazarus, R. S. (1985). The psychology of stress and coping. *Issues in Mental Health Nursing, 7*, 399–418.

2. Wissow, L. S. (1995). Child abuse and neglect. *New England Journal of Medicine, 332*, 1425–1431.

3. US Department of Health and Human Services. (2008). *Child maltreatment 2006.* Washington, DC: US Government Printing Agency.

4. Dube, S. R., Anda, R. F., Whitfield, C. L. *et al.* (2005). Long-term consequences of childhood sexual abuse by gender of victim. *American Journal of Preventive Medicine, 28*, 430–438.

5. Heim, C. and Nemeroff, C. B. (2001). The role of childhood trauma in the neurobiology of mood and anxiety disorders. *Biological Psychiatry, 49*, 1023–1039.

6. Arborelius, L., Owens, M. J., Plotsky, P. M. and Nemeroff, C. B. (1999). The role of corticotropin-releasing factor in depression and anxiety disorders. *Journal of Endocrinology, 160*, 1–12.

7. Carrasco, G. A. and van der Kar, L. D. (2003). Neuroendocrine pharmacology of stress. *European Journal of Pharmacology, 463*, 235–272.

8. LeDoux, J. E. (2000). Emotion circuits in the brain. *Annual Review of Neuroscience, 23*, 155–184.

9. Springs, F. E. and Friedrich, W. N. (1992). Health risk behaviors and medical sequelae of childhood sexual abuse. *Mayo Clinical Proceedings, 67*, 527–532.

10. Tyrka, A. R., Wier, L., Price, L. H., Ross, N. S. and Carpenter, L. L. (2008). Childhood parental loss and adult psychopathology. *International Journal of Psychiatry and Medicine, 38*, 329–344.

11. Mullen, P. E., Martin, J. L., Anderson, J. C., Romans, S. E. and Herbison, G. P. (1996). The long-term impact of the physical, emotional, and sexual abuse of children. *Child Abuse & Neglect, 20*, 7–21.

12. Hatzinger, M. (2000). Neuropeptides and the hypothalamic–pituitary–adrenocortical (HPA) system. *World Journal of Biological Psychiatry, 1*, 105–111.

13. Newport, D. J., Heim, C., Owens, M. J. *et al.* (2003). Cerebrospinal fluid corticotropin-releasing factor (CRF) and vasopressin concentrations predict pituitary response in the CRF stimulation test. *Neuropsychopharmacology, 28*, 569–576.

14. Merali, Z., Du, L., Hrdina, P. *et al.* (2004). Dysregulation in the suicide brain. *Journal of Neuroscience, 24*, 1478–1485.

15. Bissette, G., Klimek, V., Pan, J., Stockmeier, C. and Ordway, G. (2003). Elevated concentrations of CRF in the locus coeruleus of depressed subjects. *Neuropsychopharmacology, 28*, 1328–1335.

16. Tyrka, A. R., Carpenter, L. L., McDougle, C. J. *et al.* (2004). Increased cerebrospinal fluid CRF concentrations during tryptophan depletion in healthy adults. *Biological Psychiatry, 56*, 531–534.

17. Curtis, G. C., Abelson, J. L. and Gold, P. W. (1997). ACTH and cortisol responses to CRH: Changes in panic disorder and effects of alprazolam treatment. *Biological Psychiatry, 41*, 76–85.

18. Bremner, J. D. (2006). Stress and brain atrophy. *CNS Neurological Disorders and Drug Targets, 5*, 503–512.

19. Newport, D. J. and Nemeroff, C. B. (2000). Neurobiology of posttraumatic stress disorder. *Current Opinion in Neurobiology, 10*, 211–218.

20. Young, E. A., Abelson, J. L. and Cameron, O. G. (2004). Effect of comorbid anxiety disorders on the HPA axis response to a social stressor in major depression. *Biological Psychiatry, 56*, 113–120.

21. Southwick, S. M., Morgan, C. A., III Charney, D. S. and High, J. R. (1999). Yohimbine use in a natural setting. *Biological Psychiatry, 46*, 442–444.

22. Ladd, C. O., Owens, M. J. and Nemeroff, C. B. (1996). Persistent changes in CRF neuronal systems induced by maternal deprivation. *Endocrinology, 137*, 1212–1218.

23. Plotsky, P. M. and Meaney, M. J. (1993). Early, postnatal experience alters hypothalamic CRF mRNA, median eminence CRF content and stress-induced release in adult rats. *Brain Research, Molecular Brain Research, 18*, 195–200.

24. van Oers, H. J., de Kloet, E. R. and Levine, S. (1998). Early vs. late maternal deprivation differentially alters the endocrine and hypothalamic responses to stress. *Brain Research, Developmental Brain Research, 111*, 245–252.

25. Liu, D., Diorio, J., Tannenbaum, B. *et al.* (1997). Maternal care, hippocampal glucocorticoid receptors, and HPA responses to stress. *Science, 277*, 1659–1662.

26. Caldji, C., Tannenbaum, B., Sharma, S. *et al.* (1998). Maternal care during infancy regulates the development of neural systems mediating the expression of fearfulness in the rat. *Proceedings of the National Academy of Sciences of the United States of America, 95*, 5335–5340.

27. Fahlke, C., Lorenz, J. G., Long, J. *et al.* (2000). Rearing experiences and stress-induced plasma cortisol as early risk factors for excessive alcohol consumption in nonhuman primates. *Alcoholism, Clinical and Experimental Research, 24*, 644–650.

28. Lyons, D. M., Yang, C., Mobley, B. W., Nickerson, J. T. and Schatzberg, A. F. (2000). Early environmental regulation of glucocorticoid feedback sensitivity in young adult monkeys. *Journal of Neuroendocrinology, 12*, 723–728.

29. Coplan, J. D., Trost, R. C., Owens, M. J. *et al.* (1998). CSF concentrations of somatostatin and biogenic amines in grown primates reared by mothers exposed to manipulated foraging conditions. *Archives of General Psychiatry, 55*, 473–477.

30. Maestripieri, D., Higley, J. D., Lindell, S. G. *et al.* (2006). Early maternal rejection affects the development of

monoaminergic systems and adult abusive parenting in rhesus macaques. *Behavioral Neuroscience*, **120**, 1017–1024.

31. Carlson, M. and Earls, F. (1997). Psychological and neuroendocrinological sequelae of early social deprivation in institutionalized children in Romania. *Annals of the New York Academy of Sciences*, **807**, 419–428.

32. Carrion, V. G., Weems, C. F., Ray, R. D. *et al.* (2002). Diurnal salivary cortisol in pediatric posttraumatic stress disorder. *Biological Psychiatry*, **51**, 575–582.

33. De Bellis, M. D., Chrousos, G. P., Dorn, L. D. *et al.* (1994). HPA axis dysregulation in sexually abused girls. *Journal of Clinical Endocrinology and Metabolism*, **78**, 249–255.

34. Kaufman, J., Birmaher, B., Perel, J. *et al.* (1997). The CRH challenge in depressed abused, depressed nonabused, and normal control children. *Biological Psychiatry*, **42**, 669–679.

35. Meyer, S. E., Chrousos, G. P. and Gold, P. W. (2001). Major depression and the stress system. *Developmental Psychopathology*, **13**, 565–580.

36. Goenjian, A. K., Yehuda, R., Pynoos, R. S. *et al.* (1996). Basal cortisol, dexamethasone suppression of cortisol, and MHPG in adolescents after the 1988 earthquake in Armenia. *American Journal of Psychiatry*, **153**, 929–934.

37. Weller, E. B., Weller, R. A., Fristad, M. A. and Bowes, J. M. (1990). Dexamethasone suppression test and depressive symptoms in bereaved children. *Journal of Neuropsychiatry and Clinical Neuroscience*, **2**, 418–421.

38. De Bellis, M. D., Baum, A. S., Birmaher, B. *et al.* (1999). A. E. Bennett Research Award. Developmental traumatology. Part I: Biological stress systems. *Biological Psychiatry*, **45**, 1259–1270.

39. Kaufman, J., Birmaher, B., Perel, J. *et al.* (1998). Serotonergic functioning in depressed abused children. *Biological Psychiatry*, **44**, 973–981.

40. Lemieux, A. M. and Coe, C. L. (1995). Abuse-related PTSD: Evidence for chronic neuroendocrine activation in women. *Psychosomatic Medicine*, **57**, 105–115.

41. Tyrka, A. R., Wier, L., Price, L. H. *et al.* (2008). Childhood parental loss and adult HPA function. *Biological Psychiatry*, **63**, 1147–1154.

42. Heim, C., Ehlert, U. and Hellhammer, D. H. (2000). The potential role of hypocortisolism in the pathophysiology of stress-related bodily disorders. *Psychoneuroendocrinology*, **25**, 1–35.

43. Heim, C., Newport, D. J., Heit, S. *et al.* (2000). Pituitary-adrenal and autonomic responses to stress in women after sexual and physical abuse in childhood. *Journal of the American Medical Association*, **284**, 592–597.

44. Heim, C., Newport, D. J., Bonsall, R., Miller, A. H. and Nemeroff, C. B. (2001). Altered pituitary-adrenal axis responses to provocative challenge tests in adult survivors of childhood abuse. *American Journal of Psychiatry*, **158**, 575–581.

45. Rinne, T., Westenberg, H. G., den Boer, J. A. and van den Brink, W. (2000). Serotonergic blunting to meta-chlorophenylpiperazine highly correlates with sustained childhood abuse in impulsive and autoaggressive female borderline patients. *Biological Psychiatry*, **47**, 548–556.

46. Sjoberg, R. L., Nilsson, K. W., Nordquist, N. *et al.* (2006). Development of depression: Sex and the interaction between environment and a promoter polymorphism of the serotonin transporter gene. *The International Journal of Neuropsychopharmacology*, **9**, 443–449.

47. Kim, J. M., Stewart, R., Kim, S. W. *et al.* (2007). Interactions between life stressors and susceptibility genes on depression in Korean elders. *Biological Psychiatry*, **62**, 423–428.

48. Liu, Z., Zhu, F., Wang, G. *et al.* (2006). Association of CRHR1 gene SNP and haplotype with major depression. *Neuroscience Letters*, **404**, 358–362.

49. Binder, E. B., Bradley, R. G., Liu, W. *et al.* (2008). Association of FKBP5 polymorphisms and childhood abuse with risk of PTSD symptoms in adults. *Journal of the American Medical Association*, **299**, 1291–1305.

# Chapter

# 16

# Long-lasting effects of childhood abuse on neurobiology

J. Douglas Bremner, Eric Vermetten and Ruth A. Lanius

## Introduction

As several of the previous chapters have demonstrated, extreme, repetitive or abnormal patterns of stress such as abuse and related adverse experiences during critical or circumscribed periods of childhood brain development can impair, perhaps permanently, the activity of major neuroregulatory systems, with profound and lasting neurobehavioral consequences. These changes, in turn, have profound effects on the physical and mental health and the quality of life of affected individuals throughout their lifespan (see also Chs. 6–8) [1]. Based on studies of the effects of stress on animals and on the emerging work in clinical neuroscience of concerning post-traumatic stress disorder (PTSD), a working model for a neural circuitry [2,3] and neurobiology [4] of traumatic stress that is applicable to PTSD has been described [5]. This chapter will present this working model and discuss relevant findings from the neuroimaging and stress hormone literature concerning patients who have experienced childhood abuse. The last section of the chapter will address the issue of causation in reference to epidemiological studies and neuropsychiatric investigations.

## A working model for a neural circuitry of traumatic stress

An effective model applicable to traumatic stress describes mechanisms that underlie afferent input to assess fear-producing events. It explains how the integration of these data into a coherent image, grounded in space and time, is achieved and activates memory traces of similar past experience with their appropriate emotional valence. This is necessary to assess the threat potential from prior experience. The model also has to take into account the efferent projections from the brain required to mediate an individual's

neuroendocrine, autonomical and motor responses such that an adequate stress response is mounted and appropriate and adaptive behaviors are instituted, for example, defense or flight. Critical brain structures involved in mediating fear behavior resulting from traumatic stress include the locus ceruleus (LC), hippocampus, amygdala, prefrontal cortex, thalamus and hypothalamus, and periaqueductal gray. These structures contribute to neural mechanisms of fear conditioning, extinction and behavioral sensitization in case of persistent symptoms of traumatic stress.

## Afferent input to assess fear-producing events

Afferent sensory input data relating to a threatening stimulus occur through sight, hearing, smell, touch, interoceptive visceral information or any combination of these. These sensory inputs are relayed through the dorsal thalamus to cortical brain areas, such as primary visual (occipital), auditory (temporal) or tactile (postcentral gyrus) cortical areas. Olfactory sensory input, however, has direct inputs to the amygdala and entorhinal cortex [6]. Input from visceral organs is relayed in the brainstem to the LC, site of the majority of the brain's noradrenergic neurons, and from here to central brain areas. These brain areas have projections to multiple areas including amygdala, hippocampus, entorhinal cortex, orbitofrontal cortex and cingulate, which are involved in mediating memory and emotion [7, 8].

## Cognitive appraisal

Cognitive appraisal of potential threat involves placing the threatening object accurately in space and time. This task involves specific brain functions: visuospatial processing, memory, cognition, action and planning. The anterior cingulate gyrus (Brodmann area [BA] 32) assists the selection of action responses as well as an

*The Impact of Early Life Trauma on Health and Disease: The Hidden Epidemic*, ed. Ruth A. Lanius, Eric Vermetten and Clare Pain. Published by Cambridge University Press. Copyright © Cambridge University Press 2010.

accurate emotional response [9]. This area and other medial portions of the prefrontal cortex, including Brodman's area 25 and orbitofrontal cortex, modulate emotional and physiological responses to stress. If the perceived threat is of another person, it is necessary to determine whether the person's face is familiar or not. Also, it is important to place the situation in time and place. Entering a dark alleyway may trigger prior memories of being assaulted, with attendant physiological arousal and associated negative emotions. Such memories have survival value, in that an individual will avoid or usefully anticipate with better preparation a situation where previous negative events took place; arousal will be stimulated and appropriate action undertaken. If, however, memory retrieval of previously threatening circumstances occurs repeatedly in non-threatening situations, either desensitization can occur or the individual becomes sensitized, which is usually maladaptive.

## Formation of memory traces

Usually the formation of memory traces related to a potential threat is highly adaptive because they assist the individual to prevent, defend against or avoid similar types of threat in the future. However, there are also situations where an individual exposed to chronic childhood abuse, for example by a primary caregiver, can develop dissociative amnesia, understood as a defensive mental escape from the otherwise inescapable (see also Chs. 3, 17, 20 and 21) [10–12]. In the case of the former, the hippocampus and adjacent cortex mediate declarative memory function (e.g., recall of facts and lists) and play an important role in the integration of memory elements at the time of retrieval and in assigning significance for events within space and time [13]. The hippocampus also regulates the neuroendocrine response to the stress through its role in glucocorticoid negative feedback.

The function of the amygdala in the processing of fear involves conditioning and the addition of an emotional valence to the situation. The amygdala also has direct connections that initiate motor responses to fear [14]. When fearful experiences are stored in long-term memory, they are shifted first through hippocampal synaptic plasticity by protein synthesis, and then from the hippocampus to the neocortical areas where the sensory impressions are stored with them [15,16]. In situations of extreme fear, the memory is sufficiently different to be understood as fulfilling a different "category" which entails the implicit (probably unconscious) learning and storage of information about the emotional significance of events. The amygdala and the structure with which it is connected underlie emotional memory; afferent inputs from the sensory-processing areas of the thalamus and cortex mediate emotional learning in situations involving specific sensory cues, whereas learning about the emotional significance of more general contextual cues involves projections to the amygdala from the hippocampal formation [17].

Associative processes can occur during the process of fear conditioning, and these may underlie the long-term associative plasticity that constitutes memory of the conditioning experience [18]. Fear conditioning to explicit and contextual cues has been proposed as a model for intrusive memories that in a kindling-like process are reactivated by trauma-related stimuli and hyperarousal, respectively [19]. Clinicians commonly report that "traumatic cues" such as a particular sight or sound reminiscent of the original traumatic event trigger a cascade of anxiety and fear-related symptoms in a patient, quite often without conscious recall of the original traumatic event [20].

## Modulation of responsiveness

Frontal cortical areas modulate emotional responsiveness through the inhibition of amygdala function. It has been hypothesized that dysfunction in these regions may underlie the pathological emotional responses in patients with PTSD and possibly other anxiety disorders. Medial prefrontal cortex (BA 25, subcallosal gyrus) has projections to the amygdala that are involved in the suppression of amygdala responsiveness to fearful cues. Dysfunction of this area may be responsible for the failure of extinction to fearful cues, which is an important part of the anxiety response [21,22]. With regard to extinction, the aversive association in the amygdala is inhibited rather than removed; fear can be rapidly reinstated even long after extinction either by the presentation of the conditioned stimulus in a different context or by a single stimulus–shock pairing [23]. The medial prefrontal cortex is involved in regulating the peripheral responses to stress, including heart rate, blood pressure and cortisol response [24]. Finally, case studies of humans with brain lesions (e.g., the famous case of Phineas Gage) have implicated the medial prefrontal cortex (including orbitofrontal cortex, BA 25, and anterior cingulate, BA 32) in emotional and socially appropriate interactions [25]. Auditory association areas (temporal lobe) have also been implicated in animal studies as mediating extinction to fear responses [26].

Functional neuroimaging studies from various groups have examined the emotional modulation of responsiveness to trauma-related stimuli in patients with PTSD related to childhood abuse. For example, functional neuroimaging studies have measured blood flow following exposure to traumatic cues in the form of traumatic scripts in women with childhood sexual abuse-related PTSD. These studies found decreased blood flow in the medial prefrontal cortex/anterior cingulate, including BA 25 and BA 32, as well as decreased blood flow in the parietal cortex and inferior frontal gyrus [27–29]. One of the studies additionally found decreased function in hippocampus and visual association cortex [27], while the other found increased function for the superior temporal gyrus [29]. There were mixed findings for posterior cingulate and parahippocampal gyrus [27,29]. A separate study of men and women with childhood physical and/or sexual abuse found increased amygdala function measured with functional imaging during recall of traumatic words [30].

Bremner and colleagues [31] have also used a variety of other probes to assess neural circuits in women with childhood sexual abuse-related PTSD. Retrieval of emotionally valenced words (e.g., "rape-mutilate") in women with PTSD from early abuse resulted in decreased blood flow in an extensive area, which included orbitofrontal cortex, anterior cingulate and medial prefrontal cortex (BA 25, 32, 9), left hippocampus and fusiform gyrus/inferior temporal gyrus. Increased activation was found in the posterior cingulate, left inferior parietal cortex, left middle frontal gyrus and visual association and motor cortex [32]. Another study found a failure of medial prefrontal cortical/anterior cingulate activation and decreased visual association and parietal cortex function in women with abuse and PTSD, relative to women with abuse without PTSD, during performance of the emotional Stroop task (i.e., naming the color of a word such as "rape") [33]. Women with childhood sexual abuse-related PTSD had increased amygdala activation with classical fear conditioning (pairing a shock and a visual stimulus) and decreased medial prefrontal cortex function with extinction compared with healthy non-abused women [34].

A recent study has also reported a direct inhibitory influence of the medial prefrontal cortex on the amygdala [35]. Specifically, a negative correlation between blood flow in the left ventromedial prefrontal cortex and the amygdala during emotional tasks, and negative correlations between medial prefrontal cortex and the amygdala during exposure to fearful faces, has been observed [36]. Thus, the low activation of medial prefrontal regions is consistent with failed inhibition of limbic reactivity and may be associated with reexperiencing and hyperarousal symptoms often observed in PTSD patients (please see Ch. 17 for further discussion). These findings point to a network of related regions mediating symptoms of PTSD, including medial prefrontal cortex/anterior cingulate and amygdala as described in the model above [37].

# Preparation for a stress response: central and peripheral responses

A final component of the stress response concerns preparation for a response to potential threat. This requires the integration of brain areas involved in assessing and interpreting the potentially threatening stimulus with brain areas involved in mounting a response. For instance, the prefrontal cortex and anterior cingulate play an important role in the planning of action and in holding multiple pieces of information in "working memory" during the execution of a response [38]. The parietal cortex and posterior cingulate are involved in visuospatial processing, which is a critical component of the stress response. The motor cortex may represent the neural substrate of planning for action. The cerebellum has a well-known role in motor movement, which would suggest that this region is involved in planning for action. However, recent imaging studies are consistent with a role in cognition as well [39].

Connections between the parietal and prefrontal cortices are required in order to permit the organism to rapidly and effectively execute motor responses to threats. It is, therefore, not surprising that these brain areas have important innervations to the precentral (motor) cortex, which is responsible for skeletal motor responses to threat, thus facilitating survival. The striatum (caudate and putamen) modulates motor responses to stress. The dense innervation of the striatum and prefrontal cortex by the amygdala indicates that the amygdala can regulate both these systems. These interactions between the amygdala and the extrapyramidal motor system may be necessary for generating motor responses to threatening stimuli, especially those related to prior adverse experiences [40,41].

The need for the organism to rapidly effect peripheral responses to threat is mediated by the stress hormone cortisol and by the sympathetic and para-sympathetic systems. Stimulation of the lateral hypo-thalamus results in sympathetic system activation, corticotrophin-releasing factor (CRF) producing increases in blood pressure and heart rate, sweating, piloerection, and pupil dilatation. Stress stimulates release of CRF from the hypothalamic paraventricular nucleus, which, in turn, increases peripheral adreno-corticotropic hormone (ACTH) and cortisol levels. The middle prefrontal cortex, as mentioned above, also mediates increased blood pressure and pulse as well as elevations in cortisol in response to stress. Striatum, amygdala and bed nucleus of the stria terminalis also affect peripheral responses to threat through the lateral nucleus of the hypothamalus [42,43].

The vagus and splanchnic nerves are major projec-tions of the parasympathetic nervous system. Afferents to the vagus include the lateral hypothalamus, par-aventricular nucleus, LC and the amygdala. Efferent connections to the splanchnic nerves from the LC have been described [44].

As described in the model above, the pathophysi-ology of PTSD can be linked to several neurobiologi-cal mechanisms related to stress. Preclinical studies that investigated the effects of stress on neural proc-esses such as learning and memory retention were initially used to model PTSD as humans experience it. These studies suggested that an altered fear response mechanism, behavioral sensitization and failure of the extinction of fear play an important role in the patho-physiology of PTSD [3]. Furthermore, it has been shown that patients with PTSD show significant defi-cits in memory [45–48] with social and occupational consequences [49]. Below, we will describe how spe-cific neurobiological mechanisms related to stress are altered in patients who suffer from childhood trauma-related stress disorders.

## Memory dysfunction in childhood abuse-related post-traumatic stress disorder

There is considerable interest in alterations in mem-ory function of patients with childhood abuse-related PTSD [50]. The brain areas involved include the hip-pocampus, medial prefrontal cortex and amygdala, noted above as central to the neural circuitry of trau-matic stress [51].

### Hippocampus

The hippocampus, a brain area involved in verbal declarative memory, is very sensitive to the effects of stress. Stress in animals has been associated with dam-age to neurons in the CA3 region of the hippocam-pus (which may be mediated by hypercortisolemia, decreased brain-derived neurotrophic factor [BDNF] and/or elevated glutamate levels) and inhibition of neurogenesis [52–57]. High levels of glucocorticoids seen with stress were also associated with deficits in new learning [58,59].

The animal studies referenced above provided a rationale to measure hippocampal volume in patients with PTSD and depression. A number of studies have shown decreased hippocampal volume in adults with PTSD related to a range of traumas [60]. In an early study comparing 17 male and female patients with PTSD related to early childhood physical and/or sex-ual abuse with 17 matched controls, there was a 12% reduction in left hippocampal volume ($p < 0.05$) [61]. Another study showed smaller hippocampal volume in women with early sexual abuse, most of whom met criteria for PTSD [62]. We recently found a reduc-tion in bilateral hippocampal volume in women with early childhood sexual abuse and PTSD, compared with abused women without PTSD and non-abused non-PTSD women [63]. We also found that smaller left hippocampal volume was observed in women with depression and a history of childhood abuse, but not in depressed women without childhood abuse [64].

In a 2005 meta-analysis study [65], data were pooled from all the published studies on hippocampal volume. There were smaller hippocampal volumes for both the left and the right sides, equally in adult men and women with chronic PTSD, and no change in children. Another meta-analysis published the same year had similar find-ings [66]. One study showed that women with abuse-related PTSD had deficits in hippocampal activation while performing a verbal declarative memory task [63]. Both hippocampal atrophy and hippocampal-based memory deficits were reversed with treatment with the selective serotonin reuptake inhibitor paroxet-ine, which has been shown to promote neurogenesis in the hippocampus in preclinical studies [67]. It has been hypothesized that stress-induced hippocampal dys-function may mediate many of the symptoms of PTSD that are related to memory dysregulation, including both explicit memory deficits and fragmentation of memory, in abuse survivors [68].

Neuropsychological tests of long-term memory function such as the verbal Selective Reminding Test (vSRT) and percentage retention during paragraph recall on the Wechsler Memory Scale (WMS) can also be used as probes of hippocampal function. Studies in children with PTSD from a variety of traumas have shown deficits in verbal memory and verbal intelligent quotient [69–71]. Bremner *et al.* [45] found deficits in verbal declarative memory as measured by the WMS and vSRT in male and female adults with childhood physical and/or sexual abuse-related PTSD in comparison with controls. Deficits in verbal memory were significantly correlated with severity of childhood sexual abuse in those with a childhood abusehistory. One study in women with sexual abuse-related PTSD showed deficits in verbal declarative memory compared with that in women with abuse without PTSD or non-abused non-PTSD women [72]. In another study of women with early childhood sexual abuse in which some but not all of the patients had PTSD, no difference was found between abused and non-abused women [73]. Taken together, these results suggest that early abuse with associated PTSD results in deficits in verbal declarative memory.

The hippocampus demonstrates an unusual capacity for plasticity, or ability of neurons to change and regenerate in response to environmental inputs. Changes in the environment (e.g., social enrichment), can modulate generation of neurons in the dentate gyrus of the hippocampus, thus slowing the normal age-related decline in neurogenesis [74]. This has led to an examination of how certain treatment interventions may lead to neuroplasticity and alleviation of memory deficits and other symptoms in patients with PTSD.

For example, BDNF is a neuropeptide that has important nutritional effects on the hippocampus and other brain regions. Stress has been shown to result in a reduction in mRNA for BDNF in the hippocampus, suggesting that stress reduces the brain's ability to grow and thrive. There is also a direct effect of CRF on the hippocampus in early development [75]. Antidepressant drugs and electroconvulsive therapy increased BDNF levels in two regions (CA3 and CA1) of the hippocampus, probably reversing the effects seen from stress [55]. Serotonin reuptake inhibitors also increase dendritic branching and neurogenesis within the hippocampus [76]. Phenytoin, a medication used to treat epilepsy, inhibits excitatory amino acid transmission and blocks the effects of stress on the hippocampus [77]. These findings have implications for treatment of PTSD and depression and have stimulated clinical trials of these agents to look at their effects on memory and hippocampal volume in patients with PTSD and depression. There may be potential to treat

or perhaps even reverse some of the detrimental memory effects of child abuse.

### Medial prefrontal cortex and amygdala

As noted above in the traumatic stress neural circuitry model, brain structures such as the amygdala and prefrontal cortex in addition to the hippocampus have been implicated in the neural circuitry of stress. The medial prefrontal cortex has been shown to be a major target area of the neurotransmitters dopamine and norepinephrine. The prefrontal cortex has been suggested to play a role in "working memory" in conjunction with other brain areas such as the hippocampus. A critical range of dopamine and norepinephrine turnover is necessary for keeping this "working memory system" active and ready for optimal cognitive functioning [78], a situation that is impaired in situations of extreme or chronic stress [79]. The mesofrontal dopaminergic system also plays a role in emotional responses as well as in selective information processing and coping with the external world [9,80]. The medial prefrontal cortex has inhibitory inputs to the amygdala that have been hypothesized to play a role in the extinction of fear responses [81,82]. Findings from functional imaging studies on patients with a history of childhood abuse implicate dysfunction of medial prefrontal cortex, as reviewed above.

# New directions in neuroimaging research: the medial prefrontal cortex and the default mode network of the brain

Most functional neuroimaging studies to date have focused on specific cognitive tasks to examine brain functioning in various psychiatric disorders. However, the idea that the brain has an intrinsic mode of functioning has received increasing attention over the past few years [83]. Some researchers have hypothesized that the brain maintains this "default mode network" [84–86], possibly in order to facilitate a state of readiness to respond to environmental changes [87]. Other authors link default mode network activity to self-referential processing, as key regions such as the medial prefrontal cortex and the posterior cingulate cortex have been shown to subserve introspective mental imagery, self-reflection and self-awareness [88–90], processes that are often impaired in patients with childhood trauma-related PTSD [91,92].

For example, patients with childhood abuse have shown to have decreased emotional awareness as measured by the Levels of Emotional Awareness Scale as well as the Toronto Alexithymia Scale. Furthermore, alexithymia scores during trauma script-driven imagery were positively correlated with response in the insula, posterior cingulate cortex and thalamus, and negatively correlated with response in the anterior cingulate cortex. These brain regions as a group have been associated with conscious awareness and focused attention of affective- and arousal-related bodily experiences [91]. Bluhm *et al.* [93] therefore, investigated the integrity of the default network in childhood abuse-related PTSD and reported that spontaneous low-frequency activity in the posterior cingulate/precuneus at rest was more strongly correlated with activity in other areas of the default network in healthy control subjects than in subjects with PTSD. Direct comparison of the two groups showed that posterior cingulate/precuneus connectivity was also greater in healthy comparison subjects than in patients with PTSD in a number of brain areas previously associated with PTSD, including the right amygdala and the hippocampus/ parahippocampal gyrus. In this patient population, the observed alterations may be associated with the disturbances in self-referential processing often observed in PTSD related to childhood abuse.

## Childhood abuse-related post-traumatic stress disorder and the hypothalamic–pituitary–adrenal axis

In addition to its role in extinction of fear responses, the medial prefrontal cortex also plays a critical role in regulation of peripheral neurohormonal responses to stress [94]. In addition to the amygdala and the hypothalamus, portions of the medial prefrontal cortex (infralimbic, ventral prelimbic) project to the nucleus solitarius and nucleus ambiguous in the brainstem, where they regulate heart rate and blood pressure responses to stress. Lesions to the dorsal part of this region (anterior cingulate) result in increased heart responses to conditioned stimuli, suggesting that this region decreases heart rate response to stress, while lesions in the ventral portion decrease heart response, suggesting that this region increases heart rate response to stress [95]. Lesions of the medial prefrontal cortex are associated with a blunted cortisol and ACTH response to stress, with no effect on resting cortisol [96].

The long-term effects of early childhood sexual abuse on the hypothalamic–pituitary–adrenal (HPA) axis have been assessed in a series of studies of adult women with childhood sexual abuse-related PTSD, abused women without PTSD, and healthy women without a history of abuse [68,97]. Women were assessed using the Early Trauma Inventory (ETI), a reliable and validated measure of early abuse [98,99]. Women with abuse-related PTSD had decreased baseline cortisol based on 24 hour diurnal assessments of plasma, increased pulsatility of cortisol [100], and exaggerated cortisol response to stressors (traumatic stressors [101] more than neutral cognitive stressors [36]). Lower cortisol was correlated with increased symptoms of PTSD [100].

Other studies have also shown long-term alterations in HPA function in abused women with PTSD and depression. Adult women with a history of childhood abuse showed increased suppression of cortisol with low dose (0.5 mg) dexamethasone [102], while women with childhood abuse-related PTSD had hypercortisolemia [103]. Adult women with depression and a history of early childhood abuse had an increased cortisol response to a stressful cognitive challenge relative to controls [104] and a blunted ACTH response to CRF challenge [105]. These findings suggest that early abuse is associated with long-term changes to the HPA axis and call for studies examining specific interventions that specifically target the HPA axis in the treatment of childhood abuse-related PTSD.

## The issue of causation in studies examining the neurobiology of traumatic stress and epidemiological research

There is a striking convergence of recent findings from studies of the neurobiology of traumatic stress and those from large epidemiological studies of the long-term effects of early life trauma. Therefore, the question arises of causation or contribution of these traumatic stresses to later life problems. Anda *et al.* [1] have suggested criteria for establishing an argument for causation in the context of the converging evidence between neuroscience and epidemiology.

*Demonstration of a consistent strong association between the causative agent and the outcome*  The strength of the relationship between adverse childhood experiences and numerous outcomes is consistently strong, as reported in this chapter.

*Consistency of findings across research sites and methods*   Numerous studies using different study populations and measures of abuse, neglect and related experiences have shown relationships of adverse childhood experiences to a wide variety of symptoms and behaviors.

*Specificity*   In the context of the converging evidence from epidemiology and neurobiology, specificity is lacking, but this does not detract from the argument of causation.

*Temporal sequence*   Most of the outcomes presented here occurred during adulthood; the exposures (childhood experiences) clearly antedate the outcomes in these cases.

*Biological gradient*   The dose–response relationship between the number of adverse childhood experiences and each of the outcomes (as well as the number of comorbid outcomes) is strong and graded. This is consistent with cumulative effects of childhood stress on the developing brain.

*Biological plausibility*   The strength of the convergence between epidemiology and neurobiology is most evident here. Recent studies from the neurosciences show that childhood stress can affect numerous brain structures and functions, providing convincing biological plausibility for the epidemiological findings.

*Coherence*   "The term coherence implies that a cause and effect interpretation for an association does not conflict with what is known about the natural history and biology of the disease" [106]. In fact, recent research shows that childhood maltreatment interacts with a common functional polymorphism in the promoter region of the gene for the serotonin transporter, resulting in higher risk of depression and suicidality [107], both of which are associated with the ACE score in the Adverse Childhood Experiences Study (Chs. 8 and 15). This information is consistent with an effect of early maltreatment on monoamine pathways known to be involved in depressive disorders.

*Experimental evidence*   This is the most persuasive evidence, but for ethical reasons randomized experiments depend on animal studies. Evidence from studies in rodents and primates show that stressful exposures induce neuroanatomical and neurophysiological differences as well as aggression and drug-seeking behaviors.

*Analogous evidence*   A widely acknowledged analogy for an exposure causing a multitude of outcomes (as seen with adversive childhood experiences, including a dose–response relationship) is the causal relationship of cigarette smoking with cardiovascular diseases, neoplasms, lung disease and other health problems.

## Conclusions

Studies show that early childhood abuse has causative long-term effects on brain areas involved in memory and emotion, including the hippocampus, amygdala and medial prefrontal cortex. Brain circuits mediating the stress response including norepinephrine neurons, and the HPA axis also play a role. Childhood abuse-related PTSD is characterized by specific symptoms, including intrusive thoughts, hyperarousal, flash-backs, nightmares and sleep disturbances, changes in memory and concentration, and startle responses. Symptoms of PTSD are hypothesized to represent the behavioral manifestation of stress-induced changes in brain structure and function. Stress leads to acute and chronic changes to neurochemical systems and specific brain regions, resulting in long-term changes to brain "circuits" involved in the stress response [108–111]. Changes in these circuits and systems have been hypothesized to underlie some of the symptoms of PTSD.

There are important public health implications of biological changes associated with childhood abuse. If childhood stress and maltreatment leads to an inhibition of neuronal growth and/or damage to brain areas such as the hippocampus that are critical for new learning and memory, this could have detrimental effects on the ability of children to succeed academically. Also, if stress results in dysfunction of brain areas such as the medial portion of the prefrontal cortex, which are involved in the regulation of social behavior, early stress could lead to a biological vulnerability to future acts of dysfunctional behavior, thus contributing to a vicious cycle of repeated violence and abuse. As Anda *et al.* [1] argued: "… the original traumatic pathophysiological insults may be 'silent' until much later in life, when they are likely to be overlooked by investigators and clinicians who are understandably prone to focus on proximate determinants of human well-being. This leads to treatment of symptoms without a full understanding of their potential origins in the disruptive effects of adverse childhood experiences on childhood neurodevelopment."

## Acknowledgements

The work presented in this chapter was supported by grants from the NIMH (MH56120), the Emory Conte Center for Early Life Stress, and the Department of Veterans Affairs.

## References

1. Anda, R. F., Felitti, V. J., Bremner, J. D. *et al.* (2006). The enduring effects of abuse and related adverse experiences in childhood. A convergence of evidence from neurobiology and epidemiology. *European Archives of Psychiatry and Clinical Neuroscience,* **256**, 174–186.

2. Bremner, J. D., Krystal, J. H., Southwick, S. M. and Charney, D. S. (1995). Functional neuroanatomical correlates of the effects of stress on memory. *Journal of Trauma and Stress,* **8**, 527–553.

3. Charney, D. S., Deutch, A. Y., Krystal, J. H., Southwick, S. M. and Davis, M. (1993). Psychobiologic mechanisms of posttraumatic stress disorder. *Archives of General Psychiatry,* **50**, 295–305.

4. Heim, C. and Nemeroff, C. B. (2009). Neurobiology of posttraumatic stress disorder. *CNS Spectrums,* **14** (Suppl. 1), 13–24.

5. Vermetten, E. and Lanius, R. (2009). Brain circuits in PTSD. In D. Nutt, J. Zohar and M. Stein (eds.), *Post traumatic stress disorder: diagnosis, management and treatment,* 2nd edn (pp. 70–88). London: Informa Healthcare.

6. Turner, B. H., Gupta, K. C. and Mishkin, M. (1978). The locus and cytoarchitecture of the projection areas of the olfactory bulb in Macaca mulatta. *Journal of Comparative Neurology,* **177**, 381–396.

7. van Hoesen, G. W., Pandya, D. N. and Butters, N. (1972). Cortical afferents to the entorhinal cortex of the Rhesus monkey. *Science,* **175**, 1471–1473.

8. Vogt, B. A. and Miller, M. W. (1983). Cortical connections between rat cingulate cortex and visual, motor, and postsubicular cortices. *Journal of Comparative Neurology,* **216**, 192–210.

9. Devinsky, O., Morrell, M. J. and Vogt, B. A. (1995). Contributions of anterior cingulate cortex to behaviour. *Brain,* **118**, 279–306.

10. Bremner, J. D., Krystal, J. H., Charney, D. S. and Southwick, S. M. (1996). Neural mechanisms in dissociative amnesia for childhood abuse: Relevance to the current controversy surrounding the "false memory syndrome." *American Journal of Psychiatry,* **153**(Suppl. 7), 71–82.

11. Chu, J. A., Frey, L. M., Ganzel, B. L. and Matthews, J. A. (1999). Memories of childhood abuse: Dissociation, amnesia, and corroboration. *American Journal of Psychiatry,* **156**, 749–755.

12. van der Hart, O., Bolt, H. and van der Kolk, B. A. (2005). Memory fragmentation in dissociative identity disorder. *Journal of Trauma and Dissociation,* **6**, 55–70.

13. Squire, L. R. and Zola-Morgan, S. (1991). The medial temporal lobe memory system. *Science,* **253**, 1380–1386.

14. Sarter, M. and Markowitsch, H. J. (1985). Involvement of the amygdala in learning and memory: A critical review, with emphasis on anatomical relations. *Behavioral Neuroscience,* **99**, 342–380.

15. Neves, G., Cooke, S. F. and Bliss, T. V. (2008). Synaptic plasticity, memory and the hippocampus: A neural network approach to causality. *Nature Reviews of Neuroscience,* **9**, 65–75.

16. Bekinschtein, P., Cammarota, M., Igaz, L. M. *et al.* (2007). Persistence of long-term memory storage requires a late protein synthesis- and BDNF-dependent phase in the hippocampus. *Neuron,* **53**, 261–277.

17. LeDoux, J. E. (1993). Emotional memory: In search of systems and synapses. *Annals of the New York Academy of Sciences,* **702**, 149–157.

18. Rogan, M. T., Staubli, U. V. and LeDoux, J. E. (1997). Fear conditioning induces associative long-term potentiation in the amygdala. *Nature,* **390**, 604–607.

19. Grillon, C., Southwick, S. M. and Charney, D. S. (1996). The psychobiological basis of posttraumatic stress disorder. *Molecular Psychiatry,* **1**, 278–297.

20. Vermetten, E. and Bremner, J. D. (2003). Olfaction as a traumatic reminder in posttraumatic stress disorder: Case reports and review. *Journal of Clinical Psychiatry,* **64**, 202–207.

21. Morgan, M. A., Romanski, L. M. and LeDoux, J. E. (1993). Extinction of emotional learning: Contribution of medial prefrontal cortex. *Neuroscience Letters,* **163**, 109–113.

22. Anderson, K. C. and Insel, T. R. (2006). The promise of extinction research for the prevention and treatment of anxiety disorders. *Biological Psychiatry,* **60**, 319–321.

23. Myers, K. M. and Davis, M. (2007). Mechanisms of fear extinction. *Molecular Psychiatry,* **12**, 120–150.

24. Roth, R. H., Tam, S. Y., Ida, Y., Yang, J. X. and Deutch, A. Y. (1988). Stress and the mesocorticolimbic dopamine systems. *Annals of the New York Academy of Sciences,* **537**, 138–147.

25. Damasio, H., Grabowski, T., Frank, R., Galaburda, A. M. and Damasio, A. R. (1994). The return of Phineas Gage: Clues about the brain from the skull of a famous patient. *Science,* **264**, 1102–1105.

26. Quirk, G. J., Armony, J. L. and LeDoux, J. E. (1997). Fear conditioning enhances different temporal components of tone-evoked spike trains in auditory cortex and lateral amygdala. *Neuron,* **19**, 613–624.

27. Bremner, J. D., Narayan, M., Staib, L. H. *et al.* (1999). Neural correlates of memories of childhood sexual

abuse in women with and without posttraumatic stress disorder. *American Journal of Psychiatry, 156,* 1787–1795.

28. Lanius, R. A., Williamson, P. C., Densmore, M. *et al.* (2001). Neural correlates of traumatic memories in posttraumatic stress disorder: A functional MRI investigation. *American Journal of Psychiatry, 158,* 1920–1922.

29. Shin, L. M., McNally, R. J., Kosslyn, S. M. *et al.* (1999). Regional cerebral blood flow during script-driven imagery in childhood sexual abuse-related PTSD: A PET investigation. *American Journal of Psychiatry, 156,* 575–584.

30. Protopopescu, X., Pan, H., Tuescher, O. *et al.* (2005). Differential time courses and specificity of amygdala activity in posttraumatic stress disorder subjects and normal control subjects. *Biological Psychiatry, 57,* 464–473.

31. Bremner, J. D., Soufer, R., McCarthy, G. *et al.* (2001). Gender differences in cognitive and neural correlates of remembrance of emotional words. *Psychopharmacology Bulletin, 35,* 55–87.

32. Bremner, J. D., Vythilingam, M., Vermetten, E. *et al.* (2004). Neural correlates of declarative memory for emotionally valenced words in women with posttraumatic stress disorder (PTSD) related to early childhood sexual abuse. *Biological Psychiatry, 53,* 289–299.

33. Bremner, J. D., Vermetten, E., Vythilingam, M. *et al.* (2004). Neural correlates of the classical color and emotional Stroop in women with abuse-related posttraumatic stress disorder. *Biological Psychiatry, 55,* 612–620.

34. Bremner, J. D., Vermetten, E., Schmahl, C. *et al.* (2005). Positron emission tomographic imaging of neural correlates of a fear acquisition and extinction paradigm in women with childhood sexual abuse-related posttraumatic stress disorder. *Psychological Medicine, 35,* 791–806.

35. Shin, L. M., Wright, C. I., Cannistraro, P. A. *et al.* (2005). A functional magnetic resonance imaging study of amygdala and medial prefrontal cortex responses to overtly presented fearful faces in posttraumatic stress disorder. *Archives of General Psychiatry, 62,* 273–281.

36. Bremner, J. D., Vythilingam, M., Vermetten, E. *et al.* (2003). Cortisol response to a cognitive stress challenge in posttraumatic stress disorder (PTSD) related to childhood abuse. *Psychoneuroendocrinology, 28,* 733–750.

37. Bremner, J. D. (2002). Neuroimaging studies in post-traumatic stress disorder. *Current Psychiatric Reports, 4,* 254–263.

38. Goldman-Rakic, P. S. (1988). Topography of cognition: Parallel distributed networks in primate association cortex. *Annual Review of Neuroscience, 11,* 137–156.

39. Katz, D. B. and Steinmetz, J. E. (2002). Psychological functions of the cerebellum. *Behavioral and Cognitive Neuroscience Reviews, 1,* 229–241.

40. Berretta, S. (2005). Cortico-amygdala circuits: Role in the conditioned stress response. *Stress, 8,* 221–232.

41. Charney, D. S. and Deutch, A. (1996). A functional neuroanatomy of anxiety and fear: Implications for the pathophysiology and treatment of anxiety disorders. *Critical Reviews in Neurobiology, 10,* 419–446.

42. Walker, D. L., Toufexis, D. J. and Davis, M. (2003). Role of the bed nucleus of the stria terminalis versus the amygdala in fear, stress, and anxiety. *European Journal of Pharmacology, 463,* 199–216.

43. Grillon, C. (2008). Models and mechanisms of anxiety: Evidence from startle studies. *Psychopharmacology, 199,* 421–437.

44. Clark, F. M. and Proudfit, H. K. (1991). The projection of locus coeruleus neurons to the spinal cord in the rat determined by anterograde tracing combined with immunocytochemistry. *Brain Research, 538,* 231–245.

45. Bremner, J. D., Randall, P., Scott, T. M. *et al.* (1995). Deficits in short-term memory in adult survivors of childhood abuse. *Psychiatry Research, 59,* 97–107.

46. Bremner, J. D., Scott, T. M., Delaney, R. C. *et al.* (1993). Deficits in short-term memory in posttraumatic stress disorder. *American Journal of Psychiatry, 150,* 1015–1019.

47. Golier, J. A., Yehuda, R., Lupien, S. J. *et al.* (2002). Memory performance in Holocaust survivors with posttraumatic stress disorder. *American Journal of Psychiatry, 159,* 1682–1688.

48. Vasterling, J. J., Duke, L. M., Brailey, K. *et al.* (2002). Attention, learning, and memory performances and intellectual resources in Vietnam veterans: PTSD and no disorder comparisons. *Neuropsychology, 16,* 5–14.

49. Geuze, E., Vermetten, E., de Kloet, C. S. *et al.* (2009). Neuropsychological performance is related to current social and occupational functioning in veterans with posttraumatic stress disorder. *Depression and Anxiety, 26,* 7–15.

50. Elzinga, B. M. and Bremner, J. D. (2002). Are the neural substrates of memory the final common pathway in PTSD? *Journal of Affective Disorders, 70,* 1–17.

51. Bremner, J. D. (2003). Functional neuroanatomical correlates of traumatic stress revisited 7 years later, this time with data. *Psychopharmacology Bulletin, 37*(2), 6–25.

52. Gould, E., Tanapat, P., McEwen, B. S., Flugge, G. and Fuchs, E. (1998). Proliferation of granule cell precursors in the dentate gyrus of adult monkeys is diminished by stress. *Proceedings of the National Academy of Sciences of the United States of America, 95,* 3168–3171.

53. Magarinos, A. M., McEwen, B. S., Flugge, G. and Fluchs, E. (1996). Chronic psychosocial stress causes apical dendritic atrophy of hippocampal CA3 pyramidal neurons in subordinate tree shrews. *Journal of Neuroscience,* **16,** 3534–3540.

54. McEwen, B. S., Angulo, J., Cameron, H. *et al.* (1992). Paradoxical effects of adrenal steroids on the brain: Protection versus degeneration. *Biological Psychiatry,* **31,** 177–199.

55. Nibuya, M., Morinobu, S. and Duman, R. S. (1995). Regulation of BDNF and trkB mRNA in rat brain by chronic electroconvulsive seizure and antidepressant drug treatments. *Journal of Neuroscience,* **15,** 7539–7547.

56. Sapolsky, R. M., Uno, H., Rebert, C. S. and Finch, C. E. (1999). Hippocampal damage associated with prolonged glucocorticoid exposure in primates. *Journal of Neuroscience,* **10,** 2897–2902.

57. Sapolsky, R. M. (1996). Why stress is bad for your brain. *Science,* **273,** 749–750.

58. Luine, V., Villages, M., Martinex, C. and McEwen, B. S. (1994). Repeated stress causes reversible impairments of spatial memory performance. *Brain Research,* **639,** 167–170.

59. Diamond, D. M., Fleshner, M., Ingersoll, N. and Rose, G. M. (1996). Psychological stress impairs spatial working memory: Relevance to electrophysiological studies of hippocampal function. *Behavioral Neuroscience,* **110,** 661–672.

60. Bremner, J. D. (2006). Stress and brain atrophy. *CNS Neurological Disorders Drug Targets,* **5,** 503–512.

61. Bremner, J. D., Randall, P. R., Vermetten, E. *et al.* (1997). MRI-based measurement of hippocampal volume in posttraumatic stress disorder related to childhood physical and sexual abuse: A preliminary report. *Biological Psychiatry,* **41,** 23–32.

62. Stein, M. B., Koverola, C., Hanna, C., Torchia, M. G. and McClarty, B. (1997). Hippocampal volume in women victimized by childhood sexual abuse. *Psychological Medicine,* **27,** 951–959.

63. Bremner, J. D., Vythilingam, M., Vermetten, E. *et al.* (2003). MRI and PET study of deficits in hippocampal structure and function in women with childhood sexual abuse and posttraumatic stress disorder (PTSD). *American Journal of Psychiatry,* **160,** 924–932.

64. Vythilingam, M., Heim, C., Newport, C. D. *et al.* (2002). Childhood trauma associated with smaller hippocampal volume in women with major depression. *American Journal of Psychiatry,* **159,** 2072–2080.

65. Kitayama, N., Vaccarino, V., Kutner, M., Weiss, P. and Bremner, J. D. (2005). Magnetic resonance imaging (MRI) measurement of hippocampal volume in posttraumatic stress disorder: A meta-analysis. *Journal of Affective Disorders,* **88,** 79–86.

66. Smith, M. E. (2005). Bilateral hippocampal volume reduction in adults with post-traumatic stress disorder: A meta-analysis of structural MRI studies. *Hippocampus,* **15**(6), 798–807.

67. Vermetten, E., Vythilingam, M., Southwick, S. M., Charney, D. S. and Bremner, J. D. (2003). Long-term treatment with paroxetine increases verbal declarative memory and hippocampal volume in posttraumatic stress disorder. *Biological Psychiatry,* **54,** 693–702.

68. Bremner, J. D. (2005). The neurobiology of childhood sexual abuse in women with posttraumatic stress disorder. In K. A. Kendall-Tackett (ed.), *Handbook of women, stress and trauma* (pp. 181–206). New York: Brunner-Routledge.

69. Moradi, A. R., Doost, H. T., Taghavi, M. R., Yule, W. and Dalgleish, T. (1999). Everyday memory deficits in children and adolescents with PTSD: Performance on the Rivermead Behavioural Memory Test. *Journal Child Psychology and Psychiatry,* **40,** 357–361.

70. Saigh, P. A., Yasik, A. E., Oberfield, R. A., Halamandaris, P. V. and Bremner, J. D. (2006). The intellectual performance of traumatized children and adolescents with or without posttraumatic stress disorder. *Journal of Abnormal Psychology,* **115,** 332–340.

71. Saltzman, K. M., Weems, C. F. and Carrion, V. G. (2006). IQ and posttraumatic stress symptoms in children exposed to interpersonal violence. *Child Psychiatry and Human Development,* **36,** 261–272.

72. Bremner, J. D., Vermetten, E., Nafzal N. and Vythilingam, M. (2004). Deficits in verbal declarative memory function in women with childhood sexual abuse-related posttraumatic stress disorder (PTSD). *Journal of Nervous and Mental Disorders,* **192,** 643–649.

73. Stein, M. B., Hanna, C., Vaerum, V. and Koverola, C. (1999). Memory functioning in adult women traumatized by childhood sexual abuse. *Journal of Trauma and Stress,* **12,** 527–534.

74. Kempermann, G., Kuhn, H. G. and Gage, F. H. (1998). Experience-induced neurogenesis in the senescent dentate gyrus. *Journal of Neuroscience,* **18,** 3206–3212.

75. Brunson, K. L., Eghbal-Ahmadi, M., Bender, R., Chen, Y. and Baram, T. Z. (2001). Long-term, progressive hippocampal cell loss and dysfunction induced by early-life administration of corticotropin-releasing hormone reproduce the effects of early-life stress. *Proceedings of the National Academy of Sciences of the United States of America,* **98,** 8856–8861.

76. Malberg, J. E., Eisch, A. J., Nestler, E. J. and Duman, R. S. (2000). Chronic antidepressant treatment increases neurogenesis in adult rat hippocampus. *Journal of Neuroscience,* **20,** 9104–9110.

77. Watanabe, Y. E., Gould, H., Cameron, D., Daniels, D. and McEwen, B. S. (1992). Phenytoin prevents stress

and corticosterone induced atrophy of CA3 pyramidal neurons. *Hippocampus,* **2**, 431–436.

78. Horger, B. A. and Roth, R. H. (1996). The role of mesoprefrontal dopamine neurons in stress. *Critical Reviews in Neurobiology,* **10**, 395–418.

79. Arnsten, A. F. (2000). Stress impairs prefrontal cortical function in rats and monkeys: Role of dopamine D1 and norepinephrine alpha-1 receptor mechanisms. *Progress in Brain Research,* **126**, 183–192.

80. Pani, L., Porcella, A. and Gessa, G. L. (2000). The role of stress in the pathophysiology of the dopaminergic system. *Molecular Psychiatry,* **5**, 14–21.

81. Morgan, C. A. and LeDoux, J. E. (1995). Differential contribution of dorsal and ventral medial prefrontal cortex to the acquisition and extinction of conditioned fear in rats. *Behavioral Neuroscience,* **109**, 681–688.

82. Milad, M. R. and Quirk, G. J. (2002). Neurons in medial prefrontal cortex signal memory for fear extinction. *Nature,* **420**, 70–73.

83. Buckner, R. L., Andrews-Hanna, J. R. and Schacter, D. L. (2008). The brain's default network: Anatomy, function, and relevance to disease. *Annals of the New York Academy of Sciences,* **1124**, 1–38.

84. Raichle, M. E., MacLeod, A. M., Snyder, A. Z. *et al.* (2001). A default mode of brain function. *Proceedings of the National Academy of Sciences of the United States of America,* **98**(2), 676–682.

85. Gusnard, D. A. and Raichle, M. E. (2001). Searching for a baseline: Functional imaging and the resting human brain. *Nature Reviews in Neuroscience,* **2**, 685–694.

86. Gusnard, D. A., Akbudak, E., Shulman, G. L. and Raichle, M. E. (2001). Medial prefrontal cortex and self-referential mental activity: Relation to a default mode of brain function. *Proceedings of the National Academy of Sciences of the United States of America,* **98**, 4259–4264.

87. Raichle, M. E. and Gusnard, D. A. (2005). Intrinsic brain activity sets the stage for expression of motivated behavior. *Journal of Comparative Neurology,* **493**, 167–176.

88. Schneider, F., Bermpohl, F., Heinzel, A. *et al.* (2008). The resting brain and our self: Self-relatedness modulates resting state neural activity in cortical midline structures. *Neuroscience,* **157**, 120–131.

89. Northoff, G., Heinzel, A., de Greck, M. *et al.* (2006). Self-referential processing in our brain: A meta-analysis of imaging studies on the self. *Neuroimage,* **31**, 440–457.

90. Johnson, S. C., Baxter, L. C., Wilder, L. S. *et al.* (2002). Neural correlates of self-reflection. *Brain,* **125**, 1808–1814.

91. Frewen, P. A., Lanius, R. A., Dozois, D. J. A. *et al.* (2008). Clinical and neural correlates of alexithymia in PTSD. *Journal of Abnormal Psychology,* **117**, 171–181.

92. Frewen, P. A., Lane, R., Neufeld, R. W. J. *et al.* (2008). Neural correlates of levels of emotional awareness during trauma script-imagery in posttraumatic stress disorder. *Psychosomatic Medicine,* **70**, 27–31.

93. Bluhm, R. L., Williamson, P. C., Osuch, E. A. *et al.* (2009). Alterations in default network connectivity in posttraumatic stress disorder related to early-life trauma. *Journal of Psychiatric Neuroscience,* **34**, 187–194.

94. Feldman, S., Conforti, N. and Weidenfeld, J. (1995). Limbic pathways and hypothalamic neurotransmitters mediating adrenocortical responses to neural stimuli. *Neuroscience and Biobehavioral Reviews,* **19**, 235–240.

95. Frysztak, R. J. and Neafsey, E. J. (1994). The effect of medial frontal cortex lesions on cardiovascular conditioned emotional responses in the rat. *Brain Research,* **643**, 181–193.

96. Diorio, D., Viau, V. and Meaney, M. J. (1993). The role of the medial prefrontal cortex (cingulate gyrus) in the regulation of hypothalamic–pituitary–adrenal responses to stress. *Journal of Neuroscience,* **13**, 3839–3847.

97. Bremner, J. D., Elzinga, B., Schmahl, C. and Vermetten, E. (2008). Structural and functional plasticity of the human brain in posttraumatic stress disorder. *Progress in Brain Research,* **167**, 171–186.

98. Bremner, J. D., Vermetten, E. and Mazure, C. M. (2000). Development and preliminary psychometric properties of an instrument for the measurement of childhood trauma: The Early Trauma Inventory. *Depression and Anxiety,* **12**, 1–12.

99. Bremner, J., Bolus, R. and Mayer, E. (2007). Psychometric properties of the Early Trauma Inventory-Self Report. *Journal of Nervous and Mental Disorders,* **195**, 211–218.

100. Bremner, J. D., Vermetten, E. and Kelley, M. E. (2007). Cortisol, dehydroepiandrosterone, and estradiol measured over 24 hours in women with childhood sexual abuse-related posttraumatic stress disorder. *Journal of Nervous and Mental Disorders,* **195**, 919–927.

101. Elzinga, B. M., Schmahl, C. S., Vermetten, E., van Dyck, R. and Bremner, J. D. (2003). Higher cortisol levels following exposure to traumatic reminders in abuse-related PTSD. *Neuropsychopharmacology,* **28**, 1656–1665.

102. Stein, M. B., Yehuda, R., Koverola, C. and Hanna, C. (1997). Enhanced dexamethasone suppression of plasma cortisol in adult women traumatized by childhood sexual abuse. *Biological Psychiatry,* **42**, 680–686.

103. Lemieux, A. M. and Coe, C. L. (1995). Abuse-related posttraumatic stress disorder: Evidence for chronic neuroendocrine activation in women. *Psychosomatic Medicine,* **57**, 105–115.

104. Heim, C., Newport, D. J., Heit, S. *et al.* (2000). Pituitary–adrenal and autonomic responses to stress in women after sexual and physical abuse in childhood.

*Journal of the American Medical Association,* **284,** 592–597.

105. Heim, C., Newport, D. J., Bonsall, R., Miller, A. H. and Nemeroff, C. B. (2001). Altered pituitary–adrenal axis responses to provocative challenge tests in adult survivors of childhood abuse. *American Journal of Psychiatry,* **158,** 575–581.

106. Rothman, K. J. and Greenland, S. (1998). *Modern epidemiology.* Philadelphia, PA: Lippincott Raven.

107. Caspi, A., Sugden, K., Moffitt, T. E. *et al.* (2003). Influence of life stress on depression: Moderation by a polymorphism in the 5-HTT gene. *Science,* **301**(5631), 386–389.

108. Vermetten, E. and Bremner, J. D. (2002). Circuits and systems in stress. II. Applications to neurobiology and treatment of PTSD. *Depress Anxiety,* **16,** 14–38.

109. Bremner, J. D. (2002). *Does stress damage the brain? Understanding trauma-related disorders from a mind–body perspective.* New York: Norton.

110. Pitman, R. K. (2001). Investigating the pathogenesis of posttraumatic stress disorder with neuroimaging. *Journal of Clinical Psychiatry,* **62,** 47–54.

111. Vermetten, E. and Bremner, J. D. (2002). Circuits and systems in stress. I. Preclinical studies. *Depression and Anxiety,* **15,** 126–147.

# Biological framework for traumatic dissociation related to early life trauma

Christian Schmahl, Ruth A. Lanius, Clare Pain and Eric Vermetten

## Introduction

Symptoms of dissociation are an important part of the psychopathological response to traumatic stress. While dissociation may provide the appearance of emotional control over the arousing impact of life-threatening stress, it can have the paradoxical effect of transforming physical helplessness at the time of the trauma into psychological helplessness over the periodic incursions of traumatic memories and associations into consciousness. While some individuals have a sense of numbed-out terror during overwhelming experience (e.g., rape), some individuals can feel strangely in control of events at the time of the trauma – denying their fundamental helplessness at times of being physically overwhelmed – but subsequently experience intrusive thoughts, flashbacks, nightmares, numbing and amnesia as a kind of re-traumatization. In this instance, these symptoms seem to sensitize rather than produce habituation to traumatic experiences, perpetuating further acute stress, post-traumatic stress and dissociative symptoms. For others, the mechanism is not the sensitization but instead symptoms of numbing, amnesia and detachment states are triggered by reminders of the traumatic event and act to prevent the processing of the traumatic events(s).

Dissociation typically involves a disruption in the usually integrated function of consciousness, memory, identity, body awareness and/or perception of the environment [1]. Dissociation has been shown to be etiologically connected to psychological and physical trauma by several authors [2–7]. Chapter 5 of this book also points to the important relationship between emotional neglect (i.e., parental psychological unavailability) and dissociation. Specifically, Bureau *et al.* in Ch. 5 cite two prospective longitudinal studies [8,9] where neither childhood physical nor childhood sexual abuse per se was associated with dissociation in young adulthood, after controlling for parental psychological unavailability during the first 2 years of life. Instead, parental emotional neglect in infancy and, to a lesser extent, infant disorganized attachment were the two strongest predictors of dissociation in young adulthood. It should also be noted that dissociation has been shown to be related to other factors, for example genetic influences [10] or affect dysregulation in patients with borderline personality disorder (BPD) [11,12], which, in turn, may be related to emotional neglect and/or disorganized attachment patterns.

Dissociation may involve the protective activation of altered states of consciousness related to acute changes in a variety of brain systems in response to immediate danger. Several studies of individuals experiencing danger and/or life threat have shown specific peri-traumatic dissociative changes, including alterations in time sense, perception, attentional focus and awareness of pain. In addition, depersonalization occurs in a significant number of individuals facing acute life threat (reviewed by Loewenstein and Putnam [13]). Information related to the trauma may be encoded in these altered states, resulting in decreased access to information about the trauma once the person returns to his/her baseline state. This may give a subjective sense of "compartmentalization" of the traumatic experience and/or a sense of detachment from the experience, adaptively sparing as much normal function as possible, although over time this defense may prevent the normal integration of the event(s) into the autobiographical narrative.

The altered state of consciousness at the time of the trauma, along with the incongruity of trauma with ordinary experience, tends to produce memories that are discontinuous yet remain associated with the strong emotions that accompanied the original experiences. The loss of physical control associated with the trauma may be reproduced by the mental experience of involuntariness and loss of control over memories of trauma, which are either intrusive (unbidden recollections, flashbacks and/or nightmares) or unavailable (amnesia, numbing, derealization of memory and/or avoidance of reminders). These dissociative processes can also be associated with changes in bodily perceptions, such as feeling the physical pain of the trauma again or feeling as if part of the body does not belong, leading to a kind of "somatic estrangement" [14,15].

As a result, the traumatic experience is not integrated into a unitary whole or into an integrated sense of self, partly because of a failure of integration of episodic and autobiographical memory [7]. Several authors [7,16,17] (reviewed by Lowenstein and Putnam [13] and Vermetten *et al.* [17]) view this disruption of memory and associated personal identity as serving a protective function, at least in response to acute stress. However, over time, these defenses may interfere with the necessary cognitive and affective processes of integrating traumatic experiences.

Other forms of dissociation may include derealization, depersonalization, disorganized behavior, fugue states, dense dissociative amnesia for a variety of aspects of autobiographical memory, disruption of identity with loss of awareness of personal identity and/or creation of alternative identities [13]. In addition, dissociation can produce a variety of somatoform conditions such as pseudoneurological conversion symptoms, pain disorders and somatization disorder [13]. Individuals with repeated early life trauma such as dissociative identity disorder (DID) or BPD may show all of these symptoms, leading to a particularly complex and variable clinical picture.

By comparison with observation, psychological assessment data from a large sample of individuals with DID and related forms of dissociative disorder not otherwise specified postulate that chronic early life dissociation can also serve as a developmental protective and resilience factor [13, 17], which allows for as normal development as possible of cognitive function (capacity for abstract and complex thought) some capacity for attachment to others (despite attachment schemas that may be disrupted), a sense of humor and artistic and creative abilities, among others [17].

## Animal defensive responses as a model of dissociation

The analysis described above has led several investigators to note striking similarities between certain animal

defensive responses and trauma-induced dissociative psychopathology in humans [6], and the endogenous opioid system has been suggested to underlie some of these processes [6,18,19]. Animal threat behavior is considered to have four stages: (a) pre-encounter defense (involving heightened orientation and diminished interest in food), (b) post-encounter defensive behavior (the animal can manifest flight, freeze and fight responses), (c) circa-strike defense, the stage when an animal is about to be attacked (involving analgesia, emotional numbing and a startle response); and (d) post-strike behavior, involving the presumed experience of pain if the animal was injured, and recuperation [20]. During the pre-encounter defense stage, it appears that an animal's eating pattern varies with the risk of predation, and meal frequency has usually been shown to decrease as risk increases. When an animal is threatened by a predator (post-encounter defensive behavior), a flight response is often observed, assuming there is a reasonable chance of successful escape. However, freezing responses, which involve behavioral immobility, are the dominant post-encounter response patterns in some species. Freezing responses have been observed in situations with and without the availability of physical escape and are thought to increase the chance of survival because (a) predators detect immobile prey less easily than mobile prey, (b) predators may be encouraged to shift their attention to other moving stimuli and (c) movement cues are critical triggers for predatory behavior, and freezing responses usually involving hyperarousal are able to eliminate these cues. Critical anatomical structures for the post-encounter defensive behavior described above include the amygdala, the ventral periaqueductal gray and the hypothalamus. The central nucleus of the amygdala mediates transfer of information about the threat level to the ventral periaqueductal gray, which, in turn, is involved in the mediation of freezing responses through opioid-mediated neurotransmission [21,22].

During the circa-strike defense (that is, at the moment of attack), freezing responses tend to be combined with analgesia, allowing the animal to focus on defensive concerns rather than attending to the perception of pain (e.g., from injury). Analgesia has been shown to occur in response to recognized predator odors, other related danger signals, pinching of the scruff of the neck and dorsal constraint [23]. Analgesia under these conditions is mediated by the release of endogenous opioids [23–25] as well as by non-opioid mechanisms [23]. Important anatomical structures involved in the circa-strike defensive behavior include the superior colliculus and the dorsolateral periaqueductal gray, which receives nociceptive input from the spinal cord and the trigeminal nucleus [26]. Pain perception returns during the post-strike phase and allows the animal to attend to recuperative behaviors, including taking care of injuries, grooming behavior and resting behavior, allowing baseline physiological re-stabilization and healing to take place [27].

Inescapable shock, subjecting the animal to inescapable experimental traumatization such as different rates of electrical shocks, starvation and cold-water swim, has been used to model all natural stages of animal defense behavior [24]. Inescapable shock is normally followed by a state of helplessness, hypoarousal, freezing and analgesia. Even when animals are presented with a possibility of escape, they remain helpless and passively endure continued shock [28,29].

A remarkable analogy between certain animal defensive responses, including freezing responses and analgesia, and aspects of dissociative sympotmatology in humans has been noted. For example, freezing responses have been proposed to be closely related to dissociative symptomatology, and several studies have reported that a substantial number of women have reported freezing and paralysis during rape [29–30]. Clinical observations [31] have also indicated that patients with early life trauma will often exhibit freezing responses during dissociative states. In terms of analgesia, both male and female patients suffering from dissociative symptomatology related to early life trauma have been shown to present with analgesia in the face of painful stimuli [2,33]. Moreover, during World War II, 75% of severely wounded soldiers on the Italian front exhibited significant analgesia in that they did not require morphine, suggesting that "strong emotions can block pain" [33]. The hypothesis that re-exposure to a stimulus resembling the original trauma will lead to an endogenous opioid response can be indirectly measured by administration of naloxone (opioid antagonist) after patients with post-traumatic stress disorder (PTSD) have been exposed to reminders of their traumatic event. Specifically, reversible analgesia was tested in patients suffering from combat-related PTSD [34,35]. Eight Vietnam veterans with PTSD and eight matched veterans without PTSD viewed a combat videotape 20 years after the original trauma exposure under naloxone and placebo conditions in a randomized double-blind crossover design. In the placebo condition, but not after naloxone, the subjects with PTSD reported a 30% decrease in pain intensity ratings of standardized heat stimuli after the combat videotape. Derealization and depersonalization are possibly mediated by a dysregulation of κ-opioid receptors, as agonists at these receptors can cause depersonalization [36,37].

These studies resemble the analgesia responses described in the animal literature during the circa-strike defense stages. It has been hypothesized that emotional responses accompanying these reactions rely on prefrontal–amygdala cortex pathways [38]. This pathway has also been hypothesized to play an important role in the neural circuitry underlying dissociative states in humans [39–41] and states of analgesia in response to thermal pain stimuli in patients with PTSD and BPD [42–44] as described below.

Aspects of animal analogues of dissociation related to circa-strike behavior are thought to be mediated by the superior colliculus and the dorsolateral periaqueductal gray, both receiving nociceptive input from the spinal cord and the trigeminal nucleus [25]. In phylogenetically more recent species such as humans, these systems can be assumed to be under the control of higher cortical regions and activated under high levels of stress. It could be hypothesized that secondary dissociation is the representation of animal post-encounter defense modes in humans, activated during (traumatic) stress and its subsequent reminders, comprising analgesia states in the circa strike phase of defense but experienced subjectively by humans as depersonalization, derealization, emotional numbing and the other symptoms noted to occur in dissociation.

## Neurological etiologies of dissociative symptomatology in humans

### Levels of corticolimbic inhibition as a model for modulations of emotion

Bremner [45] has hypothesized that there may be two subtypes of acute trauma response – one primarily involving dissociative symptoms and the other predominantly intrusive and hyperaroused – that represent unique pathways to chronic stress-related psychopathology. These two subtypes of dissociation can be referred to as primary and secondary dissociation, as defined by van der Kolk and colleagues [46]. Primary dissociation refers to the re-experiencing/hyperaroused variant of dissociation commonly associated with cluster B symptoms of PTSD such as unbidden recollections, flashbacks and nightmares. In contrast, secondary dissociation is characterized by such symptoms as numbness, amnesia, detachment states, depersonalization, derealization, freezing, analgesia responses and subjective distance from emotional experience, to which the term dissociation is more commonly applied [46].

In studies by Lanius *et al.* [39,40,47–49], the neuronal circuitry underlying re-experiencing/hyperarousal (primary dissociation) and depersonalization/derealization dissociative (secondary dissociation) responses in PTSD predominantly related to childhood abuse was studied using the script-driven, symptom-provocation paradigm. Patients constructed a narrative of their traumatic experience, including as many sensory details as possible. Later these narratives were read back to patients, who were instructed to recall the traumatic memory as vividly as possible during functional magnetic resonance imaging (fMRI). Approximately 70% of patients relived their traumatic experience showing a predominant re-experiencing/hyperarousal response with an increase in heart rate while recalling the traumatic memory [47], while the remaining 30% had a predominant secondary dissociative response with no concomitant increase in heart rate [39,40]. In comparison with control subjects, patients who had a hyperarousal response and relived their traumatic experience after being exposed to the traumatic script showed significantly less activation of the thalamus, anterior cingulate gyrus (Bradmann area [BA] 32) and medial frontal gyrus (BA 10, BA 11), occipital lobe (BA 19) and inferior frontal gyrus (BA 47) [48]. Lower levels of anterior cingulate activation and medial prefrontal activation were consistent with several positron emission tomography (PET) script-driven imagery studies of sexual abuse and combat-related PTSD [50–54]. These brain activation patterns differ strikingly from those observed in patients who exhibited secondary dissociation in response to the traumatic script [39]. These patients exhibited *higher* levels of activation in the superior and middle temporal gyri (BA 38), the medial prefrontal cortex (BA 9), the anterior cingulate gyrus (BA 24 and BA 32), the inferior frontal gyrus (BA 47), the occipital lobe (BA 19) and the parietal lobe (BA 7). The neural correlates of re-experiencing/hyperarousal states and depersonalization/derealization dissociative states, respectively, in patients with PTSD show *opposite* patterns of brain activation in brain regions that are implicated in arousal modulation and emotion regulation. In particular, these differential patterns are found in the medial prefrontal cortex, the anterior cingulate cortex and the limbic system.

## Failure of corticolimbic inhibition

The re-experiencing/hyperaroused PTSD group exhibited abnormally *low* activation in the medial prefrontal and the anterior cingulate cortex, brain regions that are implicated in arousal modulation and emotion regulation more generally [49,55]. Consistent with impaired cortical modulation, increased activation of the limbic system, especially the amygdala (a brain structure that has been shown to play a key role in fear conditioning) has often been observed in patients with PTSD after exposure to traumatic reminders and to masked fearful faces [55]. Studies in patients with PTSD have also reported direct inhibitory influence of the prefrontal cortex on the emotional limbic system. For example, PET studies have shown a negative correlation between blood flow in the left ventromedial prefrontal cortex and the amygdala during emotional tasks, and negative correlations between the medial prefrontal cortex and the amygdala during exposure to fearful faces [51]. Therefore, the *low* activation of medial prefrontal regions described in the re-experiencing/hyperaroused PTSD subgroup is consistent with failed inhibition of limbic reactivity and is associated with re-experiencing/hyperaroused emotional undermodulation. We conceptualize this group as experiencing emotional undermodulation in response to traumatic reminders such as a subjective reliving experience of the traumatic events, including flashbacks and reliving nightmares. These symptoms can be viewed as a form of emotion dysregulation that involves emotional undermodulation, mediated by failure of prefrontal inhibition of limbic regions.

Further support for this model stems from studies that take a dimensional approach (examining different symptom severities and associated neural activation patterns within each response subtype) to individual differences in re-experiencing symptoms in response to trauma memory recall. This method examines correlations between severity of state re-experiencing to trauma scripts and brain activity in regions associated with awareness and regulation of arousal and emotions, such as the anterior cingulate cortex, the medial prefrontal cortex and the insula [56]. Results have shown that the severity of state re-experiencing was *positively* correlated with activation in the right anterior insula, a brain region that is involved in the neural representation of somatic aspects of emotional states and interoception of feeling states. In contrast, state re-experiencing was *negatively* correlated with activation of the rostral portion of the anterior cingulate cortex, a brain region that plays an important role in arousal and emotion regulation. These findings are consistent with the phenomenology and clinical presentations of patients with PTSD who exhibit pathological emotional undermodulation during re-experiencing/hyperarousal flashback states, including a variety of negative emotional states such as irritability and anger and associated bodily experiences.

## Excessive corticolimbic inhibition

In contrast to the re-experiencing/hyperaroused group, the group experiencing secondary dissociative symptoms exhibited abnormally *high* activation in the anterior cingulate cortex and the medial prefrontal cortex [39]. The patients with depersonalization/derealization dissociative PTSD can, therefore, be conceptualized as emotionally overmodulating in response to exposure to traumatic memory recall. This often involves subjective disengagement from the emotional content of the memory through depersonalization, derealization or other secondary dissociative responses, which are hypothesized to be mediated by midline prefrontal inhibition of the limbic regions.

Dimensionally, the depersonalization/derealization-type of dissociative response to trauma reminders was *negatively* correlated with right anterior insula activation and *positively* correlated with activation in the medial prefrontal cortex and dorsal anterior cingulate cortex [56]. It is interesting to note that the medial

prefrontal cortex cluster that was *positively* correlated with state re-experiencing/hyperaroused symptoms was *negatively* correlated with amygdala activity during script-driven imagery [57]. This finding provides further support for hypothesized hyperinhibition of limbic regions by medial prefrontal areas in states of pathological overmodulation, that is, during secondary dissociative states such as states of depersonalization and derealization in response to traumatic memory recall (Fig 17.1).

A recent study by Felmingham *et al.* [58] provides additional evidence for the corticolimbic inhibition model. In this study, the investigators used fMRI to examine the impact of dissociation as measured by the Clinician Administered Dissociative State Scale on fear processing in two groups of patients with PTSD, one with high and the other with low dissociation scores. Brain activation was compared during the processing of consciously and non-consciously perceived fear stimuli. Patients with high dissociation scores showed enhanced activation in the ventral prefrontal cortex during conscious fear processing, as compared with patients with low dissociation scores. The authors suggested that these data support the theory that secondary dissociation is a regulatory strategy invoked to cope with extreme arousal in PTSD through hyperinhibition of limbic regions, and that this strategy is most active during conscious processing of threat.

The neurobiology literature on pain also provides additional support for the hyperinhibition of the limbic system – including the amygdala – during dissociative states. For example, Roeder *et al.* [59] reported

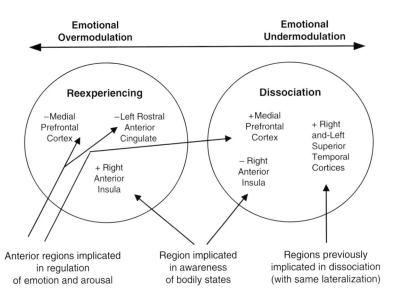

**Fig. 17.1.** Extremes of impaired emotion regulation in post-traumatic stress disorder (Adapted from Hopper *et al.* 2007 [56]).

decreased amygdala activity in response to painful stimulation during hypnosis-induced states of depersonalization in healthy subjects. In patients with PTSD and BPD, amygdala deactivation was also observed in response to thermal pain stimuli [42–44]. Most recently, we used the script-driven imagery paradigm to specifically induce secondary dissociative states in patients with BPD, while also assessing pain sensitivity in response to thermal pain stimuli [41]. For this study, individual situations eliciting secondary dissociative symptoms were depicted for each patient. During the presentation of these scripts, higher levels of secondary dissociation as determined by the Dissociation-Tension Scale [60] were found in comparison to levels with a neutral script. In addition, pain sensitivity was significantly lower during the dissociative script compared with the neutral script. On a neural level, higher activity in the dorsolateral prefrontal cortex was found during secondary dissociative states. In a subgroup analysis of 10 patients with both BPD and PTSD, increased activity was found in right insula and left cingulate cortex, thus providing further evidence for the corticolimbic inhibition model.

Experimental studies examining emotional memory suppression in healthy subjects added further support for the corticolimbic inhibition model. Results showed that memory suppression was associated with increased frontal and decreased hippocampal activity [61]. In addition, memory suppression was significantly associated with bilateral hippocampal inhibition. The authors suggested that these findings provide a possible neurobiological model involving corticolimbic inhibition as underlying the suppression of unwanted memories and that this inhibition may also play a role in dissociative amnesia [61].

Finally, studies of depersonalization disorder provide additional evidence for the corticolimbic inhibition model. Hollander *et al.* [62] reported a case study of a patient with primary depersonalization disorder, using brain electrical mapping. Results showed left frontal overactivation, indicated by increased anteriorized alpha activity. They also demonstrated with single photon emission computed tomography (SPECT) that this patient showed impaired perfusion in the left caudate and increased activity in posterior frontal areas. A subsequent investigation of a group of patients with depersonalization disorder examined event-related fMRI in response to neutral, mild, intensely happy and sad facial expressions, with simultaneous measurements of skin conductance levels [63]. Compared with healthy controls, those with depersonalization disorder showed a decrease in subcortical limbic activity to increasingly intense happy and sad facial expressions. Moreover, for both happy and sad facial expressions, patients with depersonalization disorder but not healthy controls exhibited negative correlations between skin conductance measures and activation in the bilateral dorsal prefrontal cortices. These studies support the hypothesis that those with depersonalization disorder exhibit increased prefrontal activity and/or decreased limbic activity, resulting in the hypoemotionality frequently reported in these patients and thus adding weight to the overmodulation model to explain secondary dissociative states.

The findings described above support the corticolimbic inhibition model of excessive limbic inhibition resulting in secondary dissociation symptoms in PTSD as well as in other trauma spectrum disorders such as BPD, DID and depersonalization disorders; they are consistent with the phenomenology and clinical presentation of these patients, with significant depersonalization/derealization, amnesias, pain dysregulation and other secondary dissociation symptomatology. The corticolimbic inhibition model suggests that, once a threshold of anxiety and hyperarousal is reached, the medial prefrontal cortex inhibits emotional processing in limbic structures including the amygdala, leading to a significant dampening of sympathetic output and reduced emotional experiencing, thus resulting in a variety of secondary dissociative symptoms. In contrast, in the subgroup exhibiting secondary dissociative symptoms, increased activation of medial prefrontal structures is consistent with the idea of hyperinhibition of those same limbic regions and pathological emotional overmodulation in response to trauma-related emotions [64].

## The temporal lobe and dissociation: levels of corticolimbic inhibition

Historically, much work has been done exploring psychological phenomenology stemming from temporal lobe lesions. Failure of corticolimbic inhibition or excessive corticolimbic inhibition may be one underlying mechanism that leads to altered temporal lobe and limbic system functioning.

Typically, dissociative symptoms in neurological disorders have been reported to result from lesions in the limbic system, specifically the temporal lobe or the temporoparietal junction. The lesions have included seizures, migraines, neoplasms, arteriovenous malformations and post-traumatic brain damage [65–69].

Penfield and Rasmussen [70] have also reported depersonalization-like symptoms in response to stimulation of the superior and middle temporal gyrus during neurosurgery. Moreover, psychiatric patients with significant dissociative symptomatology have also been noted to be prone to experience temporal lobe-like epilepsy symptoms. In contrast to investigating physical lesions, Teicher et al. [71] explored the relationship between early abuse and limbic system dysfunction as measured by the Limbic System Checklist-33 (LSCL-33). Results showed that LSCL-33 scores correlated well with the Dissociative Experiences Scale scores [71,72].

Altered activation in the superior and middle temporal gyri during script-driven imagery-induced depersonalization/derealization dissociative states in PTSD is consistent with temporal lobe abnormalities underlying some forms of dissociation [39], as are studies examining the neural correlates of depersonalization disorder. With regard to DID, Saxe et al. [73] investigated regional cerebral blood flow using SPECT in a patient with DID. They conducted four separate scans, with the patient in a different personality state for each scan. They found that the left temporal lobe was consistently significantly active in comparison with whole brain activity and that the level of activation of this region varied in each scan. In another SPECT study, Sar et al. [74] examined regional cerebral blood flow in 17 patients with DID. Compared with a group of healthy controls, the patients with DID exhibited increased blood flow in the left lateral temporal region and lower blood flow bilaterally in the orbitofrontal region. More recently, Reinders et al. [75] examined a group of patients with DID in two identity states, a neutral state that inhibits access to the traumatic memories, and thus enables daily life functioning, and a traumatic state that has access to the traumatic memories. Results revealed different patterns of regional cerebral blood flow in response to neutral and traumatic scripts in the two dissociative identity states. Specifically, the traumatic identity state exhibited alterations in the temporal lobe (amygdala), insula, precuneus (BA 19) and parietal area BA 7. Finally, hippocampal and amygdala volume has been examined in patients with DID [76]. Hippocampal volume was found to be 19% smaller and amygdalar volume 32% smaller in patients with DID compared with healthy controls.

Simeon et al. [77] measured resting regional cerebral blood flow using PET in eight patients with depersonalization disorder and in 24 healthy volunteers. The subjects with depersonalisation disorder showed significantly lower metabolic activity in the right superior and middle temporal gyri (BA 21, BA 22). Similarly, in a case study of a patient with primary depersonalisation disorder, Hollander et al. [62] found increased theta activity and increased evoked potential negatives in the left temporal lobe using brain electrical mapping.

It is interesting to note that studies examining the mechanisms underlying dissociative phenomena in PTSD and in dissociative disorders reported altered activation in the limbic system of the temporal lobe. These results, therefore, lend further support to the notion of altered limbic system activity in this disorder and may help to explain the pseudopsychotic/temporal epilepsy-like symptoms or limbic system dysfunction often observed clinically in this patient population [71,78] and may prove useful in providing diagnostic clarification for complex trauma disorders that can at times present similarly to psychotic disorders.

In summary, the previous sections of this chapter have shown that the normal integration of systems that regulate emotion (dorsolateral and medial prefrontal cortex, anterior cingulate and amygdala), autonomic nervous system activity (insula, thalamus), sensation and sensory processing (temporal, parietal, occipital cortex and cerebellum), attention (thalamus, anterior cingulate, frontal cortex), movement (periaqueductal gray), pain (anterior cingulate, insula, periaqueductal gray) and the endogenous opioid system and memory (hippocampus) can be disrupted in specific ways that compromise integration of identity, memory and consciousness after the occurrence of traumatic experiences. They may, therefore, play a key role in maintaining the pathophysiology of unresolved traumatic experience as well as generating the underlying dissociative symptomatology.

## Dissociative states and the effect on learning: implications for treatment

In several psychiatric disorders, it has been demonstrated that secondary dissociation has a profoundly negative impact on psychotherapy outcome [79–81]. Since most psychological treatments rely on basic learning processes to promote changes in psychopathology, it is important to investigate the interaction between learning and dissociation on an experimental level. The influence of secondary dissociation on implicit learning processes was demonstrated by the results of a startle response experiment in patients with BPD [82]. Patients with high levels of dissociation had significantly lower startle responses than patients with low levels of dissociation. Since the startle response can be directly modified by the central nucleus of the amygdala, this finding may be interpreted in the light of reduced amygdala activity during secondary dissociative states, as suggested by Sierra and Berrios [64] as well as by excessive corticolimbic inhibition as described above. In a recent study in patients with BPD, a dampening influence of dissociative experience on amygdala activity could also be demonstrated during a working memory task (Krause-Utz *et al.*, unpublished data), thus providing further evidence for this model.

The results of a classical conditioning study using a conditioning task that included an aversive sound (baby cry) as an unconditioned stimulus and two neutral inkblots as a conditioned stimulus in BPD highlights the effect of dissociation on conditioning and emotional learning processes [83]. Classical conditioning and emotional learning are largely dependent on neural pathways connecting the amygdala and the prefrontal cortex, and selective damage of the amygdala in humans has been shown to be associated with impaired emotional learning: no acquisition of skin conductance responses during conditioning. When patients with BPD were retrospectively separated into two groups (with and without secondary dissociation during conditioning, as determined by the Dissociation-Tension Scale), only those without state dissociation revealed normal conditioning processes, whereas dissociative patients did not show normal conditioning processes as determined by emotional valence ratings and acquisition of skin conductance responses.

These results suggest that emotional, amygdala-based learning processes seem to be affected by state dissociation through altering acquisition and extinction processes via frontolimbic pathways. These findings have important implications for both assessment and treatment of patients with significant secondary dissociative symptomatology. As described above, secondary dissociation has been shown to negatively predict psychotherapy outcome. Jaycox *et al.* [84] have suggested that dissociative symptoms, including numbing symptoms in PTSD, can prevent emotional engagement with trauma-related information and thereby reduce treatment effectiveness. These findings suggest the importance not only of assessing the extent of secondary dissociative psychopathology but also of providing targeted treatments to reduce dissociative symptoms, including symptoms

of depersonalization, derealization and numbing, before commencing exposure-based treatments. Failure to do so can lead to an increase in PTSD symptoms, including secondary dissociation, emotion dysregulation and an increase in the patient's overall distress and functional impairment.

Cloitre *et al.* [85] have included a stabilization phase in their empirically supported model of desensitization treatment for adults suffering from childhood abused-related PTSD. In the stabilization phase of treatment, Cloitre and colleagues focus on emotional regulation and target the development of interpersonal relational skills and grounding skills, thus reducing overall vulnerability to dissociation. Patients are assisted to identify and modify disordered attachment schemas learned in childhood, and to improve competence and confidence in social interactions, again reducing their tendency for secondary dissociation and increasing their likelihood to benefit from desensitization in the second stage of treatment (see Chs. 24, 26 and 27).

## Conclusion
Future treatment outcome research should focus on complex childhood abuse-related disorders with substantial secondary dissociative symptomatology. This will help to develop interventions that are most effective for treatment of secondary dissociation but assist our understanding of how specific interventions can be optimally timed in a phase-oriented treatment model.

## References
1. American Psychiatric Association (2000). *Diagnostic and statistical manual of mental disorders*, 4th edn, text revision. Washington, DC: American Psychiatric Press.
2. Boon, S. and Draijer, N. (1993). Multiple personality disorder in the Netherlands: A clinical investigation of 71 patients. *American Journal of Psychiatry,* **150,** 489–494.
3. Coons, P. M., Bowman, E. S. and Milstein, V. (1988). Multiple personality disorder: A clinical investigation of 50 cases. *Journal of Nervous and Mental Disease,* **176,** 519–527.
4. Kluft, R. P. (1995). The natural history of multiple personality disorder. In R. P. Kluft ( ed.), *Childhood antecedents of multiple personality* (pp. 197–238). Washington, DC: American Psychiatric Press.
5. Lewis, D. O., Yaeger, C. A., Swica, Y., Pincus, J. H. and Lewis, M. (1997). Objective documentation of child abuse and dissociation in 12 murderers with dissociative identity disorder. *American Journal of Psychiatry*, **154,** 1703–1710.

6. Nijenhuis, E. R., Vanderlinder, J. and Spinhoven, P. (1998 ). Animal defense reactions as a model for trauma-induced dissociative reactions. *Journal of Trauma and Stress,* **11**, 243–260.

7. van der Kolk, B. A., van der Hart, O. and Marmar, C. R. (1996). *Dissociation and information processing in posttraumatic stress disorder.* In B. A. van der Kolk, A. V. McFarlane and L. Weisaeth (eds.), *Traumatic stress* (pp. 303–327). New York: The Guilford Press.

8. Ogawa, J. R., Sroufe, L. A., Weinfeld, N. S., Carlson, E. A. and Egeland, B. (1997). Development and the fragmented self: Longitudinal study of dissociative symptomatology in a non-clinical sample. *Development and Psychopathology,* **9**, 855–879.

9. Dutra, L., Bureau, J.-F., Holmes, B., Lyubchik, A. and Lyons-Ruth, K. (2009). Quality of early care and childhood trauma: A prospective study of developmental pathways to dissociation. *Journal of Nervous and Mental Disease,* **197**, 383–390.

10. Jang, K. L. Paris, J. , Zweig-Frank, H. and Livesley, W. J. (1998). Twin study of dissociative experience. *Journal of Nervous and Mental Health,* **186**, 345–351.

11. Stiglmayr, C. E., Shapiro, D. A., Stieglitz, R. D., Limberger, M. F. and Bohus, M. (2001). Experience of aversive tension and dissociation in female patients with borderline personality disorder: A controlled study. *Journal of Psychiatric Research,* **35**, 111–118.

12. Stiglmayr, C. E., Ebner-Priemer, U. W., Bretz, J. *et al.* (2008). Dissociative symptoms are positively related to stress in borderline personality disorder. *Acta Psychiatrica Scandinavica,* **117**, 139–147.

13. Loewenstein, R. J. and Putnam, F. W. (2004). The Dissociative Disorders. In B. J. Sadock and V. A. Sadock (eds.), *Comprehensive textbook of psychiatry,* 8th edn, Vol. 1 (pp. 1844–1901). Baltimore, Williams & Wilkins.

14. Nemiah, J. C. (1993). Dissociation, conversation and somatization. In D. S. Spiegel and M. D. Lutherville (eds.), *Dissociative disorders: A clinical review* (pp. 104–117). Baltimore, MD: Sidran Press.

15. Spiegel, D. (1990). Hypnosis, dissociation and trauma: hidden and overt observers. In J. L. Singer (ed.), *Repression and dissociation* (pp. 121–142). Chicago, IL: University of Chicago Press.

16. Spiegel, D., Hunt, T. and Dondershine, H. E. (1988). Dissociation and hypnotisability in post-traumatic stress disorder. *American Journal of Psychiatry,* **145**, 301–305.

17. Vermetten, E., Dorahy, M. J. and Spiegel, D. (eds.) (2007). *Traumatic dissociation neurobiology and treatment.* Washington, DC: American Psychiatric Press.

18. Ludwig, A. M. (1983). The psychobiological functions of dissociation. *American Journal of Clinical Hypnosis,* **26**, 93–99.

19. Krystal, H. (1988). *Integration and self-healing. Affect, trauma, alexithymia.* Hillsdale NJ: Lawrence Erlbaum.

20. Bolles, R. C. and Fanselow, M. S. (1980). A perceptual–defensive–recuperation model of fear and pain. *Behavioral and Brain Sciences,* **3**, 291–301.

21. Fanselow, M. S. and Gale, G. D. (2003). The amygdala, fear, and memory. *Annals of the New York Academy of Sciences,* **985**, 125–134.

22. LeDoux, J. E. (1996). *The emotional brain: The mysterious underpinnings of emotional life.* New York: Simon & Schuster.

23. Siegfried, B., Frischknecht, H. R. and Nunez de Souza, R. (1990). An ethological model for the study of activation and interaction of pain, memory, and defensive systems in the attacked mouse: Role of endogenous opioids. *Neuroscience and Biobehavioral Reviews,* **14**, 481–490.

24. Fanselow, M. S., Lester, L. S. and Helmstetter, F. J. (1988). Changes in feeding and foraging patterns as an antipredator defensive strategy: A laboratory simulation using aversive stimulation in a closed economy. *Journal of the Experimental Analysis of Behavior,* **50**, 361–374.

25. Krystal, J. H., Kosten, T. R., Southwick, S. *et al.* (1989). Neurobiologic aspects of PTSD: Review of clinical and preclinical studies. *Behavior Therapy,* **20**, 177–198.

26. Blomqvist, A. and Craig, A. D. (1991). Organization of spinal and trigeminal input to the PAG. In A. Depaulis and R. Bandler (eds.), *The midbrain periaqueductal grey matter: Functional, anatomical and immunohistochemical organization* (pp. 345–363). *NATO ASI Series A*, Vol. 213. New York: Plenum.

27. Garber, J., Fencil-Morse, E., Rosellini, R. A. and Seligman, M. E. (1979). 'Abnormal fixations' and 'learned helplessness': Inescapable shock as a weanling impairs adult discrimination learning in rats. *Behaviour Research and Therapy,* **17**, 197–206.

28. Seligman, M. E. (1972). Learned helplessness. *Annual Review of Medicine,* **23,** 407–412.

29. Brickman, J. and Briere, J. (1989). Incidence of rape and sexual assault in an urban Canadian population. *International Journal of Women's Studies,* **7,** 195–206.

30. Burgess, A. W. and Holmstrom, A. L. L. (1976). Coping behaviour of the rape victim. *American Journal of Psychiatry,* **133,** 413–418.

31. Putnam, F. W. (1989). *Diagnosis and treatment of multiple personality disorder.* New York: Guilford.

32. Loewenstein, R. J. and Putnam, F. W. (1990). The clinical phenomenology of males with MPD: A report of 21 cases. *Dissociation,* **3,** 135–143.

33. Beecher, H. K. (1946). Pain in men wounded in battle. *Annals of Surgery,* **123,** 96–105.

34. van der Kolk, B. A., Greenberg, M. S., Orr, S. P. and Pitman, R. K. (1989). Endogenous opioids and stress induced analgesia in post traumatic stress disorder. *Psychopharmacology Bulletin,* **25,** 108–112.

35. Pitman, R. K., van der Kolk, B. A., Orr, S. P. and Greenberg, M. S. (1990) Naloxone reversible stress

induced analgesia in post traumatic stress disorder. *Archives of General Psychiatry, 47*:541–547.

36. Pfeiffer, A., Brantl, V., Herz, A. *et al.* (1986). Psychotominesis mediated by κ opiate receptors. *Science,* **233,** 774–776.

37. Walsh, S. L., Geter-Douglas, B., Strain, E. C. *et al.* (2001). Enadoline and butorphanol: Evaluation of κ-agonists oncocaine pharmacodynamics and cocaine self-administraion in humans. *Journal of Pharmacology and Experimental Therapeutics,* **299,** 147–158.

38. LeDoux, J. (2002). *Synapic self.* New York: Penguin Books.

39. Lanius, R. A., Williamson, P. C., Boksman, K. *et al.* (2002). Brain activation during script-driven imagery induced dissociative responses in PTSD: A functional magnetic resonance imaging investigation. *Biological Psychiatry,* **52,** 305–311.

40. Lanius, R. A., Williamson, P. C., Bluhm, R. L. *et al.* (2005). Functional connectivity of dissociative responses in posttraumatic stress disorder: A functional magnetic resonance imaging investigation. *Biological Psychiatry,* **57,** 873–884.

41. Ludaescher, P., Valerius, G., Stiglmayr, C. *et al.* (2010). Pain sensitivity and neural processing during dissociative states in patients with borderline personality disorder with and without comorbid PTSD: A pilot study. *Journal of Psychiatry and Neuroscience,* **35,** 000–000.

42. Schmahl, C., Bohus, M., Esposito, F. *et al.* (2006). Neural correlates of antinociception in borderline personality disorder. *Archives of General Psychiatry,* **63,** 659–667.

43. Geuze, E., Westenberg, H. G. M., Jochims, A. *et al.* (2007). Altered pain processing in veterans with posttraumatic stress disorder. *Archives of General Psychiatry,* **64,** 76–85.

44. Kraus, A., Esposito, F., Seifritz, E. *et al.* (2009). Amygdala deactivation as a neural correlate of pain processing in patients with borderline personality disorder and co-occurrent posttraumatic stress disorder. *Biological Psychiatry,* **65,** 819–822.

45. Bremner, J. D. (1999). Acute and chronic responses to psychological trauma: Where do we go from here?. *American Journal of Psychiatry,* **156,** 349–351.

46. van der Kolk, B. A., Pelcovitz, D., Roth, S. *et al.* (1996). Dissociation, somatization, and affect dysregulation: the complexity of adaptation of trauma. *American Journal of Psychiatry,* **153,** 83–93.

47. Lanius, R. A., Williamson, P. C., Densmore, M. *et al.* (2001). Neural correlates of traumatic memories in posttraumatic stress disorder: A functional MRI investigation. *American Journal of Psychiatry,* **158,** 1920–1922.

48. Lanius, R. A., Williamson, P. C., Densmore, M. *et al.* (2004). The nature of traumatic memories: A 4-T FMRI functional connectivity analysis. *American Journal of Psychiatry,* **161**, 36–44.

49. Lanius, R. A., Bluhm, R., Lanius, U. and Pain, C. (2006). A review of neuroimaging studies in PTSD: Heterogeneity of response to symptom provocation. *Journal of Psychiatric Research,* **40,** 709–729.

50. Shin, L. M., McNally, R. J., Kosslyn, S. M. *et al.* (1999). Regional cerebral blood flow during script-driven imagery in childhood sexual abuse-related PTSD: A PET investigation. *American Journal of Psychiatry,* **156,** 575–584.

51. Shin, L. M., Wright, C. I., Cannistraro, P. A. *et al.* (2005). A functional magnetic resonance imaging study of amygdala and medial prefrontal cortex responses to overtly presented fearful faces in posttraumatic stress disorder. *Archives of General Psychiatry,* **62,** 273–281.

52. Bremner, J. D., Narayan, M., Staib, L. H. *et al.* (1999). Neural correlates of memories of childhood sexual abuse in women with and without posttraumatic stress disorder. *American Journal of Psychiatry,* **156,** 1787–1795.

53. Bremner, J. D., Staib, L. H., Kaloupek, D. *et al.* (1999b). Neural correlates of exposure to traumatic pictures and sound in Vietnam combat veterans with and without posttraumatic stress disorder: A positron emission tomography study. *Biological Psychiatry,* **45,** 806–816.

54. Britton, J. C., Phan, K. L., Fig, L. M. and Taylor, S. F. (2005). Corticolimbic blood flow in posttraumatic stress disorder during script-driven imagery. *Biological Psychiatry,* **57,** 832–840.

55. Etkin, A. and Wager, T. D. (2007). Functional neuro-imaging of anxiety: A meta-analysis of emotional processing in PTSD, social anxiety disorder, and specific phobia. *American Journal of Psychiatry,* **164,** 1476–1488.

56. Hopper, J. W., Frewen, P. A., van der Kolk, B. A. and Lanius, R. A. (2007). Neural correlates of reexperiencing, avoidance, and dissociation in PTSD: Symptom dimensions and emotion dysregulation in responses to script-driven trauma imagery. *Journal of Trauma and Stress,* **20,** 713–725.

57. Shin, L. M., Orr, S. P., Carson, M. A., *et al.* (2004). Regional cerebral blood flow in the amygdale and medial prefrontal cortex during traumatic imagery in male and female Vietnam veterans with PTSD. *Archives of General Psychiatry,* **61,** 168–176.

58. Felmingham, K., Kemp, A. H., Williams, L. *et al.* (2008). Dissociative responses to conscious and non-conscious fear impact underlying brain function in post-traumatic stress disorder. *Psychological Medicine,* **38,** 1771–1780.

59. Roeder, C. H., Michal, M., Overbeck, G., van de Ven, V. G. and Linden, D. E. J. (2007). Pain response in depersonalization: A functional imaging study using

hypnosis in healthy subjects. *Psychother Psychosom,* **76**, 115–121.

60. Stiglmayr, C., Schmahl, C., Bremmer, J. D., Bohus, M. and Ebner-Priemer, U. (2009). Developement and pshycometric chracteristics of the DSS-4 as a short instrument to assess state dissociative experience during neurophycological experiments. *Psychopathology,* **42**, 370–374.

61. Anderson, M. C., Ochsner, K. N., Kuhl, B. *et al.* (2004). Neural systems underlying the suppression of unwanted memories. *Science,* **303**, 232–235.

62. Hollander, E., Carrasco, J. L., Mullen, L. S. *et al.* (1992). Left hemispheric activation in Depersonalization Disorder: A case report. *Biological Psychiatry,* **31**, 1157–1162.

63. Lemche, E., Surguladze, S. A., Giampietro, V. P., *et al.* (2007). Limbic and prefrontal responses to facial emotion expressions in depersonalization. *Neuroreport,* **18**, 473–477.

64. Sierra, M. and Berrios, G. E. (1998). Depersonalization: Neurobiological perspectives. *Biological Psychiatry,* **44**, 898–908.

65. Lippman, C. W. (1953). Hallucinations of physical duality in migraine. *Journal of Nervous and Mental Disorders,* **117**, 345–350.

66. Green, J. B. (1968). Treatment of epilepsy. *Journal of the Indiana State Medical Association,* **61**, 1118–1119.

67. Devinsky, O., Putnam, F., Grafman, J. *et al.* (1989). Dissociative states and epilepsy. *Neurology,* **39**, 835–840.

68. Blanke, O. (2004). Out of body experiences and their neural basis. *British Medical Journal,* **329**, 1414–1415.

69. Blanke, O. and Arzy, S. (2005). The out-of-body experience: Disturbed self-processing at the temporoparietal junction. *Neuroscientist,* **11**, 16–24.

70. Penfield, W. and Rasmussen, T. (1950). *The cerebral cortex of man: A clinical study of localization of function* (pp. 157–181). New York: Macmillan.

71. Teicher, M. H., Ito, Y., Glod, C. A., Anderson, N. D. and Ackerman, E. (1997). Preliminary evidence for abnormal cortical development in physically and sexually abused children using EEG coherence and MRI. In R. Yehuda and A. C. McFarlane (eds.), *Psychobiology of posttraumatic stress disorder,* Vol. 821 (pp. 160–175). New York: New York Academy of Sciences.

72. Bernstein, E. M. and Putnam, F. W. (1986). Development, reliability, and validity of a dissociation scale. *Journal of Nervous and Mental Disease,* **174**, 727–734.

73. Saxe, G. N., Vasile, R. G., Hill, T. C. *et al.* (1992). SPECT imaging and multiple personality disorder. *Journal of Nervous and Mental Disorders,* **180**, 662–663.

74. Sar, V., Unal, S. N. and Ozturk E. (2007). Frontal and occipital perfusion changes in dissociative identity disorder. *Psychiatry Research,* **156**, 217–223.

75. Reinders, A. A., Nijenhuis, E. R., Quak, J. *et al.* (2006). Psychobiological characteristics of dissociative identity disorder: A symptom provocation study. *Biological Psychiatry,* **60**, 730–740.

76. Vermetten, E., Schmahl, C., Lindner, S., Loewenstein, R. J. and Bremner, J. D. (2006). Hippocampal and amygdalar volumes in dissociative identity disorder. *American Journal of Psychiatry,* **163**, 630–636.

77. Simeon, D., Guralnik, O., Hazlett, E. A. *et al.* (2000). Feeling unreal: A PET study of depersonalization disorder. *American Journal of Psychiatry,* **157**, 1782–1788.

78. Kluft, R. P. (1987). First-rank symptoms as a diagnostic clue to multiple personality disorder. *American Journal of Psychiatry,* **144**, 293–298.

79. Rufer, M., Held, D., Cremer, J. *et al.* (2006).Dissociation as a predictor of cognitive behavior therapy outcome in patient with obsessive-compulsive disorder. *Psychother and Psychosom,* **75**, 40–46.

80. Spitzer, C., Barnow, S., Freyberger, H. J. and Grabe, H. J. (2007). Dissociation predicts symptom-related treatment outcome in short-term inpatient psychotherapy. *Australian and New Zealand Journal of Psychiatry* **41**, 682–687.

81. Kleindienst, N., Limberger M. F., Ebner-Priemer, U. W. *et al.* (2010). Dissociation predicts poor response to dialectical behavioral therapy in female patients with borderline personality disorder. *Journal of Personality Disorders,* in press.

82. Ebner-Priemer, U. W., Badeck, S., Beckmann, C. F. *et al.* (2005).Affective dysregulation and dissociative experience in female patients with borderline personality disorder: A startle response study. *Journal of Psychiatric Research,* **39**, 85–92.

83. Ebner-Priemer, U. W., Mauchnik, J., Kleindienst, N. *et al.* (2009). Emotional learning during dissociative states in borderline personality disorder. *Journal of Psychiatry and Neruoscience,* **34**, 24–22.

84. Jaycox, L. H., Foa, E. B. and Morral, A. R. (1998). Influence of emotional engagement and habituation on exposure therapy for PTSD. *Journal of Consulting and Clinical Psychology,* **66**, 185–192.

85. Cloitre, M., Koenen, K. C., Cohen, L. R. and Han, H. (2002). Skills training in affective and interpersonal regulation followed by exposure: A phase-based treatment for PTSD related to childhood abuse. *Journal of Consulting and Clinical Psychology,* **70**, 1067–1074.

# Chapter 18

# Neurobiological factors underlying psychosocial moderators of childhood stress and trauma

Fatih Ozbay, Vansh Sharma, Joan Kaufman, Bruce McEwen, Dennis Charney and Steven Southwick

## Introduction

Researchers in the field of traumatic stress have traditionally focused on behavioral and neurobiological alterations associated with trauma-related psychopathology. More recently, however, their focus has expanded to include the concept of resilience to extreme stress. The precise definition of stress resilience is a subject of ongoing debate among mental health researchers, in part because defining resilience as the mere absence of psychopathology following exposure to trauma may not capture all aspects of resilience as a multidimensional and complex psychological construct. According to one alternative definition, psychological resilience refers to the ability to maintain a stable equilibrium in the face of adversity [1]. As more fully described below, this ability is actually the product of multiple interacting factors, including genetic, developmental, social, psychological and neurobiological factors. This chapter will discuss resilience as a psychological construct, and then describe some of the neurobiological and psychosocial features that are believed to characterize stress-resilient individuals.

Although many definitions of resilience exist in the literature, one of the most commonly encountered definitions is based on the absence of a diagnosis of post-traumatic stress disorder (PTSD) despite trauma exposure. However, PTSD is not the sole outcome of exposure to traumatic stress [2]. A traumatized individual may develop an anxiety disorder other than PTSD, depression or substance abuse as a result of their exposure. Consequently, equating absence of PTSD with resilience may overestimate resilience.

The quest to understand resilience began approximately three decades ago by developmental psychopathology researchers [3,4] who tried to understand the protective factors moderating the impact of childhood

trauma on mental health outcomes. Childhood maltreatment is known to be associated with a variety of negative outcomes. However, the effects of maltreatment can be reduced by a variety of psychosocial interventions, such as social support, which seem to help to moderate the complex genetic and environmental risk factors for psychopathology.

A number of studies have been conducted to study the protective factors associated with resilience [5]. There is a growing interest in elucidating the mechanisms underlying these moderators and how they attenuate the vulnerabilities caused by trauma exposure in early life. While it has been suggested that there may be developmental periods during which trauma exposure is more likely to cause adverse outcomes [6], there is no evidence that indicates that these outcomes are unavoidable.

In the following sections, we will review the current understanding regarding the neurobiology of stress resilience, including neurocircuitry, neurochemistry and the role of gene–environment interactions. The chapter will conclude with a consideration of information-processing theory and a discussion of the neurobiological basis of social support in the development of stress resilience.

## Neurocircuitry of stress resilience

When an organism detects a threat in its environment, a variety of specific brain structures become activated in order to generate adaptive behavioral responses [7]. Prolonged or repetitive exposure to such threats is known to cause structural changes in the human brain [8]. These changes have been shown to be associated with psychopathology such as memory impairment, anxiety and vulnerability to substance abuse, and also with biochemical changes involving circulating

*The Impact of Early Life Trauma on Health and Disease: The Hidden Epidemic*, ed. Ruth A. Lanius, Eric Vermetten and Clare Pain. Published by Cambridge University Press. Copyright © Cambridge University Press 2010.

hormones and endogenous mediators such as neurotransmitters and neurotropins. The key structures that are thought to be involved in these changes are the amygdala, hypothalamus, hippocampus and prefrontal cortex.

The hypothalamus serves as a regulatory center for maintaining an organism's important homeostatic systems, including complex stress responses [9], and links the central nervous system with the endocrine system via the pituitary gland. The amygdala's role in processing fear and aggression by facilitating endocrine and autonomic responses to stress has been well established [10]. These signals are associated with behavioral responses to stress, including "freezing" in response to danger [11]. Repeated stress is known to cause physical changes in the amygdala, including the remodeling of dendrites and synaptic connections. Interestingly, even a single exposure to traumatic stress may trigger new synapse formation or retraction in the amygdala and cause aggressive and anxious behavior [12]. For example, a single acute immobilization stress in a rat model causes increased density of spine synapses in the amygdala and increased anxiety-like behaviors that can be detected for up to 10 days [13]. Studies conducted in rats exposed to a natural predator (i.e., cat) had similar results [14] and implicated long-lasting changes in behavioral, autonomic and hormonal parameters [15].

The hippocampus is a brain structure that is essential to memory. The hippocampus works together with the amygdala to store information about situational cues ("where we were and what we were doing") present at the time of an emotionally charged event. The hippocampus also plays a key role in spatial navigation and memory, as well as in memories of events in daily life. When an individual is exposed to chronic stress, the hippocampus undergoes structural remodeling; hippocampal cells demonstrate changes in spine synapse density, dendrite branching and length [16]. These changes are accompanied by deficits in hippocampal-dependent memory [17].

The prefrontal cortex acts as a master control region for both autonomic and neuroendocrine responses to stress. Prefrontal cortical processes also serve to limit impulsive behavior and support so-called "executive functions" such as decision making and the shifting of attention to newly relevant stimuli that predict reward or punishment [18]. Repeated stress causes remodeling of prefrontal neuronal dendrites and synaptic connections; these changes are accompanied by

impairment in tests of mental flexibility and attention shifting [19–21]. Dendrites and spines in the prefrontal cortex may even respond rapidly to acute stressors [22]. Although the predominant effect of repeated stress is retraction of dendrites and spines, there is also evidence for stress-induced expansion of dendrites in the orbitofrontal cortex [21].

In addition to the dendritic and other neurohistochemical effects described above, stress also appears to contribute to changes in gross brain structure and volume. Neuroimaging studies of adult brains more than 3 years after September 11, 2001 showed that adults with closer geographical proximity to the site of the disaster had lower gray matter volume in the amygdala, hippocampus, insula, anterior cingulate and medial prefrontal cortex, after controlling for age, gender and total gray matter volume [23].

Repeated exposure to unavoidable stress can lead to "learned helplessness," which can be understood as an acquired sense of futility as opposed to control over one's situation. Learned helplessness is associated with specific neurochemical and structural alterations. For example, recent work has highlighted the importance of downstream inhibitory control of the serotonin system in the midbrain, overactivity of which is a key feature of learned helplessness. Specifically, lesions of the medial prefrontal cortex in rats cause serotonin hyperactivity and learned helplessness behavior even when rats are given the option to control the stressor stimulus [24]. Research in this area suggests that the prefrontal cortex plays an important role in mediating subjective sense of control, which, in turn, appears to be a critical feature of resilience to stress. In the following section, we will consider this and other findings relevant to the neurobiological basis of resilience to stress.

# Neurochemistry of stress resilience

## Autonomic nervous system responses to stress

The autonomic nervous system is responsible for regulating involuntary functions such as heart rate, blood pressure and digestion. When activated by stress, the sympathetic nervous system (SNS) increases heart rate and blood pressure. Some people are prone to demonstrating an unusually strong SNS response to stress; however, the amplitude of SNS activation does not necessarily correspond to greater ability to tolerate adversity. In fact, Dienstbier [25] has suggested that optimal performance under conditions of high stress is associated with relatively low baseline levels of epinephrine in combination with robust challenge-induced increases in epinephrine and norepinephrine, followed by a rapid return to baseline levels.

Neuropeptide Y, an amino acid that is co-released with norepinephrine when the SNS is strongly activated, is thought to play an important role in maintaining SNS activity within this optimal activation range (reviewed by Southwick *et al.* [26]). Morgan *et al.* [27,28] demonstrated that high levels of neuropeptide Y are associated with better performance in highly resilient special operations soldiers (Special Forces) undergoing extremely stressful training procedures. In comparison, combat veterans diagnosed with PTSD showed reduced levels of neuropeptide Y [29].

Another peptide that is involved in neuroendocrine control, cardiovascular regulation and anxiety is galanin, which may also be associated with resilience to stress. Like neuropeptide Y, galanin is coreleased with norepinephrine during periods of high SNS activity. In rats, central administration of galanin reduces neuronal activity at the locus ceruleus, the principal site of norepinephrine synthesis in the brain. When injected into the amygdala, galanin has been shown to block the anxiogenic effects of stress [30,31]. The balance between norepinephrine, neuropeptide Y and galanin helps to determine the overall net effects of SNS hyperactivity, supporting the notion that the regulation of noradrenergic activity within an optimal window may be a neurobiological characteristic of resilience to stress [32].

## Hypothalamic–pituitary–adrenal axis responses to stress

As outlined above, the hypothalamus helps to link the nervous and endocrine systems and plays an important role in physiological responses to stress. As is the case in other endocrine organs, maintenance of a well-regulated homeostatic balance is one of the key functions of the hypothalamus, with dysregulation of this balance potentially contributing to pathology. One such link is hypothalamic–pituitary–adrenal (HPA) axis. The hypothalamus secretes corticotrophin-releasing factor (CRF) in response to acute and chronic stress, and the resultant stimulation of CRF type 1 receptors may cause anxiety-like responses. In contrast, the activation of CRF type 2 receptors has anxiolytic effects

[33,34]. The optimal regulation of these two different types of CRF receptors appears to moderate behavioral and neurobiological responses to stress and may facilitate psychobiological resilience to stress-related disorders such as PTSD and depression.

In addition, CRF stimulates the anterior pituitary gland to synthesize and release adrenocorticotropic hormone (ACTH), which leads to release of adrenal cortisol and dehydroepiandrosterone (DHEA). Cortisol mobilizes and replenishes energy stores, contains the immune response and affects behavior through actions on multiple neurotransmitter systems and brain regions [35]. However, if stress remains chronic, prolonged elevations of cortisol may cause hippocampal damage, as evidenced by reductions in dendritic branching, a loss of dendritic spines and a reduction in the growth of new granule cell neurons in the dentate gyrus [36]. Damage to the hippocampus may weaken its ability to reduce HPA activation, resulting in even greater glucocorticoid levels, and a vicious cycle may ensue.

In contrast to cortisol, DHEA exerts antiglucocorticoid and antiglutamatergic activity in the brain and may confer neuroprotection [37]. The administration of DHEA has an antidepressant effect in patients diagnosed with major depression [38], and numerous studies indicate that DHEA may also play an important role in stress resilience. For example, Morgan *et al.* [39] found a negative relationship between the DHEA/cortisol ratio and dissociation, and a positive correlation between DHEA/cortisol ratio and performance among elite Special Forces soldiers during intensive survival training. Lower DHEA levels have also been shown to be associated with more severe symptoms in women with PTSD [40]. Similarly, allopregnanolone, another neuroactive steroid, exerts negative feedback inhibition on the HPA axis, in addition to its direct anxiolytic effect through interaction with gamma-aminobutyric acid (GABA) type A receptors. Rasmusson *et al.* [41] have demonstrated lower cerebrospinal fluid levels of allopregnanolone in those diagnosed with PTSD compared with controls. In summary, DHEA and allopregnanolone may contribute to stress resilience by helping to terminate HPA activation [42].

Inhibition of the HPA system may underlie another important resilience mechanism termed "stress inoculation," which refers to the "steeling" effects of mild and controlled stress on an individual's capacity to cope with future and possibly harsher stressors. There is a body of animal literature suggesting the protective effects of early exposure to controllable stress in rodents, as evidenced by its association with reduced fear responses to threatening stimuli (reviewed by Dienstbier [43]). Parker et al. [44] showed that stress inoculation via intermittent maternal separation during postnatal weeks 17–27 leads to lower basal plasma ACTH and cortisol, lower stress-induced cortisol levels and diminished anxiety responses upon exposure to a novel environment. Upon reaching 18 months of age, these stress-inoculated monkeys were administered a response inhibition test and were found to have superior prefrontal cortex function as a group compared to non-stress-inoculated monkeys [44]. A study of rescue and recovery workers at the World Trade Center site after September 11, 2001 found a much lower prevalence of PTSD among police officers than in unaffiliated volunteers [45]. One interpretation of these results is that, in contrast to unaffiliated volunteers, police officers were protected from developing PTSD through a stress-inoculation effect conferred by their line of work and training. Taken together, these studies suggest that exposure to mild and controlled stress may moderate the effects of future life stressors via activation of the prefrontal cortex and subsequent inhibition of the HPA system.

While some degree of low-level exposure to stress seems to confer a protective advantage, it is now well established that prolonged or excessive maternal separation leads to hyperactivity of the brain regions and neurotransmitter systems that have been implicated in the pathophysiology of depression and PTSD [46]. For example, prolonged and variable maternal separation causes chronic hyperresponsiveness of the HPA axis and the locus ceruleus/noradrenergic system, which may lead to exaggerated "emotional" reactivity to stress [47]. Exaggerated emotional reactivity during childhood may increase the risk of developing stress-related disorders such as depression and PTSD in adulthood [48]. Consequently, it appears that the "manageability" of stress during development is critical. Uncontrollable stress associated with early deprivation may promote future exaggerated neurobiological stress reactivity (stress sensitization), whereas mild to moderate controllable stress may dampen future stress reactivity (stress inoculation) by influencing the development of stress-related neurobiological systems in distinct ways. Of note, animal adoption studies have shown that even after stress-induced neurobiological and behavioral alterations have occurred, it may still be possible to modify these alterations by subsequent supportive maternal caregiving and/or pharmacological interventions [49,50].

## Stress resilience and gene–environment interactions

The importance of gene–environment interactions in the pathogenesis of mental illness was first conceptualized by Zubin and Spring [51] with their diathesis-stress model, which was developed with an eye toward understanding the etiological factors involved in schizophrenia. According to this model, environmental stressors were considered triggering agents that had the potential to activate disease processes in genetically vulnerable subjects. In order to quantify the extent of genetic vulnerability for a given disorder, the term "heritability" was coined. In statistical genetics, heritability refers to the proportion of variation in a trait that is directly explained by genetic factors. Since the early twentieth century, researchers have used twin studies to ascertain the heritability of schizophrenia and major affective disorders, and these studies have established a firm genetic basis for these syndromes. Several twin studies focusing on Vietnam War veterans have shown that genetic factors play a significant role in PTSD as well. True et al. [52] found that heritability accounted for 32% of the variance in liability for PTSD symptoms in 4042 twin pairs who served in the Vietnam era. In a smaller civilian sample, Stein et al. [53] found an overall heritability estimate for PTSD of 38%. Interestingly, these researchers also reported that many of the genes that modulate susceptibility to PTSD symptoms also appear to influence the likelihood of exposure to assaultive trauma.

The development of commercially available technologies to analyze variations in DNA (genetic polymorphisms) enabled molecular geneticists to begin investigating the associations between specific genes and mental disorders. However, the field of psychiatric genetics, which was once enthusiastically predicted to elucidate the molecular basis of psychiatric illness, has so far largely failed to deliver on this promise. The literature is marked by an abundance of studies with conflicting results. Comings et al. [54] reported an association between combat-related PTSD and the A1 allele of a dopamine $D_2$ receptor gene (DRD2) polymorphism. However, Gelernter et al. [55] were unable to replicate this finding in a larger Vietnam-related PTSD sample and reported a negative association between DRD2 "A" system alleles or DRD2 haplotypes and PTSD. Later on, Young *et al.* [56] reported a significant association between *DRD2* and PTSD with comorbid harmful drinking. A group of investigators focusing on another dopaminergic system gene, the dopamine transporter I, demonstrated an association between the 9-repeat allele of the variable number tandem repeat (VNTR) polymorphism at the SLC6A3 locus and PTSD in a sample of 102 patients with chronic PTSD and 104 trauma survivors who did not develop PTSD [57].

Genetic heterogeneity is thought to complicate the study of specific genetic factors in the pathogenesis of PTSD. According to this view, PTSD is a heterogeneous illness: a syndrome encompassing clinically indistinguishable yet pathophysiologically different disorders. A recent article reporting on a husband–wife couple who were both diagnosed with PTSD after they had been in a car accident illustrates this issue remarkably well by describing their unique symptom presentations and differential brain activation patterns in response to script-driven imagery of the traumatic event [58]. The use of endophenotypes has been suggested when different susceptibility factors are suspected to be associated with the same clinical phenotype. Endophenotypes are constructed to delineate the genetic component of psychopathology by focusing on the dimensional or biological aspects of the disorder, which may be genetically less heterogeneous than the disorder itself. For example, in a study of 100 healthy twin female pairs, investigators showed that the heart rate, skin conductance and blood pressure responses, to socially stressful films were moderately heritable [59]. One example of a genetically mediated variation in sympathetic activity was reported by Finley *et al.* [60], who found that a polymorphism in the gene for the $\alpha_2$-adrenoceptor was associated with autonomic hyperresponsiveness in healthy subjects. Similarly, neuropeptide Y levels during stress exposure have been shown to be affected by a polymorphism in the gene that encodes that molecule [61].

These conflicting results are not unusual in the study of genetically complicated disorders, which are understood to represent the product of environmental factors and a large number of genes, each with a small effect size. The interaction between environmental and genetic factors in the expression of disease is complex, and the true mechanisms underlying these interactions are largely unknown. The environment may affect the expression of genes at different levels. One oft-cited example is phenylketonuria, a hereditary metabolic disorder caused by mutations in the gene that codes for the enzyme responsible for metabolizing the amino acid phenylalanine. One could argue that the heritability estimate of phenylketonuria is 100%, since individuals who are carrying two defective copies of the gene are bound to express the phenotype (autosomal recessive heritance pattern). However, if the individual's diet is devoid of phenylalanine, then the mutation will have no effect in practice. In this case, both the genetic vulnerability (mutation) and the environmental factor (phenylalanine) are required for the full expression of the phenotype.

Unfortunately, the field of molecular genetics has only recently begun to investigate gene–environment interactions as they pertain to psychiatric disorders. The findings of Caspi *et al.* [62] indicating that serotonin transporter promotor polymorphism influences liability for major depression by increasing a person's susceptibility to stressful life events were initially received with great enthusiasm. Consistent with the stress-diathesis model, Caspi *et al.* [62] showed that the long allele of the *5-HTTLPR*, encoding the promotor region, attenuated the effects of stressful life events by decreasing the risk for major depression and suicide attempts. However, a recently published meta-analysis of similar studies that have been conducted since then failed to show that such a relationship between *5-HTTLPR* and stressful life events exists [63]. Focusing on childhood maltreatment, Kaufman *et al.* [64] reported that polymorphisms in the genes for the brain-derived neurotrophic factor (BDNF) and the serotinin transporter, in conjunction with strong social support, cumulatively decrease the risk of developing depression in maltreated children. Maltreatment during childhood increases risk for PTSD later in life, and investigators have recently found that polymorphisms in the FK506 binding protein 5 gene (*FKBP5*) may mediate this risk by enhancing glucocorticoid receptor sensitivity [65], which had previously been reported to be a risk factor for PTSD [66].

These preliminary findings are consistent with the stress-diathesis theory, which proposes that environmental stressors cause psychiatric symptoms only in the presence of genetic or developmental vulnerabilities. Individuals who carry certain alleles may be resilient to the effects of stress and its psychological sequelae. This inherited biological resilience may be considered a first-line defense against the effects of stress and trauma. With the identification of additional resilience genes and description of the mechanisms by which they counter environmental stress, we may be able to conceptualize new biological interventions that can be administered in the immediate aftermath of trauma in order to increase the victim's resilience. To date, the non-selective $\beta$-adrenergic antagonist propranolol is the only medication that has been studied as a prophylactic agent in prevention of PTSD. Two small clinical trials showed that short-term treatment with propranolol following acute trauma was associated with lower incidence of subsequent development of PTSD. Further research is needed to test the efficacy of this and other interventions in secondary prophylaxis of trauma-related psychopathology.

In summary, genetic factors contribute to an individual's capacity to cope with stressful experiences by way of their interaction with environmental factors. The literature suggests that personality traits, trauma exposure history and psychophysiological reactivity may be useful in predicting responses to traumatic experiences. Genetic factors are implicated in the tremendous variation within all of these domains. However, the specific mechanisms that mediate resilience-promoting genes are largely unknown in humans. For example, the resilience-conferring polymorphism in the gene for BDNF (causing Val66Met) has been shown to be associated with superior neuronal integrity in the hippocampus and better performance in episodic memory tests [67]. Future genetic studies focusing on intermediate or endophenotypes of pathology and resilience may better elucidate the gene–environment interactions underlying the biological aspects of resilience.

## Stress resilience and information processing theory

If a neutral stimulus (e.g., an auditory tone) is co-administered with a fear-inducing stimulus (e.g., an electrical shock), the neutral stimulus then becomes a conditioned stimulus and acquires the property of inducing a fear response on its own [68]. Known as "fear conditioning," this process is thought to be a central mechanism in the development of psychopathology following exposure to traumatic stress. For example, driving through a tunnel or under a bridge is normally a neutral stimulus that does not induce fear in the majority of people. However, if a soldier is ambushed under a bridge during combat, the act of driving under a bridge may acquire the property of inducing a strong fear response at a later time. Ordinarily, continued

exposure to a conditioned stimulus (driving under a bridge) in the absence of a naturally fear-inducing stimulus (getting ambushed) will lead to the formation of a new memory, which will abolish the fear response to the conditioned stimulus. This is known as "fear extinction" and serves as the basis for exposure-based therapies in the treatment of a variety of anxiety disorders, including phobias and PTSD [69].

Resilience may be conceptualized as a tendency to be resistant to fear conditioning and/or a propensity to acquire fear extinction quickly and efficiently after exposure to a traumatic event. Various animal models have been studied in order to explore the neuroanatomical basis of fear conditioning. Currently, the hippocampus, amygdala and anterior cingulate cortex are considered the key brain structures involved in processing fear conditioning and extinction in humans [70,71]. Upon exposure to conditioned stimuli, the central nucleus of the amygdala sends information to the brainstem and thereby initiates certain stereotyped fear responses, such as freezing, elevated heart rate and increased skin conductance. LeDoux and Gorman [72] have posited that active coping with the reminders of a traumatic event may dampen the conditioned fear response by engaging a different part of the amygdala, the basal nucleus, which sends information to the ventral striatum as opposed to the brainstem. Based on this view, it can be surmised that optimal activation of the basal amygdala is associated with resilience and with active coping rather than the display of disabling conditioned fear responses.

Using a laboratory-based fear conditioning and extinction paradigm, investigators recently found that unmedicated subjects with PTSD more easily acquire and more slowly extinguish conditioned fear responses than control subjects [73]. Guthrie and Bryant [74] followed a cohort of police officers during their training and first 2 years of service and prospectively showed that faster extinction of a conditioned fear response predicted a reduced risk for post-traumatic stress. These results are consistent with the hypothesis that efficient fear extinction may protect an individual against the psychological sequelae of trauma and serve to enhance resilience.

Another putative resilience mechanism in the information-processing domain may be cognitive flexibility. Positive reframing, or reappraisal, refers to the ability to reinterpret an adverse or negative event so as to find meaning and opportunity, and it has been linked to decreased likelihood of developing PTSD in combat veterans [75], better adjustment after loss of a family member [76], and reductions in plasma concentrations of the stress hormone cortisol among women in the early stages of breast cancer [77].

# The neurobiological basis of social support in stress resilience

Social support has been studied extensively in relation to both stress and resilience. Theoretical models providing a conceptual understanding of social support are complex and well beyond the scope of this chapter. However, structural (i.e., network size) and functional dimensions are more readily described and utilized in the description of social support [78]. Numerous studies have shown that social support is associated with positive mental and physical health outcomes in diverse populations, including unemployed workers, caregivers of patients with Alzheimer's disease, and parents of seriously ill children. Mitchinson *et al.* [79] found that people with more active friendship networks had less preoperative anxiety and required less postoperative analgesic medication.

Clinical studies focusing on traumatic stress clearly demonstrate the beneficial effects of social support on current mental health. For example, Boscarino [80] found that, after controlling for trauma exposure, veterans with high social support were 1.8 times less likely to develop PTSD compared with those with low social support. Elucidating the biological basis of the effects of social support is crucial to understanding the neural underpinnings of resilience. The following section aims to provide a neurobiological framework with which to approach social support based on existing preclinical and translational studies. We will first briefly review the literature on the neurochemistry of formation and maintenance of social attachment and then look at the effects of social support on stress-induced changes at the behavioral and neuroendocrinological levels. Finally, we will speculate on ways in which the neurobiology underlying these effects can be exploited in order to enhance resilience.

The neuropeptides oxytocin and vasopressin have been extensively studied regarding their role in regulation of social attachment and promotion of positive social interactions [81]. The type and duration of social attachments formed by voles (field mice) heavily depend on differential oxytocin and vasopressin receptor expression patterns in the ventral pallidum and medial amygdala. For example, montane voles

native to mountainous regions of the western USA typically avoid social contact except while mating, and have lower levels of oxytocin receptors in the nucleus accumbens compared with prairie voles, which are highly social and typically monogamous [82]. Oxytocin is critical for learning social cues and enhances maternal care in rats [83]. Furthermore, oxytocin has anxiolytic effects that are associated with attenuated secretion of ACTH and corticosterone in lactating rodents and humans alike [84]. A recent study showed that oxytocin potentiated the calming effects of social support in healthy men undergoing the Trier Social Stress Test [85]. Thus, neuropeptides such as oxytocin and vasopressin appear not only to promote social attachment but also to mediate the anxiolytic effects of social support.

In contrast, preclinical studies suggest that social isolation is associated with elevated heart rate and blood pressure, hypercortisolemia and atherosclerosis [86]. Results from human studies are consistent with these results: low social support has been shown to be associated with exaggerated cardiovascular and neuroendocrine responses to laboratory stressors [87]. There is also a vast animal literature supporting a critical role for social support in normal development and moderation of early life stressors (for a thorough review see Kaufman *et al.* [48]). It has been well established in rodent and primate models that early maternal separation is associated with heightened stress sensitivity, as evidenced by enhanced release of ACTH and cerebrospinal norepinephrine [88] in response to acute stress, in addition to decreased inhibitory GABAergic tone [49]. In rhesus monkeys, early social deprivation induces cognitive impairment and enhanced anxiety in adult life [89]. Interestingly, subsequent supportive maternal caregiving may reverse neurobiological and behavioral alterations induced by early social deprivation. These alterations, most notably HPA axis sensitization, may also be reversed by a variety of psychotropic agents including selective serotonin reuptake inhibitors. Cross-fostering experiments indicate that increased handling and maternal care may also reduce stress sensitivity associated with heritable factors in rats. Taken together, these studies suggest that social support is an important resilience factor that may moderate the gene–environment interactions in the expression of stress response and the ensuing allostatic load.

The literature suggests that neurobiological factors play a role both in forming social attachments and in mediating the beneficial effects of social support on reversing stress-related behavioral and neuroendocrine changes. Moreover, it may be possible to enhance resilience in at-risk individuals by providing nurturing environments and/or by administering pharmacological agents that stabilize HPA axis functioning. For example, following exposure to traumatic stress, blockade of CRF overdrive with CRF antagonists may contain the allostatic load and prevent stress-related psychopathology.

## Conclusions

In this chapter we have traced the concept of stress resilience to its origins in the developmental psychopathology literature and have seen how resilience has come to be understood as the ability to maintain equilibrium in the face of adversity, as opposed to merely avoiding the development of psychopathology. The neurocircuitry of stress resilience consists of a variety of brain structures intimately involved in mediating the stress response, including the amygdala, hypothalamus, hippocampus and prefrontal cortex. The neurochemistry of stress resilience can be understood in terms of two major endogenous mechanisms for responding to stress: the autonomic nervous system along with its various neuropeptide modulators, and the HPA axis. Gene–environment interactions, as typified by the diathesis-stress model of illness, are important factors in the development of stress resilience, and further research is needed to begin to elucidate the specific mechanisms underlying resilience-promoting genes.

5. Charney, D. S. and Manji, H. K. (2004). Life stress, genes, and depression: Multiple pathways lead to increased risk and new opportunities for intervention. *Science's STKE,* (2004) 225, re5.

6. McClellan, J., McCurry, C., Ronnei, M. *et al.* (1996). Age of onset of sexual abuse: Relationship to sexually inappropriate behaviors. *Journal of the American Academy of Child and Adolescent Psychiatry,* **35,** 1375–1383.

7. Mesches, M. H., Fleshner, M., Heman, K. L., Rose, G. M. and Diamond, D. M. (1999). Exposing rats to a predator blocks primed burst potentiation in the hippocampus in vitro. *Journal of Neuroscience,* **19,** RC18.

8. Vyas, A., Mitra, R., Shankaranarayana Rao, B. S. and Chattarji, S. (2002). Chronic stress induces contrasting patterns of dendritic remodeling in hippocampal and amygdaloid neurons. *Journal of Neuroscience,* **22,** 6810–6818.

9. Ehlert, U., Gaab, J. and Heinrichs, M. (2001). Psychoneuroendocrinological contributions to the etiology of depression, posttraumatic stress disorder, and stress-related bodily disorders: The role of the hypothalamus–pituitary–adrenal axis. *Biological Psychology,* **57,** 141–152.

10. Goldstein, L. E., Rasmusson, A. M., Bunney, B. S. and Roth, R. H. (1996). Role of the amygdala in the coordination of behavioral, neuroendocrine, and prefrontal cortical monoamine responses to psychological stress in the rat. *Journal of Neuroscience,* **16,** 4787–4798.

11. LeDoux, J. E. (1996). *The emotional brain: The mysterious underpinnings of emotional life.* New York: Simon & Schuster.

12. McEwen, B. S. and Chattarji, S. (2004). Molecular mechanisms of neuroplasticity and pharmacological implications: The example of tianeptine. *European Neuropsychopharmacology,* **14**(Suppl 5), S497–S502.

13. Mitra, R., Jadhav, S., McEwen, B. S., Vyas, A. and Chattarji, S. (2005). Stress duration modulates the spatiotemporal patterns of spine formation in the basolateral amygdala. *Proceedings of the National Academy of Sciences USA,* **102,** 9371–9376.

14. Adamec, R. E., Burton, P., Shallow, T. and Budgell, J. (1998). NMDA receptors mediate lasting increases in anxiety-like behavior produced by the stress of predator exposure: Implications for anxiety associated with posttraumatic stress disorder. *Physiology & Behavior,* **65,** 723–737.

15. Korte, S. M., Koolhaas, J. M., Wingfield, J. C. and McEwen, B. S. (2005). The darwinian concept of stress: Benefits of allostasis and costs of allostatic load and the trade-offs in health and disease. *Neuroscience and Biobehavioral Reviews,* **29,** 3–38.

16. McEwen, B. S. (1999). Stress and hippocampal plasticity. *Annual Review of Neuroscience,* **22,** 105–122.

processes in development. *American Psychologist,* 56, 227–238.

17. Conrad, C. D., LeDoux, J. E., Magariños, A. M. and McEwen, B. S. (1999). Repeated restraint stress facilitates fear conditioning independently of causing hippocampal CA3 dendritic atrophy. *Behavioral Neuroscience,* **113,** 902–913.

18. Damasio, A. R. (1997). Towards a neuropathology of emotion and mood. *Nature,* **386,** 769–770.

19. Wellman, C. L. (2001). Dendritic reorganization in pyramidal neurons in medial prefrontal cortex after chronic corticosterone administration. *Journal of Neurobiology,* **49,** 245–253.

20. Radley, J. J., Rocher, A. B., Janssen, W. G. M. *et al.* (2005). Reversibility of apical dendritic retraction in the rat medial prefrontal cortex following repeated stress. *Experimental Neurology,* **196,** 199–203.

21. Liston, C., Miller, M. M., Goldwater, D. S. *et al.* (2006). Stress-induced alterations in prefrontal cortical dendritic morphology predict selective impairments in perceptual attentional set-shifting. *Journal of Neuroscience,* **26,** 7870–7874.

22. Izquierdo, A., Wellman, C. L. and Holmes, A. (2006). Brief uncontrollable stress causes dendritic retraction in infralimbic cortex and resistance to fear extinction in mice. *Journal of Neuroscience,* **26,** 5733–5738.

23. Ganzel, B. L., Kim, P., Glover, G. H. and Temple, E. (2008). Resilience after 9/11: Multimodal neuroimaging evidence for stress-related change in the healthy adult brain. *Neuroimage,* **40,** 788–795.

24. Amat, J., Baratta, M. V., Paul, E. *et al.* (2005). Medial prefrontal cortex determines how stressor controllability affects behavior and dorsal raphe nucleus. *Nature Neuroscience,* **8,** 365–371.

25. Dienstbier, R. A. (1991). Behavioral correlates of sym-pathoadrenal reactivity: The toughness model. *Medicine and Science in Sports and Exercise,* **23,** 846–852.

26. Southwick, S. M., Bremner, J. D., Rasmusson, A. *et al.* (1999). Role of norepinephrine in the pathophysiology and treatment of posttraumatic stress disorder. *Biological Psychiatry,* **46,** 1192–1204.

27. Morgan, C. A. III, Rasmusson, A. M., Wang, S. *et al.* (2002). Neuropeptide-Y, cortisol, and subjective distress in humans exposed to acute stress: Replication and extension of previous report. *Biological Psychiatry,* **52,** 136–142.

28. Morgan, C. A., III, Wang, S., Southwick, S. M. *et al.* (2000). Plasma neuropeptide-Y concentrations in humans exposed to military survival training. *Biological Psychiatry,* **47,** 902–909.

29. Rasmusson, A. M., Hauger, R. L., Morgan, C. A., III *et al.* (2000). Low baseline and yohimbine-stimulated plasma neuropeptide Y (NPY) levels in combat-related PTSD. *Biological Psychiatry,* **47,** 526–539.

30. Bing, O., Moller, C., Engel, J. A., Soderpalm, B. and Heilig, M. (1993). Anxiolytic-like action of centrally administered galanin. *Neuroscience Letters,* **164,** 17–20.

31. Möller, C., Sommer, W., Thorsell, A. and Heilig, M. (1999). Anxiogenic-like action of galanin after intra-amygdala administration in the rat. *Neuro-psychopharmacology,* **21,** 507–512.

32. Yehuda, R., Brand, S. and Yang, R. K. (2006). Plasma neuropeptide Y concentrations in combat exposed veterans: Relationship to trauma exposure, recovery from PTSD, and coping. *Biological Psychiatry,* **59,** 660–663.

33. Bale, T. L., Contarino, A., Smith, G. W. *et al.* (2000). Mice deficient for corticotropin-releasing hormone receptor-2 display anxiety-like behaviour and are hypersensitive to stress. *Nature Genetics,* **24,** 410–414.

34. Bale, T. L., Picetti, R., Contarino, A. *et al.* (2002). Mice deficient for both corticotropin-releasing factor receptor 1 (CRFR1) and CRFR2 have an impaired stress response and display sexually dichotomous anxiety-like behavior. *Journal of Neuroscience,* **22,** 193–199.

35. Yehuda, R. (2002). Current status of cortisol findings in post-traumatic stress disorder. *Psychiatric Clinics of North America,* **25,** 341–368.

36. Sapolsky, R. M. (2003). Stress and plasticity in the limbic system. *Neurochemical Research,* **28,** 1735–1742.

37. Charney, D. S. (2004). Psychobiological mechanism of resilience and vulnerability: Implications for successful adaptation to extreme stress. *American Journal of Psychiatry,* **161,** 195–216.

38. Wolkowitz, O. M., Reus, V. I., Keebler, A. *et al.* (1999). Double-blind treatment of major depression with dehydroepiandrosterone. *American Journal of Psychiatry,* **156,** 646–649.

39. Morgan, C. A., III, Southwick, S., Hazlett, G. *et al.* (2004). Relationships among plasma dehydroepian-drosterone sulfate and cortisol levels, symptoms of dissociation, and objective performance in humans exposed to acute stress. *Archives of General Psychiatry,* **61,** 819–825.

40. Rasmusson, A. M., Vasek, J., Lipschitz, D. S. *et al.* (2004). An increased capacity for adrenal DHEA release is associated with decreased avoidance and negative mood symptoms in women with PTSD. *Neuropsychopharmacology,* **29,** 1546–1557.

41. Rasmusson, A. M., Pinna, G., Paliwal, P. *et al.* (2006). Decreased cerebrospinal fluid allopregnanolone levels in women with posttraumatic stress disorder. *Biological Psychiatry,* **60,** 704–713.

42. Yehuda, R., Brand, S. R., Golier, J. A. and Yang, R. K. (2006). Clinical correlates of DHEA associated with post-traumatic stress disorder. *Acta Psychiatrica Scandinavica,* **114,** 187–193.

43. Dienstbier, R. A. (1989). Arousal and physiological toughness: Implications for mental and physical health. *Psychological Review,* **96,** 84–100.

44. Parker, K. J., Buckmaster, C. L., Schatzberg, A. F. and Lyons, D. M. (2004). Prospective investigation of stress

inoculation in young monkeys. *Archives of General Psychiatry, 61*, 933–941.

45. Perrin, M. A., DiGrande, L., Wheeler, K. *et al.* (2007). Differences in PTSD prevalence and associated risk factors among world trade center disaster rescue and recovery workers. *American Journal of Psychiatry, 164*, 1385–1394.

46. Southwick, S. M., Vythilingam, M. and Charney, D. S., III (2005). The psychobiology of depression and resilience to stress: Implications for prevention and treatment. *Annual Review of Clinical Psychology, 1*, 255–291.

47. Bremner, J. D. and Vermetten, E. (2001). Stress and development: Behavioral and biological consequences. *Development and Psychopathology, 13*, 473–489.

48. Kaufman, J., Plotsky, P. M., Nemeroff, C. B. and Charney, D. S. (2000). Effects of early adverse experiences on brain structure and function: Clinical implications. *Biological Psychiatry, 48*, 778–790.

49. Caldji, C., Tannenbaum, B., Sharma, S., *et al.* (1998). Maternal care during infancy regulates the development of neural systems mediating the expression of fearfulness in the rat. *Proceedings of the National Academy of Sciences USA, 95*, 5335–5340.

50. Kuhn, C. M. and Schanberg, S. M. (1998). Responses to maternal separation: Mechanisms and mediators. *International Journal of Developmental Neuroscience, 16*, 261–270.

51. Zubin, J. and Spring, B. (1977). Vulnerability: A new view of schizophrenia. *Journal of Abnormal Psychology, 86*, 103–126.

52. True, W. R., Rice, J., Eisen, S. A. *et al.* (1993). A twin study of genetic and environmental contributions to liability for posttraumatic stress symptoms. *Archives of General Psychiatry, 50*, 257–264.

53. Stein, M. B., Jang, K. L., Taylor, S., Vernon, P. A. and Livesley, W. J. (2002). Genetic and environmental influences on trauma exposure and posttraumatic stress disorder symptoms: A twin study. *American Journal of Psychiatry, 159*, 1675–1681.

54. Comings, D. E., Muhleman, D. and Gysin, R. (1996). Dopamine D2 receptor (DRD2) gene and susceptibility to posttraumatic stress disorder: A study and replication. *Biological Psychiatry, 40*, 368–372.

55. Gelernter, J., Southwick, S., Goodson, S. *et al.* (1999). No association between D2 dopamine receptor (DRD2) "A" system alleles, or DRD2 haplotypes, and posttraumatic stress disorder. *Biological Psychiatry, 45*, 620–625.

56. Young, R. M., Lawford, B. R., Noble, E. P. *et al.* (2002). Harmful drinking in military veterans with posttraumatic stress disorder: Association with the D2 dopamine receptor A1 allele. *Alcohol and Alcoholism, 37*, 451–456.

57. Segman, R. H., Cooper-Kazaz, R., Macciardi, F. *et al.* (2002). Association between the dopamine transporter gene and posttraumatic stress disorder. *Molecular Psychiatry, 7*, 903–907.

58. Lanius, R. A., Hopper, J. W. and Menon, R. S. (2003). Individual differences in a husband and wife who developed PTSD after a motor vehicle accident: A functional MRI case study. *American Journal of Psychiatry, 160*, 667–669.

59. Lensvelt-Mulders, G. and Hettema, J. (2001). Genetic analysis of autonomic reactivity to psychologically stressful situations. *Biological Psychology, 58*, 25–40.

60. Finley, J. C. Jr., O'Leary, M., Wester, D. *et al.* (2004). A genetic polymorphism of the alpha2-adrenergic receptor increases autonomic responses to stress. *Journal of Applied Physiology: Respiratory, Environmental and Exercise Physiology, 96*, 2231–2239.

61. Kallio, J., Pesonen, U., Kaipio, K. *et al.* (2001). Altered intracellular processing and release of neuropeptide Y due to leucine 7 to proline 7 polymorphism in the signal peptide of preproneuropeptide Y in humans. *FASEB Journal, 15*, 1242–1244.

62. Caspi, A., Sugden, K., Moffitt, T. E. *et al.* (2003). Influence of life stress on depression: Moderation by a polymorphism in the 5-HTT gene. *Science, 301*, 386–389.

63. Risch, N., Herrell, R., Lehner, T. *et al.* (2009). Interaction between the serotonin transporter gene (5-HTTLPR), stressful life events, and risk of depression: A meta-analysis. *Journal of the American Medical Association, 301*, 2462–2471.

64. Kaufman, J., Yang, B. Z., Douglas-Palumberi, H. *et al.* (2006). Brain-derived neurotrophic factor-5–HTTLPR gene interactions and environmental modifiers of depression in children. *Biological Psychiatry, 59*, 673–680.

65. Binder, E. B., Bradley, R. G., Liu, W. *et al.* (2008). Association of FKBP5 polymorphisms and childhood abuse with risk of posttraumatic stress disorder symptoms in adults. *Journal of the American Medical Association, 299*, 1291–1305.

66. Yehuda, R., Golier, J. A., Yang, R. K. and Tischler, L. (2004). Enhanced sensitivity to glucocorticoids in peripheral mononuclear leukocytes in posttraumatic stress disorder. *Biological Psychiatry, 55*, 1110–1116.

67. Egan, M. F., Kojima, M., Callicott, J. H. *et al.* (2003). The BDNF Val66Met polymorphism affects activity-dependent secretion of BDNF and human memory and hippocampal function. *Cell, 112*, 257–269.

68. Lavond, D. G. and Steinmetz, J. E. (2003). *Handbook of classical conditioning.* Boston, MA: Kluwer Academic.

69. Hermans, D., Craske, M. G., Mineka, S. and Lovibond, P. F. (2006). Extinction in human fear conditioning. *Biological Psychiatry, 60*, 361–368.

70. Bremner, J. D., Vermetten, E., Schmahl, C. *et al.* (2005). Positron emission tomographic imaging of neural

correlates of a fear acquisition and extinction paradigm in women with childhood sexual-abuse-related post-traumatic stress disorder. *Psychological Medicine, 35*, 791–806.

71. Buchel, C., Dolan, R. J., Armony, J. L. and Friston, K. J. (1999). Amygdala-hippocampal involvement in human aversive trace conditioning revealed through event-related functional magnetic resonance imaging. *Journal of Neuroscience, 19*, 10869–10876.

72. LeDoux, J. E. and Gorman, J. M. (2001). A call to action: Overcoming anxiety through active coping. *American Journal of Psychiatry, 158*, 1953–1955.

73. Orr, S. P., Metzger, L. J., Lasko, N. B. *et al.* (2000). De novo conditioning in trauma-exposed individuals with and without posttraumatic stress disorder. *Journal of Abnormal Psychology, 109*, 290–298.

74. Guthrie, R. M. and Bryant, R. A. (2006). Extinction learning before trauma and subsequent posttraumatic stress. *Psychosomatic Medicine, 68*, 307–311.

75. Aldwin, C. M., Levenson, M. R. and Spiro, A., III. (1994). Vulnerability and resilience to combat exposure: Can stress have lifelong effects? *Psychology and Aging, 9*, 34–44.

76. Davis, C. G., Wortman, C. B., Lehman, D. R. and Silver, R. C. (2000). Searching for meaning in loss: Are clinical assumptions correct. *Death Studies, 24*, 497–540.

77. Cruess, D. G., Antoni, M. H., McGregor, B. A., *et al.* (2000). Cognitive-behavioral stress management reduces serum cortisol by enhancing benefit finding among women being treated for early stage breast cancer. *Psychosomatic Medicine, 62*, 304–308.

78. Travis, L. A., Lyness, J. M., Shields, C. G., King, D. A. and Cox, C. (2004). Social support, depression, and functional disability in older adult primary-care patients. *American Journal of Geriatric Psychatry, 12*, 265–271.

79. Mitchinson, A. R., Kim, H. M., Geisser, M., Rosenberg, J. M. and Hinshaw, D. B. (2008). Social connectedness and patient recovery after major operations. *Journal of the American College of Surgeons, 206*, 292–300.

80. Boscarino, J. A. (1995). Post-traumatic stress and associated disorders among vietnam veterans: The significance of combat exposure and social support. *Journal of Traumatic Stress, 8*, 317–336.

81. Bartz, J. A. and Hollander, E. (2006). The neuroscience of affiliation: Forging links between basic and clinical research on neuropeptides and social behavior. *Hormones and Behavior, 50*, 518–528.

82. Insel, T. R. and Shapiro, L. E. (1992). Oxytocin receptor distribution reflects social organization in monogamous and polygamous voles. *Proceedings of the National Academy of Sciences USA, 89*, 5981–5985.

83. Francis, D. D., Champagne, F. C. and Meaney, M. J. (2000). Variations in maternal behaviour are associated with differences in oxytocin receptor levels in the rat. *Journal of Neuroendocrinology, 12*, 1145–1148.

84. Neumann, I. D., Torner, L. and Wigger, A. (2000). Brain oxytocin: Differential inhibition of neuroendocrine stress responses and anxiety-related behaviour in virgin, pregnant and lactating rats. *Neuroscience, 95*, 567–575.

85. Heinrichs, M., Baumgartner, T., Kirschbaum, C. and Ehlert, U. (2003). Social support and oxytocin interact to suppress cortisol and subjective responses to psychosocial stress. *Biological Psychiatry, 54*, 1389–1398.

86. Rozanski, A., Blumenthal, J. A. and Kaplan, J. (1999). Impact of psychological factors on the pathogenesis of cardiovascular disease and implications for therapy. *Circulation, 99*, 2192–2217.

87. Phillips, A. C., Gallagher, S. and Carroll, D. (2009). Social support, social intimacy, and cardiovascular reactions to acute psychological stress. *Annals of Behavioral Medicine, 37*, 38–45.

88. Ladd, C. O., Thrivikraman, K. V., Huot, R. L. and Plotsky, P. M. (2005). Differential neuroendocrine responses to chronic variable stress in adult Long Evans rats exposed to handling–maternal separation as neonates. *Psychoneuroendocrinology, 30*, 520–533.

89. Sanchez, M. M., Hearn, E. F., Do, D., Rilling, J. K. and Herndon, J. G. (1998). Differential rearing affects corpus callosum size and cognitive function of rhesus monkeys. *Brain Research, 812*, 38–49.

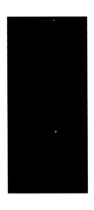

# Part 4 synopsis

Sonia J. Lupien

## Overview

A colleague of mine once told me a story that keeps coming to my mind each time I read or work on the topic of early adversity on psychobiology, brain development and cognitive process. He was at a cocktail party with family members and friends and, while talking to a group of people, he overheard his brother talking about his parents and family life to another group of people. His brother was describing how difficult his childhood had been, and how sometimes neglectful his parents had been. He stated that this has had a serious impact on his capacity to regulate his emotions and was attributing the presence of his anxiety disorder to the parenting style of his parents. My colleague told me that, when he heard his brother's story, he felt that his brother was not describing their parents accurately, as he had a completely different experience of his early childhood. He considered his parents to be good, close to their children and attentive to their needs. He had never seen his parents neglectful or harsh with his brothers and sisters, and he did not understand his bother's point of view. He finished his story by telling me that he could not understand how two brothers growing up in the same family could have such different interpretations of their experience.

Without knowing it, my colleague was summarizing in a short story the intricate relationships that exist between genes, environment and development. The five chapters in this section provide a thorough examination of the biological, developmental and cognitive processes that can result from exposure to adverse environments.

In Ch. 14, Skelton and colleagues emphasize the importance of using a developmental neurobiological model in understanding gene environment ($G \times E$) interactions. Here, they state that there is a general tendency in the genetic literature to organize data primarily on the bases of specific candidate genes rather than on key neural systems and/or related developmental neurobiology. Yet, it is clear from their review of the literature that different expression of genes from exposure to different environments may also depend on the timing of exposure to these various environments. This results in a broadening of the $G \times E$ model, to a $G \times E \times$ development model. Indeed, exposure to a stressful environment in a very young child may have a different effect on the expression of a given gene when compared with exposure to the *same* environment in an older child. Almost no studies to this day have assessed this important factor and yet the various studies reported in Ch. 14 would tend to suggest that such a dissociation of $G \times E$ effects may strongly depend on the developmental stage of the individual being exposed to the stressful environment.

The authors of Ch. 14 go on to remind us that at each developmental stage there may be an epigenetic mechanism by which environmental cues can alter gene expression. Studies on developmental cognitive processes in children demonstrate that the interpretation of events depend on the age of the child. Consequently, it may be possible that the impact (negative or positive) of a given environmental factor has different epigenetic effects as a function of the developmental stage of the child when exposed to the event. The addition of a developmental factor into the $G \times E$ equation of early adversity on neurobiology and behavior could explain how two brothers raised in the same family environment can experience such strikingly different outcomes (and/or interpretations) as a result of their early childhood experiences. This could also occur because the neurobiological systems that respond to stressful life events may be differentially sensitive as a function of the developmental stage at which these events occur.

*The Impact of Early Life Trauma on Health and Disease: The Hidden Epidemic*, ed. Ruth A. Lanius, Eric Vermetten and Clare Pain. Published by Cambridge University Press. Copyright © Cambridge University Press 2010.

The utilization of a $G \times E \times$ development model could also help shed light on the intriguing study reported in Ch. 14 in which children's cortisol response to an intervention aiming at improving parenting skills in mothers was shown to be dependent upon the presence of the 7-repeat allele in the *DRD4* gene (encoding a dopamine receptor) in a group of children [1]. In this study, many children were exposed to the same situation/environment (here, the intervention) and yet only some of them benefited from this positive environment, an effect that seemed to depend upon the presence of a genetic variation. Here again, I think of my colleague's story. Two brothers with potentially different genes and raised in a similar environment and yet one of them becomes an adult with severe anxiety disorder and the other is resilient.

However, there is an important difference between growing up in an "ordinary family environment" (with parents who are often stressed out by their jobs, in a family where there can sometimes be conflicts or separation, and with brothers and sisters that can be stressors by themselves) and growing up in a highly adverse environment characterized by emotional, physical and/or sexual abuse. In Ch. 15 LaPrairie and colleagues show that exposure to such levels of adversity can effect the neurobiology of the endocrine systems responding to stress/threat (hypothalamic–pituitary–adrenal [HPA] system, the autonomic system and the corticotropin–releasing factor [CRF] system), and can influence mental health. What is interesting to note in this chapter is the implication of the corticotrpin-relating factor (CRF) involvement in the etiology of mental health disorders resulting from childhood trauma (depression, and anxiety/post-traumatic stress disorder [PTSD]). The authors note that most human studies, for ethical reasons, are correlational by nature. However, the involvement of the CRF system in the development of these stress-related disorders in adulthood has been well described in rodent and primate studies using experimental models, lending credence to the importance of the CRF system in the etiology of these disorders. In most of these animal and human studies, results point toward a pituitary CRF receptor downregulation subsequent to hypersecretion of CRF from the hypothalamus in response to exposure to chronic early adversity.

What is interesting to note here is the report that children reared by mothers diagnosed with a psychiatric illness also exhibit this pattern of exaggerated adrenocorticotropic hormone activation in response to CRF challenge, compared with children raised by mothers with no psychiatric illness [2]. Although growing up in a family in which a parent suffers from a serious mental health disorder may be quite stressful, it is unclear at this point whether this by itself constitutes an adverse experience that can be of similar magnitude to physical or sexual abuse or whether the neuroendocrine pattern observed in the children of psychiatrically ill individuals may also be associated with genetic susceptibility. As underlined by the authors themselves, there is a great need at this point to study the nature (rather than just the magnitude) of exposure to early adverse experiences on the patterns of neuroendocrine dysruptions in children and adults.

Since the early 1990s, researchers working on the effects of early adversity on neuroendocrine function, brain development and cognition have provided a wealth of empirical data on the effects of early adversity on these diverse functions. Consequently, we now have a large database on this issue, but we are in great need of a model to explain (and then predict) the different outcomes that can result from exposure to early adversity. In order to be able to predict outcomes with good efficacy, this model should integrate the neurobiology of the stress system, along with the cognitive processes that develop over time and that can be affected by increased production of stress hormones. Chapters 16 and 17 provide two very interesting models that integrate these different factors.

In Ch. 16, Bremner and colleagues propose a model describing the neural circuitry of traumatic stress, a model that also integrates cognitive processes. What is very interesting about this model is that it proposes a chronological process by which information can be cognitively processed as being potentially "dangerous," leading to neurobiological activation and behavioral consequences. For each of these steps, Bremner and colleagues propose different brain regions that could be involved in this process. The authors' model suggests that the first step in the process underlying the neural circuitry of traumatic stress is the cognitive appraisal of a situation as being threatening. Here again, it is important to note that the nature and/or magnitude of cognitive appraisal, as suggested in Ch. 15, can be modulated by the age of the child and/or by early exposure to adverse events. Ch. 16 describes once the threat information is encoded, the formation of a memory trace, a process that is sustained by complex interactions between the amygdala, the hippocampus and the prefrontal cortex. At this point, the frontal regions will modulate the emotional responsiveness through inhibition of amygdala function. Failure to do so, as suggested in Chs. 16 and 17, can result in a hypersensitivity or hyposensitivity to emotional cues. Based on this evaluation, there will then be the preparation of the stress response, involving both central and peripheral processes. Here, it is interesting to note the recent paper of Pruessner and colleagues [3] who have shown that cognitive appraisal of a stress within the scanning environment leads to inhibition of frontal regions. The authors state that this inhibition can be the triggering factor inducing activation of the HPA response, given the inhibitory role-played by the prefrontal cortex on activity of the HPA axis. These data support the neural circuit of traumatic stress proposed by Bremner and colleagues in Ch. 16.

The second model is proposed by Schmahl and colleagues in Ch. 17. This model proposes a biological framework for traumatic dissociation related to early life trauma. This is a very interesting model based on the interaction between the cortical region (particularly frontal regions) and limbic regions (particularly the amygdala). The authors base the first part of their model on Bremner's assumption that there are two subtypes of acute trauma response that can lead to two different types of dissociative process. The first one, called primary dissociation, involves intrusions and hyperarousal, while the second one, called secondary dissociation, involves mostly symptoms such as numbness, amnesia, detachment states, depersonalization, subjective distance and others. The main point made by Schmahl and colleagues is that the occurrence of one or the other type of dissociative process in any given individual exposed to an acute trauma could be related to the close connections that exist between frontal and amygdala regions. As stated above, the frontal cortex usually acts by inhibiting amygdala function. Here, the authors suggest that primary dissociation, where there is the presence of hyperarousal and vigilance, could result from a failure of this corticolimbic inhibition such that a hypoactive frontal cortex fails to inhibit amygdala activity adequately, which results in increased amygdala function and hyperarousal toward potentially threatening information. In contrast, in cases of secondary dissociation, there may be excessive corticolimbic inhibition such that a hyperactive frontal cortex acts by overinhibiting the activity of the amygdala, leading to feelings of numbness and detachment states. This model could have the potential to explain and predict vulnerability to primary or secondary dissociative

disorder in response to acute trauma. It will be important to further test this model and determine potential modulator factors (age, gender, etc.) that could act on this corticolimbic inhibition process.

Another very interesting point made by Schmahl and colleagues is the fact that in some cases the development of a dissociative process in the face of acute trauma could serves as a developmental protective and resilience factor. There could be some neurobiological and/or cognitive mechanisms that act at the time of trauma to protect the developing system. I think about the story of my colleague. Although it is possible that my colleague's brother was indeed treated more harshly by their parents than my colleague realized, their descriptions of their parent's attitudes were painted as being quite markedly diverse. Who was right in this story? My colleague or his brother? Both of them? It is possible that the parents of my colleague used harsh parenting and neglected their children and, by being exposed to these stressful events, my colleague's brother developed an increased vulnerability to anxiety disorder later in life. If this is the case, then the resilience shown by my colleague who grew up in the same family with no objective psychological sequelae could indeed that reflect the fact upon exposure to these "adverse events," he developed a dissociative process that modified the encoding and/or consolidation and/or recall process of these events. By not remembering these familial events the same way that his brother did, my colleague appeared more resilient. Or else, these familial "adverse events" were not as extreme as remembered by my colleague's brother, who processed them in a negative way (because of genetic make up, cognitive process or both) and developed an increased vulnerability to anxiety disorders later in life. Yet again, it may be possible that the parents treated siblings differently, leading to different outcomes in each child.

As stated by Ozbay and colleagues in the Ch. 18, as long as there are no longitudinal studies to follow children in adverse family environments, we cannot tease out the influence of genes and environment in the development of resilience in face of adversity. However, the authors propose in this chapter a very interesting avenue to take in order to improve our understanding of the factors that can predict resilience. Here, they are using a cognitive processing approach to understand resilience using basic principles of fear conditioning. In a fear conditioning response, a neutral stimulus is co-administered with a fear-inducing stimulus. When this happens, the neutral stimulus becomes a conditioned stimulus and acquires the property of inducing a fear response on its own. This process has been used to describe the development of psychopathology following exposure to traumatic stress. If one uses this model for the study of resilience, then it becomes clear that resilience can be seen either as an increased resistance to fear conditioning or as a greater propensity to acquire fear extinction. Interestingly, both of these processes have been shown to rely on corticolimbic circuitry as described in Ch. 17 and it is interesting to think that the higher capacity to resist fear conditioning or to acquire fear extinction could also result from individual differences in corticolimbic connections, which could be rooted in genes, early life events or even cognitive processes.

## Future directions

New data in the field of cognitive science suggest that individual differences in brain volumes can predict differences in the nature of the information that is processed by any given individual. Intrusive recollections are the manifestation of strong emotional memories upon exposure to stressful and/or emotional events that persist and often intrude into thoughts; this describes cluster B symptoms of PTSD. Previous studies, however, have shown that intrusive recollections are associated with the presence of persistent depression or anxiety, poor psychological adjustment, and poorer quality of life [4,5]. A recent paper published by Matsuoka et al. [6] has provided some evidence for the suggestion that small hippocampal volumes predict intrusive recollection of emotional information. The authors had reported in past studies that women with a history of cancer-related intrusive recollections had a smaller left hippocampal volume compared with those without intrusive recollection. In order to determine whether smaller left hippocampal volumes in these women represented the neurotoxic effects of several years of persistent stress-inducing intrusive recollections, or whether predetermined small hippocampal volumes predisposed these women to pathological stress reactions to cancer experience, they assessed the association between intrusive recollection and hippocampal volumes in a group of healthy young women with no history of cancer. The results revealed the presence of a strong negative correlation between left hippocampal volumes and intrusive recollections as assessed by the recall of an emotional story learned

1 week earlier. Healthy young women with no previous history of trauma with a small left hippocampal volume presented increased intrusive recollections compared with young healthy women with larger left hippocampal volumes. These results, obtained in a group of healthy young women, revealed that predetermined small hippocampal volumes may predispose women to develop intrusive recollections when faced with stressful experiences.

We have recently reported that about 25% of young healthy adults with no previous history of trauma present hippocampal volumes as small as individuals aged 60 to 75 years of age [7]. This result suggests that genes and/or environmental factors during development may be good predictor of hippocampal volume. Variations in hippocampal volumes could modify the nature of the cognitive processing of environmental cues and potentially lead to increased vulnerability to developed mental health disorders in the face of adversity. Here again, this suggestion entails a complex relationship between genes, environment and development and, based on the conclusions of the five chapters presented in this section, it becomes clear that future studies assessing the intricate relationship between genes and environment in the development of mental health disorders in response to early adversity will have to include the developmental stage of the individual exposed to the adverse event into the equation.

## References

1. Bakermans-Kranenburg, M. J., van Ijzendoorn, M. H., Mesman, J., Alink, L. R. and Juffer, F. (2008). Effects of an attachment-based intervention on daily cortisol moderated by dopamine receptor D4: A randomized control trial on 1- to 3-year-olds screened for externalizing behavior. *Developmental Psychopathology*, **20**, 805–820.
2. Meyer, S. E., Chrousos, G. P. and Gold, P. W. (2001). Major depression and the stress system: A life span perspective. *Developmental Psychopathology*, **13**, 565–580.
3. Pruessner, J. C., Dedovic, K., Khalili-Mahani, N. *et al.* (2008). Deactivation of the limbic system during acute psychosocial stress: Evidence from positron emission tomography and functional magnetic resonance imaging studies. *Biological Psychiatry*, **63**, 234–240.
4. Matsuoka, Y., Yamawaki, S., Inagaki, M., Akechi, T. and Uchitomi, Y. (2003). A volumetric study of amygdala in cancer survivors with intrusive recollections. *Biological Psychiatry*, **54**, 736–743.
5. Nakano, T., Wenner, N., Inagaki, M. *et al.* (2002). Relationship between distressing cancer-related

recollections and hippocampal volume in cancer survivors. *American Journal of Psychiatry,* **159**, 2087–2093.

6. Matsuoka, Y., Negamine, M., Mori, E. *et al.* (2007). Left hippocampal volume inversely correlates with enhanced emotional memory in healthy middle-aged women. *Journal of Neuropsychiatry and Clinical Neuroscience,* **19**, 335–338.

7. Lupien, S. J., Eveans, A., Lord, C. *et al.* (2007). Hippocampal volume is as variable in young as in older adults: implications for the notion of hippocampal atrophy in humans. *NeuroImage,* **34**, 479–485.

# Clinical perspectives: assessment and treatment of trauma spectrum disorders

# Assessment of the impact of early life trauma: clinical science and societal effects
# Assessing the effects of early and later childhood trauma in adults

John Briere and Monica Hodges

## Introduction

A wide range of potentially adverse events have been associated with psychological disturbance in adults [1], with most studies indicating that interpersonal trauma has the most negative long-term impacts [2]. Significantly, although victimization experienced in adulthood (e.g., rape, physical assault) can result in major psychological disturbance, a review of the clinical and empirical literature strongly suggests that abuse and/or neglect experienced in childhood is particularly toxic [3].

The critical role of childhood abuse and neglect in many instances of non-organic adult psychological disturbance was, in many ways, predicted by early clinicians and attachment theorists. Noteworthy are the earlier (pre-oedipal) writings of Freud [4] as well as Ferenczi [5] and other writers of the early twentieth century. Bowlby later famously articulated the effects of being raised by neglectful or psychologically disattuned caretakers in the early years of life [6]. More recently, clinical writers have suggested that early childhood maltreatment (especially childhood sexual abuse and psychological neglect/parental disattunement) can (a) disturb or dysregulate early parent–child attachment, (b) lead to dysfunctional relational schemata, and (c) condition negative emotional states to implicit infantile memories, thereby engendering specific problems in identity, affect regulation and interpersonal relatedness [7,8].

## Early versus later trauma

Despite the fact that most clinical writings predict the heightened role of early childhood trauma on later adult functioning, modern research on child maltreatment has generally examined the effects of sexual or physical abuse without reference to time of onset. This non-specific focus likely reflects the limitations of retrospective research methodologies, wherein adults are asked to report on their memories of childhood maltreatment. This approach, although helpful in demonstrating the adverse effects of childhood victimization, is inherently constrained by the relative unavailability of early childhood memories to later autobiographical recall [9]. Since the first years of life cannot be recollected by adults, it is generally impossible to use retrospective methodologies to investigate the effects of maltreatment that occurred during these years. Further, because such studies rely on accurate recall of exactly when an instance of abuse or neglect first occurred, it often difficult to correlate time of maltreatment and later symptomatology.

There are, however, two sources of information suggesting that negative early experiences may, in fact, be especially injurious: research on young children who have experienced significant child abuse and/or neglect, and longitudinal research. In the former, various studies indicate that early maltreatment may markedly affect childhood physical, neurological and psychological development [10,11], and, by inference, potentially impact adult psychosocial functioning in ways that later victimization typically may not. Similarly, longitudinal research, wherein children are first studied early in life and then followed up as they mature into adulthood, generally indicates that early abuse and/or neglect can be especially psychologically deleterious in the long term [12]. Unfortunately, prospective research is costly and, by definition, time consuming. As a result, the total number of available studies in this area is small.

*The Impact of Early Life Trauma on Health and Disease: The Hidden Epidemic*, ed. Ruth A. Lanius, Eric Vermetten and Clare Pain. Published by Cambridge University Press. Copyright © Cambridge University Press 2010.

In summary, based on the clinical literature and the results of both retrospective and longitudinal research, there is strong support for the notion that childhood trauma, especially interpersonal victimization and/or neglect, is a risk factor for later psychological difficulties and symptoms in adulthood – a risk that in many cases even exceeds the effects of more recent traumas. In light of this accumulated work, the remainder of this chapter will address the known effects of childhood interpersonal trauma and outline assessment approaches that may explicate these impacts in adult clients. Further, where the literature indicates a special role of earlier trauma on the development of specific psychological symptoms, this relationship will be noted.

## Complex outcomes

Much of the early research on the effects of childhood victimization and other traumas on adults tended to focus on anxiety, depression, interpersonal problems and, later, post-traumatic stress. More recent research, however, suggests that the repetitive and chronic nature of many instances of childhood maltreatment is likely to be associated with more complex, multisymptom presentations [3]. Although early studies focused primarily on physical and sexual abuse, recent research suggests that psychological neglect also has major impacts and may be especially relevant to early-onset, complex psychological outcomes [13]. Further, childhood maltreatment may not only produce complex long-term symptoms, but also can be associated with a greater risk of being revictimized in the future [14], potentially resulting in even more outcome complexity. Finally, there is some evidence that childhood victimization may lead the victim to respond to later trauma exposure with more extreme symptomatology [15], further complicating the clinical picture. In some cases, this wide range of maltreatment-related symptomatology has been described as "complex post-traumatic stress disorder (PTSD)" [16] or "disorders of extreme stress not otherwise specified" (DESNOS [3]). Other writers, however, have questioned whether there is a specific complex trauma syndrome per se, as opposed to a broad range of potential symptoms that vary in type, frequency and severity as a function of any given individual's specific trauma history (including age at onset, chronicity and types of victimization), sex, biology, attachment history and culture [e.g., Briere and Spinazzola [17].

## Assessment

Because childhood maltreatment can result in a number of symptoms and problems, any assessment of adults exposed to early trauma must address a variety of potential clinical outcomes. These effects are divided into two overlapping categories in the current chapter: *general abuse* and *early trauma* outcomes. As noted above, however, this division is somewhat arbitrary, in that (a) it is likely that in many studies the outcomes of child maltreatment actually varied as a function of time of onset, yet this variation was unmonitored or inadequately assessed because of the retrospective self-report nature of the investigations and (b) some of the hypothesized effects of early trauma have relatively limited empirical support, based on the small number of longitudinal studies currently available and the lack of follow-up in many attachment studies regarding the actual continuation of early symptoms or disturbance (however profound) into the long term.

## General abuse outcomes

Adult symptoms associated with childhood sexual, physical and psychological abuse include a number of difficulties, any combination of which may be present simultaneously, as described above. These include anxiety and depression [18,19], post-traumatic stress and PTSD [20], dissociation [21], cognitive distortions such as low self-esteem or self-blame [22], somatization [23], sexual concerns or conflicts [24], suicidality [25] and substance abuse or dependence [26]. In addition, several other difficulties commonly described in the abuse literature without reference to age are linked by others to earlier-onset child maltreatment. These include problems in close or intimate relationships; "tension-reduction behaviors" such as bingeing and purging, self-mutilation and compulsive sexual behavior; problems with identity and affect regulation; and, more generally, personality disorders [3, 27–30]. Although these issues are mentioned here to reflect their presence in the general abuse literature, they are described in more detail in the section on earlier trauma outcomes below. Finally, although these symptoms are presented here as general abuse outcomes, certain symptoms are more commonly linked to specific forms of maltreatment (e.g., sexual symptoms with sexual abuse, and anger and aggression with physical abuse [31]), although almost all possible symptoms have been linked to more than one form of abuse.

### Assessment approach

General abuse outcomes often can be evaluated with standardized psychological tests, although many of these measures were initially developed without reference to child abuse or neglect [32]. Ideally, the initial interview is supplemented with one or more generic, multiscale tests that, together, assist the clinician in choosing additional psychometric measures that further explore specific abuse-related disturbance. Not all symptoms found in a given client will necessarily be related to abuse or neglect, of course, despite their often clinically pressing aspects. This is a central notion in the assessment of abuse-related trauma: the entire clinical picture must be evaluated for any given client, not just those thought to arise from trauma [32].

## Generic broadband measures

### Broadband measures

As noted in several trauma assessment texts [32,33], a number of standardized, multiscale measures can be used in the initial screening of individuals who have been exposed to childhood maltreatment. The most common of these broadband tests are the Minnesota Multiphasic Personality Inventory, 2nd edition (MMPI-2) [34]; the Psychological Assessment Inventory (PAI) [35]; the Millon Clinical Multiaxial Inventory, 3rd edition (MCMI-III) [36] and the Symptom Checklist-90-Revised (SCL-90-R) [37]. A projective test, the Rorschach [38], may also yield data on a range of constructs relevant to complex post-traumatic distress, such as psychological defenses, ego strength, reality testing, aggression and bodily concerns [39], as well as, more indirectly, post-traumatic stress, dissociation and other more abuse-specific issues [40]. Although this chapter is more focused on self-report measures, standardized clinical interviews such as the Structured Clinical Interview for SCID-I and II (versions I and II) of the *Diagnostic and Statistical Manual*, 4th edition (DSM-IV) [41] also may be helpful in evaluating a range of trauma-related disorders.

Most of the tests mentioned above contain specific scales covering potentially maltreatment-related anxiety, depression, suicidality and interpersonal problems. A subset directly assesses anger or aggression (PAI, SCL-90-R), somatization (PAI, MCMI-III, SCL-90-R), post-traumatic stress (PAI, MMPI-2, MCMI-III) and substance abuse (PAI, MCMI-II and, more indirectly, MMPI-2). Most also yield some information on axis II and self-capacity difficulties frequently associated with complex abuse- or neglect-related post-traumatic outcomes, more fully described in the section on Earlier trauma outcomes, below.

### Focused non-broadband tests

When assessment with multiscale measures indicates specific problems or the clinician has otherwise determined the presence of certain clinical issues, additional, more specific, tests may also be applied. These include measures of suicidality (Adult Suicidal Ideation Questionnaire [ASIQ; 42]), aggression (State-Trait Anger Expression Inventory-2 [43]), general interpersonal problems (Inventory of Interpersonal Problems [IIP; 44]), eating disorders (Eating Disorders Inventory [EDI-3; 45]), cognitive distortions (Cognitive Distortion Scales [CDS; 46]) and substance abuse (Addiction Severity Index [ASI; 47]).

### Trauma-specific measures

In addition to generic assessment measures both broadband and non-broadband, a number of more trauma-specific instruments can be used to evaluate childhood trauma effects. In most cases, these measures were developed to assess trauma symptoms irrespective of when the adverse event was thought to have occurred: in adulthood as well as earlier in life. However, as noted above, many trauma symptoms in adults have childhood etiologies, and child maltreatment is often associated with later re-victimization; in the latter case, even adult-onset symptoms may be relevant to child abuse and neglect.

As is true for generic measures, trauma-specific assessment instruments may be divided into broadband tests, which survey a range of symptom clusters, and focused non-broadband tests, which evaluate specific trauma symptoms.

### Broadband measures

There are two standardized, normed, multiscale tests of trauma response available to the clinician, the Trauma Symptom Inventory (TSI) [48] and the Detailed Assessment of Post-traumatic Stress (DAPS) [49]. The TSI in particular has been used to evaluate the lasting effects of childhood trauma, whereas the DAPS has often been applied more to adult-onset events.

The TSI taps the overall level of post-traumatic symptomatology experienced by an individual in the previous 6 months. It has three validity scales (Response Level, Atypical Response and Inconsistent Response) and 10 clinical scales (Anxious Arousal, Depression, Anger/irritability, Intrusive Experiences, Defensive Avoidance, Dissociation, Sexual Concerns, Dysfunctional Sexual Behavior, Impaired Self-Reference and Tension Reduction Behavior). Various studies indicate that the TSI is reliable and valid in a range of contexts, e.g., McDevitt-Murphy *et al.* [50], and, because of the number of symptom clusters it evaluates, may serve as a general proxy for complex post-traumatic disturbance [51].

The DAPS has two validity scales and 10 scales that evaluate (a) exposure to childhood or adult traumatic events; (b) general response style; (c) immediate cognitive, emotional and dissociative responses to a specified trauma; (d) symptoms related to PTSD- and acute stress disorders; and (e) associated features of post-traumatic stress: trauma-specific dissociation, suicidality, and substance abuse. Its various scales have been found to be reliable and valid, and to have acceptable specificity and sensitivity in the diagnosis of PTSD [49].

### Focused non-broadband tests

There are a variety of specific tests available for the assessment of post-traumatic stress and dissociation. Most of those described below are standardized and/or normed, and all have been shown in multiple studies to be psychometrically reliable and valid.

Measures of post-traumatic stress typically assess the three symptom clusters used as criteria for PTSD in DSM-IV (reexperiencing, avoidance/numbing and hyperarousal), and in some cases provide a provisional diagnosis. The most widely used of these are the Post-traumatic Stress Diagnostic Scale (PDS) [52] and the Clinician-Administered PTSD Scale (CAPS) [53], a standardized clinical interview. In addition, the Impact of Event Scale [54] is a widely used research measure of post-traumatic stress symptoms that has been correlated with childhood trauma in adults [55]. In the absence of full standardization data, however, this measure may not be appropriate for clinical use.

Dissociation, which can be described as a defensive alteration in awareness [32], has been associated with both adult and childhood trauma exposure. Many clinicians, however, particularly link dissociative symptoms to childhood abuse [21] and some additionally implicate abuse- and neglect-related affect dysregulation, as described in the section. Earlier trauma outcomes, below. There are four major tests of dissociative symptoms available to clinicians and researchers. The first, the Dissociative Experiences Scale (DES) [56], has been used to study many traumatized populations, including adults abused as children [57], although its lack of normative data constrains its clinical use to some extent. Two other measures, the Multiscale Dissociation Inventory (MDI) [58] and the Multidimensional Inventory of Dissociation (MID) [59], were developed as clinical tests and have

been shown to have good reliability and validity in a variety of contexts [60]. Finally, the Structured Clinical Interview for DSM-IV Dissociative Disorders (SCID-D) [61] has been shown to be a helpful clinical tool, with good reliability and validity. In all three of these last tests, dissociation is measured as a multidimensional construct, with different scales measuring different symptom clusters (e.g., depersonalization versus memory disturbance).

## Earlier trauma outcomes

As described at the outset of this chapter, a number of clinicians and researchers have suggested that, in addition to the effects described above that are not onset specific, there are a number of symptoms, problems and disorders that can be linked specifically to early childhood abuse or neglect. These outcomes and associated assessment approaches are outlined below.

### Effects of disrupted attachment

Central to most clinical theories of early trauma effects is the notion of disrupted attachment. Generally following on the work of Bowlby [6], it is suggested that early abuse and/or neglect may alter a child's normal attachment to parents or caretakers, especially if these relational figures were directly or indirectly involved in the child's maltreatment. The child's resultant fear, anger and insecurity may become conditioned to relational stimuli, as well as leading to implicit, negative inferences about self and others [7,8]. The overwhelming quality of these negative internal states and schema is further thought to disrupt developmental processes that would otherwise support the acquisition of important early skills or capacities [8]. The altered developmental trajectory may result in problems in self-definition, negative perceptions of and interactions with others, and reduced abilities to regulate negative emotional states [62]. Such impaired "self-capacities" are viewed by many as representing the core impacts of early interpersonal trauma, above and beyond the post-traumatic stress, dysphoria and cognitive effects of child maltreatment per se [17,63]. Problems in these areas are, in fact, often viewed as the central aspects of complex PTSD and DESNOS, as well as more classical diagnoses such as borderline personality disorder, which is increasingly understood as potentially related to abuse or neglect [64].

### Identity

The identity capacity reflects the ability to maintain a sense of personal existence, self-awareness and self-other boundaries that is relatively stable across affects, situations and interactions with other people. Most modern views of identity development stress the importance of positive early relationships with attachment figures, wherein the caretaker(s) provide security, positive regard and emotional attunement [8,65]. In contrast, negative early childhood environments are by definition unlikely to involve these experiences. They also may interfere with identity development by reinforcing hypervigilance and "other-directedness," while at the same time punishing internal awareness to the extent that awareness means greater contact with painful internal states [2,7].

### Relatedness

The interpersonal impacts of early childhood abuse and neglect have been described widely, partially because caretaker–child attachment is implicitly relational, and, therefore, its dysregulation is likely to include relational difficulties. In fact, the notion of *insecure attachment* most basically involves ongoing fear, avoidance and/or ambivalence regarding self–other relationships, based on altered "internal working models" [6] or relational schema [66] that have been distorted by early negative interpersonal experiences. As a result, there may be difficulties in (a) forming or maintaining meaningful interpersonal relationships, (b) viewing self as worthy and entitled to positive treatment and others as potentially non-dangerous and non-abandoning and (c) recognizing and negotiating self–other boundaries [67].

### Affect regulation

Affect (or emotional) regulation difficulties generally refer to an inability to modulate and/or tolerate negative emotional states. Individuals with problems in affect regulation are often subject to emotional instability or mood swings, problems in inhibiting the expression of strong affect and difficulties in terminating dysphoric internal states [68,69]. Research into both the psychological and the biological components of affect regulation indicates a central role for positive early attachment experiences [70]. Conversely, various studies suggest that child abuse and neglect may be specifically associated with later problems in emotional regulation [30].

In the absence of sufficient internal affect regulation skills, some individuals with histories of child maltreatment may respond with external behaviors that distract, soothe, numb or otherwise reduce internal distress [7]. Examples of such tension reduction behaviors include deliberate self-injury (e.g., self-cutting), dysfunctional

sexual behavior, bingeing and/or purging eating behavior and impulsive aggressive behavior. Abuse-related affect dysregulation may also play a role in some instances of substance abuse [71], dissociation [72] and suicidality [73]. Growing clinical awareness that early childhood maltreatment and inadequate affect regulation may be implicated in "acting out," "self-destructive" or "addictive" behaviors has supported the growing use of treatments that specifically include affect regulation development and trauma processing in their approach to these problems [2,29,68,69].

### Assessment measures

Assessment of early childhood trauma effects usually focuses on sustained attachment disturbance (i.e., insecure adult attachment styles) or the altered relational schema, "object relations" and/or self-capacities widely thought to arise from childhood maltreatment.

### Attachment-specific instruments

Typically, attachment measures do not seek to assign clinical labels to individuals; in fact, to date, almost all instrumentation in this area has been limited to research studies. As a result, these measures generally lack the norms and level of standardization typically expected of modern clinical tests. As the importance of attachment disturbance becomes clearer to practicing clinicians, however, it is likely that measures will be developed with demonstrated reliability, validity and normative/standardization information. Until then, clinicians should use the currently available measures with caution, since their clinical psychometrics may not yet be known.

Attachment measures designed for use with adults may be divided in two general categories: narrative or interview-based assessment versus self-report. The Adult Attachment Interview (AAI) [74] is a semi-structured interview based on a set of standard questions concerning participants' childhood attachment relationships, loss and separation from attachment figures, and perceptions of how these relationships have shaped development and personality [75]. The adult attachment classifications (Secure–Autonomous, Dismissing, Preoccupied, Unresolved–Disorganized) are based on the coherence of responses with respect to consistency, relevance and manner of responses, among other considerations. These classifications have been theoretically [76] and empirically related to corresponding infant attachment status for participants' own children [reviewed by van Ijzendoorn [77]].

Several self-report measures of adult attachment have been described in the literature. Some argue that self-report of attachment style is unlikely to evaluate the construct at the level achieved by the AAI, and/or that defensive responding will often result in inaccurate self-report [10]. Nevertheless, the rapidity with which these measures can be applied and the wealth of data available on their relevance to attachment issues suggest important future roles in the clinical assessment of early trauma effects.

Perhaps the most well-known and brief measure of probable attachment style is Bartholomew and Horowitz's Relationship Questionnaire (RQ) [78]. The RQ categorizes individuals into one of four attachment representations (secure, dismissing, preoccupied and fearful), based on ratings of how accurately descriptions of each classification fit them. More psychometrically complex than the RQ are two inventories often used in attachment research: the Experiences in Close Relationships-Revised (ECR-R) Questionnaire [79] and the Revised Adult Attachment Scale (AAS-R) [80]. The ECR-R evaluates two dimensions associated with attachment status: attachment anxiety and attachment avoidance. Cross-referencing these two scales produces the typical four adult attachment dimensions (secure, preoccupied, dismissing and fearful avoidance). The AAS-R evaluates underlying dimensions associated with attachment styles, yielding three subscales: Close (comfort with intimacy and closeness), Depend (comfort with depending/relying on others) and Anxiety (worries about rejection and abandonment).

### Tests of disturbed object relations, self-capacities and schema

Beyond measures of disturbed or insecure attachment per se are several clinically validated and standardized measures that assess identity, affect regulation, relational functioning, self-other schema and other assumed sequelae of early trauma. These include two free-standing self-report tests (the Bell Object Relations and Reality Testing Inventory [BORRTI; 81] and the Inventory of Altered Self Capacities [IASC; 82]), a measure of disrupted schemata (the Trauma and Attachment Belief Scale [TABS; 83], specific scales from three broadband instruments (the PAI, MCMI-III and TSI), scoring approaches to two projective tests (the Rorschach and the Thematic Apperception Test [TAT; 84]) and a structured interview for complex post-traumatic disturbance (the Structured Interview for Disorders of Extreme Stress [SIDES; 85]).

The BORRTI is grounded in object relations theory [86] and contains scales that yield data on four related constructs (alienation, insecure attachment, egocentricity and social incompetence), as well as indices of poor reality testing, including the presence of hallucinations and delusions. The BORRTI object relation scales have been shown to predict and potentially explain relational dysfunction in individuals thought to have some form of personality disorder, as well as underlying risk factors for substance abuse and eating disorders [81].

The IASC was developed without reference to any particular theoretical or diagnostic perspective, but rather was based on the empirical literature on the lasting effects of childhood maltreatment and victimization on self-functioning. This standardized test evaluates difficulties in the areas of relatedness, identity and affect regulation and contains the following scales: Interpersonal Conflicts, Idealization–Disillusionment, Abandonment Concerns, Identity Impairment, Susceptibility to Influence, Affect Dysregulation and Tension Reduction Activities. Elevated scores on IASC scales have been shown in various samples to predict adult attachment style, childhood trauma history, relational functioning, suicidality and substance abuse history, as well as borderline and antisocial personality traits, PTSD and dissociation [30,67,87].

The TABS is a self-report, standardized test that measures disrupted cognitive schemata associated with complex trauma exposure, especially childhood maltreatment, that alters attachment-related needs and cognitions. In contrast to more symptom-based tests, the TABS measures the self-reported needs and expectations of trauma survivors as they predict self in relation to others. It evaluates disturbance using five scales: Safety, Trust, Esteem, Intimacy and Control. There are reliable subscales for each of these domains, rated both for "self" and "other."

Three broadband instruments described earlier in this chapter have scales that tap psychological disturbance often linked to early abuse and/or neglect during childhood. The TSI includes the Impaired Self-Reference (ISR) Scale, intended to evaluate identity confusion, self-other disturbance and a relative lack of self-support; the Dysfunctional Sexual Behavior (DSB) scale, tapping sexual behavior that is indiscriminate, potentially self-harming or used to accomplish nonsexual goals; and the Tension Reduction Behavior (TRB) Scale, which assesses involvement in external methods of reducing internal tension or distress, such as self-mutilation, angry outbursts and suicide threats. The PAI contains two scales especially relevant to early trauma (the Borderline Features and Antisocial Features Scales), as well as four six-item subscales of the Borderline Features Scale that tap self-capacity-related phenomena (i.e., Affective Instability, Identity Problems, Negative Relationships and Self-Harm). Finally, the MCMI-III includes scales that assess antisocial and borderline personality features, as well as "facet" scales developed to examine specific aspects of these two types of personality disturbance.

Two projective tests, the Rorschach and TAT, have been used to assess the effects of traumas thought to occur early in development, as well as more general constructs of impaired identity and relational functioning. Modern scoring approaches to the Rorschach yield information about various constructs relevant to early and complex trauma, such as "primitive" psychological defenses, lack of ego strength, impaired reality testing, disturbed self-capacities, aggression and excessive bodily concerns [39], as well as post-traumatic stress and dissociation [88].

Less broadly used than the Rorschach, the Social Cognition and Object Relations Scale (SCORS) [89] can be applied to TAT narratives to generate information on eight object relations constructs: Complexity of Representations, Affective Quality of Representation, Emotional Investment in Relationships, Emotional Investment in Values and Moral Standards, Understanding of Social Causality, Experience and Management of Aggressive Impulses, Self-Esteem, and Identity and Coherence of Self. Various studies indicate that SCORS variables are predictive of attachment style, interpersonal functioning, personality disorder and relational expectations [90].

In contrast to specific measures of attachment styles, self-capacities and object relations, the SIDES evaluates the broader notion of early-onset, complex post-traumatic disturbance. This interview measures the current and lifetime presence of six symptom clusters that were proposed for the diagnosis of DESNOS in DSM-IV: Affect Dysregulation, Somatization, Alterations in Attention or Consciousness, Self-Perception, Relationships with Others, and Systems of Meaning. The SIDES interview has good interrater reliability and internal consistency and has been shown to predict the various features of complex post-traumatic disturbance outlined in this chapter [85]. We suggest that the SIDES be used not as a measure of DESNOS per se but rather as an interview-based review of the various symptoms and difficulties that have been linked to trauma early in development.

## Conclusions

This chapter has briefly reviewed the impacts of childhood trauma and has described the various assessment methodologies that may be helpful in evaluating such effects. Early abuse and neglect appear to be significant risk factors for disrupted parent–child attachment and, as a result, the development of a wide variety of symptoms and problems that traditionally have not been viewed as particularly trauma related. Growing awareness of the childhood etiology of many of these more complex outcomes is likely not only to reconfigure clinical understanding of many axis II or "personality disorder" presentations but also to assist in the development of more trauma-focused treatment approaches to such outcomes. In order for treatment to be effectively targeted, the clinician must correctly assess the pychological impacts involved, generally by administering the appropriate psychological tests and interpreting them based on the current complex trauma literature.

## References

1. Reyes, G., Elhai, J. and Ford, J., eds. (2008). *Encyclopedia of psychological trauma*. New York: Wiley.

2. Briere, J. and Scott, C. (2006). *Principles of trauma therapy: A guide to symptoms, evaluation, and treatment*. Thousand Oaks, CA: Sage.

3. van der Kolk, B. A., Roth, S., Pelcovitz, D., Sunday, S. and Spinazzola, J. (2005). The disorders of extreme stress: The empirical foundation of complex adaptation to trauma. *Journal of Traumatic Stress*, **18**, 389–399.

4. Freud, S. (1962). The aetiology of hysteria. In F. J. Strachey (ed.), *The standard edition of the complete psychological works of Sigmund Freud* (pp. 189–221). Vol. 3. London: Hogarth Press.

5. Ferenczi, S. (1955). Confusion of tongues between adults and the child. In S. Ferenczi (ed.), *Final contributions to the problems and methods of psychoanalysis* (pp. 156–167), London: Hogarth Press.

6. Bowlby, R. (1973). *Attachment and loss,* Vol. 2. *separation.* New York: Basic Books.

7. Briere, J. (2002). Treating adult survivors of severe childhood abuse and neglect: Further development of an integrative model. In J. E. B. Myers, L. Berliner, J. Briere *et al.*(eds.), *APSAC handbook on child maltreatment* (pp. 175–202), 2nd edn. Newbury Park, CA: Sage.

8. Pearlman, L. A. and Courtois, C. A. (2005). Clinical applications of the attachment framework: Relational treatment of complex trauma. *Journal of Traumtic Stress*, **18**, 449–459.

9. Nelson, C. A. (1998). The nature of early memory. *Preventive Medicine*, **27**, 172–179.

10. Cassidy, J. and Shaver, P. R. (eds.). (2008). *Handbook of attachment: Theory, research, and clinical implications.* New York: Guilford Press.

11. Cichetti, D. and Toth, S. L. (1995). A developmental psychopathology perspective on child abuse and neglect. *Journal of the American Academy of Child and Adolescent Psychiatry,* **34**, 541–565.

12. Sroufe, L. A., Egeland, B, Carlson, E. A. and Collins W. A. (2005). *The development of the person: The Minnesota study of risk and adaptation from birth to adulthood.* New York: Guildford.

13. Erickson, M. F. and Egeland B. (2002).Child neglect. In J. E. B. Myers, L. Berliner, J. Briere, *et al.* (eds.), *APSAC handbook on child maltreatment*, 2nd edn. (pp. 3–20), Newbury Park, CA: Sage Publications.

14. Classen, C. C., Palesh, O. G. and Aggarwal, R. (2005). Sexual revictimization: A review of the empirical literature. *Trauma, Violence and Abuse,* **6**, 103–129.

15. Bremner, J. D., Southwick, S. M., Johnson, D. R., Yehuda, R. and Charney, D. S. (1993). Childhood physical abuse and combat-related posttraumatic stress disorder in Vietnam veterans. *American Journal of Psychiatry*, **150**, 235–259.

16. Herman, J. L. (1992). Complex PTSD: A syndrome in survivors of prolonged and repeated trauma. *Journal of Traumatic Stress*, **5**, 377–391.

17. Briere, J. and Spinazzola, J. (2005). Phenomenology and psychological assessment of complex posttraumatic states. *Journal of Traumatic Stress*, **18**, 401–412.

18. Heim, C. and Nemeroff, C. B. (2001). The role of childhood trauma in the neurobiology of mood and anxiety disorders: Preclinical and clinical studies. *Biological Psychiatry* **49**, 1023–1039.

19. Putnam, F. W. (2003). Ten-year research update review: Child sexual abuse. *Journal of the American Academy of Child and Adolescent Psychiatry*, **43**, 269–278.

20. Zlotnick, C., Johnson, J., Kohn, R. *et al.* (2008). Childhood trauma, trauma in adulthood, and psychiatric diagnoses: Results from a community sample. *Comprehensive Psychiatry*, **49**, 163–169.

21. Chu, J. A., Frey, L. M., Ganzel, B. L. and Matthews, J. A. (1999). Memories of childhood abuse: Dissociation, amnesia, and corroboration. *American Journal of Psychiatry*, **156**, 749–755.

22. Foa, E. B., Ehlers, A., Clark, D. M., Tolin, D. F. and Orsillo, S. M. (1999). The Posttraumatic Cognitions Inventory (PTCI): Development and validation. *Psychological Assessment*, **11**, 303–314.

23. Dietrich, A. M. (2003). Characteristics of child maltreatment, psychological dissociation, and somatoform dissociation of Canadian inmates. *Journal of Trauma and Dissociation*, **4**, 81–100.

24. van Bruggen, L. K., Runtz, M. G. and Kadlec, H. (2006). Sexual revictimization: The role of sexual self-esteem and dysfunctional sexual behaviors. *Child Maltreatment,* **11**, 131–145.

25. Fergusson, D. M., Boden, J. M. and Horwood, L. J. (2008). Exposure to childhood sexual and physical abuse and adjustment in early adulthood. *Child Abuse & Neglect*, **32**, 607–619.

26. Najavits, L. M. (2002). *Seeking safety: A treatment manual for PTSD and substance abuse.* New York: Guilford Press.

27. Allen, B. (2008). An analysis of the impact of diverse forms of childhood psychological maltreatment on emotional adjustment in early adulthood. *Child Maltreatment*, **13**, 307–312.

28. Bandelow, B., Krause, J., Wedekind, D. *et al.* (2005). Early traumatic life events, parental attitudes, family history, and birth risk factors in patients with borderline personality disorder and healthy controls. *Psychiatry Research*, **134**, 169–179.

29. Berenbaum, H., Thompson, R. J., Milandek, M. E., Boden, M. T. and Bredemeier, K. (2008). Psychological trauma and schizotypal personality disorder. *Journal of Abnormal Psychology*, **117**, 502–519.

30. Briere, J. and Rickards, S. (2007). Self-awareness, affect regulation, and relatedness: Differential sequelae of childhood versus adult victimization experiences. *Journal of Nervous and Mental Disorders*, **195**, 497–503.

31. Briere, J. and Runtz, M. (1990). Differential adult symptomatology associated with three types of child abuse histories. *Child Abuse & Neglect,* **14**, 357–364.

32. Briere, J. (2004). *Psychological assessment of adult posttraumatic states: Phenomenology, diagnosis, and measurement*, 2nd edn. Washington, DC: American Psychological Association.

33. Carlson, E. B. (1997). *Trauma assessments: A clinician's guide.* New York: Guilford.

34. Butcher, J. N., Dahlstrom, W. G., Graham, J. R., Tellegen, A. and Kaemmer, B. (1989). *Minnesota multiphasic personality inventory (MMPI-2). Manual for administration and scoring.* Minneapolis: University of Minnesota Press.

35. Morey, L. C. (1991). *Personality assessment inventory professional manual.* Odessa, FL: Psychological Assessment Resources.

36. Millon, T. (1994). *Millon clinical multiaxial inventory-III: Manual for the MCMI-III.* Minneapolis, MN: National Computer Systems.

37. Derogatis, L. R. (1983) *SCL-90-R administration, scoring, and procedures manual II for the revised version*, 2nd edn. Towson, MD: Clinical Psychometrics Research.

38. Rorschach, H. (1981/1921). *Psychodiagnostics: A diagnostic test based upon perception,* 9th edn. P. Lemkau, B. and Kronemberg (eds.), New York: Grune & Stratton.

39. Exner, J. E. (1986). *The rorschach: A comprehensive system,* 2nd edn. New York: Wiley.

40. Luxenberg, T. and Levin, P. (2004). The utility of the Rorschach in the assessment and treatment of trauma. In J. Wilson and T. Keane (eds.), *Assessing psychological trauma and PTSD* 2nd edn. (pp. 190–225), New York: Guilford.

41. First, M. B., Spitzer, R. L. and Gibbon, M. (1997). *Structured clinical interview for DSM-III-R personality disorders (SCID-II).* Washington, DC: American Psychiatric Press.

42. Reynolds, W. M. (1991). Psychometric characteristics of the Adult Suicidal Ideation Questionnaire in college students. *Journal of Personality Assessment,* **56,** 289–307.

43. Spielberger, C. D., Sydeman, S. J., Owne, A. E. and Marsh, B. J. (1999). Measuring anxiety and anger with the State-Trait Anxiety Inventory (STAI) and the State-Trait Anger Expression Inventory (STAXI). In M. E. Maruish (ed.), *The use of psychological testing for treatment planning and outcomes assessment,* 2nd edn. (pp. 993–1021), Mahwah, NJ: Lawrence Erlbaum.

44. Horowitz, L. M., Alden, L. E., Wiggins, J. S. and Pincus, A. (2000). *Inventory of interpersonal problems manual.* Odessa, FL: Psychological Corporation.

45. Garner, D. M. (2004). *Eating disorder inventory-3 professional manual.* Odessa, FL: Psychological Assessment Resources.

46. Briere, J. (2000). *Cognitive distortion scales (CDS).* Odessa, FL: Psychological Assessment Resources.

47. McClellan, A. T., Kushner, H., Metzger, D. *et al.* (1992). The fifth edition of the Addiction Severity Index. *J Substance Abuse and Treatment,* **9,** 199–213.

48. Briere, J. (1995). *Trauma symptom inventory (TSI).* Odessa, FL: Psychological Assessment Resources.

49. Briere, J. (2001). *Detailed assessment of posttraumatic stress (DAPS).* Odessa, FL: Psychological Assessment Resources.

50. McDevitt-Murphy, M. E., Weathers, F. W. and Adkins, J. W. (2005) The use of the Trauma Symptom Inventory in the assessment of PTSD symptoms. *Journal of Traumatic Stress,* **18,** 63–67.

51. Resick, P. A., Nishith, P. and Griffin, M. G. (2003). How well does cognitive-behavioral therapy treat symptoms of complex PTSD? An examination of child sexual abuse survivors within a clinical trial. *CNS Spectrums,* **8,** 351–355.

52. Foa, E. B. (1995). *Posttraumatic stress diagnostic scale.* Minneapolis MN: National Computer Systems.

53. Blake, D. D., Weathers, F. W., Nagy, L. M. *et al.* (1995). The development of a clinician-administered PTSD scale. *Journal of Traumatic Stress,* **8,** 75–90.

54. Horowitz, M. D., Wilner, N. and Alvarez, W. (1979). Impacts of Event Scale: A measure of subjective stress. *Psychosomatic Medicine,* **41,** 209–218.

55. Briere, J. and Elliott, D. M. (1998). Clinical utility of the Impact of Event Scale: Psychometrics in the general population. *Assessment,* **5,** 135–144.

56. Bernstein, E. M. and Putnam, F. W. (1986). Development, reliability, and validity of a dissociation scale. *Journal of Nervous and Mental Disorders,* **174,** 727–735.

57. van Ijzendoorn, M. H. and Schuengel, C. (1996). The measurement of dissociation in normal and clinical populations: Meta-analytic validation of the Dissociative Experiences Scale (DES). *Clinical Psychology Review,* **16,** 365–382.

58. Briere, J. (2002). *Multiscale dissociation inventory.* Odessa, FL: Psychological Assessment Resources.

59. Dell, P. F. (2006). The Multidimensional Inventory of Dissociation (MID): A comprehensive measure of pathological dissociation. *Journal of Trauma and Dissociation,* **7,** 77–106.

60. Briere, J. and Armstrong, J. (2007). Psychological assessment of posttraumatic dissociation. In E. Vermetten, M. Dorahy and D. Spiegel (eds.), *Traumatic dissociation: Neurobiology and treatment* (pp. 259–274). Washington, DC: American Psychiatric Press.

61. Steinberg, M. (1994). *Interviewer's guide to the structured clinical interview for DSM-IV dissociative disorders (SCID-D),* revised edn. Washington, DC: American Psychiatric Press.

62. Cloitre, M., Stovall-McClough, K. C., Zorbas, P. and Charuvastra, A. (2008). Attachment organization, emotion regulation, and expectations of support in a clinical sample of women with childhood abuse histories. *Journal of Traumatic Stress,* **21,** 282–289.

63. McCann, I. L. and Pearlman, L. A. (1990). *Psychological trauma and the adult survivor: Theory, therapy, and transformation.* New York: Brunner/Mazel.

64. Ogata, S., Silk, K., Goodrich, S. *et al.* (1990). Childhood sexual and physical abuse in adult patients with borderline personality disorder. *American Journal of Psychiatry,* **147,** 1008–1013.

65. Stern, D. (1985). *The interpersonal world of the infant: A view from psychoanalysis and developmental psychology.* New York: Basic Books.

66. Baldwin, M. W., Fehr, B., Keedian, E., Seidel, M. and Thompson, D. W. (1993). An exploration of the relational schemata underlying attachment styles: Self-report and lexical decision approaches. *Personality and Social Psychology Bulletin,* **19,** 746–754.

67. Briere, J. and Runtz, M. R. (2002). The inventory of Altered Self-Capacities (IASC): A standardized measure of identity, affect regulation, and relationship disturbance. *Assessment,* **9,** 230–239.

68. Cloitre, M., Cohen, L. R. and Koenen, K. C. (2006). *Treating survivors of childhood abuse: Psychotherapy for the interrupted life.* New York: Guilford.

69. Linehan, M. M. (1993). *Cognitive-behavioral treatment of borderline personality disorder.* New York: Guilford.

70. Schore, A. N. (1994). *Affect regulation and the origin of the self: The neurobiology of emotional development.* Hillsdale, NJ: Lawrance Erlbaum.

71. Khantzian, E. J. (1997). The self-medication hypothesis of substance use disorders: A reconsideration and recent applications. *Harvard Review of Psychiatry, 4,* 231–244.

72. Briere, J. (2006). Dissociative symptoms and trauma exposure: Specificity, affect dysregulation and post-traumatic stress. *Journal of Nervous and Mental Disorders,* **194,** 78–82.

73. Koenen, K. C. (2006). Developmental epidemiology of PTSD: Self-regulation as a central mechanism. In R. Yehuda (ed.), Psychobiology of posttraumatic stress disorders: A decade of progress. *Annals of the New York Academy of Sciences,* **1071,** 255–266.

74. George, C., Kaplan, N. and Main, M. (1985). *Adult attachment interview.* Berkeley, CA: Department of Psychology, University of California, Berkeley.

75. Main, M. (1996). Introduction to the special section on attachment and psychopathology: Overview of the field of attachment. *Journal of Consulting and Clinical Psychology,* **64,** 237–243.

76. Main, M. and Goldwyn, R. (1985). *Adult attachment scoring and classification system.* Berkeley, CA: Department of Psychology, University of California.

77. van Ijzendoorn, M. (1995). Adult attachment representations, parental responsiveness, and infant attachment: A meta-analysis on the predictive validity of the Adult Attachment Interview. *Psychology Bulletin,* **117,** 387–403.

78. Bartholomew, K. and Horowitz, L. M. (1991). Attachment styles among young adults: A test of a four-category model. *Journal of Personality and Social Psychology,* **61,** 226–244.

79. Fraley, R. C., Waller, N. G. and Brennan, K. A. (2000). An item response theory analysis of self-report measures of adult attachment. *Journal of Personality and Social Psychology,* **78,** 350–365.

80. Collins, N. L. (1996). Working models of attachment: Implications for explanation, emotion, and behavior. *Journal of Personality and Social Psychology,* **71,** 810–832.

81. Bell, M. D. (1985). *Bell object relations and reality testing inventory.* Los Angeles, CA: Western Psychological Services.

82. Briere, J. (2000). *Inventory of altered self-capacities (IASC).* Odessa, FL: Psychological Assessment Resources.

83. Pearlman, L. A. (2003). *Trauma and attachment belief scale.* Los Angeles, CA: Western Psychological Services.

84. Murray, H. A. (1943). *Thematic apperception test manual.* Cambridge, MA: Harvard University Press.

85. Pelcovitz, D., van der Kolk, B. A., Roth, S. *et al.* (1997). Development of a criteria set and a structured interview for disorders of extreme stress (SIDES). *Journal of Traumatic Stress,* **10,** 3–16.

86. Kernberg, O. F. (1976). Technical considerations in the treatment of borderline personality organization. *Journal of the American Psychoanalytic Association,* **24,** 795–829.

87. Bornstein, R. F., Languirand, M. A., Geiselman, K. J. *et al.* (2003). Construct validity of the Relationship Profile Test: A self-report measure of dependency-detachment. *Journal of Personality Assessment,* **80,** 64–74.

88. Levin, P. and Reis, B. (1997). Use of the Rorschach in assessing trauma. In J. P. Wilson and T. M. Keane (eds.), *Assessing psychological trauma and PTSD* (pp. 529–543). New York: Guilford.

89. Westen, D. (1995). *Social cognition and object relations scale: Q-sort for projective stories (SCORS–Q).* Boston, MA: Harward Medical School.

90. Hilsenroth, M. and Segal, D. (eds.) (2004). Personality assessment. In M. Hersen (ed.), *Comprehensive handbook of psychological assessment,* Vol. 2 (pp. 283–296). Hoboken, NJ: Wiley.

# Chapter 20

# Memory and trauma: examining disruptions in implicit, explicit and autobiographical memory

Melody D. Combs and Anne P. DePrince

Amongst the many deleterious correlates of trauma exposure, disruptions in memory functioning have been among the most challenging and controversial to study (for a historical review, see Brewin [1]). Challenges arise from the need to reconcile seemingly inconsistent reports of both hyper- and hypo-memory for trauma-related information, as well as improved and impoverished performance on laboratory tasks. Controversy has centered on if, how and why memory impairment for trauma-related autobiographical memories occurs. While it is beyond the scope of this chapter to do justice to all of these issues, we review data on disruptions in explicit and implicit memory associated with post-traumatic stress disorder (PTSD) and dissociation in laboratory research. Drawing on this memory literature, we then discuss several biological and cognitive mechanisms proposed to account for autobiographical memory impairment.

## Laboratory studies of explicit and implicit memory

### Explicit memory and post-traumatic stress disorder

Laboratory-based studies of memory offer opportunities for better understanding of basic memory functioning in trauma-exposed individuals. A large body of research now demonstrates associations between trauma exposure and explicit memory deficits (e.g., in neutral, standardized memory tasks) as a function of PTSD status. Individuals diagnosed with PTSD stemming from traumas that are combat or non-combat related (e.g., physical and sexual abuse) show deficits

in basic explicit memory performance on standardized neuropsychological tests relative to peers without PTSD and without trauma exposure [2–4]. For example, adult women diagnosed with childhood sexual abuse-related PTSD performed worse on explicit memory tasks than sexually abused women without PTSD and non-abused women [5]. Still other studies assessing explicit memory through working memory tasks have shown links between trauma exposure and poorer explicit performance [6], including among women exposed to intimate partner violence [7]. Although fewer studies have examined basic memory functioning in children, at least one study has demonstrated that children diagnosed with maltreatment-related PTSD show deficits in memory relative to a no-trauma control group [8]. DePrince et al. [9] found that children exposed to familial traumas (sexual abuse, physical abuse or witnessing domestic violence) showed worse explicit memory (as measured by a working memory task) relative to peers exposed to either non-familial traumas (e.g., motor vehicle accidents) or no trauma. While additional research is needed with child populations, these two studies suggest that trauma and/or PTSD-related explicit memory deficits may occur fairly early in development among children exposed to interpersonal violence, such as abuse.

Given that hypervigilance to threat is characteristic of PTSD, several studies have examined attention to, and explicit memory for, trauma-related stimuli, revealing that memory for trauma-relevant information may actually be heightened relative to other information [10,11]. For example, Golier et al. [12] reported that Holocaust survivors diagnosed with PTSD recalled fewer paired-associates overall (consistent with the literature on poor explicit memory reviewed above) but more Holocaust-related word pairs than neutral word pairs, relative to Holocaust-exposed control participants without PTSD, whose recall was unaffected by word type. Similarly, crime victims (including rape and physical assault) diagnosed with acute PTSD recalled significantly more trauma-related words in a free recall task than a control group without crime exposure or PTSD [10]. Therefore, PTSD is associated with both general deficits in explicit memory performance and heightened memory for trauma-related stimuli.

## Implicit memory and post-traumatic stress disorder

Although much of the laboratory research on trauma and memory has emphasized explicit memory, implicit memory (believed to be an automatic process) may be particularly important for understanding those PTSD symptoms that appear involuntary and automatic, such as intrusive thoughts, flashbacks and nightmares. Individuals diagnosed with PTSD may have implicit biases for trauma-related information or cues that trigger re-experiencing and intrusions; however, these individuals may remain unaware of the cues.

To date, research on implicit memory for trauma-related stimuli in PTSD is mixed [10,12–14], perhaps in part a consequence of the particular methods of assessment. For example, Golier et al. [12] found no differences between Holocaust survivors with PTSD and controls on the tendency to use Holocaust-related words in a word-stem completion task. Conversely, Zeitlin and McNally [14] found that Vietnam combat veterans with PTSD demonstrated a greater implicit bias for using combat-related words in a word completion task compared with combat veterans without PTSD. Some researchers have attributed these inconsistencies to the use of word-stem completion tasks to assess implicit memory (see MacLeod & McLaughlin [15]), suggesting that word-stem completion is affected by explicit memory. In a study using a relatively pure measure of implicit memory, combat veterans with PTSD showed greater implicit memory biases for combat-related sentences in a noise judgment task compared with combat veterans without PTSD [13].

Alterations in implicit memory have also been examined in conditioned fear paradigms, allowing for an assessment of implicit memory that is not reliant on language processes. Using the eyeblink reflex as a measure of startle responsiveness, participants diagnosed with PTSD do not show increased baseline

startle responsiveness [16,17]; but do show heightened fear response to threatening contexts (e.g., threat of shock) and normal startle responsiveness to threatening stimuli (e.g., the shocks) compared with control participants [16,18]. In this study, increased startle responses appear to be elicited by fear-inducing environments rather than stemming from a general, increased baseline level of startle responsiveness [19].

Conditioned fear responding has also been assessed using heart rate, skin conductance and electromyography measures. Participants diagnosed with PTSD demonstrate greater increases in heart rate and skin conductance in response to the auditory startle paradigm compared with controls [20]. In addition, Gulf War combat veterans with PTSD exhibited increased skin conductance and electromyograph responses compared with controls while imagining and listening to an audio recording of the Gulf War's missile alarm [21]. Survivors of non-war related traumatic events who had chronic PTSD or who had recently experienced severe trauma demonstrated increased heart rate in response to traumatic pictures [22]. Importantly, however, not all studies document increases in reactivity with PTSD. For example, Pole and colleagues [23] reported that the experience of childhood trauma alone without the presence of PTSD was associated with increased physiological responses to threat stimuli and startling sounds compared with adults without reported childhood trauma. Further research is needed to tease out the role that trauma exposure and PTSD each play in dysregulation (either increases or decreases) of physiological reactivity in response to threat.

In sum, PTSD is often associated with increased startle responsiveness during threatening contexts, as well as increases in physiological responsiveness to trauma-related stimuli. These findings, in conjunction with implicit priming effects for traumatic stimuli, demonstrate that individuals with PTSD, or who have experienced childhood trauma, have alterations in implicit memory functioning in the context of threatening information. These patterns of heightened implicit memory and response to traumatic stimuli and contexts in individuals diagnosed with PTSD may underlie these individuals' involuntary memory (i.e., intrusions, flashbacks, sensory re-experiencing) for traumatic events.

## Explicit memory and dissociation

In addition to PTSD, researchers have been interested in connections between dissociation and memory performance. Dissociation, defined as a lack of integration in typically connected aspects of information processing [24], has been proposed to provide one route by which individuals may keep threatening information from awareness (e.g., Freyd [25]). To the extent that their cognitive styles are characterized by avoidant encoding strategies [26], individuals with high dissociation should show poorer recall for trauma-relevant stimuli relative to neutral stimuli than do those with low dissociation. However, several investigators have instead reported that higher dissociation is associated with heightened memory function and improved recall for traumatic or emotional stimuli [27–29]. To account for these somewhat counter-intuitive findings, deRuiter et al. [28] proposed that heightened attention, working memory capacity and episodic memory in highly dissociative individuals may serve as risk factors for pathological dissociation if coupled with particular traumatic experiences. In this view, dissociative experiences result from a combination of cognitive style, characterized by enhanced attention and memory, and trauma exposure.

Still others have argued that dissociation may be associated with impaired recall for trauma-related stimuli *under certain attention conditions*. Indeed, several studies now point to interesting links between dissociation and attention performance, such that highly dissociative individuals (determined either by scores above the pathological cut point on a measure of dissociation or by diagnostic group) appear to perform better under divided attention [30,31] or greater cognitive load conditions [32], relative to other conditions. For example, DePrince and Freyd [30] reported that highly dissociative individuals exhibited more interference under standard selective attention demands and less interference under divided attention demands of a modified Stroop task relative to those with low dissociation, who showed the opposite pattern. Further, highly dissociative individuals recalled fewer emotionally charged words and more neutral words relative to those with low dissociation, who showed the opposite pattern. Using the directed forgetting task, highly dissociative individuals recalled fewer trauma-related words and more neutral words under divided attention conditions than those with low dissociation, who again showed the opposite pattern [33–35]. Similarly, preschool-aged children who had been abused and had high dissociation scores recalled fewer emotionally charged pictures under divided attention conditions compared with non-abused children with low dissociation scores [36].

Taken together, the above findings suggest that highly dissociative individuals may be at a cognitive advantage under certain attentional conditions, raising important areas for future research. For example, do these findings reflect a coherent dissociative cognitive style, and if so, is that dissociative cognitive style a risk factor for or a consequence of dissociation (and trauma exposure)? Further, to the extent that dissociation is associated with poorer recall of trauma-related stimuli relative to other conditions under some attentional demands, are these differences in memory a result of encoding or inhibitory mechanisms?

# Autobiographical memories for trauma

Building on the laboratory-based literature reviewed above, we address two key questions about trauma-related autobiographical memories. First, to what extent are traumatic memories like or unlike non-traumatic memories? Second, what mechanisms may help to explain how impairment in trauma-related autobiographical memories develops?

We begin with the assumption that memory impairment for trauma does happen, based on the large extant literature documenting reports of memory impairment in a range of populations using both prospective [37,38] and retrospective [39–43] methods. Notably, reports of memory impairment are not constrained to abuse (reviewed by Freyd et al. [44]), although impairment in abuse-related memories has garnered the most controversy. With a literature stretching back to the beginning of modern trauma studies with combat veterans (e.g., Sargant and Slater, [45]) that validates the phenomenon of memory impairment, we focus attention on issues central to understanding impaired trauma-related autobiographical memories.

The question of whether autobiographical memory for trauma is, in fact, different from non-traumatic autobiographical memories is a matter of current debate [46,47]. In a recent review, Brewin [46] described this controversy and discussed research on voluntary (intentional, conscious recollection) and involuntary (memory intrusions and flashbacks) autobiographical memory for trauma in clinical and non-clinical populations, concluding that, at least for clinical populations, involuntary traumatic and non-traumatic memories appear to be different. Traumatic memories appear more vivid, involve a greater degree of sensory experience and are likely to be reexperienced as happening in the present. In addition, Brewin highlighted emerging evidence that voluntary traumatic and non-traumatic memories differ in organization and content, but he also called for more systematic studies. Data from neuroimaging studies add to the complexity of these issues. For example, the underlying neural circuitry associated with traumatic memories appears to vary as a function of PTSD and dissociative [48] symptoms, leading to the question of whether trauma memories differ generally from non-trauma memories, or only differ in the context of particular trauma-related symptoms (i.e., in conjunction with the experience of memory intrusions or flashbacks).

## How and why might impoverished autobiographical memory come about?

Among the mechanisms proposed to account for autobiographical memory deficits for traumatic experiences, three general categories emerge: (a) compromises to brain structures that result in changes in function, (b) cognitive mechanisms and (c) consequences of post-traumatic symptoms. Importantly, these mechanisms are not mutually exclusive and in fact may operate simultaneously.

### Compromises to brain structures

Impoverished autobiographical memory may arise from the compromised integrity of brain regions involved in memory functioning, such as the hippocampus [49–51]. Several structures in the medial temporal lobe, including the hippocampus, are critical to the formation and consolidation of episodic memories [52]. Reduced hippocampal volume has been observed in both combat veterans [49] and adult survivors of childhood physical and sexual abuse [50,53], suggesting some fundamental disruption in the function of this region among adults exposed to trauma. In spite of the importance of these findings, the specific consequences of reduced brain volume for autobiographical memory remain unclear.

While the direction of causal relationships between reduced brain volume and the development of PTSD and/or memory deficits was long unclear, recent twin studies inform our understanding of directionality. For example, Pitman et al. [54] observed lower hippocampal volume and other neurological abnormalities in combat veterans diagnosed with PTSD and their unexposed twins compared with veterans without PTSD and their unexposed twins. These findings suggest that lower hippocampal volume and other neurological irregularities may be risk factors for (rather than consequences of)

PTSD. Notably, however, observations of hippocampal volume reductions have not been consistently replicated in children, although maltreated children (particularly those diagnosed with PTSD) appear to have smaller total brain and/or cerebral volumes than their peers (reviewed by Watts-English et al. [55]).

Nadel and Jacobs [56] demonstrated differential effects of stress on brain structures involved in autobiographical memory. Specifically, stress enhances amygdala function, which is involved in memory for emotionally charged events, but impairs hippocampal function, which is involved in episodic memory. These differential effects may help to explain otherwise counter-intuitive impairments in episodic memory for the traumatic event *and* enhanced fear response to traumatic stimuli [56,57].

In sum, disruptions in autobiographical and more general explicit memories could come about as a result of alterations in the functioning of brain structures, such as the hippocampus and amygdala, that are crucial to memory processes. Preexisting vulnerabilities, such as smaller hippocampal volume, could contribute to alterations in the formation and integration of memories, thus resulting in retrieval impairments for autobiographical memories as well as the explicit memory deficits observed in the laboratory. Of particular note are findings suggesting that stress may result in enhanced and impaired functioning of brain regions (e.g., amygdala and hippocampus) in ways that contribute to the seemingly inconsistent patterns of enhanced emotional memory and impoverished episodic memory.

### Cognitive processes

Memory impairment may also arise via cognitive processes rooted in psychological motivations. For example, betrayal trauma theory [25,44] proposes that if the abuse is perpetrated by a caregiver upon whom the victim relies for survival, *unawareness* about the abuse may be adaptive. Freyd et al. [44] have argued that unawareness, or "the phenomenon of information inaccessibility" (p. 296), may help a child to maintain necessary attachments with abusive caregivers. The theory implicates dissociation as a potential route to unawareness, although acknowledging that information can become inaccessible via many routes (e.g., everyday forgetting, encoding failures [44]).

In addition to passive cognitive processes (e.g., encoding failures, everyday forgetting), non-passive cognitive mechanisms such as active inhibitory processes may also contribute to impaired autobiographical memory. Anderson and colleagues [58,59] have proposed that executive control processes are involved in preventing unwanted explicit memories from entering awareness. When individuals continually inhibit cues for unwanted memories, recall of the unwanted memory becomes more difficult. Experimental studies have shown that individuals recalled fewer response words when they had previously inhibited the words' corresponding cues [59,60]. These results support the existence of an active inhibitory cognitive process that impairs recall of unwanted memories when they are kept out of awareness. Paradoxically, the more cues one encounters to an unwanted memory, the less accessible that memory may become. Therefore, active inhibitory processes may provide a mechanism by which forgetting occurs more often for betrayal traumas than for traumas inflicted by strangers [58].

Memory impairments for traumatic events may also arise from changes in meta-awareness (explicit awareness of our experiences). Schooler [61] proposed that memory for trauma is not entirely forgotten; rather, the experience of "discovering" a traumatic memory occurs because of a change in meta-awareness for the memory that was intentionally or non-intentionally avoided. In this view, conscious recollection of an experience is dissociated from one's appraisal of that experience. According to Schooler, changing, re-accessing, or gaining a new meta-awareness for the meaning of (or emotions surrounding) a traumatic experience may be confused with first-time access of the memory and, therefore, someone may be led to believe that they are remembering the event for the first time.

In sum, autobiographical memory impairment could occur via active or involuntary cognitive processes. Active inhibitory processes contribute to difficulty retrieving trauma-related memories because of repeated inhibition of event-related cues. Alternatively, changes to meta-awareness may alter one's beliefs about access to trauma-related memories. Importantly, these explanations are not incompatible; for example, repeated deliberate inhibition of traumatic memories suppresses retrieval and perhaps decreases reflection and other processes that lead to gaining meta-awareness for the event.

## Post-traumatic symptoms

Autobiographical memory impairments for trauma may also be consequences of information-processing changes associated more generally with post-traumatic symptoms, as evidenced by studies documenting autobiographical memory impairments in relation to both PTSD and dissociation [62–64]. For example, Briere and Conte [62] found that current psychological symptoms were among the factors most predictive of amnesia for childhood sexual abuse in an adult sample. Notably, though, evidence for links between impairments in autobiographical memory and PTSD/dissociation symptoms has been inconsistent in the literature, with some studies failing to find relationships between PTSD and disruptions in either memory for details or coherence of autobiographical memories for trauma [65,66]. Given such inconsistencies, associations between symptoms and memory impairment may be better explained by correlated factors, such as the compromises to brain structure and function, or cognitive processes reviewed above.

Associations between autobiographical memory impairments for trauma and PTSD/dissociation symptoms are difficult to reconcile with laboratory findings. As reviewed above, PTSD is associated with explicit memory impairments for neutral stimuli and heightened memory for trauma stimuli in the laboratory; dissociation is associated with impoverished memory for trauma stimuli (relative to neutral stimuli) under certain attentional conditions compared with controls. Further, PTSD and dissociation are interrelated (reviewed by DePrince et al. [67]). Therefore, while these symptoms are associated with very different patterns of explicit memory performance in the laboratory, both are (sometimes) related to autobiographical memory impairments.

Several hypotheses generated from the complex and at times contradictory findings that emerge inside and outside the laboratory warrant further investigation. First, memory systems tapped in the laboratory may not relate to those responsible for trauma-related memory impairment outside the laboratory, bringing us back to questions about the very nature of traumatic memories: to what extent is memory (or memory impairment) for trauma outside the laboratory similar to or different from memory (or memory impairment) for non-traumatic events/stimuli in the laboratory [46]. Second, memory findings in the laboratory mark more general risk/protective factors that may not relate directly to autobiographical memory. For example, the general explicit deficits associated with PTSD in the laboratory may be a risk factor for developing PTSD [54] while enhanced explicit memory for neutral stimuli may be a risk factor for developing dissociation [28]. In turn, disruptions in autobiographical memory are then associated with PTSD and dissociation through a third variable (e.g., compromises in brain function caused by traumatic stress). Third, memory performance in the laboratory may be relevant to understanding impairments in autobiographical memory for trauma outside the laboratory, pointing to multiple routes to memory disruption. That is, the differences in memory patterns associated with PTSD and dissociation in the laboratory may imply that PTSD and dissociation contribute to autobiographical memory impairment via different mechanisms.

## Conclusions

This review highlights several puzzles that remain to be solved. For example, how do laboratory-based findings relate to and help us to understand trauma survivors' reports of disruptions in trauma-related explicit memories? How do interrelated symptoms of dissociation and PTSD, which are associated with different patterns of performance on laboratory memory tasks, both relate to reports of impoverished trauma-related explicit memories? We hope that future research aimed at untangling these puzzles will bring together the best of advances in prospective, twin, neuropsychological and neuroimaging methods to examine memory across multiple domains and contexts.

## References

1. Brewin, C. R. (2003). *Posttraumatic stress disorder: Malady or myth?* New Haven, CT: Yale University Press.
2. Bremner, J. D., Randall, P., Scott, T. M. *et al.* (1995). Deficits in short-term memory in adult survivors of childhood abuse. *Psychiatry Research*, **59**, 97–107.
3. Sutker, P. B., Winstead, D. K., Galina, Z. H. and Allain, A. N. (1991). Cognitive deficits and psychopathology among former prisoners of war and combat veterans of the Korean conflict. *American Journal of Psychiatry*, **148**, 67–72.
4. Yehuda, R., Keefe, R. S.E., Harvey, P. and Levengood, R. A. (1995). Learning and memory in combat veterans with posttraumatic stress disorder. *American Journal of Psychiatry*, **152**, 137–139.
5. Bremner, J. D., Vermetten, E., Afzal, N. and Vythilingam, M. (2003). Deficits in verbal declarative memory function in women with childhood sexual abuse-related posttraumatic stress disorder. *Journal of Nervous and Mental Disease*, **192**, 643–649.
6. El-Hage, W., Gaillard, P., Isingrini, M. and Belzung, C. (2006). Trauma-related deficits in working memory. *Cognitive Neuropsychiatry*, **11**, 33–46.
7. Stein, M. B., Kennedy, C. M. and Twamley, E. W. (2002). Neuropsychological function in female victims of intimate partner violence with and without posttraumatic stress disorder. *Biological Psychiatry*, **52**, 1079–1088.
8. Beers, S. R. and De Bellis, M. D. (2002). Neuro-psychological function in children with maltreatment-related posttraumatic stress disorder. *American Journal of Psychiatry*, **159**, 483–486.
9. DePrince, A. P., Weinzierl, K. M. and Combs, M. D. (2009). Executive function performance and trauma exposure in a community sample of children. *Child Abuse and Neglect*, **33**, 353–361.
10. Paunovic, N., Lundh, L.-G. and Öst, L.-G. (2002). Attentional and memory bias for emotional information in crime victims with acute posttraumatic stress disorder (PTSD). *Journal of Anxiety Disorders*, **16**, 675–692.
11. Vrana, S. R., Roodman, A. and Beckham, J. C. (1995). Selective processing of trauma-relevant words in posttraumatic stress disorder. *Journal of Anxiety Disorders*, **9**, 515–530.
12. Golier, J. A., Yehuda, R., Lupien, S. J. and Harvey, P. D. (2003). Memory for trauma-related information in Holocaust survivors with PTSD. *Psychiatry Research*, **121**, 133–143.
13. Amir, N., McNally, R. J. and Wiegartz, P. S. (1996). Implicit memory bias for threat in posttraumatic stress disorder. *Cognitive Therapy and Research,* **20**, 625–635.
14. Zeitlin, S. B. and McNally, R. J. (1991). Implicit and explicit memory bias for threat in post-traumatic stress disorder. *Behaviour Research and Therapy*, **29**, 451–457.
15. MacLeod, C. and McLaughlin, K. (1995). Implicit and explicit memory bias in anxiety: A conceptual replication. *Behaviour Research and Therapy*, **33**, 1–14.
16. Grillon, C., Morgan, C. A., III, Davis, M. and Southwick, S. M. (1998). Effects of experimental context and explicit threat cues on acoustic startle in Vietnam veterans with posttraumatic stress disorder. *Society of Biological Psychiatry*, **44**, 1027–1036.
17. Grillon, C., Morgan, C. A., III, Southwick, S. M., Davis, M. and Charney, D. S. (1996). Baseline startle amplitude and prepulse inhibition in Vietnam veterans with posttraumatic stress disorder. *Psychiatry Research*, **64**, 169–178.
18. Morgan, C. A., III, Grillon, C., Southwick, S. M., Davis, M. and Charney, D. S. (1995). Fear-potentiated startle in post traumatic stress disorder. *Biological Psychiatry*, **38**, 378–385.
19. Morgan, C. A., III and Grillon, C. (1998). Acoustic startle in individuals with posttraumatic stress disorder. *Psychiatric Annals*, **28**, 430–434.
20. Shalev, A. Y., Orr, S. P., Peri, T., Schreiber, S. and Pitman, R. K. (1992). Physiologic responses to loud

tones in Israeli patients with posttraumatic stress disorder. *Archives of General Psychology*, **49**, 870–875.

21. Shalev, A. Y., Peri, T., Gelpin, E., Orr, S. P. and Pitman, R. K. (1997). Psychophysiological assessment of mental imagery of stressful events in Israeli civilian posttraumatic stress disorder patients. *Comprehensive Psychiatry*, **38**, 269–273.

22. Elsesser, K., Sartory, G. and Tackenberg, A. (2004). Attention, heart rate, and startle response during exposure to trauma-relevant pictures: A comparison of recent trauma victims and patients with posttraumatic stress disorder. *Journal of Abnormal Psychology*, **113**, 289–301.

23. Pole, N., Neylan, T. C., Otte, C. *et al.* (2007). Associations between childhood trauma and emotion-modulated psychophysiological responses to startling sounds: A study of police cadets. *Journal of Abnormal Psychology*, **116**, 352–361.

24. American Psychiatric Association (1994). *Diagnostic and statistical manual of mental disorders,* 4th edn. Washington, DC: American Psychiatric Press.

25. Freyd, J. J. (1996). *Betrayal trauma: The logic of forgetting child abuse.* Cambridge, MA: Harvard University Press.

26. Cloitre, M. (1992). Avoidance of emotional processing: A cognitive science perspective. In D. J. Stein and J. E. Young (eds.), *Cognitive science and clinical disorders* (pp. 19–41). San Diego, CA: Academic Press.

27. Cloitre, M., Cancienne, J. Brodsky, B., Dulit, R. and Perry, S. W. (1996). Memory performance among women with parental abuse histories: Enhanced directed forgetting or directed remembering? *Journal of Abnormal Psychology*, **105**, 204–211.

28. de Ruiter, M. B., Elzinga, B. M. and Phaf, R. H. (2006). Dissociation: Cognitive capacity or dysfunction? *Journal of Trauma and Dissociation*, **7**, 115–134.

29. Elzinga, B. M., de Beurs, E., Sergeant, J. A., Van Dyck, R. and Phaf, R. H. (2000). Dissociative style and directed forgetting. *Cognitive Therapy and Research*, **24**, 279–295.

30. DePrince, A. P. and Freyd, J. J. (1999). Dissociative tendencies, attention, and memory. *Psychological Science*, **10**, 449–452.

31. Simeon, D., Knutelska, M. E., Putnam, F. *et al.* (2006). Attention and memory in dissociative disorders, posttraumatic stress disorder, and healthy volunteers. In *Proceeding of the Annual Meeting of the International Society for Traumatic Stress Studies*, Hollywood, CA, abst 158865.

32. Elzinga, B. M., Ardon, A. M., Heijnis, M. K. *et al.* (2006). Neural correlates of enhanced working memory performance in dissociative disorder: A functional MRI study. *Psychological Medicine*, **37**, 235–245.

33. DePrince, A. P. and Freyd, J. J. (2001). Memory and dissociative tendencies: The roles of attentional context

and word meaning in a directed forgetting task. *Journal of Trauma and Dissociation*, **2**, 67–82.

34. DePrince, A. P. and Freyd, J. J. (2004). Forgetting trauma stimuli. *Psychological Science*, **15**, 488–492.

35. DePrince, A. P., Freyd, J. J. and Malle, B. F. (2007). A replication by another name: A response to Devilly *et al.* (2007). *Psychological Science*, **18**, 218–219.

36. Becker-Blease, K. A., Freyd, J. J. and Pears, K. C. (2004). Preschoolers' memory for threatening information depends on trauma history and attentional context: Implications for the development of dissociation. *Journal of Trauma and Dissociation*, **5**, 113–131.

37. Williams, L. M. (1994). Recall of childhood trauma: A prospective study of women's memories of child sexual abuse. *Journal of Consulting and Clinical Psychology*, **62**, 1167–1176.

38. Williams, L. M. (1995). Recovered memories of abuse in women with documented child sexual victimization histories. *Journal of Traumatic Stress*, **8**, 649–673.

39. Edwards, V. J., Fivush, R., Anda, R. F., Felitti, V. J. and Nordenberg, D. F. (2001) Autobiographical memory disturbances in childhood abuse survivors. *Journal of Aggression, Maltreatment and Trauma*, **4**, 247–264.

40. Feldman-Summers, S. and Pope, K. S. (1994). The experience of "forgetting" childhood abuse: A national survey of psychologists. *Journal of Consulting and Clinical Psychology*, **62**, 636–639.

41. DePrince, A. P., Freyd, J. J. and Zurbriggen, E. L. (2001). Self-reported memory for abuse depends upon victim-perpetrator relationship. *Journal of Trauma and Dissociation*, **2**, 5–16.

42. Schultz, T., Passmore, J. L. and Yoder, C. Y. (2003). Emotional closeness with perpetrators and amnesia for child sexual abuse. *Journal of Child Sexual Abuse*, **12**, 67–88.

43. van der Hart, O., Hilde, B. and van der Kolk, B. A. (2006). Memory fragmentation in dissociative identity disorder. *Journal of Trauma and Dissociation*, **6**, 55–70.

44. Freyd, J. J., DePrince, A. P. and Gleaves, D. H. (2007). The state of betrayal trauma theory: Reply to McNally (2006), conceptual issues, and future directions. *Memory*, **15**, 295–311.

45. Sargant, W. and Slater, E. (1941). Amnestic syndromes of war. *Proceedings of the Royal Society of Medicine*, **34**, 757–764.

46. Brewin, C. R. (2007). Autobiographical memory for trauma: Update on four controversies. *Memory*, **15**, 227–248.

47. Shobe, K. K. and Kihlstrom, J. F. (1997). Is traumatic memory special? *Current Directions in Psychological Science*, **6**, 70–74.

48. Lanius, R. A., Williamson, P. C., Boksman, K. *et al.* (2002). Brain activation during script-driven imagery

induced dissociative responses in PTSD: A function magnetic resonance imaging investigation. *Biological Psychiatry*, **52**, 305–311.

49. Bremner, J. D., Randall, P., Scott, T. M. and Bronen, R. A. (1995). MRI-based measurement of hippocampal volume in patients with combat-related posttraumatic stress disorder. *American Journal of Psychiatry*, **152**, 973–981.

50. Bremner, J. D., Randall, P., Vermetten, E. and Staib, L. (1997). Magnetic resonance imaging-based measurement of hippocampal volume in posttraumatic stress disorder related to childhood physical and sexual abuse: A preliminary report. *Biological Psychiatry*, **41**, 23–32.

51. Uno, H., Tarara, R., Else, J. G., Suleman, M. A. and Salpolsky, R. M. (1989). Hippocampal damage associated with prolonged and fatal stress in primates. *Journal of Neuroscience*, **9**, 1705–1711.

52. Zola-Morgan, S. and Squire, L. R. (1993). Neuro-anatomy of memory. *Annual Review of Neuroscience*, **16**, 547–563.

53. Stein, M. B., Koverola, C., Hanna, C., Torchia, M. G. and McClarty, B. (1997). Hippocampal volume in women victimized by childhood sexual abuse. *Psychological Medicine*, **27**, 951–959.

54. Pitman, R. K., Gilbertson, M. W., Gurvits, T. V. *et al.* (2006). Clarifying the origin of biological abnormalities in PTSD through the study of identical twins discordant for combat exposure. In R. Yehuda (ed.), *Psychobiology of post-traumatic stress disorder: A decade of progress* (pp. 242–254). Malden, MA: Blackwell.

55. Watts-English, T., Fortson, B. L., Gibler, N., Hooper, S. R. and De Bellis, M. D. (2006). The psychobiology of maltreatment in childhood. *Journal of Social Issues*, **62**, 717–736.

56. Nadel, L. and Jacobs, W. J. (1998). Traumatic memory is special. *Current Directions in Psychological Science*, **7**, 154–157.

57. Jacobs, W. J. and Nadel, L. (1998). Neurobiology of reconstructed memory. *Psychology, Public Policy, and Law*, **4**, 1110–1134.

58. Anderson, M. C. (2001). Active forgetting: Evidence for functional inhibition as a source of memory failure. *Journal of Aggression, Maltreatment and Trauma*, **4**, 185–210.

59. Anderson, M. C. and Green, C. (2001). Suppressing unwanted memories by executive control. *Nature*, **410**, 366–369.

60. Anderson, M. C., Ochsner, K. N., Kuhl, B. *et al.* (2004). Neural systems underlying the suppression of unwanted memories. *Science*, **303**, 232–235.

61. Schooler, J. W. (2001). Discovering memories of abuse in the light of meta-awareness. *Journal of Aggression, Maltreatment and Trauma*, **4**, 105–136.

62. Briere, J. and Conte, J. (1993). Self-reported amnesia for abuse in adults molested as children. *Journal of Traumatic Stress*, **6**, 21–31.

63. Carlson, E. B., Armstrong, J., Loewenstein, R. and Roth, D. (1998). Relationships between traumatic experiences and symptoms of posttraumatic stress, dissociation, and amnesia. In J. D. Bremner and C. R. Marmar (eds.), *Trauma, memory, and dissociation* (pp. 205–228). Washington, DC: American Psychiatric Press.

64. Bremner, J. D., Vermetten, E., Southwick, S. M., Krystal, J. H. and Charney, D. S. (1998). Trauma, memory, and dissociation: An integrative formulation. In J. D. Bremner and C. R. Marmar (eds.), *Trauma, memory, and dissociation* (pp. 365–402). Washington, DC: American Psychiatric Press.

65. Berntsen, D., Willert, M. and Rubin, D. C. (2003). Splintered memories or vivid landmarks? Reliving and coherence of traumatic memories in PTSD. *Applied Cognitive Psychology*, **17**, 675–693.

66. Rubin, D. C., Feldman, M. E. and Beckham, J. C. (2004). Reliving, emotions, and fragmentation in the autobiographical memories of veterans diagnosed with PTSD. *Applied Cognitive Psychology*, **18**, 17–35.

67. DePrince, A. P., Chu, A. and Visvanathan, P. (2006). Dissociation and posttraumatic stress disorder. *PTSD Research Quarterly*, **17**, 1–8.

# Chapter 21

# Scientific progress and methodological issues in the study of recovered and false memories of trauma

Constance J. Dalenberg and Oxana G. Palesh

## Introduction

Given the history of the recovered memory (RM) as a centerpiece in battles regarding the nature of science and evidence, it may be surprising for some to learn that the science of RM is rich and long standing, based on increasingly sophisticated methods with consensually accepted results. Since the time of Ebbinghaus's publication of the forgetting curve in 1885 [1], a sizable literature has developed on "simple inhibition," in which "some specific target (a list of nonsense syllables, some dreadful event, a taboo desire) is inhibited or subtracted out of consciousness" ([2], p. 502). Following the Ebbinghaus methodology, early research also repeatedly established that the intensive focus on *retrieval* of a memory can have a profoundly hypermnesiac (memory increasing) effect [2]. Anecdotal examples of recovered memory have also been described by many experimental memory experts (e.g., Loftus [3]), including those who would later emerge as dismissive of the concept. A clear articulation of the meaning of terms is important in evaluating the current state of science in this area, particularly in light of the disparate conclusions set forth by the relevant researchers.

## Is it a memory? Is it recovered?

In rejecting the concept of RM, those proposing false memory (FM) often make the argument that the apparent recovery of a memory may not be what it appears. First, and most obviously, it could be false (produced by suggestion or deduction, not memory), even if historically accurate. Second, the apparent recovered memory experience could be an example of conscious withholding followed by disclosure. Third, the victim may be misunderstanding the recovery question, referring only to the fact that s/he went through periods of not thinking about the trauma.

Less frequently, critics of FM research note similar problems [4,5]. When the participant in a FM experiment reports that s/he *does* remember the allegedly false event provided by a trusted other, the individual may be (a) subjectively "remembering," (b) reporting a false belief or (c) pretending to recall in order to meet social demands. Furthermore, how do we know that the memory is indeed false? In Hyland's dissertation [6], when the researcher returned to the mother, armed with details regarding the "false" memory, the mother frequently claimed to remember that the child was indeed right. She *had* lost a pet when she was 8 years old. Alternative hypotheses must be carefully addressed by those working in both FM and RM areas.

## What about anecdotal evidence?

In making their case, both (trauma research) often turn to the dreaded anecdote, precisely because it is these individual cases that present the best proof of their phenomenon. Simultaneously, each group occasionally chastises the other for the use of illustrative examples. How do we know that the retractors who move from suggestive therapists to suggestive FM support groups are reporting their therapy accurately? How do we know that RM victims who claim to have recently recalled their trauma, even if it is proven true, are not ashamed to tell us that they had simply lacked the will to disclose?

Anecdotes offer examples of individuals who recovered provably accurate memories outside of therapy in the absence of suggestion (e.g., the first victim of a multiple abuser), and who describe vague memories that become clearer over time (e.g., Frank Fitzpatrick, the first accuser of Father Porter, and Ross Cheit [7], the Director of the Recovered Memory Archives). Added to these public personages are disguised case studies [8], in which well-described RM accounts are supported by perpetrator confession. Such evidence is hard to deny, and many skeptical researchers acknowledge the power of these anecdotes in passing. After a critical review of the existing published case studies, Brenneis [9] concluded that the existence of traumatic experiences unrelated to head trauma that are selectively lost to conscious memory and later recovered has been "conclusively demonstrated" (p. 73). Corroborated case studies were also offered by Schooler [8] and Dalenberg [10], among many others.

The anecdotes offered by FM researchers tend not to include external verification from others. However, de Rivera [11] presented "Ann," who accused her family of abusing her during what she describes as manipulative psychotherapy. Supportive of the FM conclusion is the fact that "Ann" wrote a letter to her parents, accusing them of abuse, that she was allegedly not familiar with FM literature and that she does not report any counter-suggestion (beyond that provided by her family).

Both groups complain that there is an absence of "well-documented" cases for the other's position, with the retractor group particularly understudied in relation to the alleged availability of thousands or millions of cases. Studies of RM are more available and larger in scope, but those studies gathering information about mechanism of recovery and corroboration of abuse are smaller and less frequent (but see Melchert [12]). Given the complexity of the alternative hypotheses that each group wishes to rule out, the further presentation and publication of well-documented anecdotes with evidence related to mechanisms of memory loss and recovery and verification of abuse history appear essential.

## Corroboration of recovered memories

Researchers in the early FM studies were adamant in their rejection of the possible accuracy of recovered abuse memories. Pope and Hudson [13] stated that they had never seen a confirmed case of "noncontrived amnesia" among neurologically intact individuals over age 6 who experienced traumatic events that "no one would be expected to simply forget" (p. 716). Merskey [14] referred to recovered memories in general as "implausible memories without corroboration."

One of the first studies of RM accuracy was published by Herman and Schatzow in 1987 [15], who studied 53 women in psychotherapy. The majority of these women lacked full recall of their abuse, and over one-quarter (28%) showed "severe amnesia." Three-quarters of the women claimed external confirmation of their sexual abuse, and corroboration was not related to amnesia status.

Careful attention to corroboration has been seen in the literature after 1995, beginning with Williams' seminal research [16]. In her work, 129 women were interviewed in a 17 year follow-up to a study on child victimization. At the time of the abuse, the women had been 12 years old or younger. When details recalled were matched with records, RM and continuous memory victims were equally accurate (78–79% correct detail).

Dalenberg [10] investigated the question of RM accuracy with 17 women who had completed individual psychotherapy. By using repeated measures methods (within women experiencing both RM and continuous memories), variables that confounded the comparison of memory types could be ruled out, and the question of whether RM evidence is inherently unreliable could be investigated. The survivors and their alleged perpetrators (many of whom confessed) collected and disclosed evidence about the abuse. Dalenberg found equal (approximately 75%) corroboration of RM and continuous memories. Kluft [17] and Pope and Tabachnick [18] also reported high rates of corroboration.

An interesting exception to this pattern is the study by Geraerts et al. [19], who found 55% patient-reported corroboration in continuous memory victims, 63% corroboration in those who recovered memories outside of therapy, and 0% corroboration in those who recovered memories in therapy. The results of Pope and Tabachnick [18] suggested that corroboration rates could be related to the nature of therapy. Non-psychodynamic therapists reported that 61% of the RM clients found external validation, while psychodynamic therapists reported a 28% rate. These results may reflect a lesser push for external evidence among psychodynamic theorists (in service of "neutrality") or greater use of suggestion (e.g., dream interpretation).

Experimental FM research is another source for corroboration of RM. In the study by Hyman et al. [20], 25% of false events were reported in later interviews. The probability that a true and non-remembered event would be "recovered" in later interviews was 0.57, over double the recovery rate for false events. Just as in the clinical studies above, the majority of recovered events were (to the best of the researcher's knowledge) true.

## Phenomenology of recovered memory experiences

From the earliest surveys of RM survivors, researchers have noted that recovery often comes with a surge (or recurrence) of symptoms. Elliott and Briere [21] noted that RM victims tend to be more symptomatic than continuous survivors, a finding also reported by Herman and Schatzow [15] and Dalenberg [10]. McNally and colleagues, in partial contrast, found that the groups did not differ on clinical measures of distress [22], but did differ on measures of dissociation and absorption [23]. This surge of emotion is probably one source for the interpretation of some theorists that they were dealing with "de-repression," or a release of some defensive barrier. Andrews *et al.* [24] found some degree of reliving of emotion (with fear being the most common) with memory return in 83% of cases.

Andrews *et al.* [24] also found that 62% of RM returned as fragments, with only one-third of these eventually filling in sufficiently to be called "whole" memories. Fragmentation in trauma memory is also reported frequently by clinical writers (e.g., Roe and Schwartz [25]). Of note, Brenneis [9], who has argued that the best-documented cases of RM were less fragmented, quite reasonably posited that hazy and disjointed memories provide the most opportunity for misinterpretation by therapists.

Timing and triggers for recovery have been studied by numerous researchers, with fairly consistent findings, as predicted by FM and trauma research perspectives. Therapy tends to be among the triggers for recovery but it does not account for the majority of memory returns [12,16,26]. Triggers that are common across studies include events involving children or family, reminders from others describing similar abuse, media coverage and contact with the perpetrator or danger to self or others [16,24,26]. Timing of recovery in therapy does not appear to be related to use of "risky" techniques such as hypnosis or dream interpretation. Sensory triggers (visual, olfactory, sensorimotor or auditory) are more frequently noted than are verbal cues.

While sexual abuse is the most common recovered memory studied, the content of the memories is quite broad. Recovered memories of rape, child physical abuse and car accidents [12,21] have been reported. Within sexual abuse samples, violent abuse is sometimes reported as more frequently lost to memory [15], but this finding is not consistent across studies [16]. The finding of greater likelihood of loss and recovery of memory for parent perpetration appears to be more reliable [16,27,28]. Weak maternal support was a predictor in the research by Williams [16,27] just as avoidant maternal behavior is a predictor of lost detail for traumatic medical procedures in child eyewitness literature [29].

The age at the time of the original trauma appears to vary over a wide span, although later traumas (particularly those lasting into adolescence) are less likely to be lost and recovered [15,16,26,27]. Duration of the lost and recovered memories has been less well studied, with most literature contradicting by Terr [30] original prediction that lost memory would be more common for repeated than single-instance trauma. The occasional finding that repeated trauma is more often lost might be an artifact of the correlation between number of instances of abuse and parent status.

## Mechanisms of recovered memory

The research on mechanisms of RM experiences has generally centered in five areas: FM, repression and dissociation, state dependency, ordinary memory loss and recovery, and not-thinking.

### False memory

The method of the Lost in the Mall technique, and others to follow, was to engage a trusted figure in the role of dispensing authoritative misinformation to a research participant about childhood events, and asking the participants to think about or imagine the event. Loftus and Pickrell [31] found that approximately 25% of participants claim to remember the event. Since the study involved a common event, perhaps not false in entirety, Hyman and Billings [32] confirmed the finding with plausible but more unusual events. However, Pezdek *et al.* [33] found that no participant accepted the FM of an *implausible* traumatic event. This amendment to the "ease" of implanting FM has been largely accepted in later work, so that most cognitive researchers now state that it is difficult (but not impossible) to "implant" an implausible memory. In measuring individual differences, Hyman and Billings [32] found that dissociation correlated with the acceptance of the FM and with the level of detail in the true memory. Imagination inflation studies also have shown that FMs are held with greater confidence after repeated visualization [34], although alternative explanations for research effects are not always ruled out.

The Deese–Roediger–McDermott (DRM) paradigm is also used to study FM [35]. In this paradigm, individuals might be presented a series of words (e.g., nap, doze, dream, blanket), all of which related to a nonpresented word (sleep). Geraerts *et al.* [36] reported that FM production in this paradigm was related to fantasy proneness but not to trauma experience or dissociation, while Watson, Bunting *et al.* [37] found a relationship to working memory capacity and ability to exercise cognitive control.

Very little information exists on the relationship of FM of word lists to FM of trauma [38]. The results of the paradigm should not be ignored, however, and it is possible that memory phenomena that apply at a more trivial level also apply to more salient life events and could yield data that would help to differentiate accurate and false memories of trauma. For instance, the research above might suggest that a person low in fantasy proneness and high on working memory capacity would not be a strong candidate for application of the FM hypothesis, while a fantasy-prone individual with poor working memory might be likely to fit into this explanatory niche.

Researchers into FM often recommend "clarification interviews" for recovered memory studies, but such actions are ethically difficult to justify. For instance, Pope *et al.* [39] suggest that Williams [27] should have confronted her allegedly amnestic sexually abused women, disclosing their abuse and asking them to explain their lack of memory. Typically, the critique is presented with the counter-example from the study by Femina *et al.* [40]. In the description of this study by Pope *et al.* [39], Femina and colleagues contacted and re-interviewed eight individuals who had originally denied abuse, finding that all were consciously withholding; "in no case" did repression apply. In fact, Femina *et al.* contacted all non-disclosers in their study and most refused to be interviewed. They concluded that their sample was too small to make generalizations as to mechanisms for the change of report but stated that some individuals were "suppressing awareness" [40].

Clarification interviews are ethically less problematic in the FM literature but are rarely included, showing that each group of researchers tends to "trust" their own subjects and question those of the opposing researchers. For instance, when FM subjects do remember that they were lost in the mall, researchers seldom confront the parent (who had initially denied this) with the details of the child's recall. As mentioned earlier, Hyland [6] found that parents often affirmed that the memories their children recovered were not fully false (and were at times wholly true), but were forgotten by the parents until reminded by the detailed description.

The distinction between FM and false beliefs also is not clear in most research. Many of those who falsely remember the non-presented word in the DRM paradigm are unsure of their memory (seemingly recognizing that they are deducing rather than remembering). The social desirability pressure in the typical memory study is quite pronounced, as authority figures push participants to "remember" an allegedly established fact. Certainly a proportion of subjects might simply yield to the pressure and would admit lack of memory if given a minimal counter-pressure. In the study by Leichtman and Ceci [41] of FMs produced by 3- and 5-year-old children about a non-existent "crime," 100% of the 5 year olds (but not all 3 year olds) gave up their false accusations when an interviewer gently questioned the memory. De Rivera [42], examining 56 retractors and found that only 37.5% endorsed the option that the original FM "formed a coherent story with concrete details and feelings that seemed like a real memory." Others described the experience more as an imagined story, a set of connected or disconnected imagery, a feeling that abuse had occurred, a belief endorsed only by the therapist, or a "faked" description. Importantly, however, false beliefs might become FM over time, particularly if repeated visualization techniques are used and no questioning of the memories occurs.

## Repression and dissociation

As described above, the hypothesis that repression or dissociation are mechanisms responsible for the RM phenomenon has often been confused with the question of whether the phenomenon itself exists. Clinicians are often weary of defending "repression" against its critics, since the match between the current use of the term and Freud's description of it [43] lacks immediate clinical importance. Modern researchers appear to agree on three criteria for repression – inaccessibility (lack of conscious access), existence (some memory representation exists) and motivation (ongoing motivational forces prevent awareness). Dissociation requires a form of inaccessibility and existence, but motivation is debated. Although dissociation is thought to be defensive, the consequent poor encoding of material (perhaps through narrowing of attention [44] may then lead to inaccessibility without the need for ongoing motivational forces impeding access [4]. In Janet's original description [45], dissociated traumatic memory was thought to be inflexible and fixed (i.e., not adaptable to present circumstances), fragmented (consisting largely of feelings and bodily sensation) and responsive to automatic evocation by reminders (rather than voluntarily accessed). Therefore, the inaccessibility of the dissociating individual is at least partially state dependent.

Motivational forces are implicated in the directed forgetting/remembering literature, which now includes more than 200 peer-reviewed studies. In such research, words or word lists are shown to participants with a remember or forget instruction, with a finding that the to-be-forgotten words are recalled with lower frequency (theoretically an inhibition of accessibility) in later unexpected tests [46]. The generalization that abuse victims often wish to forget is not controversial, nor is the finding that emotional autobiographical information can be inhibited in a directed forgetting paradigm.

Most recently, the think/no think procedure has been developed by Anderson and colleagues (reviewed by Anderson [47]) and applied to the concept of motivated forgetting and repression. In this paradigm, participants learn unrelated word pairs and then practice retrieving certain paired words (think) and inhibiting retrieval of others (no think). Results of memory testing indicate that the no-think pairs are remembered more poorly than are unpractised words. Anderson and colleagues have argued that victims might purposely practice more acceptable memories of a feared family member (think) and inhibit memories of abuse (no-think).

If motivated forgetting can produce loss of memory for autobiographical events, as seems clear, FM and loss of memory for an important and salient event (such as child abuse) through directed forgetting still may be rare. However, if active attempts are being made to avoid and forget traumatic material, avoidant cognitive processes can become automatic. It is also well documented that threat-associated cues can be recognized without conscious mediation (e.g. individuals will show enhanced autonomic arousal to a feared stimulus presented too quickly to be consciously perceived [48]). Therefore, attention can be withdrawn unconsiously from reminders, and/or behaviors can be instituted to distance from reminders before cognitive awareness is triggered, thus maintaining traumatic amnesia.

Some evidence supports the role of dissociation in traumatic amnesia and RM. Goodman et al. [49] found a relationship between dissociation and alleged lack of memory for sexual trauma in a documented sample of victims, and Melchert [12] reported a correlation between dissociation and RM in a survey sample. Further, rape victims with reported amnesia very shortly after trauma had greater levels of peritraumatic dissociation than did non-amnestic victims [50]. Repression as measured by social desirability and anxiety measures was not related to memory loss or recovery in samples collected by Melchert [12] but was related to recall of rape by Krahe [51].

It is, of course, problematic to interpret low correlations between recovered amnesia and repression/dissociation after memories have been recovered. If dissociativity, for instance, is related to the capacity for traumatic amnesia, then return of memory may occur in periods of lower dissociation. It is, therefore, relevant to the argument for dissociation as a mechanism for RM that: (a) dissociative individuals are known to use avoidant coping [52]; (b) dissociation is associated with numbing and loss of affect [53], which is, in turn, related to memory loss [54]; and (c) dissociation has been related to errors of commission in memory work [55]. The role of dissociation in the prediction of traumatic amnesia and memory recovery is, therefore, likely to be quite complex.

## State dependency

Dissociation theory incorporates a type of state dependency, as highly dissociative individual may organize memories around emotional themes [56]. However, the general theory of state dependency does not require defensive or motivational features. Mood state dependency theory would argue that memories included in an unusual and extreme emotional state if "forgotten" through directed forgetting or normal decay may return in the context of another highly specific emotional state [26]. Fear state dependency has been studied by Lang et al. [57]. In general, however, mood state-dependency research tends to produce weak and methods-specific results and is an unsatisfying full explanation for RM in most instances (although it may be part of the equation in many).

## Ordinary memory and not-thinking

Infantile amnesia, one well-accepted feature of normal or ordinary memory, has been offered by theorists from all perspectives as one source for loss of trauma memory. The limitations of memory before age 3 [58] virtually guarantee high error rates in autobiographical accounts that were generated without external aid. Ordinary memory also plays into the RM discussion when critics argue that certain sexual abuse events are minor and, therefore, are simply forgotten. The frequently stated argument that the event, once remembered, could be re-interpreted (in adult consciousness) in a new way, turning a noxious event into a trauma [59], is non-controversial. It is less clear that a continuously-remembered event, if re-interpreted, could feel subjectively like a recovery.

Consequently, the debate about the role of ordinary memory as an explanation of RM events is not whether some events may be lost and recovered through decay and focused attention. Rather, debate centers on whether ordinary memory can constitute a full explanation of accurate RM events. Here, the evidence for the position is weak. At least three repeated findings are problematic for the ordinary memory hypothesis. First, amnesia appears to be more likely in situations in which the perpetrator is well known [28]. Second, amnesia following severe trauma seems to be more pronounced shortly after the incident than several months later in a subset of subjects [50]. Third, the intensity and reliving after return of memory is not experienced by survivors or their therapists as "ordinary" [24].

A variant of the ordinary memory explanation, the suggestion of not-thinking as an alternative understanding of RM phenomena, is offered by more recent reviewers (e.g., McNally [59]). As an example, Briere and Conte [60] asked participants if there was ever a time when they could not remember their abuse. As McNally [59] pointed out, a "yes" answer to this question could be interpreted in many ways, including that the individual simply did not wish to think about the incident. Not thinking about an event constantly, critics point out, is quite different than not being able to recall it.

Again, this explanation is likely to cover some subset of RM victims. However, arguing against the proposition that not-thinking explains all such accounts are the points that (a) studies discussing mechanisms with participants find descriptions of both not-thinking and failure to recall [12,16], (b) control groups reporting unpleasant non-traumatic events claim few RM experiences [26] and (c) not-thinking is difficult to square with the sense of surprise and increase in symptoms that often follows a RM experience [10,19].

# Conclusions and further issues

## Acknowledging bias
As articulated above, it is a common argument in the FM literature to state that while forgetting of negative events has been proven in the laboratory and related to trauma-relevant personality measures this constitutes "no evidence" for "robust repression" of trauma. However, the same researchers state that implanting of negative events in the laboratory *is* evidence for false memories of trauma. If we use the same standard of evidence for both sets of research, there is good (but imperfect) laboratory evidence for FM and RM of negative experiences. The field would be well served to give up the idea of my side, the objective scientists, versus your side, the biased advocates.

## Complex study of recovered memory samples
Many studies of RM have had fairly small sample sizes. Given the biases above, it is quite possible that these small samples will constitute quite different groups across researchers in FM and trauma. McNally *et al.* [22,23], who define RM as including those who report not thinking about a continuously remembered event, may be studying a population that does not overlap with that of Dalenberg [10], who included only clients who were subjectively experiencing a new and non-remembered event. At this point, the field would be advanced by a more clear description of the sample being offered. Symptom changes and treatment progress for the RM individual is another understudied area.

## Complex study of false memory samples
To date, most FM research has focused on laboratory analogues to the aggressive overzealous therapist who pushes an agenda on the hapless client. Further research is needed on those individuals who more spontaneously adopt a past event as their own, and those retractors with false beliefs versus those with false memories.

## Further study of lost, forgotten, repressed or dissociated memories
McNally *et al.* [22,23] and Geraerts *et al.* [19,36] have gathered data on the "repressed memory" group, defined as those who believe that they have been abused but do not know that this is so. No major trauma researcher is on record accepting that repressed memory can be

defined in this way. While there is value to these data, more central to the questions before us here would be the results from a group of individuals who claim that they do not now recall a trauma that has been documented as experienced.

## Deep study of individuals

The continued citation and clear influence of prominent FM and RM cases on the developing literature is at times acknowledged as "compelling existence of proof for our side" or "meaningless anecdote for your side." There is enormous value in careful and critical description, such that the critical distinction between FM (which could be confused with RM) and false belief (which is more likely to be distinguishable) can be made.

## Forensic evaluation

A glaring omission in the literature is in the area of malingering within RM cases against alleged perpetrators and FM cases against therapists. The biases that both groups deny are most evident here, as neither group wishes to acknowledge that in some cases malingering is a third alternative explanation for allegations of extreme and unusual memory, whether or not followed by retraction. The malingering research on PTSD would provide an excellent foundation.

## A return to civility

It is difficult to expect that one might be grateful to those who would attack and seek to undermine our strongly held theories. The indisputable fact that there are dozens of highly reputable and highly published critical thinkers who reject and accept the findings of most of the FM or RM studies above argues against simple dismissal of either FM or RM of trauma as always a fad, myth or dishonest attempt to avoid (or enable) prosecution or to garner clients. We are studying a phenomenon in an arena in which the stakes are high and the complexity is great enough to guarantee that our fellow scientists will design important but imperfect experiments. Our time can be spent solely in criticism, or in improvement and extension of design and expanded examination of alternative hypotheses.

## References

1. Ebbinghaus, H. (1885/1913). *Memory: A contribution to experimental psychology*. [Trans. H. Ruger and C. Bussenuis]. New York: Columbia University Press.
2. Erdelyi, M. (2006). The unified theory of repression. *Behavioral and Brain Sciences*, **29**, 499–551.
3. Loftus, E. (1988). *Memory: Surprising new insights into how we remember and why we forget.* New York: Ardsley House.
4. Dalenberg, C. (2006). Recovered memory and the Daubert Criteria: Recovered memory as professionally tested, peer reviewed, and accepted in the relevant scientific community. *Trauma, Violence and Abuse*, 7, 274–310.
5. DePrince, A., Allard, C., Oh., H. and Freyd, J. (2004). What's in a name for memory errors? Implications and ethical issues arising for the use of the term "false memory" for errors in memory for details. *Ethics & Behavior*, **14**, 201–233.
6. Hyland, K. (2000). *Pathways to false memory production: The role of content, individual differences, and citations of parental authority*. Ph.D. Thesis. Alliant International University, San Diego.
7. Cheit, R. (1998). Consider this, skeptics of recovered memory. *Ethics & Behavior*, **8**, 141–160.
8. Schooler, J. (1994). Seeking the core: The issues and evidence surrounding recovered accounts of sexual trauma. *Consciousness and Cognition*, 3, 452–469.
9. Brenneis, C. (2000). Evaluating the evidence: Can we find authenticated recovered memory? *Psychoanalytic Psychology*, **17**, 61–77.
10. Dalenberg, C. (1996). Accuracy, timing, and circumstances of disclosure in therapy of recovered and continuous memories of abuse. *Journal of Psychiatry & Law*, **24**, 229–275.
11. de Rivera, J. (1997). The construction of false memory syndrome: The experience of retractors. *Psychological Inquiry*, **8**, 271–292.
12. Melchert, T. (1999). Relations among childhood memory, a history of abuse, dissociation, and repression. *Journal of Interpersonal Violence*, **14**, 1172–1192.
13. Pope, H. and Hudson, J. (1995). Can individuals "repress" memories of childhood sexual abuse? An examination of the evidence. *Psychiatric Annals*, **25**, 715–719.
14. Merskey, H. (1996). Ethical issues in the search for repressed memories. *American Journal of Psychotherapy*, **50**, 323–325.
15. Herman, J. and Schatzow, E. (1987). Recovery and verification of memories of childhood sexual abuse. *Psychoanalytic Psychology*, **4**, 1–14.
16. Williams, L. (1995). Recovered memories of abuse in women with documented child abuse sexual victimization histories. *Journal of Traumatic Stress*, **8**, 649–673.
17. Kluft, R. (1997). The argument for the reality of delayed recall of trauma. In P. Appelbaum, L. Uyehara and M. Elin (eds.), *Trauma and memory: Clinical and legal controversies* (pp. 25–59). New York: Oxford University Press.

18. Pope, K. and Tabachnick, B. (1995). Recovered memories of abuse among therapy patients: A national survey. *Ethics and Behavior*, **5**, 237–248.

19. Geraerts, E., Schooler, J., Merckelbach, H. *et al.* (2007). The reality of recovered memories: Corroborating continuous and discontinuous memories of childhood sexual abuse. *Psychological Science*, **18**, 564–568.

20. Hyman, I., Husband, T. and Billings, F. (1995). False memories of childhood experiences. *Applied Cognitive Psychology*, **9**, 181–187.

21. Elliott, D. and Briere, J. (1995). Posttraumatic stress associated with delayed recall of sexual abuse: A general population study. *Journal of Traumatic Stress*, **8**, 629–647.

22. McNally, R., Perlman, C., Ristuccia, C. and Clancy, S. (2006). Clinical characteristics of adults reporting repressed, recovered, or continuous memories of childhood sexual abuse. *Journal of Consulting and Clinical Psychology*, **74**, 237–242.

23. McNally, R., Clancy, S., Schachter, D. and Pitman, R. (2000). Personality profiles, dissociations, absorption in women reporting repressed, recovered and continuous memories of childhood sexual abuse. *Journal of Consulting and Clinical Psychology*, **68**, 1033–1037.

24. Andrews, B., Brewin, C., Ochera, J. *et al.* (2000). Timing, triggers, and qualities of recovered memories in therapy. *British Journal of Clinical Psychology*, **39**, 11–26.

25. Roe, C. and Schwartz, M. (1996). Characteristics of previously forgotten memories of sexual abuse: A descriptive study. *Journal of Psychiatry & Law*, **24**, 289–206.

26. Albach, F., Moormann, P. and Bermond, B. (1996). Memory recovery of childhood sexual abuse. *Dissociation*, **9**, 261–272.

27. Williams, L. (1994). Recall of childhood trauma: A prospective study of women's memories of child sexual abuse. *Journal of Consulting and Clinical Psychology*, **62**, 1167–1176.

28. Freyd, J. (1996). *Betrayal trauma: The logical of forgetting childhood abuse.* Cambridge, MA: Harvard University Press.

29. Alexander, K., Goodman, G., Schaaf, J. *et al.* (2002). The role of attachment and cognitive inhibition in children's memory and suggestibility for a stressful event. *Journal of Experimental Child Psychology*, **83**, 262–290.

30. Terr, L. (1991). Childhood traumas: An outline and overview. *American Journal of Psychiatry*, **148**, 10–20.

31. Loftus, E. and Pickrell, J. (1995). The formation of false memories. *Psychiatric Annals*, **25**, 720–725.

32. Hyman, I. and Billings, F. (1998). Individual differences and the creation of false childhood memories. *Memory*, **6**, 1–20.

33. Pezdek, K., Finger, K. and Hodge, D. (1997). Planting false childhood memories: The role of event plausibility. *Psychological Science*, **8**, 437–441.

34. Garry, M., Manning, C., Loftus, E. and Sherman, S. (1996). Imagination inflation: Imagining a childhood event inflates confidence that it occurred. *Psychonomic Bulletin & Review*, **3**, 206–214.

35. Roediger, H. and McDermott, K. (1995). Creating false memories: Remembering words not presented in lists. *Journal of Experimental Psychology: Learning, Memory, and Cognition*, **21**, 803–814.

36. Geraerts, E., Smeets, E., Jelicic, M., van Heerden, J. and Merckelbach, H. (2005). Fantasy proneness, but not self-reported trauma is related to DRM performance of women reporting recovered memories of childhood sexual abuse. *Consciousness and Cognition*, **14**, 602–612.

37. Watson, J., Bunting, M., Poole, B. and Conway, A. (2005). Individual differences in susceptibility to false memory in the Deese–Roediger–McDermott paradigm. *Journal of Experimental Psychology: Learning, Memory, and Cognition*, **31**, 76–85.

38. Freyd, J. and Gleaves, D. (1996). "Remembering" words not presented in lists: Relevance to the current recovered/false memory controversy. *Journal of Experimental Psychology: Learning, Memory, and Cognition*, **22**, 811–813.

39. Pope, H., Oliva, P. and Hudson, J. (1999). The scientific status of repressed memories. In D. Faigman, D. Kaye, M. Saks and J. Sanders (eds.), *Modern scientific evidence: The law and science of expert testimony* (pp. 115–155). St. Paul: West Publishing.

40. Femina, D., Yeager, C. and Lewis, D. (1990) Child abuse: adolescent records vs. adult recall. *Child Abuse & Neglect*, **14**, 227–231.

41. Leichtman, M. and Ceci, S. (1995). The effects of stereotypes and suggestions in preschoolers' reports. *Developmental Psychology*, **31**, 568–578.

42. De Rivera, J. (2000). Understanding those who repudiate memories recovered in therapy. *Professional Psychology: Research & Practice*, **31**, 378–386.

43. Freud, S. (1914) Remembering, repeating and working-through. (1914). In S. James (ed.), *The standard edition of the complete psychological works of Sigmund Freud.* Vol. 7. New York: Norton.

44. Christianson, S. and Nilsson, L. (1984). Functional amnesia as induced by a psychological trauma. *Memory & Cognition*, **12**, 142–155.

45. Janet, P. (1904). L'Amnesie et la dissociation des souvenirs par l'emotion. *Journal de Psychologie*, **1**, 417–453.

46. Bjork, R. and Bjork, R. (1996). Continuing influences of to-be-forgotten information. *Consciousness and Cognition*, **5**, 176–196.

47. Anderson, M. (2003). Rethinking interference theory: Executive control and the mechanisms of

forgetting. *Journal of Memory and Language*, **49**, 415–445.

48. Parra, C., Esteves, F., Flykt, A. and Ohman, A. (1997). Pavolovian conditioning to social stimuli: Backward masking and dissociation of implicit and explicit cognitive processes. *European Psychologist*, **2**, 106–117.

49. Goodman, G., Ghetti, S., Quas, J. *et al.* (2003). A prospective study of memory for child sexual abuse: New findings relevant to the repressed memory controversy. *Psychological Science*, **14**, 113–118.

50. Mechanic, M., Resick, P. and Griffin, M. (1998). A comparison of normal forgetting, psychopathology, and information-processing models of reported amnesia for recent sexual trauma. *Journal of Consulting and Clinical Psychology*, **66**, 948–957.

51. Krahe, B. (1999). Repression and coping with the threat of rape. *European Journal of Personality*, **13**, 15–26.

52. Marmar, C., Weiss, D., Metzler, T. and Delucchi, K. (1996). Characteristics of emergency services personnel related to peritraumatic dissociation during critical incident exposure. *American Journal of Psychiatry*, **153**, 94–102.

53. Feeny, N., Zoellner, L., Fitzgibbons, L. and Foa, E. (2000). Exploring the roles of emotional numbing, depression, and dissociation in PTSD. *Journal of Traumatic Stress*, **13**, 489–498.

54. Richards, J. and Gross, J. (2000). Emotional regulation and memory: the cognitive cost of keeping one's cool. *Journal of Personality and Social Psychology*, **79**, 410–424.

55. Merckelbach, H., Zeles, G., van Bergen, S. and Giesbrecht, T. (2007). Trait dissociation and commission errors in memory reports of emotional events. *American Journal of Psycology*, **120**, 1–14.

56. Putnam, F. (1997). *Dissociation in children and adolescents: A developmental perspective*. New York: Guilford.

57. Lang, A., Craske, M., Brown, M. and Ghaneian, A. (2001). Fear-related state dependent memory. *Cognition and Emotion*, **15**, 695–703.

58. Bauer, P. (2002). Early memory development. In: H. Goswami (ed.), *Handbook of cognitive development* (pp. 127–145). Oxford: Balckwell

59. McNally, R. (2003). Progress and controversy in the study of posttraumatic stress disorder. *Annual Review of Psychology*, **54**, 229–252.

60. Briere, J. and Conte, J. (1993). Self-reported amnesia for abuse in adults molested as children. *Journal of Traumatic Stress*, **6**, 21–31.

# The psychosocial consequences of organized violence on children

Felicia Heidenreich, Mónica Ruiz-Casares and Cécile Rousseau

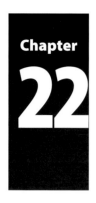

## Introduction

Research on the mental health consequences of organized violence on children is not new. After World War II, Anna Freud studied the impact of the concentration camp trauma on child survivors; likewise, the effects of bombings and parental separation were documented in children living in London [1]. Since then, numerous studies have explored the associations between exposure to organized violence and psychopathology in children. Although most studies have focused on post-traumatic stress disorder (PTSD) as a specific mental health consequence of exposure to trauma, research is increasingly emphasizing the strengths manifested by children, thus shifting the interest toward the understanding of resilience. The study of organized violence is structured around numerous disciplines in the social sciences, such as anthropology, political science and sociology, as well as the mental health disciplines. Their different perspectives and methods determine in large part the relative emphasis on culture, context and psychological phenomena of the research focusing on the consequences of organized violence for children.

Organized violence is defined as any form of violence perpetrated directly by the state or its organs against people because of their political opinion, ethnic origin, gender, sexual orientation or religious orientation [2]. This applies also to situations where the state does not protect its citizens from violence or when it does not grant basic human rights, leading to a form of structural violence.

This chapter reviews recent research about the consequences of organized violence on children and proposes an update on treatment approaches. The first part will summarize the literature on the determinants of risk and protection for children in situations of organized violence, reviewing research undertaken in both countries still at war and in post-conflict situations,

including studies with child soldiers, refugee children and unaccompanied minors in Western countries. We will then focus on the transgenerational transmission of trauma, its implications for symptom expression and the appearance of paradoxical outcomes in relation to the notions of resilience, vulnerability and risk for generations to come. Finally, the advances and limitations of classical and innovative therapeutic approaches will be discussed and recommendations for future research.

## Assessment methodology

Research into organized violence and children displays large heterogeneity in regards to methods and underlying research questions. Some studies examine the prevalence of PTSD, depression and anxiety disorders in children. Others go a step further and explore associations between trauma experiences, cumulative risk factors such as family situation, and psychopathological outcomes. The study of resiliency and risk factors has received increased interest since they seem to translate into prevention and intervention measures. Two sets of limitations need to be noted about a majority of studies: the problematic utilization of screening instruments in intercultural contexts and the question of the limited applicability of the PTSD category in traumatized children of different developmental levels and cultural backgrounds. Most of the children experiencing organized violence come from non-Western countries and they speak languages for which many instruments have not been formally validated. Cultural considerations invite us to be prudent in applying Western diagnostic criteria (i.e., *Diagnostic and Statistical Manual of Mental Disorders* [3]) to non-Western populations [4]. The construction of these criteria is in itself deeply cultural, as has been shown for PTSD in the USA [5]. Moreover, the diagnostic

*The Impact of Early Life Trauma on Health and Disease: The Hidden Epidemic*, ed. Ruth A. Lanius, Eric Vermetten and Clare Pain. Published by Cambridge University Press. Copyright © Cambridge University Press 2010.

criteria for PTSD, which are centered on fear and reexperiencing, are fit to adults, and direct transposition to children is not always adequate. Children exposed to trauma report different emotions, such as helplessness, depression, shame, grief and mental collapse, which are not accounted for by PTSD criteria [6]. Learning difficulties, loss of previously acquired developmental skills, separation anxiety and new phobias are possible reactions to trauma that are not accounted for in some standard screening instruments [7].

Psychological outcomes vary depending on the age at exposure illustrating how the effect of trauma depends on the developmental stage of the child [8]. In spite of this, only very few studies specify the age at time of exposure. For example, in a study of Israeli children who had experienced the First Gulf War between the ages of 3 and 5 years, the younger children showed more correlation between own and maternal post-traumatic symptoms 3 years later whereas this correlation could not be found in the older children [9]. In situations of organized violence, both children and their primary attachment figures might have been repeatedly exposed; this triggers a complex response to trauma and makes it difficult to draw clear correlates between trauma response and a certain age group.

# Determinants of risk and protection

## Country at war or post-conflict situation

A growing number of studies assess children in their country of origin either in their families or in camps for internally displaced persons in order to evaluate needs or the efficacy of proposed interventions. Most of the studies find very high prevalence of PTSD and depressive symptoms. Different epidemiological studies in countries with ongoing violent situations have shown high prevalence of psychological symptoms in the general population of children, including somatization, PTSD, anxiety disorders and depression, for example, in Gaza [10]; Mosul, Iraq [11]; Southern Darfur [12]; Bosnia-Herzegovina [13]; and Sri Lanka [14].

There is consensus on the importance of attachment figures for very young children and on the fact that the traumatization of mother or father can be as damaging for an infant as direct exposure [13,15]. In a review of 17 studies on the relational context of PTSD in very young children, Scheeringa and Zeanah [16] consistently found a relation between psychopathology in parents and maladaptive outcomes in children. A few studies have also underlined the importance of

the family environment and its relation to the severity of children's symptoms. Family violence in Sri Lanka was found to be linked to war violence exposure and substance abuse in parents and to contribute to higher scores in PTSD and depression scores in children [14]. Qouta and his colleagues [17] studied the relation between war experience and aggressive behavior in children in Gaza and found that supportive parenting was a determining factor for children not to be aggressive. A study with children in Bosnia who had all experienced war trauma found higher PTSD scores in children who had lost one or both parents [18]. Children living with both parents showed lower psychological disturbances, whereas those living with the surviving parent scored high on depression. Family can thus be seen both as a protective factor when it manages to provide a "safe haven" within the upheaval of the surrounding organized violence and also as a risk factor when it fails to protect the child from the disorganization and violence in the outside world.

As a result of war and displacement, thousands of children must grow in the absence of one or both parents, and separated from siblings and other family members. The disruption of attachment is often compounded by poverty, lack of access to schooling, stigma and marginalization [19,20]. Researchers have found elevated levels of psychological distress in orphans, including depressive symptoms and suicidality [21,22]. Although fostering of children within the extended family can reduce the impact of orphanhood, child- and youth-headed households have emerged as a result of abuses by relatives, families' inability or unwillingness to take children in and children's own choice [23].

Several in-depth studies have documented the importance of culture in the understanding of the consequences of organized violence. A qualitative study on traumatic events in the Mozambique civil war found that one of the most traumatic situations for parents and children was the necessity to hide in earth holes, which put the individuals hiding in a position equivalent to the dead and thus represented a major transgressive act with respect to cultural values [24]. This shows how situations usually considered as providing protection might in fact be more traumatizing in a specific cultural context. Ethnographic research with women in Bosnia during the war explored the particular awareness of mothers of their children's needs and vulnerabilities plus it allowed for the expression of the protective strategies they used [25]. This type of research questions the utilization of standard screening instruments across cultures and underlines the need to include ethnographic research in the development of mental health surveys.

Public health studies have shown the negative impact of long periods of conflict on the nutritional status and general health of children under 5 years in Afghanistan [26]. The same study found high rates (52%) of PTSD among mothers who had experienced at least one event related to armed conflict and also that food security mitigated the occurrence of PTSD symptoms. Some studies insist on the importance of cumulative risks such as natural disasters or aggravating factors such as socioeconomic hardship [14,26]. In fact, chronic food shortages, malnutrition and lack of healthcare in countries at war can leave durable marks on children in the form of physical handicaps or intellectual disabilities, and it can add to the psychological sequelae of violence exposure. In this context, it is important to point to the insecurity, instability and potential retraumatization linked to the living conditions of intenrnally displaced persons in camps and the negative effect of this on the family's well-being.

Several studies have addressed the plight of child soldiers, who are considered as a group particularly at risk; they enumerate the atrocities these children went through and document the psychological outcomes [27,28]. Kohrt and his colleagues [29] compared child soldiers with non-conscripted children in Nepal and, as one would expect, found psychiatric symptoms to be more prevalent and more severe in child soldiers than in children who were not abducted into armies, even when controlled for the higher trauma exposure in child soldiers. This was particularly the case especially for girls, which led the authors to suspect a high level of sexual violence. There is a need for future studies to consider the specific situation and hardships of girls in contexts of organized violence, as well as the effects of gender-specific violence [30].

Bayer and colleagues [31] studied the relation between PTSD symptoms and feelings of revenge or openness to reconcile in former child soldiers in the Great Lakes Area in Africa. They found that over a third of child soldiers met PTSD symptom criteria, with higher levels of PTSD symptoms clearly related to more feelings of revenge and less openness to reconcile. Results did not confirm the frequent association between traumatic experiences and PTSD symptoms. Even though this study does not explain the pathways between PTSD and the youths' capacity to reconcile, it does highlight the need for psychosocial interventions for children affected by violence in all peace-building efforts.

## Refugee children in Western countries

There is a growing body of literature on refugee children in Western countries [32]. As for the studies in the countries of origin, most of them assess prevalence of psychiatric symptoms, mostly PTSD, depression and anxiety.

Research shows that the family may act as a buffer or as a risk factor for child mental health. A study by Daud et al. [33] linked child psychopathology to parental mental health, and in particular to the presence of PTSD in the adults in the family. However, not all children of traumatized parents show PTSD-related symptoms and those who are non-symptomatic seem to maintain adequate family and peer relations. Several studies on the mental health of refugee youth highlight their resilience and the apparently paradoxical strengths that can stem from adversity [34]. In a longitudinal study of Khmer refugee children in Montreal, the Khmer adolescents did not report more internalizing symptoms than their Canadian peers and reported much less risk behavior. Within the Khmer study subjects, the adolescents whose families had experienced more traumas reported fewer externalizing symptoms and displayed better school performance. Community informants and qualitative data suggested that the children of very traumatized families felt compelled to compensate for the family losses, and this mission, although also a burden, proved to be protective [35]. A longitudinal qualitative study with Congolese refugee families in Montreal investigated the ways in which families make sense of separation and reunion, which are part of the refugee experience for many families. This study showed how refugee families need to develop new strategies and rely on previous experiences of loss and separation in order to make sense of the plights they experience in exile [36].

In the context of resettlement, many different issues relating to the pre-, peri- or post-migratory situation come into play, and the complexity of the situation needs to be taken into account. Having previously emphasized pre-migratory variables, more and more studies are focusing on post-migratory stressors that could contribute to child vulnerability, such as detention [37], instability and frequent relocation [38], or discrimination [39]. A study by Montgomery [40] concluded that of refugee youths who had been in Denmark for 8 to 9 years concluded that aspects of social life, maternal education and stressful life context in exile were better predictors of psychological problems than were traumatic experiences before arrival. These results question the simple models associating traumatic events prior to migration with mental health problems after resettlement. In spite of the persisting association between the number of traumatic events and the severity of PTSD symptoms [41], there is compelling evidence that psychosocial factors in the aftermath of organized violence play a role of utmost importance in the mental health of refugee children. Newman and Steele [37] have underscored the political dilemmas clinicians face when working with asylum-seeking families detained in Australia, and they have called for an ethical stance of professionals as advocates and witnesses of governmental structural violence. Restricted access of refugee children to healthcare or rehabilitation services has been documented in numerous Western countries [42]. These studies suggest that there is a discrepancy between the official discourse of protection of refugee children, which denounces the traumatic events the children experienced in their country of origin, and the political position taking a stance for the improvement of their socioeconomic situation in Western countries. Clinicians working with refugee children are very well aware of the traumatizing effects of the social and legal situations in which refugee families live and emphasize the need for political advocacy in this domain [43]. Research should document the structural violence of the legal and social system of the host countries and advocate for policies that ensure equity for refugees in various domains of life.

Several studies have looked at unaccompanied refugee children as a particular group. Most of these children have experienced violence not only in their country of origin but also during their sometimes chaotic trajectories [44]. Traumatic separations and losses are part of their plight and often continue in the host country when they have to move from one center or foster family to another. Moreover, depending on the host country's legislation, unaccompanied refugee minors may face a whole set of new legal problems when they become adults. There are discrepancies between the manifest psychological needs of these children and the way that the political system treats them [45]. Given the importance of family as a protective factor for refugee children, we have to consider unaccompanied minors as a group particularly at risk for psychopathology and ensure their basic security, stability and care needs.

# Transgenerational transmission

From professional experience we know the importance of the transgenerational transmission of traumatic experience. The negative influence of maternal depression on child development and attachment relations has been largely documented [46]; likewise, there are case reports with compelling clinical evidence concerning maternal trauma [47]. Oftentimes developmental delay or other child psychiatric symptoms are the reason for referral, and the traumatic history of parents might be a fortuitous finding. Nonetheless, trauma transmission is not always followed by psychological problems, and population-based studies are needed to document positive outcomes.

Some of the knowledge on the transmission of trauma stems from extensive research with Holocaust survivors and their children. A review of nearly 400 publications on the transmission of trauma found that the non-clinical population of children of Holocaust survivors does not show signs of more psychopathology than the general population [48]. According to most research, children of Holocaust survivors tend to function rather well in terms of avoiding manifest psychopathology. The clinical population of these children however, tends to present a specific "psychological profile" that includes a predisposition to PTSD, various difficulties in separation–individuation and a contradictory mix of resilience and vulnerability when coping with stress.

# Paradoxical effects and social implications

From the different studies on the effects of organized violence on children, it is apparent that the trauma response is always complex and involves several frameworks of understanding and interpretation. The individual response to trauma might seem paradoxical or unexpected, even socioeconomic, political, cultural and gender issues are considered as well as actual psychological responses. Organized violence affects not only individuals but also society in its core structures and humankind in its essence. This leads us to question the practice of describing trauma outcomes only in terms of individual psychopathology. Therapy that is focused only on the individual might end up perpetuating the traumatic experience, in that it singles out the person as a victim and cuts the links to the larger societal framework and social fabric. Notions such as resiliency and vulnerability are mostly used in an individualistic manner to specify personal characteristics, making a person more or less able to support traumatic experiences. Lately, some studies on resiliency have adopted a more social approach, integrating resiliency into a larger context of protective factors [49] and introducing the notion of "family resilience" to underline the necessity to work with refugee children *and* their parents [50]. This echoes with ideas about social healing and political acts of pardoning and forgiveness, as in the issues raised in Canadian aboriginal communities who have endured the organized violence of residential schools and forced acculturation. Narrating the traumatic experiences and giving voice to those who underwent and partook in violence are indispensable parts of the healing process [51]. Eliciting children's perspectives and meanings, as well as their feelings and attitudes, about violence or separation is, therefore, paramount; children's age and (cognitive) capacity will determine how to best accomplish this. The question of meaning, which is at the center of psychodynamic, interpersonal and narrative therapeutic approaches, needs to be elaborated in the context of the individual's social and cultural network. For unaccompanied minors from Somalia, the experience of being alone in Canada made sense in the meaning framework of their nomadic culture where young men might be sent away to learn about a pastoral way of life [52]. Throughout the world, culture provides frameworks of meaning for situations of suffering and loss. In some cases of organized violence, culture in itself is attacked and loses its capacity to help in the construction of meaning. The disruption of cultural structures and systems of support is a very frequent consequence of organized violence, and there is need to assess its long-term influences on child development and societal cohesion in the years and decades after the violence [53]. In all clinical and research situations, it is essential to take into consideration the cultural and social context in which children grow up, learn to make sense of the world around them and experience love, relationships and also violence. In order to achieve this, children have to be understood not only as victims and survivors of violence who need assistance but also as individuals who engage actively in the circumstances of war [54].

## Therapeutic interventions

The studies that have evaluated therapeutic tools in countries at war or in post-conflict situations are very heterogeneous both in design and in their findings. Betancourt and Williams [55] reviewed a handful of

intervention studies conducted in recent years. Dyadic therapies with mothers and their children seem to be indicated in certain situations, and a study in Bosnia has shown a positive effect on mother–infant psychotherapy using such as approach when comparing it with medical care only [56]. Generally, interventions that include parents in the therapies and propose psychosocial interventions and changes in the children's environment, such as promoting nutrition and education [57], seem to be more effective than psychotherapy only. Others have proposed group interventions with depressed children in Uganda, although the results of a randomized controlled trial showed positive outcomes only for girls [58]. Cognitive-behavioral therapy has been considered for treatment with refugee youth and has been found effective when integrated with other services [59]. There are case reports on the use of a whole array of therapeutic interventions, such as psychodynamic therapy, interpersonal therapy, narrative therapy, relaxation, art and group therapy among others [60]. Since the mid-1990s, school-based prevention and intervention programs for children living in an organized violence context or in exile have been developed. These programs emphasize culturally adapted cognitive-behavioral therapy programs [61], creative expression programs [62] or mixed modalities [63]. Such programs are particularly promising because of their capacity to reach all children in a non-stigmatizing manner and for their transformation of the school environment – a key element in child mental health. All of these interventions underline the necessity to take into account the extremely complex situation in which children live and the interplay of individual, family and societal factors therein [43].

## Conclusions

Rousseau in 1995 [34] pointed out three avenues for future research in the field of child refugee studies. In the light of this recent review of literature, all of them are still valid. First, there is a strong need for longitudinal studies, particularly in general populations, examining the impact of trauma in relation to age at exposure and outcomes over the lifespan. Second, confronted with limited psychometric validity of survey instruments, more qualitative research is warranted. This type of research would introduce models of complexity including not only clinical variables but also cultural, social and political elements. Third, there is some literature on the documentation of therapeutic and preventive endeavors, but most of these studies explore neither the question of meaning-making in a transcultural context nor the construction of collective solidarity among children's families and communities. A growing concern for girls advocates for research on the effects of gender-based violence, and on how the specific roles ascribed to girls might affect their experience and response to organized violence. In order to move forward from looking at organized violence to focusing on "organized protection" of children, both in their countries of origin and in host countries, we need to promote research on therapeutic intervention strategies and best practices. This implies the development and evaluation of measurement instruments in transcultural contexts. Finally, as indicated above, there is a need to elucidate the mechanisms of the transmission of trauma in order to improve out understanding of the effect of trauma on very young children. Information on the pathways of influence of trauma on children would provide new directions for the design and implementation of prevention measures and early therapeutic interventions.

Because there is no simple linear model connecting exposure to organized violence in children and outcomes, clinicians and researchers have to be aware of the possibility of paradoxical reactions and of the diversity of outcomes as a function of the complex interactions of collective and individual factors. The importance of both culture and context when it comes to the impact of organized violence on children necessitates a systemic and interdisciplinary appraisal in order to adopt interventions and innovatoins in terms of prevention.

# References

1. Freud, A. and Burlingham, D. T. (1944). *War and children*. NY, International Universities Press.
2. World Health Organization (1986). *Ottawa charter for health promotion*. Geneva: World Health Organization.
3. American Psychiatric Association (1994). *Diagnostic and statistical manual of mental disorders,* 4th edn. Washington, DC: American Psychiatric Press.
4. Bracken, P. J., Giller, J. E. and Summerfield, D. (1995). Psychological responses to war and atrocity: The limitations of current concepts. *Social Science & Medicine*, **40**, 1073–1082.
5. Young, A. (1995). *The harmony of illusions. Inventing post-traumatic stress disorder*. Princeton, NJ: Princeton University Press.
6. van der Kolk, B. A. (2007). The developmental impact of childhood trauma. In L. J. Kirmayer, R. Lemelson and M. Barad (eds.), *Understanding trauma: Integrating biological, clinical, and cultural prespectives* (pp. 224–241). New York: Cambridge University Press.
7. Scheeringa, M. S., Zeanah, C. H., Myers, L. and Putnam, F. W. (2003). New findings on alternative criteria for PTSD in preschool children. *Journal of the American Academy of Child and Adolescent Psychiatry*, **42**, 561–570.
8. Pynoos, R. S., Steinberg, A. M., Ornitz, E. M. and Goenjian, A. K. (1997). Issues in the developmental neurobiology of traumatic stress. *Annals of the New York Academy of Sciences*, **821**, 176–193.
9. Wolmer, L., Laor, N., Gershon, A., Mayes, L. C. and Cohen, D. J. (2000). The mother–child dyad facing trauma: A developmental outlook. *Journal of Nervous and Mental Disease,* **188**, 409–415.
10. Thabet, A. A. M. and Vostanis, P. (2005). Child mental health problems in the Gaza Strip. *Israelian Journal of Psychiatry and Related Sciences*, **42**, 84–87.
11. Al-Jawadi, A. A. and Abdul-Rhman, S. (2007). Prevalence of childhood and early adolescence mental disorders among children attending primary health care centers in Mosul, Iraq: a cross-sectional study. *BMC Public Health*, 7, 274.
12. Morgos, D., Worden, J. W. and Gupta, L. (2007–2008). Psychosocial effects of war experiences among displaced children in southern Darfur. *OMEGA: Journal of Death and Dying*, **56**, 229–253.
13. Smith, P., Perin, S., Yule, W. and Rabe-Hesketh, S. (2001). War exposure and maternal reactions in the psychosocial adjustment of children from Bosnia–Herzegovina. *Journal of Child Psychology and Psychiatry*, **42**, 395–404.
14. Catani, C., Jacob, N., Schauer, E., Kohila, M. and Neuner, F. (2008). Family violence, war, and natural disaster: A study of the effect of extreme stress on children's mental health in Sri Lanka. *BMC Psychiatry*, **8**, 33.
15. Al-Turkait, F. A. and Ohaeri, J. U. (2008). Psychopathological status, behavior problems, and family adjustment of Kuwaiti children whose fathers were involved in the first gulf war. *Child and Adolescent Psychiatry and Mental Health*, **2**, 12.
16. Scheeringa, M. S. and Zeanah, C. H. (2001). A relational perspective on PTSD in early childhood. *Journal of Traumatic Stress*, **14**, 799–815.
17. Qouta, S., Punamäki, R.-L., Miller, T. and Eyad, E.-S. (2008). Does war beget child aggression? Military violence, gender, age and aggressive behavior in two Palestinian samples. *Aggressive Behavior*, **34**, 231–244.
18. Hasanovic, M., Sinanovic, O., Selimbasic, Z., Pajevic, I. and Avdibegovic, E. (2006). Psychological disturbances of war-traumatized children from different foster and family settings in Bosnia and Herzegovina. *Croatian Medical Journal*, **47**, 85–94.

19. Boris, N., Brown, L., Thurman, T. *et al.* (2008). Depressive symptoms in youth heads of household in Rwanda: correlates and implications for intervention. *Archives of Pediatrics & Adolescent Medicine*, **162**, 836–843.

20. Cluver, L., Gardner, F. and Operario, D. (2008). Effects of stigma on the mental health of adolescents orphaned by AIDS. *Journal of Adolescent Health,* **42**, 410–417.

21. Bhargava, A. (2005). AIDS epidemic and the psychological well-being and school participation of Ethiopian orphans. *Psychology, Health & Medicine*, **10**, 263–275.

22. Makame, V., Ani, C. and Grantham-McGregor, S. (2002). Psychological wellbeing of orphans in Dar-Es-Salaam, Tanzania. *Acta Paediatrica*, **91**, 459–465.

23. Ruiz-Casares, M. (2008). Between adversity and agency: Child and youth-headed households in Namibia. *Vulnerable Children and Youth Studies*, **4**, 238–248.

24. Igreja, V. (2003). The effects of traumatic experiences on the infant–mother relationship in the former war-zones of Central Mozambique: The case of Madzawde in Gorongosa. *Infant Mental Health Journal*, **24**, 469–494.

25. Robertson, C. L. and Duckett, L. (2007). Mothering during war and postwar in Bosnia. *Journal of Family Nursing*, **13**, 461–483.

26. Mashal, T., Takano, T., Nakamura, K. *et al.* (2008). Factors associated with the health and nutritional status of children under 5 years of age in Afghanistan: Family behaviour related to women and past experience of war-related hardships. *BMC Public Health*, **8**, 301.

27. Derluyn, I., Broekaert, E., Schuyten, G. and de Temmerman, E. (2004). Post-traumatic stress in former Ugandan child soldiers. *Lancet*, **363**, 861–863.

28. Medeiros, E. (2007). Integrating mental health into post-conflict rehabilitation. The case of Sierra Leonean and Liberian "child soldiers." *Journal of Health Psychology*, **12**, 498–504.

29. Kohrt, B. A., Jordans, M. J. D., Tol, W. A. *et al.* (2008). Comparison of mental health between former child soldiers and children never conscripted by armed groups in Nepal. *Journal of the American Medical Association*, **300**, 691–702.

30. Boothby, N. (2008). Political violence and development: An ecologic approach to children in war zones. *Child and Adolescent Psychiatric Clinics of North America*, **17**, 497–514.

31. Bayer, C. P., Klasen, F. and Adam, H. (2007). Association of trauma and PTSD symptoms with openness to reconciliation and feelings of revenge among former Ugandan and Congolese child soldiers. *Journal of the American Medical Association*, **298**, 555–559.

32. Lustig, S. L., Kia-Keating, M., Knight Grant, W. *et al.* (2004). Review of child and adolescent refugee mental health. *Journal of the American Academy of Child and Adolescent Psychiatry*, **43**, 24–36.

33. Daud, A., Klinteberg, B. and Rydelius, P.-A. (2008). Resilience and vulnerability among refugee children of traumatized and non-traumatized parents. *Child and Adolescent Psychiatry and Mental Health*, **2**, 7.

34. Rousseau, C. (1995). The mental health of refugee children. *Transcultural Psychiatric Research Review*, **32**, 299–331.

35. Rousseau, C., Drapeau, A. and Rahimi, S. (2003). The complexity of trauma response: A 4-year follow-up of adolescent Cambodian refugees. *Child Abuse & Neglect*, **27**, 1277–1290.

36. Rousseau, C., Rufagari, M., Bagilishya, D. and Measham, T. (2004). Remaking family life: Strategies for re-establishing continuity among Congolese refugees during the family reunification process. *Social Science & Medicine*, **59**, 1095–1108.

37. Newman, L. K. and Steele, Z. (2008). The child asylum seeker: Psychological and developmental impact of immigration detention. *Child and Adolescent Psychiatric Clinics of North America*, **17**, 665–683.

38. Nielsen, S. S., Norredam, M., Christiansen, K. L. *et al.* (2008). Mental health among children seeking asylum in Denmark – the effect of length of stay and number of relocations: A cross-sectional study. *BMC Public Health*, **8**, 293.

39. Ellis, B. H., MacDonald, H. Z., Lincoln, A. K. and Cabral, H. J. (2008). Mental health of Somali adolescent refugees: The role of trauma, stress, and perceived discrimination. *Journal of Consulting and Clinical Psychology*, **76**, 184–193.

40. Montgomery, E. (2008). Long-term effects of organized violence on young Middle Eastern refugees' mental health. *Social Science & Medicine*, **67**, 1596–1603.

41. Ellis, B. H., Lhewa, D., Charney, M. and Cabral, H. J. (2006). Screening for PTSD among Somali adolescent refugees: Psychometric properties of the UCLA PTSD Index. *Journal of Traumatic Stress*, **19**, 547–551.

42. Ruiz-Casares, M., Rousseau, C., Derluyn, I., Watters, C. and Crépeau, F. (2010). Right and access to healthcare for undocumented children: Addressing the gap between international conventions and disparate implementations in North America and Europe. *Social Science and Medicine*, **70**, 1–8.

43. Silove, D. (2007). Adaptation, ecosocial safety signals, and the trajectory of PTSD. In L. J. Kirmayer, R. Lemelson and M. Barad (eds.), *Understanding trauma: integrating biological, clinical, and cultural perspectives* (pp. 242–258). New York: Cambridge University Press.

44. Thomas, S., Thomas, S., Nafees, B. and Bhugra, D. (2004). "I was running away from death": The pre-flight experiences of unaccompanied asylum seeking children in the UK. *Child Care, Health and Development*, **30**, 113–122.

45. Derluyn, I. and Broekaert, E. (2008). Unaccompanied refugee children and adolescents: The glaring contrast between a legal and a psychological perspective. *International Journal of Law and Psychiatry*, **31**, 319–330.

46. Sohr-Preston, S. L. and Scaramella, L. V. (2006). Implications of timing of maternal depressive symptoms for early cognitive and language development. *Clinical Child and Family Psychology Review*, **9**, 65–83.

47. Rezzoug, D., Baubet, T., Broder, G., Taïeb, O. and Moro, M. R. (2008). Addressing the mother–infant relationship in displaced communities. *Child and Adolescent Psychiatric Clinics of North America*, **17**, 551–568.

48. Kellerman, N. (2001). Psychopathology in children of Holocaust survivors: A review of the research literature. *Israel Journal of Psychiatry and Related Sciences*, **38**, 36–46.

49. Betancourt, T. S. and Khan, K. T. (2008). The mental health of children affected by armed conflict: protective processes and pathways to resilience. *International Review of Psychiatry*, **20**, 317–328.

50. Weine, S. (2008). Family roles in refugee youth resettlement from a prevention perspective. *Child and Adolescent Psychiatric Clinics of North America*, **17**, 515–532.

51. Castellano, M., Linda Archibald, L. and DeGagné, M. (2008). *From truth to reconciliation: Transforming the legacy of residential schools.* Ottawa: The Aboriginal Healing Foundation.

52. Rousseau, C., Said, T. M., Gagné, M.-J. and Bibeau, G. (1998). Resilience in unaccompanied minors from the north of Somalia. *Psychoanalytic Review*, **85**, 615–635.

53. Igreja, V. (2004). Cultural disruption and the care of infants in post-war Mozambique. In J. Boyden and J. de Berry (eds.), *Children and youth on the front line: Ethnography, armed conflict and displacement*, Vol. 14, (pp. 24–41). New York: Berghahn Books.

54. Boyden, J. and de Berry, J. (2004). Introduction. In J. Boyden and J. de Berry (eds.), *Children and youth on the front line: Ethnography, armed conflict and displacement*, Vol. 14 ( pp. vi–xxvii). New York: Berghahn Books.

55. Betancourt, T. S. and Williams, T. (2008). Building an evidence base on mental health interventions for children affected by armed conflict. *International Journal of Mental Health, Psychosocial Work and Counseling in Areas of Armed Conflict*, **6**, 39–56.

56. Dybdahl, R. (2001). Children and mothers in war: An outcome study of a psychosocial intervention program. *Child Development*, **72**, 1214–1230.

57. Gupta, L. and Zimmer, C. (2008). Psychosocial interventions for war-affected children in Sierra Leone. *British Journal of Psychiatry*, **192**, 212–216.

58. Bolton, P., Bass, J., Betancourt, T. S. *et al.* (2007). Interventions for depression symptoms among adolescent survivors of war and displacement in Northern Uganda: a randomized controlled trial. *Journal of the American Medical Association*, **298**, 519–527.

59. Murray, L. K., Cohen, J. A., Ellis, B. H. and Mannarino, A. P. (2008). Cognitive behavioral therapy for symptoms of trauma and traumatic grief in refugee youth. *Child and Adolescent Psychiatric Clinics of North America*, **17**, 585–604.

60. Möhlen, H., Parzer, P., Resch, F. and Brunner, R. (2005). Psychosocial support for war-traumatized child and adolescent refugees: evaluation of a short-term treatment program. *Australian and New Zealand Journal of Psychiatry*, **39**, 81–87.

61. Kataoka, S. H., Stein, B. D., Jaycox, L. H. *et al.* (2003). A school-based mental health program for traumatized Latino immigrant children. *American Academy of Child & Adolescent Psychiatry*, **42**, 311–318.

62. Rousseau, C. and Guzder, J. (2008). School-based prevention programs for refugee children. *Child and Adolescent Psychiatric Clinics of North America*, **17**, 533–549.

63. Tol, W. A., Komproe, I. H., Susanty, D. *et al.* (2008). School-based mental health intervention for children affected by political violence in Indonesia. *Journal of the American Medical Association*, **300**, 655–662.

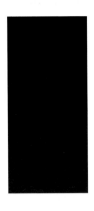

# Part 5 synopsis

David Spiegel

## Overview

There is a saying in popular psychology that "what doesn't kill us makes us stronger." Well, what almost kills us may make us weaker, or at the least, the strength required to survive the aftermath of trauma may exact a high cost in cognitive function, affect management, identity development and relationship growth. These problems are well described in the chapters of Part 5.

In Ch. 22, Heidenreich and colleagues make a number of important methodological points about the effects of trauma on children and their development. They note that age at the time of trauma exposure is often overlooked in child trauma studies, and that the younger the child is, the more likely it is that the child's trauma response will mirror that of the parent. This makes good developmental sense. In addition, the parent's trauma exposure and response may be as important in determining the aftermath for a young child as their own experience. Parental traumatization not only imposes a burden of post-traumatic symptomatology but also interferes with necessary parental bonding and support for the young developing child.

The meaning of traumatic experience in the broader culture also plays a role in the intensity of symptoms. During the Mozambique civil war, parents and children were forced to hide in earth holes, which is considered a transgression of cultural values that proscribe behaving like the dead. This added an additional burden to those forced to do this to flee the fighting. The authors also emphasize the often neglected theme of resilience. Khmer refugee children in Montreal reported less externalizing symptoms and much less risk behavior than their Canadian peers. They apparently felt they had to compensate for family losses incurred, which was a protective burden to them. They also point out that post-trauma adjustment has much

to do with family, cultural and political attitudes in its aftermath. The availability of broader social support is crucial, and, conversely, the displacement, poverty and confusion engendered by exile and emigration also compounds post-traumatic recovery.

Heidenreich and colleagues also emphasize broadening the discussion of resilience to encompass "family resilience" as a functioning social system, not just a collection of individual attributes. They extend this also to social ceremonies involving social judgment and forgiveness such as the "truth and reconciliation" process in South Africa. They note that children's culture is often also a victim of violence, and the children's displacement further removes them from stabilizing influence. In addition, some of these victims were also coerced perpetrators and have to deal with the fact of their participation in the destruction of their own family and culture, however forced it was. Most trauma victims blame themselves inappropriately for events over which they had little or not control. Some child soldiers were forced to kill their families before being abducted, as was common practice by Joseph Kony, head of the hated and feared "Lord's Resistance Army," in Uganda, Congo and Southern Sudan. Jeremy Weinstein [1] has noted that those rebel groups that receive funding from outside of their target country are more likely to inflict cruelty on the indigenous population because they depend less upon them for good will and support.

The authors of Ch. 22 call for more research on meaning-making and the collective social and cultural implications of violence in the restorative process. In particular, they note that, with the rise of collective sexual violence, the meaning and response to systematic sexual abuse of women (and, less often men) needs to be better understood and addressed. We often blame the victim, in part as a means of distancing ourselves from exposure to our own vulnerability. In some cultures, there is a formal conviction that a raped woman is a fallen woman, blamed for her own involuntary sexual contact and bringing shame upon her and her family. This travesty of justice is also a psychological burden, complicating the already heavy aftermath of violence and rape. The philosopher René Girard [2] has noted that humans suffer from two fundamental weaknesses: (a) the willingness to let others redefine pleasure for us and (b) the tendency to scapegoat – to blame others for our own misfortune. Those scapegoated are, by definition, innocent of the charge, and the more innocent, the greater the apparent power of those defining the outcasts to control the social order. Child victims of organized violence are particularly vulnerable to such unfair judgment, which can inhibit their re-incorporation into the social world, the more so if they also suffer the "slings and arrows of outrageous fortune" as displaced refugees in an alien culture. Chapter 22 usefully highlights the damage done to child victims of collective violence through its effects on child, family and social context.

Briere and Hodges, in Ch. 19, note a long-standing literature rooted initially in early psychoanalytic observations that early life trauma damages attachment and psychosocial development. The premise underlying their position that early trauma is more damaging than that occurring later in life is that its effects are more pervasive – interfering with normal development of cognition, affect and relationships; damaging the view of self and others; and establishing relationship schemas in which nurturance is commingled with abuse. This, in turn, leads to an elevated risk of subsequent victimization later in life, which compounds the effect of the early neglect and maltreatment. They note that a child's fear, anger and uncertainty may become conditioned to relational, especially intimate or caretaking, stimuli. Thus relationships that should be supportive and calming come to seem arousing and destructive, which not only impairs the development of future relationships but also triggers the "traumatic transference," in which those with serious trauma histories expect to be damaged rather than helped in psychotherapy. The very trauma focus of the treatment, necessary given the observation that exposure-based therapies have the best established track record [3], can be experienced by the patient as designed to harm again rather than help, with the therapist appearing to induce and enjoy rather than empathically work with the patient's

discomfort. This perspective is complementary to that in Ch. 22 linking developmental disruption by trauma to later relationship problems.

Chapters 20 and 21 examine effects of trauma on memory and address cognitive mechanisms of trauma-related psychopathology. Dalenberg and Palesh in Ch. 21 provide an intriguing examination of recovered memories. They begin with Erdelyi's important observation [4] that accurate recollection improves with repeated retrieval efforts. The clear implication of this well-established fact is that memory information is often accurately stored but not entirely retrievable, at least not without effort that involves tapping associative networks. Given the contentious debates about so-called false memories of abuse, they make the balanced argument that if false memories of traumatic experiences early in life are possible, so are false memories that abuse did not occur – false negatives as well as false positives. Indeed, in an often-quoted study of children's reports of receiving a (real) injection at the doctor's office, Bruck *et al.* [5] found that the nature of the debriefing of the child affected the level of pain they reported. So they would exaggerate the painfulness of the injection if asked how big the needle was, and how much it hurt. But when the questioning minimized the unpleasant aspects of the event, children tended to say "I hardly cried when I got my shot." This study, often used to underscore the malleability of children's memory and the likelihood that they are making up traumatic events, actually illustrates how social influence can lead children to minimize traumatic experiences. Abusive families are likely to coerce children to minimize or deny abuse or its after-effects. This will affect memory as well as conscious withholding.

In reviewing the evidence regarding recovered memory of abuse, Dalenberg and Palesh (Ch. 21) emphasize the comparable accuracy of recovered versus continuous memory of abuse. Perhaps the most startling aspect of Williams' classic study of a past traumatic event [6,7] was the fact that 38% of women interviewed 17 years after the event reported no conscious recollection of it. An additional 14% reported that during some period of their life they could not recall the traumatic event. Documentation of the event occurrence had been obtained from hospital emergency room records. This study as well as others provides robust evidence that major traumatic events may not be available for conscious recollection for periods up to decades after they occurred. This is not about relative accuracy but rather about the existence of traumatic amnesia. Dalenberg and Palesh note that Pope and others have insisted that "clarification interviews" should have been employed to push subjects in the Williams' study to admit that they were consciously withholding memories. Ethical concerns aside, the interviewers in Williams' study were appropriately blind to the information from the patients' medical records, which is the appropriate approach to avoiding contamination of memory in questioning. Furthermore, Williams noted that a substantial proportion of the subjects had reported other episodes of abuse, so they were not, in general, ashamed of admitting to having been abused.

Dalenberg and Palesh also note that the recovery of traumatic memory is usually accompanied by strong affect, usually fear. This provides support for the idea that affect regulation is involved in memory suppression. Indeed Koutstaal and Schacter [8] found that shortly after childhood trauma occurs, survivors engage in intentional forgetting strategies to manage their distress. Like any learned behavior, this may become more automatic over time, leading to traumatic amnesia in which conscious effort is no longer required to keep such memories out of consciousness. As Dalenberg and Palesh add, research has demonstrated that simple instructions to remember or forget will affect the frequency of later word recall. But such functional amnesia is not merely another presentation of organic amnesia. Kritchevsky *et al.* [9] studied 10 cases of documented functional amnesia and demonstrated that they indeed had retrograde but not anterograde amnesia – they could remember but did not. In the related discussion of amnesia for repeated versus single-incident memories, it is worth keeping in mind that while retroactive inhibition may play a role in amnesia, in that memory of one traumatic event may overlie or distort memory of another similar event, single-blow traumas may be more discordant with ordinary reality (in the family or other parts of the environment). There may be fewer associative cues to connect one traumatic event to the network of associations that defines the family in general, making access to a single trauma more difficult. An event that seems implausible may be less memorable, even if it happened. This is related to the discussion of "betrayal trauma" in Ch. 20. The need to maintain a relationship with an abusive parent may lead to selective inactivation of memories inconsistent with that goal.

The use of the Deese–Roediger–McDermott (DRM) paradigm as a model for "false memories" is conceptually problematic. It purports to show that subjects will incorrectly "remember" a word from a list. The lure is a word that is conceptually similar to words that were presented (e.g., sugar when words on the list included jam, candy and honey). What the paradigm really shows is that people remember the gist of the list but are mistaken about the details. They do not misidentify "vinegar" or "acid" as having been on that list of sweets. In analogy to false memories of abuse, they correctly recall being beaten, but the perpetrator may have used a brush instead of a belt.

Dissociation is closely intertwined with amnesia. Indeed, Hilgard [10] has argued that amnesic barriers are the intrinsic structure by which mental contents that would ordinarily be connected are disaggregated, to use Janet's original term [11]. Dalenberg and Palesh wonder about the existence of motivation for dissociation, since it is more clearly articulated in psychoanalytic repression theory. Yet the dissociation of identity, memory and consciousness in the aftermath of trauma would seem to provide its own evidence of motivation, especially since dissociation often occurs during traumatic events and provides a means of immediate affect regulation [12–14]. Furthermore, those with greater capacity to dissociate would be more likely to utilize the ability in the face of overwhelming threat and afterwards [15].

Dalenberg and Palesh in Ch. 21 call for a de-escalation of the war of words and memories, both recovered and false, reminiscent of Mr. Justice Frankfurter's wry comment about the "cross-sterilization of disciplines." Memory is malleable, to many purposes, and with many results, and it is useful for us to remember that.

Combs and DePrince in Ch. 20 report on a number of useful laboratory studies of individuals with posttraumatic stress disorder (PTSD), noting deficits in explicit memory performance coupled with enhanced memory for trauma-related stimuli. These effects do not occur among those with trauma exposure but no PTSD. The occurrence of PTSD is also associated with heightened sensitivity to trauma cues in implicit memory tasks, and those with PTSD show more psychophysiological responsiveness. Consequently, their trauma sensitivity is higher at many levels, but cognitive processing is poorer. The authors of Ch. 20 put forward interesting data suggesting that high dissociators, by contrast, have better cognitive function, especially in the face of demand for divided attention or directed forgetting. Therefore, dissociation, which can be problematic at times, may also preserve cognitive function in traumatic situations. They cite Brewin's observation [16] that, compared with non-traumatic memories, traumatic autobiographical memories are more likely to be vivid, sensory in nature and relived in the present tense rather than remembered in the past.

Combs and DePrince review evidence of smaller hippocampal volume and enhanced amygdala function in PTSD as a basis for cognitive and memory impairment. This could explain both memory failures and enhanced affect-related association to trauma stimuli. They also refer to Freyd's betrayal trauma theory of cognitive processing [17] in which the need to maintain relationships with abusive parents may reinforce development of cognitive means to keep dangerous information out of awareness. Cognition and memory are not impaired by unacceptable incestuous fears and wishes but rather by incompatible actions by abusive caretakers. They also note apparent inconsistencies in effects of PTSD (impaired explicit memory and enhanced trauma-related recall) and dissociation (better divided attention and reduced memory for trauma-related stimuli). One way of resolving this apparent paradox, especially given comorbidity of PTSD and dissociation, is to recognize a dissociative subtype of PTSD [18]. There is evidence for such a subtype in one-third of those with PTSD [19], associated with hyperactivation of prefrontal regions and inhibition of limbic structures on functional brain imaging [20–22]. Within PTSD itself, there are apparently paradoxical symptoms: intrusion, avoidance and hyperarousal. Trauma is a discontinuity of experience, and would likely produce discontinuity in response, with either undermodulation (intrusion, hyperarousal) or overmodulation (avoidance, dissociation) of response. Some may typically have one type of response or another; others may fluctuate between the two [23].

## Conclusions

Together these chapters indicate much growth in our understanding of the lasting effects of trauma on development, cognition, mood and relationships. We understand more about the brain basis of impairment in memory processing and hypersensitivity to trauma-related cues. We have come a long way from ignoring the effects of trauma or blaming the victim for dealing poorly with unacceptable incestuous fears and wishes. We have moved from Freud to Freyd.

## References

1. Weinstein, J. (2006). *Inside rebellion*. Cambridge, UK: Cambridge University Press.

2. Girard, R. (1986). *The scapegoat*. Baltimore, MD: Johns Hopkins University Press.

3. Institute of Medicine (2007). *Treatment of PTSD: An assessment of the evidence*. Washington, DC: Institute of Medicine, National Academy of Sciences.

4. Erdelyi, M. H. and Kleinbard, J. (1978). Has Ebbinghaus decayed with time? The growth of recall (hypermnesia) over days. *Journal of Experimental Psychology: Human, Learning, and Memory*, **4**, 275–289.

5. Bruck, M., Ceci, S. J., Francoeur, E. and Barr, R. (1995). "I hardly cried when I got my shot!" Influencing children's reports about a visit to their pediatrician. *Child Development,* **66**, 193–208.

6. Williams, L. M. (1994). Recall of childhood trauma: A prospective study of women's memories of child sexual abuse. *Journal of Consulting and Clinical Psychology*, **62**, 1167–1176.

7. Williams, L. M. (1995). Recovered memories of abuse in women with documented child victimization histories. *Journal of Traumatic Stress*, **8**, 649–673.

8. Koutstaal, W. and Schacter, D. (1997). Intentional forgetting and voluntary thought suppression: Two potential methods for coping with childhood trauma. In L. M. R. Dickstein and J. Oldham (eds.), *Review of psychiatry*. Vol. 16 (pp. II-55–II-78). Washington, DC: American Psychiatric Press.

9. Kritchevsky, M., Chang, J. and Squire, L. R. (2004). Functional amnesia: Clinical description and neuropsychological profile of 10 cases. *Learning and Memory*, **11**, 213–226.

10. Hilgard, E. (1986). *Divided consciousness: Multiple controls in human thought and action,* revised edn. New York: Wiley.

11. Janet, P. (1889). *L'automatisme psychologique*. Paris: Felix Alcan.

12. Spiegel, D. (1997). Trauma, dissociation, and memory. *Annals of the New York Academy of Sciences*, **821**, 225–237.

13. Cardeña, E. and Spiegel, D. (1993). Dissociative reactions to the San Francisco Bay Area earthquake of 1989. *American Journal of Psychiatry*, **150**, 474–478.

14. Spiegel, D. and Cardena, E. (1991). Disintegrated experience: The dissociative disorders revisited. *Journal of Abnormal Psychology*, **100**, 366–378.

15. Butler, L. D., Duran, E. F. D., Jasiukatis, P., Koopman, C. and Spiegel, D. (1996). Hypnotizability and traumatic

experience: A diathesis-stress model of dissociative symptomatology. *American Journal of Psychiatry,* **153,** 42–63.

16. Brewin, C. R. (2007). Autobiographical memory for trauma: Update on four controversies. *Memory,* **15,** 227–248.

17. Freyd, J. J. (1996). *Betrayal trauma: The logic of forgetting child abuse.* Cambridge, MA: Harvard University Press.

18. Lanius, R. A., Vermetten, E., Loewenstein, R. J. *et al.* (2010). Emotion modulation in PTSD: Clinical and neurobiological evidence for a dissociative subtype. *American Journal of Psychiatry,* in press.

19. Ginzburg, K., Koopman, C., Butler, L. D. *et al.* (2006). Evidence for a dissociative subtype of post-traumatic stress disorder among help-seeking childhood sexual abuse survivors. *Journal of Trauma and Dissociation,* **7,** 7–27.

20. Frewen, P. A. and Lanius, R. A. (2006). Neurobiology of dissociation: Unity and disunity in mind–body–brain. *Psychiatric Clinics of North America,* **29,** 113–128, ix.

21. Lanius, R. A., Bluhm, R., Lanius, U. and Pain, C. (2006). A review of neuroimaging studies in PTSD: Heterogeneity of response to symptom provocation. *Journal of Psychiatric Research,* **40,** 709–729.

22. Lanius, R. A., Williamson, P. C., Bluhm, R. L. *et al.* (2005). Functional connectivity of dissociative responses in posttraumatic stress disorder: A functional magnetic resonance imaging investigation. *Biological Psychiatry,* **57,** 873–884.

23. Horowitz, M. J. (1986). *Stress response syndromes,* 2nd edn. Northvale, NJ: Jason Aronson.

# Strategies to reduce the impact: clinical treatment
# The role of mentalizing in treating attachment trauma

Jon G. Allen, Peter Fonagy and Anthony Bateman

In agreement with Kazdin [1], who considered that treatment interventions should address core psychopathological processes, we advocate bolstering mentalizing as an optimal focus for treating trauma suffered in early attachment relationships. This chapter begins by explicating the concept of mentalizing – in brief, attending to mental states in self and others – before moving on to discuss the intergenerational transmission of mentalizing impairments in the context of attachment disturbance, illustrating how this developmental psychopathology is exemplified in borderline personality disorder (BPD). Finally, mentalizing-focused interventions for BPD and trauma-related symptoms are examined. This chapter aims to present succinctly a coherent conceptual framework for treating attachment trauma and thus entice readers to consult additional literature for more detail [2–7].

## Mentalizing

Mentalizing has a foreign ring to many ears, and the word does not appear in many dictionaries. Yet its first recorded use goes back two centuries, and mentalizing first appeared in the *Oxford English Dictionary* a century ago [3]. The term appeared in the French psychoanalytic literature in the late 1960s [8] and was introduced into the English professional literature in 1989 by Morton [9] to characterize the core deficit in autism. Shortly thereafter, Fonagy [10] extended the concept to trauma-related developmental psychopathology, as manifested in BPD, for example. Whereas autism is associated with relatively stable, neurobiologically based deficits in mentalizing capacity, BPD reflects more transient, dynamic impairments in mentalizing associated with perturbed attachment relationships.

The phrase "holding mind in mind" captures the gist of mentalizing; more elaborately, we define mentalizing as *imaginatively perceiving and interpreting the behavior of self and others as conjoined with intentional mental states*. Thus mentalizing encompasses a large territory, including not only self and others but also the full range of mental states, from desires, feelings, thoughts, beliefs and dreams, through to hallucinations, delusions, dissociative phenomena and so forth. But the complexity of mentalizing does not end there: we distinguish between mentalizing *implicitly* as an intuitive, automatic and procedural process (e.g., as in empathically adopting a demeanor appropriate to another person's distress or unthinkingly taking turns in conversation) and mentalizing *explicitly* as a conscious and deliberative process, typically involving language (e.g., putting feelings into words or constructing a narrative account to explain puzzling behavior). Furthermore, we can mentalize in relation to the present (i.e., a current mental state in oneself or another person), the past (e.g., understanding in hindsight the reasons for one's behavior) or the future (e.g., anticipating the impact of one's actions on another person). Moreover, the scope of mentalizing can be narrow (e.g., identifying a particular feeling) or broad (e.g., understanding a recurrent pattern of behavior in relation to an extended autobiographical narrative).

The term mentalizing may have a discordant ring to the uninitiated, but, referring to the fundamental capacity that makes us human, it cannot be a new idea. Therefore, we add mentalizing to a host of overlapping concepts: mindreading, theory of mind, metacognition, psychological mindedness, insight, empathy, emotional intelligence and mindfulness. Having drawn admittedly subtle distinctions among these terms elsewhere [3,11], we note here three primary reasons for employing mentalizing in clinical practice. First, although the term is multifaceted, it has optimal breadth (e.g., in balancing attention to self and others, as well as implicit

*The Impact of Early Life Trauma on Health and Disease: The Hidden Epidemic*, ed. Ruth A. Lanius, Eric Vermetten and Clare Pain. Published by Cambridge University Press. Copyright © Cambridge University Press 2010.

and explicit processes). Second, we prefer a term that has a verb form (e.g., as contrasted with theory of mind, metacognition or psychological mindedness) to underscore agency. Third, mentalizing is something we clinicians and our patients aspire *to do*. Last but perhaps most importantly, mentalizing is linked explicitly to attachment research. Regarding this last point, while "theory of mind" holds sway in developmental research, we make the following distinction: theory of mind is our folk psychological conceptual framework for explaining behavior [12] while the *activity* of mentalizing makes use of this framework.

Although we are unabashed advocates of mentalizing, we have one reservation: the word misleadingly connotes an intellectual process. However, mentalizing typically is suffused with emotion, and the mental states we are most keen to mentalize in clinical practice are emotional states. Accordingly, we devote considerable attention to mentalizing emotion [3]: in short, thinking and feeling about thinking and feeling in self and others. Mentalizing emotion has three facets [6]: *identifying* emotions (i.e., not only labeling feelings but also elaborating and articulating conflicts as well as clarifying the meaning of emotions and conflicts), *modulating* emotions (i.e., diminishing unreasonably intense emotional responses and amplifying defensively blocked emotions) and *expressing* emotions (i.e., not only outwardly to others but also inwardly, to oneself). As is all too plain in our clinical work, attachment trauma impairs the capacity to mentalize emotion, and we are challenged to promote attachment relationships that will strengthen this capacity.

## Intergenerational transmission

Developmental research has provided a solid foundation for clinical practice in a well-established relationship between attachment and mentalizing that can be passed across generations – for better or for worse.

## Secure attachment

The research of Meins and colleagues exemplifes the link between mentalizing and secure attachment. Meins [13] employed the concept of maternal *mind-mindedness* to capture the mother's "recognition of her child as a mental agent, and her proclivity to employ mental state terms in her speech" (p. 127). Meins *et al.* [14] showed that mind-minded commentary in mothers' interactions with their 6-month-old infants predicted security of attachment at 12 months, as evident in a laboratory separation–reunion paradigm, the Strange Situation [15]. Additional research has demonstrated associations between mind-mindedness for fathers and mothers [16] as well showing that maternal mind-mindedness and secure attachment in infancy predict the child's later competence in mentalizing (e.g., theory-of-mind) tasks [17–19]. As summarized by Meins *et al.* [14], "Appropriate mind-related comments at 6 months index the beginnings of mothers' and infants' joint attention to mind, in which mothers' appropriate labeling of their infant's current mental states helps draw infants' attention to the existence (and perhaps functional significance) of mental states and processes" (p. 1208).

Fonagy *et al.* [20] stimulated research on intergenerational transmission when they discovered that expectant mothers who demonstrated secure attachment to their parents in the Adult Attachment Interview [21] gave birth to infants who, at 1 year of age, were likely to be securely attached as evident in the Strange Situation. Subsequent research showed the same pattern for fathers [22], and the link between parental and infant attachment has been widely replicated [23]. Slade *et al.* [24,25] have pinpointed the role of mentalizing in mediating the intergenerational transmission of attachment: securely attached mothers who are able to mentalize in relation to their own attachment history also mentalize in relation to their 10-month-old infants; in turn, maternal mentalizing of infants predicts the infants' attachment security at 14 months. Buttressing these findings, Arnott and Meins [26] assessed mothers' and fathers' security of attachment and mentalizing in relation to their own parents (prenatally), both parents' mind-minded comments in interaction with their 6-month-old infant, and the infant's attachment to each parent at 12 months. As hypothesized, parental secure attachment was linked to infant secure attachment through high levels of parental mind-mindedness, whereas parental insecure attachment was linked to infant insecure attachment through low levels of parental mind-mindedness.

## Insecure attachment

As we have just noted, the intergenerational transmission of insecure attachment is the converse of secure attachment in being mediated by poor parental mentalizing. Pertinent to our concerns with attachment trauma, Slade *et al.* [24,25,27] proposed that parents with insecure attachment and precarious mentalizing capacities are liable to be disorganized by their child's distress-related bids for attachment, as manifested, for example, by confusing their feelings with the child's feelings (e.g., demonizing the child). At worst, the child's attachment needs can become a reminder of parental trauma, and the parent's non-mentalizing response can be viewed as a post-traumatic state [28].

Main and Hesse [29] construed parental *frightening or frightened* behavior as generating disorganized attachment – itself an indicator of attachment trauma. Consistent with Main and Hesse's proposal, Lyons-Ruth and Jacobvitz [30] identified two broad patterns of maternal behavior as being conducive to disorganized attachment in infants: hostile intrusiveness and helpless withdrawal. Both patterns are indicative of aversion to the child's attachment needs and a collapse of mentalizing when the child most needs it. Supporting Lyons-Ruth's research, Grienenberger *et al.* [27] observed several patterns of non-mentalizing parental behavior to be associated with attachment disorganization: affective communication errors, boundary confusions, fearful behavior, intrusive behavior and withdrawal.

Just as mentalizing begets mentalizing, non-mentalizing begets non-mentalizing. Fonagy *et al.* [7] summarized evidence from a number of studies consistent with impaired mentalizing in maltreated children: for example, these children engage in relatively little symbolic play, talk less about mental states, show diminished empathy, demonstrate poor understanding of emotions and, accordingly, show conspicuous problems with emotion regulation. The occurrence of BPD is an unfortunate legacy of this developmental trajectory.

# Borderline personality disorder

Befitting the sheer complexity of symptomatology, we recognize a diversity of developmental pathways to BPD. For example, genetic factors [31] potentially associated with difficult-to-manage temperaments [32] contribute to child-to-parent effects that might play a significant role in early attachment disturbance. Furthermore, neurobiological substrates are inherently intertwined with the impairments described here from a psychosocial perspective [33]. Here the focus is rather single-mindedly on mentalizing impairments in attachment relationships as providing optimal leverage in treating BPD.

## Developmental contributions

From the broad perspective of mentalizing, deficits in social cognition render individuals with BPD susceptible to interpersonal stress while simultaneously impairing their interpersonal problem-solving capacities [3]. Two key domains of deficits are linked to attachment-related mentalizing problems: affect regulation and effortful control of attention.

The high levels of negative affect and impairments of affect regulation in BPD [34] can be related to a lack of parental mentalizing. As detailed elsewhere [6,7,35], infants gradually develop the capacity to represent and regulate their affective states by virtue of caregivers responding to their affective displays in a highly contingent fashion that marks the caregiver's emotion as reflecting the infant's affect rather than expressing the caregiver's affect. For example, mirroring her infant's frustration, a mother might intermingle an expression of sympathy with one of frustration rather than merely expressing her own frustration directly. Such responsiveness depends on the caregiver's inclination and ability to mentalize, which, in turn, is intertwined with the caregiver's attachment security. Alternatively, non-contingent (mismatched) emotional responses are liable to promote poorly integrated misrepresentations of emotional states, while direct expressions of affect (e.g., the caregiver's frustration) are liable to escalate the infant's distress.

Intertwined with affect dysregulation in BPD is impaired capacity for effortful control of attention [36], as evident, for example, in the inability to suppress aversive but irrelevant thoughts [37]. Like affect regulation, the development of the ability to control attention is embedded in attachment relationships, for example in interactions entailing joint attention [38]. Hence secure attachment is predictive of better performance on attention tasks [39], and disorganized attachment is associated with impaired social-attention coordination [40]. More generally, mutual responsiveness in mother–child dyads is associated with greater self-control [41], whereas controlling parent–child interactions are associated with impaired self–control [42].

Four lines of evidence associate BPD with attachment disturbance. First, extensive evidence shows BPD to be related to preoccupied and disorganized attachment [43]. Second, problematic parenting is commonly reported in the histories of persons with BPD [44], and longitudinal research shows features of BPD to be associated with low levels of parental affection [45] and high levels of disrupted maternal communication [46]. Third, mothers with BPD interact with their infants in ways that show difficulty modulating emotional expressions [47] as well as with intrusiveness and insensitivity [48]; concomitantly, children of mothers with BPD show relatively high levels of psychiatric disturbance, including features of BPD [49]. Fourth, extensive evidence links attachment trauma to the development of BPD [28]; although the trauma literature highlights sexual abuse, it is generally embedded in a broader pattern of family dysfunction marked by neglect [50].

Acknowledging the multifarious childhood adversity associated with BPD, we construe the core traumatic experience as being the failure of attachment figures to engage in mentalizing interactions with the child in times of high emotional distress. Hence we are in accord with Linehan and colleagues' emphasis on an *invalidating* family environment as central in the development of BPD [51,52], while construing the lack of mentalizing as the core of invalidation. While focusing on acts of omission – parental underinvolvement and lack of psychological availability – we are keenly aware of the adverse impact of various acts of commission, including sexual, physical and psychological abuse. Indeed, abusing a child is itself a glaring exemplar of failure in mentalizing that poses a dual liability [53]: it evokes extreme distress and undermines the *development* of the capacity to regulate distress.

## Pre-mentalizing modes of experience

A history of early attachment trauma puts the patient with BPD at risk for impaired mentalizing in later attachment relationships insofar as the activation of attachment needs portends danger, escalates dysphoric affect and undermines mentalizing; at which point earlier modes of psychological functioning come into play. Accordingly, BPD is characterized by three pre-mentalizing modes of experience. First, in the *psychic-equivalence mode*, the individual loses a sense of mind as representing the world in various ways; rather, what is thought or imagined is real. For example, in a paranoid state, feelings and beliefs are unquestioned; alternative perspectives carry no weight. Similarly, in a post-traumatic flashback, a memory is equated with current reality insofar as reliving replaces remembering. Second, in the *pretend mode*, ideas lose their grounding in reality. Examples of pretend mode are dissociatively detached states that lack emotional reality and discussions employing psychological jargon or clichés (perhaps parroted from treatment experiences) that might give the patient and therapist the illusion of doing real work and then lead to disillusionment when the patient's functioning remains unaffected. Third, the *teleological mode* is associated with goal-directed

actions that are not linked to associated mental states. In the teleological mode, actions speak louder than words: only being hugged by the therapist counts as caring; emotional pain can be expressed adequately only by the sight of blood from self-inflicted cuts.

Non-mentalizing interactions are the bane of psychotherapy. The psychic-equivalence mode is antithetical to reflection. Flooded with negative affect, patients with BPD can find some relief through projective identification: they externalize alien parts of the self by behaving in ways that create painful experience in the other. Self-injurious behaviors in the teleological mode, for example, can be terrorizing, evoking fear and anger in others akin to feelings the patient felt when terrorized in prior attachment relationships. Hence intense counter-transference experiences are part and parcel of working with patients with BPD [54]. Therapists beset with counter-transference naturally distance themselves emotionally from their patients [55]; yet this enactment creates vicious circles by recapitulating what we construe as the core trauma: the patient feels abandoned (i.e., without a mentalizing connection) in a state of intense distress. Then the therapist will be challenged to reinstate mentalizing.

## Mentalizing interventions

Offering an attachment relationship, the psychotherapist puts the traumatized patient with BPD in a dilemma: stimulating attachment needs potentially evokes trauma-related affects and thereby inhibits the fundamental capacity on which psychotherapy depends, namely, mentalizing. Accordingly, psychotherapy can make the patient worse [56]. Whereas older follow-up studies of intensively treated patients with BPD suggested a protracted illness [57], recent longitudinal data reveal a more favorable natural course of the illness in the absence of intensive treatment [58].

How might intensive treatment go wrong? We are most concerned that patients with precarious mentalizing capacities could respond adversely to interpretive interventions that fly in the face of their conscious experience. Such interventions leave the patient with two options: dismissing the interpretation (the better option) or taking it in as an alien presence within the self (the option consistent with responses to invalidating or non-mentalizing attributions in early childhood). Mentalization-based therapy (MBT) aims to avoid this risk by single-mindedly promoting mentalizing through consistently maintaining a *mentalizing stance*: an open-minded, exploratory attitude of curiosity and inquisitiveness about mental states in oneself and others – ironically for psychotherapists, a "not-knowing" stance that recognizes the inherent opaqueness of mental states as well as their infinitely layered texture. As developmental research attests, mentalizing begets mentalizing, and the ultimate value of psychotherapy lies in strengthening the capacity to maintain mentalizing in the context of an affect-laden attachment relationship.

## Basic principles

The technique of MBT is covered in detail by Bateman and Fonagy [4,5]; here we convey some general principles. To avoid confusion at the outset, we emphasize that we consider our focus on mentalizing to be the *least novel* approach imaginable [59], simply because mentalizing is the core common factor in psychotherapy [3].

Mentalizing-focused therapy is relatively commonsensical in exploring current mental states; hence, therapists seeking training are told that they are doing it already. Perhaps most novel is our attentiveness to avoiding undermining mentalizing and our conviction that the most common non-mentalizing intervention is to confidently impute to patients mental states of which they are unaware. Rather, as therapists generally aspire to do, we strive to engage the patient in a collaborative effort to find meaning and to create a coherent narrative. We emphasize the here and now, shifting between considering mental states of the self and other. We do not encourage free association or elaboration of fantasies. Hence MBT frees therapists from the pressure to provide answers and insights; indeed, we consider therapeutic cleverness to be a cardinal sin. In short, we emphasize *process over content –* meaning-making over particular meanings.

We illustrate these principles with a straightforward approach to mentalizing within the transference, by which we refer to exploring the patient's and the therapist's mental states as they relate to each other. For example, patients who make unwarranted assumptions about therapists can be challenged to mentalize – to consider possible differences between their perspective and ours. Often this approach entails self-disclosure on the part of the therapist, not in the sense of revealing personal information but rather in the sense of letting the patient know what is on the therapist's mind for the sake of encouraging multiple perspectives. The patient declares, "I know you must be fed up with me by now!" The therapist might respond by stating "I'm interested that you're thinking I'm fed up because just a few moments ago I was thinking that you'd brought up something very useful for us to explore." Alternatively, the therapist might reply, "I wouldn't have said that I'm fed up, but you might be picking up my frustration because I have been feeling in this session that you're stonewalling me by dismissing everything I say." Such responses are consistent with a high frequency of therapist "I statements," which underscore that the therapist has no privileged access to the truth but rather is merely conveying one perspective: "When you said that, I started thinking…" "When you started talking about that, I began feeling…" "If that happened to me, I might feel…" We are mindful that focusing on the transference, even in the straightforward way we do it, can stimulate intense affect and that intense affect can undermine mentalizing. Hence, we try to avoid such interventions when the patient's mentalizing is precarious, at which time considering multiple points of view is out of reach. In all, we advocate a relatively supportive yet challenging approach.

Mentalization-based therapy has been provided systematically in partial-hospital and intensive-outpatient programs. The partial-hospital program has demonstrated positive outcomes at discharge and 18-month follow-up in comparison with treatment as usual [60,61]; recent results from an 8-year follow-up [62] also are encouraging, as is the effectiveness of the intensive outpatient program [63]. Moreover, MBT appears to be easily exportable to other treatment settings, such that a broader base of outcomes data will forthcoming. More specifically, a study of MBT as a focus for treating eating disorders is underway [64]; Fearon and colleagues are investigating mentalizing as a core technique in family therapy and in adolescence [65]; and replication by an independent group of the original studies on treating BPD is in progress.

## Trauma-related interventions

On the premise that the secure base of attachment promotes exploration of the inner as well as the outer world, Bowlby [66] elegantly articulated (p. 138) the therapist's task as providing

> the patient with a secure base from which he can explore the various unhappy and painful aspects of his life, past and present, many of which he finds it difficult or perhaps impossible to think about and reconsider without a trusted companion to provide support, encouragement, sympathy, and, on occasion, guidance.

A patient in one of our psychoeducational groups [67] brilliantly epitomized trauma therapy in this context: when the leader proposed that "the mind can be a scary place," she exclaimed, "Yes – and you wouldn't want to go in there alone!"

Emulating Bowlby, our approach to post-traumatic intrusive symptoms goes against the grain of the patient's understandable wish to keep the traumatic experience out of mind: by holding the patient's mind in mind, we enable the patient to hold the traumatic memories and emotions in mind as meaningful experiences. Mentalizing treatment simply – but not easily – helps the patient to think, feel and talk about traumatic experiences. What could be less novel? In short, we promote mentalizing in relation to the trauma in the context of an attachment relationship, on the assumption that lacking the opportunity to mentalize in the course of the traumatic events constitutes the core of the trauma.

Yet we face a dilemma: reminders of trauma evoke symptoms of post-traumatic stress disorder (PTSD), and such reminders are ubiquitous in trauma treatment. Accordingly, trauma treatments must be carefully paced [68,69] so as to balance processing with containment [28]. The Catch-22 is that the two cornerstones of containment are secure attachment relationships and emotion-regulation capacities, both of which are undermined by attachment trauma and thoroughly intertwined with mentalizing. Hence the capacity for containment is not a prerequisite for trauma treatment but rather its ideal outcome. The means to this outcome, as it is in early development, is begetting mentalizing by mentalizing. Accordingly, the spirit of mentalizing as it has been developed in MBT for BPD is consistent with trauma-focused interventions in treating PTSD.

Construing mentalizing as a common psychotherapeutic factor, we are inclined to view a wide range of trauma treatments through this lens. Empirically supported cognitive-behavioral approaches, ranging from exposure therapy [70] to eye movement desensitization and reprocessing [71] and cognitive restructuring [72], enable the patient to bring the traumatic memories to mind in the context of a safe relationship and to develop a coherent narrative of traumatic experience in the process. Therapeutic exposure to traumatic memories lies at the core of all trauma treatments, but we consider the concept of desensitization (or habituation) too passive to account for therapeutic change. Rather, when the therapy is successful, the patient is actively mastering the traumatic experience by mentalizing in the context of attachment; this mastery not only enables the patient to manage intrusive memories

(e.g., rather than being blindsided and resorting to self-injurious defensive strategies) but also provides a model of attachment that can be extended to other relationships, building emotion-regulation competence in the process.

As we hope to have made amply clear, attachment trauma goes far beyond PTSD, and psychodynamic approaches to treating trauma [69,73] are particularly adept at addressing a profoundly important facet of trauma not captured in the criteria for PTSD: reenactment of past trauma in current relationships [74]. To reiterate, PTSD symptoms are notoriously evoked by reminders of trauma, and reenactments provide powerful reminders. Indeed, we might construe the cardinal symptom of BPD – intense sensitivity to abandonment – as the post-traumatic reexperiencing of psychological unavailability (mentalizing failure) in the context of high levels of emotional distress. If ongoing reenactments are not addressed, processing post-traumatic intrusive symptoms related to past trauma will be futile. A main aspiration of MBT is to promote a sense of agency, and helping patients to become aware of their unwitting re-creation of past trauma in current relationships is a central goal of trauma treatment.

## Early intervention

Trauma therapists are liable to feel as if they are rowing upstream when their success depends on the very capacities that the patient with a history of attachment trauma has failed to develop. Psychotherapy is properly viewed as providing developmental help [75]; working with traumatized adults provides such help belatedly.

Before the advent of MBT, Fraiberg and colleagues [76] pioneered "psychotherapy in the kitchen" with a traumatized mother, focusing on her potentially traumatizing interactions with her infant daughter. In effect, the therapist functioned as a surrogate mind-minded mother, drawing the mother's attention to her baby's mental states and acting as a model for mentalizing in the process. Moreover, as a trusting relationship between the mother and the therapist began to evolve, the therapist was able to help the mother talk about her own traumatic past and to see how her baby might have similar feelings in response to her own behavior. As the mother became better able to mentalize in relation to her own history and in relation to her baby, a secure mother–infant relationship began developing.

Explicitly using the concepts of reflective functioning, mentalizing and attachment, Slade *et al.* [77–79] have now developed a systematic program for at-risk young mothers and their infants, which they have dubbed "Minding the Baby." This program relies on home visitors, who begin intervening during pregnancy and assist mothers with practical problem solving (e.g., obtaining proper medical care and social services) as well as promoting mentalizing of the infant. Initial results of this program are highly encouraging, as measured by the health of infants and mothers as well as success in forestalling the development of disorganized attachment [77].

## Conclusions

We have aspired in this chapter to provide a glimpse of the rich and burgeoning developmental science on mentalizing, and we have articulated some of the basic principles of what we consider to be mentalizing-promoting interventions for patients who have suffered trauma in attachment relationships. We conclude by noting that mentalizing in conducting therapy – actually *doing it* on a moment-to-moment basis – is an art, not a science [3]. Trying to mentalize according to scientific rules would be akin to what persons with Asperger's syndrome must do in interacting with others to compensate for their limited mentalizing capacities. We can follow some general guidelines but ultimately we are dependent on intuition; whatever skill we may have is based on our fundamental humanity.

We now make explicit what has been implicit: in trauma treatment, therapists and their patients are in the same boat: each brings to the relationship their individual attachment proclivities and mentalizing capacities; each is liable to lose mentalizing in the throes of attachment insecurity and intense emotional arousal; each will inevitably undermine the other's mentalizing by lapsing into pre-mentalizing modes; and each will promote the other's mentalizing by recovering mentalizing. We now have apt models for a trauma therapist: the mind-minded mother [13] who holds her child's mind in mind, and the trusted companion who provides a secure base for exploration [66] such that the patient need not go into that frightening mental place alone.

## References

1. Kazdin, A. E. (2003). Psychotherapy for children and adolescents. *Annual Review of Psychology*, **54**, 253–276.

2. Allen, J. G. and Fonagy, P. (eds.). (2006). *Handbook of mentalization-based treatment*. Chichester, UK: Wiley.

3. Allen, J. G., Fonagy, P. and Bateman, A. (2008). *Mentalizing in clinical practice*. Washington, DC: American Psychiatric Press.

4. Bateman, A. and Fonagy, P. (2004). *Psychotherapy for borderline personality disorder: Mentalization-based treatment*. New York: Oxford University Press.

5. Bateman, A. and Fonagy, P. (2006). *Mentalization-based treatment for borderline personality disorder: A practical guide*. New York: Oxford University Press.

6. Fonagy, P., Gergely, G., Jurist, E. L. and Target, M. (2002). *Affect regulation, mentalization, and the development of the self*. New York: Other Press.

7. Fonagy, P., Gergely, G. and Target, M. (2007). The parent–infant dyad and the construction of the subjective self. *Journal of Child Psychology and Psychiatry*, **48**, 288–328.

8. Lecours, S. and Bouchard, M.-A. (1997). Dimensions of mentalisation: Outlining levels of psychic transformation. *International Journal of Psycho-Analysis*, **78**, 855–875.

9. Morton, J. (1989). The origins of autism. *New Scientist*, **1694**, 44–47.

10. Fonagy, P. (1991). Thinking about thinking: Some clinical and theoretical considerations in the treatment of a borderline patient. *International Journal of Psychoanalysis*, **72**, 639–656.

11. Allen, J. G. (2006). Mentalizing in practice. In J. G. Allen and P. Fonagy (eds.), *Handbook of mentalization-based treatment* (pp. 3–30). Chichester, UK: Wiley.

12. Malle, B. F. (2004). *How the mind explains behavior: Folk explanations, meaning, and social interaction*. Cambridge, MA: MIT Press.

13. Meins, E. (1997). *Security of attachment and the social development of cognition*. Brighton, UK: Psychology Press.

14. Meins, E., Fernyhough, C., Fradley, E. and Tuckey, M. (2001). Rethinking maternal sensitivity: Mothers' comments on infants' mental processes predict security of attachment at 12 months. *Journal of Child Psychology and Psychiatry*, **42**, 637–648.

15. Ainsworth, M. D. S., Blehar, M. C., Waters, E. and Wall, S. (1978). *Patterns of attachment: A psychological study of the strange situation*. Hillsdale, NJ: Lawrence Erlbaum.

16. Lundy, B. L. (2003). Father– and mother–infant face-to-face interactions: Differences in mind-related comments and infant attachment? *Infant Behavior and Development*, **26**, 200–212.

17. Meins, E., Fernyhough, C., Russell, J. and Clark-Carter, D. (1998). Security of attachment as a predictor of symbolic and mentalising abilities: A longitudinal study. *Social Development*, 7, 1–24.

18. Meins, E., Fernyhough, C., Wainwright, R. *et al.* (2003). Pathways to understanding mind: Construct validity

and predictive validity of maternal mind-mindedness. *Child Development*, **74**, 1194–1211.

19. Meins, E., Fernyhough, C., Wainwright, R. *et al.* (2002). Maternal mind-mindedness and attachment security as predictors of theory of mind understanding. *Child Development*, **73**, 1715–1726.

20. Fonagy, P., Steele, H. and Steele, M. (1991). Maternal representations of attachment during pregnancy predict the organization of infant–mother attachment at one year of age. *Child Development*, **62**, 891–905.

21. Main, M. and Goldwyn, R. (1994). *Adult attachment scoring and classification systems*. Berkeley, CA: Department of Psychology, University of California, Berkeley.

22. Steele, H., Steele, M. and Fonagy, P. (1996). Associations among attachment classifications of mothers, fathers, and their infants. *Child Development*, **67**, 541–555.

23. van Ijzendoorn, M. H. (1995). Adult attachment representations, parental responsiveness, and infant attachment: A meta-analysis on the predictive validity of the Adult Attachment Interview. *Psychological Bulletin*, **117**, 387–403.

24. Slade, A. (2005). Parental reflective functioning: An introduction. *Attachment and Human Development*, **7**, 269–281.

25. Slade, A., Grienenberger, J., Bernbach, E., Levy, D. and Locker, A. (2005). Maternal reflective functioning, attachment, and the transmission gap: A preliminary study. *Attachment and Human Development*, **7**, 283–298.

26. Arnott, B. and Meins, E. (2007). Links between ante-natal attachment representations, postnatal mind-mindedness, and infant attachment security: A preliminary study of mothers and fathers. *Bulletin of the Menninger Clinic*, **71**, 132–149.

27. Grienenberger, J., Kelly, K. and Slade, A. (2005). Maternal reflective functioning, mother–infant affective communication, and infant attachment: Exploring the link between mental states and observed caregiving behaviour in the intergenerational transmission of attachment. *Attachment and Human Development*, **7**, 299–311.

28. Allen, J. G. (2001). *Traumatic relationships and serious mental disorders*. Chichester, UK: Wiley.

29. Main, M. and Hesse, E. (1990). Parents' unresolved traumatic experiences are related to infant disorganized attachment status: Is frightened and/or frightening parental behavior the linking mechanism? In M. T. Greenberg, D. Cicchetti and E. M. Cummings (eds.), *Attachment in the preschool years: Theory, research, and intervention* (pp. 161–182). Chicago, IL: University of Chicago Press.

30. Lyons-Ruth, K. and Jacobvitz, D. (1999). Attachment disorganization: Unresolved loss, relational violence, and lapses in behavioral and attentional strategies.

In J. Cassidy and P. R. Shaver (eds.), *Handbook of attachment: Theory, research, and clinical applications* (pp. 520–554). New York: Guilford.

31. Torgersen, S., Lygren, S., Oien, P. A. *et al.* (2000). A twin study of personality disorders. *Comprehensive Psychiatry*, **41**, 416–425.

32. Depue, R. A. and Lenzenweger, M. F. (2001). A neuro-behavioral dimensional model of personality disorders. In W. J. Livesley (ed.), *The handbook of personality disorders* (pp. 136–176). New York: Guilford.

33. Gabbard, G. O., Miller, L. A. and Martinez, M. (2006). A neurobiological perspective on mentalizing and internal object relations in traumatized patients with borderline personality disorder. In J. G. Allen and P. Fonagy (eds.), *Handbook of mentalization-based treatment* (pp. 123–140). Chichester, UK: Wiley.

34. Conklin, C. Z., Bradley, R. and Westen, D. (2006). Affect regulation in borderline personality disorder. *Journal of Nervous and Mental Disease*, **194**, 69–77.

35. Gergely, G. and Watson, J. S. (1996). The social biofeedback theory of parental affect-mirroring: The development of emotional self-awareness and self-control in infancy. *International Journal of Psycho-Analysis*, **77**, 1181–1212.

36. Posner, M. I., Rothbart, M. K., Vizueta, N. *et al.* (2002). Attentional mechanisms of borderline personality disorder. *Proceedings of the National Academy of Sciences of the United States of America*, **99**, 16366–16370.

37. Domes, G., Winter, B., Schnell, K. *et al.* (2006). The influence of emotions on inhibitory functioning in borderline personality disorder. *Psychological Medicine*, **36**, 1163–1172.

38. Mundy, P. and Neal, R. (2001). Neural plasticity, joint attention, and a transactional social-orienting model of autism. In L. M. Glidden (ed.), *International review of mental retardation: Autism*, Vol. **23** (pp. 139–168). San Diego, CA: Academic Press.

39. Fearon, P. and Belsky, J. (2004). Attachment and attention: Protection in relation to gender and cumulative social-contextual adversity. *Child Development*, **75**, 1677–1693.

40. Claussen, A. H., Mundy, P. C., Mallik, S. A. and Willoughby, J. C. (2002). Joint attention and disorganized attachment status in infants at risk. *Development and Psychopathology*, **14**, 279–291.

41. Kochanska, G., Coy, K. C. and Murray, K. T. (2001). The development of self-regulation in the first four years of life. *Child Development*, **72**, 1091–1111.

42. Ryan, R. M. and Deci, E. L. (2003). On assimilating identities to the self: A self-determination theory perspective on internalization and integrity within cultures. In M. R. Leary and J. P. Tangney (eds.), *Handbook of self and identity* (pp. 253–272). New York: Guilford.

43. Levy, K. N. (2005). The implications of attachment theory and research for understanding borderline personality disorder: A preliminary study. *Development and Psychopathology*, **17**, 959–986.

44. Russ, M. J., Shearin, E. N., Clarkin, J. F., Harrison, K. and Hull, J. W. (1993). Subtypes of self-injurious patients with borderline personality disorder. *American Journal of Psychiatry*, **150**, 1869–1871.

45. Johnson, J. G., Cohen, P., Chen, H., Kasen, S. and Brook, J. S. (2006). Parenting behaviors associated with risk for offspring personality disorder during adulthood. *Archives of General Psychiatry*, **63**, 579–587.

46. Lyons-Ruth, K., Yellin, C., Melnick, S. and Atwood, G. (2005). Expanding the concept of unresolved mental states: Hostile/helpless states of mind on the Adult Attachment Interview are associated with disrupted mother–infant communication and infant disorganization. *Development and Psychopathology*, **17**, 1–23.

47. Danon, G. and Graignic, R. (2003). Borderline personality disorder and mother–infant interaction. In *Proceedings of the Meeting of the Society for Research in Child Development*, Atlanta, GA.

48. Crandell, L. E., Patrick, M. P. H. and Hobson, R. P. (2003). "Still-face" interactions between mothers with borderline personality disorder and their 2-month old infants. *British Journal of Psychiatry*, **183**, 239–247.

49. Weiss, M., Zelkowitz, P., Feldman, R. B. *et al.* (1996). Psychopathology in offspring of mothers with borderline personality disorder: A pilot study. *Canadian Journal of Psychiatry*, **41**, 285–290.

50. Zanarini, M. C., Williams, A. A., Lewis, R. E. *et al.* (1997). Reported pathological childhood experiences associated with the development of borderline personality disorder. *American Journal of Psychiatry*, **154**, 1101–1106.

51. Fruzzetti, A. E., Shenk, C. and Hoffman, P. D. (2005). Family interaction and the development of borderline personality disorder: A transactional model. *Development and Psychopathology*, **17**, 1007–1030.

52. Linehan, M. M. (1993). *Cognitive-behavioral treatment of borderline personality disorder*. New York: Guilford.

53. Fonagy, P. and Target, M. (1997). Attachment and reflective function: Their role in self-organization. *Development and Psychopathology*, **9**, 679–700.

54. Gabbard, G. O. and Wilkinson, S. M. (1994). *Management of countertransference with borderline patients*. Washington, DC: American Psychiatric Press.

55. Aviram, R. B., Brodsky, B. S. and Stanley, B. (2006). Borderline personality disorder, stigma, and treatment implications. *Harvard Review of Psychiatry*, **14**, 249–256.

56. Fonagy, P. and Bateman, A. W. (2006). Progress in the treatment of borderline personality disorder. *British Journal of Psychiatry*, **188**, 1–3.

57. Stone, M. H. (1990). *The fate of borderline patients: Successful outcome and psychiatric practice.* New York: Guilford.

58. Zanarini, M. C., Frankenberg, F. R., Hennen, J. and Silk, K. R. (2003). The longitudinal course of borderline psychopathology: 6-year prospective follow-up of the phenomenology of borderline personality disorder. *American Journal of Psychiatry*, **160**, 274–283.

59. Allen, J. G. and Fonagy, P. (2006). Preface. In J. G. Allen and P. Fonagy (eds.), *Handbook of mentalization-based treatment* (pp. ix–xxi). Chichester, UK: Wiley.

60. Bateman, A. W. and Fonagy, P. (1999). Effectiveness of partial hospitalization in the treatment of borderline personality disorder: A randomized controlled trial. *American Journal of Psychiatry*, **156**, 1563–1569.

61. Bateman, A. W. and Fonagy, P. (2001). Treatment of borderline personality disorder with psychoanalytically oriented partial hospitalization: An 18-month follow-up. *American Journal of Psychiatry*, **158**, 36–42.

62. Bateman, A. and Fonagy, P. (2008). 8-year follow-up of patients treated for borderline personality disorder: Mentalization-based treatment versus treatment as usual. *American Journal of Psychiatry*, **165**, 631–638.

63. Bateman, A. and Fonagy, P. (2009). Randomized controlled trial of out-patient mentalization-based treatment versus structured clinical management for borderline personality disorder. *American Journal of Psychiatry*, **166**, 1355–1364

64. Skårderud, F. (2007). Eating one's words: Mentalisation-based psychotherapy. An outline for a treatment and training manual. *European Eating Disorders Review*, **15**, 323–339.

65. Fearon, P., Target, M., Sargent, J. *et al.* (2006). Short-term mentalization and relational therapy (SMART): An integrative family therapy for children and adolescents. In J. Allen and P. Fonagy (eds.), *Handbook of mentalization-based treatment* (pp. 201–222). Chichester, UK: Wiley.

66. Bowlby, J. (1988). *A secure base: Parent–child attachment and healthy human development*. New York: Basic Books.

67. Allen, J. G. (2005). *Coping with trauma: Hope through understanding*, 2n edn. Washington, DC: American Psychiatric Press.

68. Chu, J. A. (1992). The therapeutic roller coaster: Dilemmas in the treatment of childhood abuse survivors. *Journal of Psychotherapy: Practice and Research*, **1**, 351–370.

69. Herman, J. L. (1992). *Trauma and recovery*. New York: Basic Books.

70. Foa, E. B. and Rothbaum, B. O. (1998). *Treating the trauma of rape: Cognitive-behavioral therapy for PTSD.* New York: Guilford.

71. Shapiro, F. (1995). *Eye movement desensitization and reprocessing: Basic principles, protocols, and procedures.* New York: Guilford.

72. Resick, P. A. and Schnicke, M. K. (1993). *Cognitive processing therapy for rape victims: A treatment manual.* London: Sage.

73. Davies, J. M. and Frawley, M. G. (1994). *Treating the adult survivor of childhood sexual abuse.* New York: Basic Books.

74. van der Kolk, B. A. (1989). The compulsion to repeat the trauma: Reenactment, revictimization, and masochism. *Psychiatric Clinics of North America, 12,* 389–411.

75. Hurry, A. (1998). Psychoanalysis and developmental therapy. In A. Hurry (ed.), *Psychoanalysis and developmental therapy* (pp. 32–73). Madison, CT: International Universities Press.

76. Fraiberg, S., Adelson, E. and Shapiro, V. (1975). Ghosts in the nursery: A psychoanalytic approach to the problems of impaired infant–mother relationships. *Journal of the American Academy of Child Psychiatry, 14,* 387–421.

77. Sadler, L. S., Slade, A. and Mayes, L. C. (2006). Minding the Baby: A mentalization-based parenting program. In J. G. Allen and P. Fonagy (eds.), *Handbook of mentalization-based treatment* (pp. 271–288). Chichester, UK: Wiley.

78. Slade, A. (2002). Keeping the baby in mind: A critical factor in perinatal mental health. In A. Slade, L. Mayes and N. Epperson (eds.), *In a special issue on perinatal mental health* (pp. 10–16). Washington, DC: Zero to Three.

79. Slade, A., Sadler, L. S., Currier, J. *et al.* (2004). *Minding the baby: A manual.* New Haven, CT: Yale Child Study Center.

# Chapter 24

# Pragmatic approaches to stage-oriented treatment for early life trauma-related complex post-traumatic stress and dissociative disorders

Richard J. Loewenstein and Victor Welzant

## Introduction

In this chapter we discuss aspects of treatment of complex post-traumatic stress disorder (CPTSD). Assessment and treatment of this population has recently been definitively reviewed in a book edited by Courtois and Ford [1]. This chapter will emphasize issues that are helpful for the clinician to understand, and the reader is referred to Courtois and Ford for a comprehensive overview [1].

The concept of CPTSD was definitively formulated by Herman in 1992 [2,3], based on work from many different clinicians and researchers [4]. The construct attempted to differentiate post-traumatic disorders that arise from a single, often non-interpersonal traumatic event (PTSD), from those related to prolonged, repeated, abusive trauma (CPTSD).

Here, the PTSD concept alone was insufficient to delineate the full range of what could be best understood as chronic *adaptations* to recurring, coercive interpersonal trauma. Many of these patients reported multiple types of trauma, generally beginning in early childhood and continuing throughout development, often with repeated re-victimization in adulthood. In these survivors, major problems existed in attachments and relationships; capacity for work; views of self, others and the world; and even in spiritual domains. A similar clinical picture developed in survivors of extreme, recurrent adult traumas such as genocide, political torture and sexual trafficking.

This research, as well as data on the substantial prevalence of multiple types and episodes of early childhood trauma in many clinical populations, led to the proposal by Herman and her collaborators for the

inclusion in the upcoming fourth edition of *Diagnostic and Statistical Manual* (DSM-IV) [5] of a category that would specify diagnostic criteria for a complex post-traumatic disorder. This diagnostic construct, "disorders of extreme stress not otherwise specified" (DESNOS) [6], enumerated six dimensions of disturbed functioning in survivors of chronic traumatization: (a) regulation of affect and impulses, (b) attention or consciousness, (c) self-perception, (d) relations with others, (e) somatization, and (f) systems of meaning. Despite support for this diagnostic category from studies that were part of the DSM-IV field trials for PTSD [7], the DESNOS category was rejected as a diagnosis in the DSM-IV since, according to Herman, this construct could not be aligned with the view of PTSD as an anxiety disorder [8]. Nonetheless, the DESNOS construct and variants of it, most frequently dubbed complex PTSD, have continued to be of major clinical and research significance [1,9–12].

## Complex trauma disorders and dissociative disorders

The literature on the diagnosis and treatment of dissociative disorders (DD), particularly dissociative identity disorder (DID), has developed mostly in parallel with that on CPTSD. In general, DID has been conceptualized as a childhood-onset post-traumatic developmental disorder, related to multiple types of childhood trauma and deprivation, generally beginning before the age of 5 years [13]. In addition, patients with depersonalization disorder (DPD) frequently report high rates of severe childhood emotional abuse in their histories

*The Impact of Early Life Trauma on Health and Disease: The Hidden Epidemic*, ed. Ruth A. Lanius, Eric Vermetten and Clare Pain. Published by Cambridge University Press. Copyright © Cambridge University Press 2010.

[14]. Emotional abuse generally does not fit the DSM-IVTR criterion A for a traumatic stressor, required for the diagnosis of PTSD. However, recent research supports the view that childhood emotional/verbal abuse has psychobiological outcomes similar to recurrent childhood sexual and/or physical abuse [15].

Although often not stated explicitly in the literature, the vast majority of patients with DID, related forms of dissociative disorders not otherwise specified (DDNOS), chronic forms of dissociative amnesia, and some patients with DPD fit the DESNOS/CPTSD construct. The bulk of the "pathological dissociation" taxon described by Waller and colleagues [16,17] is made up of DID and DID-like forms of DDNOS.

## Approach to the treatment of complex post-traumatic stress disorder

Complex PTSD is a multidimensional construct that crosses a number of DSM-IV (text revision) diagnoses. General principles of treatment for CPTSD may be similar among different clinical groups, and there are many similar difficulties faced by survivors of different types of cumulative trauma. Clinical differences among those with CPTSD may depend on many factors, including the types of trauma, the age(s) at which it was experienced, genetic and epigenetic factors, social supports and restitutive experiences, and whether traumas involved betrayal by a trusted person, rather than occurring in wartime or during sociopolitical upheaval [18].

Those with CPTSD generally show disruptions in many dimensions of life. They may have a mixture of intrapsychic, interpersonal, familial, social, cultural, neuropsychiatric, addiction, medical, forensic, economic, environmental and spiritual problems, which may require a wide range of pragmatic clinical interventions, let alone skilled psychotherapeutic and/or psychopharmacological interventions [11].

### Issues for clinicians

There are factors that may predispose some clinicians to work more effectively with certain populations of patients with CPTSD than others. These may include the clinician's own personal history and life space; cross-cultural competencies; predisposition to work more effectively with certain types of patients; ability to listen to repeated reports of extreme trauma; tolerance for certain kinds of (usually negative) transferences; capacity to deal with emergencies, often involving violence to self or others; and ability to maintain therapeutic boundaries and/or to set limits on behavior that disrupts and/or interferes with treatment. Clinicians may not be prepared for the intense transference/counter-transference reactions that can occur with this population. Counter-transference reactivity may escalate into a syndrome of "secondary PTSD," which may parallel the symptoms of CPTSD. This may include affect regulation problems, social withdrawal and relational problems, intrusive preoccupation with the traumatized patient, alterations in view of the self and the world, and substance abuse, among others [19]. Also, there may be particular counter-transference problems in work with severely dissociative patients. These may relate to these patients' dissociativity, hypnotizability, traumatic transference configurations and projective identifications [20,21].

## Social and political issues

Clinicians working with patients with CPTSD/DD may experience bafflement, skepticism, hostility, or outright attempts at interference in treatment from colleagues [22]. Reactions may range from those who express bewilderment at the existence of CPTSD and DDs, to those with strong negative opinions about these diagnostic constructs and a belief that clinicians who diagnose and treat these patients should be censured and/or even sued for allegedly practicing below the standard of care [23]. Accordingly, clinicians working with patients with CPTSD/DD must recognize that there are sociopolitical aspects to controversies about this population that are much deeper, and often far more virulent, than usual professional and academic controversies [24,25].

Clinicians should understand the risk-management aspects of working with this population, including informed consent. The latter may include discussion with the patient about management of danger to self and/or others, the limits of confidentiality, the nature of treatment boundaries, the trajectory of treatment in which some symptoms may appear to worsen before improving and controversies about use of hypnosis in treatment, delayed recall of trauma memory and/or the etiology of DID [26,27]. The provision of informed consent is an ongoing process that is particularly important in this patient population because of CPTSD, patients' cognitive and memory problems, capacity for negative transference, ambivalent attachments to reported perpetrators and confusion about relational boundaries, among other issues [28].

# Phasic trauma treatment for post-traumatic disorders

It is the general consensus that effective treatment of post-traumatic disorders follows a tripartite structure [1,3,27–29]. In the first phase, the patient works towards basic safety and stability. In the second, the focus is on the detailed narrative and emotionally intense recollection and processing of trauma memories. In the third phase, the therapeutic work is directed towards "reintegration," living well in the present, with traumatic memories relegated more to the status of "bad memories" rather than flashbacks, behavioral re-experiencing phenomena and/or intense post-traumatic reactivity to current situations. These stages are heuristic, since memory material may need to be addressed in stage 1, if only in a more cognitive and distanced manner, and then worked through again from a more integrated perspective in stage 3. The entirety of trauma treatment is directed towards the patient developing a better, safe adaptation to current life.

Kluft and Loewenstein [28] put forward a treatment model for DID with nine subphases within the basic tripartite structure. The subphases of stage 1 include (in addition to establishment of safety) a variety of interventions to access, map, stabilize and promote communication and collaboration among the DID self-states. Consensus in the field, buttressed by evidence-based studies, strongly supports direct work with DID self-states. In particular, treatment models that do not involve direct interaction with self-states have been shown to have poorer overall patient outcomes [27]. The fourth phase in this model, Kluft's phase 4, "metabolism of trauma," corresponds to Herman's stage 2. The additional stages in the model of Kluft and Loewenstein relate to fusion/integration of self-states and the patient's gaining competency in living without dissociative defenses.

## Stage 1

### Safety and stability

Patients with CPTSD/DD commonly seek or are referred to treatment because of problems with safety and/or overwhelming symptoms. The clinician must logically prioritize basic life and health over other interventions. This includes management of (a) dangerousness to self and/or others, including minor children of the patient; (b) lack of food, clothing, and/or shelter; (c) substance abuse; (d) eating disorders;

(e) lack of access to adequate medical care; (f) high-risk behaviors; (g) and enmeshment in abusive/traumatizing relationships. In addition to symptoms of PTSD and dissociation, the patient may be affected by symptoms of other neuropsychiatric disorders, including mood disorders, somatoform disorders, brain injury, psychotic disorders and personality disorders. The clinician may need to resort to many different levels and types of intervention to protect the patient. These may include hospitalization specialized substance use or eating disorders programs, police assistance and shelter for victims of intimate partner violence, social service intervention to protect minor children, and assistance with housing and access to medical care, and so on. Psychiatric consultation may be needed for definitive psychopharmacological interventions for comorbid disorders [30,31]. In addition, patients may need a variety of psychotherapeutic interventions for stabilizing PTSD and dissociative symptoms. These may include psychoeducation, cognitive therapy, dialectical behavior therapy, psychodynamic interventions and techniques from family systems theory such as reframing symptoms as adaptations, among others. In addition, many patients may be taught a variety of symptom management techniques, such as relaxation, imagery and self-hypnosis [32,33].

### Trauma focus

It is helpful to begin to understand the patient's symptoms as logically related to post-traumatic reactivity, trauma scripts, trauma-based cognitive distortions, traumatic projections, projective identifications and transference [20,34–36]. The patient is invited to understand his/her reactions as potentially "triggered" by post-traumatic reminders, which set off intense reactivity, often in the form of "unconscious flashbacks" [37] or "emotional flashbacks" [33]. Here, the patient is unconsciously repeating traumatic scenarios and/or having excessively intense emotional reactions to everyday situations based on traumatic experiences or relationship schemas, respectively. This reactivity may lead to self-destructive behavior, maladaptive interactions with others and emotional dysregulation, usually accompanied by marked cognitive distortions about what is occurring. Remarkably, through powerful projective identifications, others may be drawn into interactions with the patient that seemingly replay reported traumatic situations from the past, or as one patient put it, "walking into the flashback together" [20].

259

Elucidation of the traumatic scenario that is being replayed allows the patient to begin "separation of past from present." The patient examines the extent to which current problems, maladaptive behaviors, troubled relationships, inexplicably intense emotional reactivity and/or self-destructive behaviors result from unconscious "reliving" of past trauma scenarios and/or attempts at self-protection from anticipated traumas and betrayals based on past traumatic relationships.

There is often a "method in the madness" of patients' self-destructive behavior. For example, among the manifold cognitive distortions that may drive self-injury is the idea (or variants) that "I'm going to get hurt no matter what I do, so control the timing and intensity of harm, that's all the control I get." These beliefs can be reframed as an attempt to survive the helplessness and unpredictability of repeated maltreatment. The therapeutic goal then becomes to change this "survival skill" to a "recovery skill" [38]: developing adult, non-trauma-based strategies for appraising one's current life situation and level of external danger, gaining a repertoire of skills to keep oneself safe in the present and creating overall safety and self-protection in one's current life.

Even suicidal ideation may have post-traumatic meaning [3]. Many patients will recall being suicidal as small children. Suicide seemed like the only possible control over inescapable abuse and torment. Not infrequently, beginning in childhood, these patients fantasized about a benevolent afterlife. In addition, patients may see themselves as needing euthanasia to alleviate their suffering. We sometimes reframe these ideas as the "life-affirming function of suicide," since the patient is commonly seeking control, surcease from maltreatment and diminution of suffering, not necessarily death per se.

### Affect regulation

Many CPTSD/DD symptoms can be best understood as attempts at self-regulation [10]. The patients' experience of affective states, either numbing or overwhelming intrusion, may be homologous to the numbing/intrusion cycle of PTSD. Self-harm, substance abuse, dissociation and eating disorders, among others, may be attempts to ablate intolerable, often unnameable, affective states such as extreme shame, humiliation, rage, horror, helplessness and disgust/revulsion. Conversely, self-injury may be an attempt to "feel something" when in a numb state, or to "put the pain on the outside" where it seems more real or where others may take it more seriously.

It is helpful to use strategies for education: giving names to emotions, helping the patient understand emotions as a kind of "sensory system" rather than an implacable, destructive force [39]. Patients can learn that part of early development involves assistance in self-regulation and tolerance of emotional and behavioral states [13]. Repeated early trauma, especially by caregivers, causes extreme, overstimulating emotions – terror, rage, shame, helplessness, horror and disgust – for which the child may have no words or comprehension. In addition, the traumatized child is not soothed or comforted when hurt, or is only soothed unpredictably [40]. He/she finds ways to manage emotions as best as possible, often through self-destructive means.

Through their actions, abusive adults implicitly share a model with the child that emotions and thoughts are dangerous, ineluctable equivalents to action. Yet, the child is given the message that his/her thoughts, needs and emotions are unwanted, undesirable; the child is often hurt for expressing distress: "I'll give you something to cry about!" The maltreated child internalizes the idea that if someone has a problem then harming the child's (or someone else's) body can solve it. Consequently, it is not surprising that survivors of childhood maltreatment often have major difficulties with regulation of dangerousness to themselves or others.

### Attachment, traumatic transference and the therapeutic alliance

Most patients with CPTSD/DD have been hurt in the context of early attachments. Attachment pathology has been hypothesized as an important factor in the development of dissociative defenses and complex trauma reactions [41]. In DID, one aspect of development of altered self-states may involve attempts at attachment to caregivers who are highly contradictory and/or behave differently at different times, whether as a result of substance abuse, affect dysregulation, dissociation, or combinations of these [13,42]. In the mind of the preoperational child, it is as if he/she is relating to a different person at these times, requiring the child to be a "different person" to complete the dyad. Accordingly, divided representations of self/other may take considerable therapeutic effort to resolve.

Forging a therapeutic alliance in the treatment of complex trauma is an essential but difficult long-term process. Patients with complex trauma have been hurt in the context of their most basic relationships, and therapy is a relationship. In therapy, the trauma survivor is placed in a situation that may be experienced as an excruciating, impossibly tricky trap [43]. In the survivor's development, the experience of need and dependence has been unpredictably associated with trauma, terror, abandonment, intrusion, overstimulation, rejection, mockery, sadism and humiliation, all before "big words" like the foregoing were even imagined. The solution is to dissociate all need, and even dissociate that there *are* needs [44]. Of course, this only increases the power of the needs and the reciprocal pressure to deny their existence. Dalenberg [43] describes the neediness of the survivor in therapy as having the dual quality of addiction and allergy.

Many traumatic transference/counter-transference dilemmas in treatment of patients with CPTSD/DD may result from this basic experience of the survivor: attachment, need and dependence are implicitly the source of profound humiliation. The following fictionalized patient narrative may give some idea of the patient's experience of this.

> Something good, something warm, something that you need and feel you must count on, is suddenly ripped from you like a kick in your gut. You are made to know that you are "too much," you must somehow calibrate your needs, or take care of someone big, to "get" anything. Your needs, your emotions, your body reactions prove that you are bad, disgusting, shameful, loathsome, the cause of all the bad that has happened to you. They tell you that and you feel that in your body. You become the bad. You have no control over what you need. It can appear; it can disappear. So, *you* must control you, to never show anyone this needy side of you. Perhaps you will take care of everyone else to show you have no needs. Perhaps you will withdraw, leave and stay away from everyone, so you will never be humiliated by need again. You will leave before you are left: "You can't fire me! I quit." You will hurt and humiliate yourself to show how shameful you are for your needs, and that no one can shame you better than you. You will beat them to the punch. Yet, it is still all *your* fault that you need, that you are enraged by those who come and go, oblivious to your predicament. Of course, you can't show that. Your needy, shameful rage will drive the other one away: because your emotions are wrong, your needs are wrong, showing your needs is wrong, everything about you is shameful and wrong.
>
> The therapist tells you this is "all in the past." You tell your therapist that she is wrong. It is all still right here in the present. Your therapist doesn't understand. And gets confused. And gets frustrated. And thinks you are a "borderline." And still you are the bad one.

> If you have alter personalities, they speak to you in the voice of your abuser, your parents, your siblings. They say shut up, don't talk, you are shamefully bad, you are a whore and a slut, a wimp and a loser, and the cause of everything bad that has ever happened. It isn't safe to talk, they tell you. They'll kill you if you talk. Or someone you love. Besides, you always trust too much. You get into those situations where you get hurt and humiliated, because you are too stupid to see what's coming. Of course, deep down, they are ashamed that they can't seem to stop any of this either, so they attack you, even though they are also attacking themselves. They will hurt you terribly for possibly believing (again) that someone is OK and won't hurt or abandon you. Your judgment of other people is a humiliation waiting to happen. Actually, these "parts" who shame you are your protectors and helpers who care about you, but that is a secret.

It is a wonder that any complex trauma survivor stays in therapy.

### Shame

Shame "scripts" are among the most endemic and powerful, often unrecognized, aspects of trauma responses. The work of Nathanson [39] on affect theory provides a compelling framework for understanding shame in the context of trauma treatment. Kluft [45] has developed a construct for understanding dissociative defenses and DID self-states as manifestations of shame affect. In part, the avoidance symptoms of PTSD can be conceptualized as avoidance of the shame that is an essential part of interpersonal trauma. A central feature of perpetration, of bullying, child abuse, rape, torture and sadism, is the deliberate humiliation of the victim; when we say that the perpetrator is motivated by power and control, the reciprocal is that the victim is rendered powerless, helpless, without control: profoundly humiliated.

Nathanson [39] described the "compass of shame", which includes four "poles": *self-attack*, *attack other*, *avoidance* and *withdrawal*. The self-attack pole has aspects of, "I'm worthless, I'm a loser, I'm not good enough, big enough, strong enough, a failure, not fit to be on the face of the earth." The attack-other pole derives from the perpetrator, the bully: he/she is not the helpless shamed one, but the powerful, controlling shaming one. The one who is shamed wishes to attack back, to make the bully, the perpetrator, feel the shame that the victim experiences. Unfortunately, attempts by the victim to attack back often only lead to more humiliation. In the case of the abused child, where the child is smaller, weaker and often dependent on the attacking person, this "attack other" script may become automatically turned back on the victim before it ever achieves conscious awareness [46]. In DID, the persecutory and/or "introject" self-states frequently engage in internalized attack-other scripts. Depressed, depleted, self-defeating self-states frequently embody "attack-self" scripts, which are redoubled by the attack-other scripts of the persecutory self-states. The third pole of the shame compass is avoidance. We all tend to avoid memories, reminders, triggers, situations and interactions that are associated with embarrassment or shame. The final pole is the chronic form of avoidance, withdrawal. The ashamed person may feel a need to hide, stay away from others and withdraw completely, since any interaction seems to provoke shame affect. One chronically withdrawn survivor said, "I feel too ashamed to even breathe." Common clichés about shame, such as "I was so embarrassed I could have died" or "I was so ashamed I wished the ground could've swallowed me up," may represent a significant component of the chronic suicidality and apparently refractory "depression" in patients with CPTSD/DD. To be sure, this apparent mood disorder may be a complex mixture of shame, post-traumatic grief and demoralization, among other emotions. However, the shame component is often the least explored.

Education about shame scripts, shame affect and the compass of shame can be exceptionally helpful in the treatment of patients with CPTSD/DD. Typically, these patients readily recognize themselves in every pole of the compass. They find it helpful to understand shame experiences in therapy, in intrapsychic life and in their interpersonal relationships. Some acknowledge that they have meta-shame: they are ashamed that they are ashamed. Attendance to subtly self-shaming aspects of common phrases may be helpful, such as "Why did I do that? What's wrong with me? What *is* my problem?" These may be useful questions, but we rarely say them to ourselves in the spirit of neutral enquiry. In English, these forms of speech usually are reproaches, not requests for information. Clinicians working with CPTSD/DD may find it helpful to avoid the "why" construction, since this may convey an unintended shaming message.

Generic statements of support, such as "you're such a nice person," that are meant to counter shame rarely help patients with CPTSD/DD, it is far more helpful to identify specific improvements, competencies, personal characteristics and forms of mastery to counter shame [45], for example "You took a big risk when you let your friend visit you the other night, and the two of you had a really good time, despite how afraid you were that she would see your shame and hate you."

# Stage 2

The first phase of complex trauma treatment requires rigorous attention to a variety of basic interventions to stabilize the patient and the psychotherapy. The second phase, with elements of progressive exposure, where memory material is dealt with in a detailed way accompanied by expression of strong affect, should not be undertaken without reasonably successful completion of the tasks of the first phase (see Kluft and Loewenstein [28] for a more comprehensive discussion of stage 2 work). Patients who cannot master and/or adequately apply the tasks of stage 1 should continue in a long-term supportive treatment focused on stage 1 work.

## Preparation for stage 2 work

In order for patients to give informed consent, they should be given information about the nature of the stage 2 process, including the likelihood for symptom exacerbations during it, as well as the positive outcomes that can occur with successful memory processing in order for them to give informed consent. It may be helpful to revisit discussion of controversies about the nature of "recovered" memory and the reconstructive aspect of autobiographical memory, among others.

Patients should have a rational motivation for stage 2 work. They should demonstrate a basic understanding about work on trauma memory; for example, they should understand that trauma recall is not about "getting rid of" memories, but involves mourning and integration of the reality of painful life history. In addition, logistical issues such as support and safe transportation must be adequate to support the work.

Patients with CPTSD, particularly those with dissociative disorders, are often of two minds about their own recall: believing themselves at some times and not at others. Rather than validating or discounting memoires in this context, it is far more important for the therapist to identify the conflicts the patients has about his/her own recall. It is most helpful for the therapist to focus on the process of understanding and integrating memory material, not belief versus disbelief. The goal here is to allow the patient the freedom to explore and resolve, as fully as possible, questions about what did or did not occur, without pressure to come to premature closure. Many important issues may be embedded in this uncertainty about the past. These can include, among many others, attachments to reported perpetrators, defenses against sadness and grieving over post-traumatic losses, deliberate attempts by perpetrators to confuse the victim's recall by drugs or other methods, incorporation of childhood restitutive fantasies as memory and, even, development of factitious memories by the patient.

Patients and clinicians should have the psychological, physical and life-space resources for a very difficult process. Comorbid medical and psychiatric disorders should be stabilized and medications optimally adjusted. The patient should have adequate ego strength and willingness to go forward with the work, and the therapist should have the psychological resources and sufficient education to manage a complex and difficult process, as well as the psychological wherewithal to tolerate hearing highly distressing material.

Stage 2 work should be *paced, planned* and *structured*, not allowed to "just happen." Patients with CPTSD have experienced trauma as unpredictable and inescapable. To the extent possible, the process to detoxify trauma memories should implicitly provide the opposite experience. The therapist and patient should agree *in advance* on the memory material to be worked on, the schedule for the work, the level of affective intensity, the symptom management techniques that will be used and the "disaster plan" if the work begins to decompensate the patient.

In work with DID, planning should include which self-states will be part of the memory work and which will be "contained" or in hypnotic "sleep." In DID, *all* self-states must at least be willing to tolerate undertaking work on specific memories. Majority does *not* rule in these situations. Because CPTSD/DID is a condition of being forced to submit to the intolerable, if a self-state experiences memory work as unendurable, the work should not proceed, even if other self-states implore the clinician to ignore the objection. Attempts to go forward in this situation almost invariably result in safety crises, severe symptom exacerbations and failure to complete the memory work. It is far better to explore the objections of the reluctant self-state(s). They usually have vital information to impart that must be considered if memory work is to be successful.

In patients with CPTSD but not DID, similar issues may be experienced as covert ambivalence about doing stage 2 work. The patient may be reluctant to express hesitance to go forward because of shame, not wanting to seem like a "bad patient," wanting to please the

therapist and/or distorted beliefs about the nature of memory processing. The clinician must be attentive to track significant reluctance to go forward that would necessitate additional stabilization, education about trauma processing, cognitive therapy and work to stabilize the self-state system.

Trauma therapists can model for patients with CPTSD/DD the capacity to avoid catastrophizing, and to learn from mistakes and/or events that do not go as planned. Stage 2 work is an imperfect process with a considerable likelihood of unexpected outcomes, especially when the patient is still learning to do the work and has not yet experienced the benefits of successful memory integration. For example, there are a number of factors indicating that stage 2 work is not accomplishing resolution of traumatic memories. These include increased PTSD intrusions to other memories rather than decreased affective intensity of the memories targeted for attention; failure by the patient to apply what is learned in broader therapy contexts; the patient pressing to uncover "more" rather than finish working on the index material; escalation of safety problems; and, in DID, emergence of additional self-states and/or exacerbation of conflict and internal punitiveness between self-states.

Difficulties like these indicate to the therapist that he/she must "go back to basics" to help the patient restabilize and focus again on basic tasks and goals of therapy. These difficulties should be viewed and presented to the patient as a central part of trauma resolution, rather than a shameful failure. As in scientific endeavors, early theories must be revised as more data are acquired. In memory work, apparent obstacles are indicators that essential, often hidden, issues must be addressed for stage 2 work to proceed successfully.

### The memory processing session
The therapist should be active during the memory processing work to assist with structuring the time, pacing the work and monitoring the patient for signs of impending problems. The therapist should make sure that there is adequate time for the work to proceed. If a current problem requires discussion that takes up more than the first third of the appointment, the memory work should be deferred. In addition, the therapist should alert the patient during the last third of the appointment to begin containment of the material and the process of grounding back "into the present."

The therapist should anticipate that the patient may lose "duality" and no longer be aware of current reality during the session. The patient may experience the therapist as someone from the past who is part of the memory. In DID, the patient may switch to an unknown self-state, a disoriented self-state or an angry protector self-state, and may begin to harm him/herself, attempt to leave the office, huddle in a corner or become threatening. At these times, the therapist should attempt to completely re-orient the patient: have the patient open his/her eyes, look around the room; become more grounded by using the five senses, shift position, breathe deeply; become aware of objects like a cell phone, portable computer or iPod that could not possibly exist at the time of the memory events. In DID, the therapist should ask for self-states to come forward who can assist at such times. If hypnotic symptom containment is part of the therapy, the therapist should attempt to rapidly induce a state of greater calm, containment and distance.

If the session proceeds without problems, the therapist should attempt to track all aspects of the memory: behavioral, affective, somatosensory and cognitive (BASK dimensions) [47] to monitor which aspects of the memory may be missing or attenuated. Also, the therapist should attempt to track important affects commonly associated with trauma: horror, terror, confusion, shame, humiliation, mortification, sorrow, helplessness, anguish, grief, guilt, rage, disgust and revulsion. It is important to attend to affects that are more easily reported, those that are difficult to speak of and those that appear absent, even though they would logically be experienced. Perpetrator words are often very powerfully embedded in memory material. The memory may not be resolved until these words are brought into consciousness, the emotional reactions to them experienced and the power of the words to shape the meaning of the events addressed.

As the session progresses, the therapist can address cognitive distortions, comment on misattribution of blame, clarify and name affects and address traumatic transference issues.

Trauma memories may have a kind of central node or core that determines the meaning(s) of the event for the survivor, frequently determining important aspects of the survivor's assumptive world. Commonly, these aspects of the memory involve profound humiliation and/or betrayal, yet it is important to uncover these central elements to allow full detoxification and integration of the memory. For example, an incest survivor repeatedly worked on a memory of being raped by her father, and her many feelings and reactions to her abusive father based on this and other assaults. However,

the memory did not resolve until the patient recalled that her mother witnessed the assault, turned away and left the room. At that point, the mother's role in the patient's life and her complicity in the incest became the central focus of the therapy.

During the last 10–20 minutes of the memory session, the therapist concludes by helping the patient "come back" to the present and "put away" the memory and associated affects if this is indicated, as well as working on soothing and calming. The therapist should help the patient to review the material in a cognitive summary, which can provide an overview of what has (and has not) been understood by the patient. In addition, the therapist can help to assess the extent of redissociation of the material, if any.

There should be a plan for what happens after the patient leaves the office. This should include anticipation of "aftershocks," exhaustion and/or additional intrusive symptoms, which may take the form of what occurred in the patient's life in the immediate aftermath of the rape, the beating, and so on. Therapists and patients tend to focus on the basic trauma memory, often forgetting that all events have a "before" and an "after." Recollection of the events "after" the trauma may hold powerful determinants of the patient's post-traumatic reactivity and assumptive world. Consequently, the clinician should anticipate and educate the patient that he/she may experience distress on this basis following an intensive memory session.

In many cases, it can be both humane and clinically important to plan on at least a brief telephone call to the patient to check in after a memory processing session. A planned call gives a sense of connection, predictability and support for the patient, who in the past has been abandoned to calm and soothe him/herself. As described in the prior clinical vignette, the therapist can assess the patient's stability and plan additional treatment interventions if needed.

After a memory session, additional work needs to be done in subsequent sessions to revisit the material at various levels of affective intensity to allow for additional integration of thoughts, feelings and beliefs about the trauma.

## Stage 3

Herman [3] proposed seven criteria for the resolution of a trauma disorder: (a) the physiological symptoms have been brought within manageable limits; (b) the person is able to bear the feelings associated with his or her traumatic memories; (c) the person can exercise authority over his or her memories (i.e., the person can elect both to remember the trauma and to put such memory aside); (d) the memories of the traumas have become coherent narratives, linked with feeling; (e) the person's damaged self-esteem has been restored; (f) the person's important relationships have been reestablished; and (g) the person has constructed a coherent system of meaning and belief that encompasses the story of the trauma.

In the third phase of treatment for DID, full subjective integration (fusion) of the alters commonly occurs, although this process begins in prior stages. The subjective self of the patient shifts away from multiplicity toward greater unity, and in many cases full integration occurs. Here, subjective self-division is no longer present when systematically assessed over at least 24 months [48,49].

Previously dissociated material is now experienced as available autobiographical memory. The patient can consciously tolerate discussion of subjects previously fraught with extreme emotions, particularly shame, guilt and revulsion. The patient's observing ego is improved so that he/she is more proactively aware of cognitive distortions and shame scripts. The transference shows modifications consistent with integration of dissociated autobiographical memory, and attitudes towards self and others are similarly consistent with integration of psychologically separated self–other schemata. The patient shows improved distress tolerance, affect modulation and subjective well-being. Accordingly, the patient has greater energy, enthusiasm and resilience for new relationships, life tasks and avocations. At the same time, memory material may need to be reworked, and additional grief-work done, in order to acknowledge more fully the reality of the patient's traumatic life history. The patient may return to reappraise aspects of autobiographical memory. He/she may be more able to resolve uncertainty about what did or did not occur or, in some instances, accept that a definitive conclusion may not be possible.

Adjustments in relationships and development of new ones may be a particular challenge. Intimacy and sexuality may present particular challenges requiring additional work on body awareness to give a sense, often for the first time, of having one's own body and living peaceably within it.

The patient with CPTSD/DID may need to develop non-trauma based/non-dissociative coping for medical illness, death of important others and even subsequent traumatic experiences. The last may cause relapse into active PTSD and/or multiplicity, as well as into "old" trauma-based thinking. The relapse itself must be managed, as well as the patient's fear and shame about the implications of it. Frequently, the crisis can be resolved with the patient using the hard-won skills of therapy to deal with the traumatic events and to reintegrate.

Patients with CPTSD/DID often report the fantasy that treatment ends like a movie: all is resolved, finished, the credits come up and the patient rides off into the sunset to live happily ever after. The patient is chagrined to discover that recovery is a lifelong process. Yet, despite the uncertainty that we all must accept, the patient with CPTSD/DID can find relief at the relative calm predictability of a new life. One patient declared her delight at finding that she had become "normal, average and boring." She was no longer riding what she had called the "nightmare roller coaster."

# References

1. Courtois, C. A. and Ford, J. D. (eds.) (2009). *Treating complex traumatic stress disorders: An evidence-based guide.* New York: Guilford.

2. Herman, J. L. (1992). Complex PTSD: A syndrome in survivors of prolonged and repeated trauma. *Journal of Traumatic Stress,* **5**, 377–391.

3. Herman, J. L. (1992). *Trauma and recovery.* New York: Basic Books.

4. Pelcovitz, D., van der Kolk, B. A. and Roth, S. *et al.* (1997). Development of a criteria set and a structured interview for disorders of extreme stress (SIDES). *Journal of Traumatic Stress,* **10**, 3–16.

5. American Psychiatric Association (1994). *Diagnostic and statistical manual of mental disorders,* 4th edn. Washington, DC: American Psychiatric Press.

6. Herman, J. L. (1993). Sequelae of prolonged and repeated trauma: Evidence for a complex posttraumatic syndrome (DESNOS). In J. R. T. Davidson and E. B. Foa (eds.), *Posttraumatic stress disorder: DSM-IV and beyond* (pp. 213–228). Washington, DC: American Psychiatric Press.

7. van der Kolk, B., Pelcovitz, D., Roth, S. *et al.* (1996). Dissociation, somatization, and affect dysregulation: The complexity of adaptation to trauma. *American Journal of Psychiatry,* **153**, 83–93.

8. Herman, J. L. (2009). Forward. In C. A. Courtois and J. D. Ford (eds.), *Treating complex traumatic stress disorders: An evidence-based guide* (pp. xiii–xvii). New York: Guilford.

9. Cloitre, M., Cohen, L. R. and Koenen, K. C. (2006). *Treating survivors of childhood abuse: Psychotherapy for the interrupted life.* New York: Guilford.

10. Luxenberg, T., Spinazzola, J. and van der Kolk, B. (2001). Complex trauma and disorders of extreme stress (DESNOS) Diagnosis. Part 1: Assessment. *Directions in Psychiatry*, **21**, 373–393.

11. Luxenberg, T., Spinazzola, J., Hidalgo, J., Hunt, C. and van der Kolk, B. A. (2001). Complex trauma and disorders of extreme stress (DESNOS). Part 2: Treatment. *Directions in Psychiatry*, **21**, 395–414.

12. Cloitre, M., Stovall-McClough, K. C., Miranda, R. and Chemtob, C. M. (2004). Therapeutic alliance, negative mood regulation, and treatment outcome in child abuse-related posttraumatic stress disorder. *Journal of Consulting and Cinical Psychology*, **72**, 411–416.

13. Putnam, F. W. (1997). *Dissociation in children and adolescents: A developmental model*. New York: Guilford.

14. Simeon, D., Guralnik, O., Schmeidler, J., Sirof, B. and Knutelska, M. (2001). The role of childhood interpersonal trauma in depersonalization disorder. *American Journal of Psychiatry*, **158**, 1027–1033.

15. Teicher, M. H., Samson, J. A., Polcari, A. and McGreenery, C. E. (2006). Sticks, stones, and hurtful words: Relative effects of various forms of childhood maltreatment. *American Journal of Psychiatry,* **163**, 993–1000.

16. Waller, N. G., Putnam, F. W. and Carlson, E. B. (1996). Types of dissociation and dissociative types: A taxonometric analysis of dissociative experiences. *Psychological Methods*, **1**, 300–321.

17. Waller, N. G. and Ross, C. A. (1997). The prevalence and biometric structure of pathological dissociation in the general population: Taxonmetric and behavioral genetic findings. *Journal of Abnormal Psychology,* **106**, 499–510.

18. Freyd, J. J. (1996). *Betrayal trauma: The logic of forgetting childhood abuse*. Cambridge, MA: Harvard University Press.

19. Lindy, J. D. (l988). *Vietnam: A casebook*. New York: Brunner and Mazell.

20. Loewenstein, R. J. (1993). Posttraumatic and dissociative aspects of transference and countertransference in the treatment of multiple personality disorder. In R. P. Kluft and C. G. Fine (eds.), *Clinical perspectives on multiple personality disorder* (pp. 51–85). Washington, DC: American Psychiatric Press.

21. Kluft, R. P. (1994). Countertransference in the treatment of multiple personality disorder. In J. P. Wilson and J. D. Lindy (eds.), *Countertransference in the treatment of PTSD* (pp. 122–150). New York: Guilford.

22. Dell, P. F. (1988). Professional skepticism about multiple personality. *Journal of Nervous and Mental Disorders,* **176**, 528–531.

23. Brown, D., Scheflin, A. W. and Hammond, D. C. (1998). *Memory, trauma, treatment, and the law*. New York: Norton.

24. Loewenstein, R. J. and Putnam, F. W. (2004). The dissociative disorders. In B. J. Sadock and V. A. Sadock (eds.), *Comprehensive textbook of psychiatry*, 8th edn (pp. 1844–1901). Baltimore, MD: Williams & Wilkins.

25. Loewenstein, R. J. (2007). Dissociative identity disorder: Issues in the iatrogenesis controversy. In E. Vermetten, M. Dorahy and D. Spiegel (eds.), *Traumatic dissociation* (pp. 275–299). Washington, DC: American Psychiatric Press.

26. Brown, D. W., Frischholz, E. J. and Scheflin, A. W. (1999). Iatrogenic dissociative identity disorder: An evaluation of the scientific evidence. *Journal of Psychiatric Law*, **27**, 549–638.

27. Chu, J. A., Loewenstein, R. J., Dell, P. F. *et al.* (2005). Guidelines for treating dissociative identity disorder in adults. *Journal of Trauma and Dissociation*, **6**, 69–149.

28. Kluft, R. P. and Loewenstein, R. J. (2007). Dissociative disorders and depersonalization. In G. O. Gabbard (ed.), *Gabbard's treatment of psychiatric disorders*. 4th edn. (pp. 547–572). Washington, DC: American Psychiatric Press.

29. Foa, E. B., Keane, T. M. and Friedman, M. J. (eds.) (2000). *Effective treatments for PTSD: Practice guidelines from the international society for traumatic stress studies*. New York: Guilford.

30. Loewenstein, R. J. (2005). Psychopharmacologic treatments for dissociative identity disorder. *Psychiatric Annals*, **35**, 666–673.

31. Briere, J. and Scott, C. (2006). *Principles of trauma therapy: A guide to symptoms, evaluation, and treatment*. Thousand Oaks, CA: Sage.

32. Loewenstein, R. J. and Wait, S. B. (2008). The trauma disorders unit. In S. S. Sharfstein, F. B. Dickerson and J. M. Oldham (eds.), *Textbook of hospital psychiatry* (pp. 103–118). Washington, DC: American Psychiatric Press.

33. Loewenstein, R. J. (2006). DID 101: A hands-on clinical guide to the stabilizaton phase of dissociative identity disorder treatment. *Psychiatric Clinics of North America,* **29**, 305–332.

34. Peebles-Kleiger, M. J. (1989). Using countertransference in the hypnosis of trauma victims: A model for turning hazard into healing. *American Journal of Psychotherapy*, **43**, 518–530.

35. Spiegel, D. (1986). Dissociation, double binds, and posttraumatic stress. In B. G. Braun (ed.), *The treatment of multiple personality disorder* (pp. 61–77). Washington, DC: American Psychiatric Press.

36. Kluft, R. P. (1991). Hospital treatment of multiple personality disorder: An overview. *Psychiatric Clinics of North America,* **14**, 695–720.

37. Blank, A. S. (1985). The unconscious flashback to the war in Viet Nam veterans: Clinical mystery, legal defense, and community problem. In S. M. Sonnenberg, A. S. Blank and J. A. Talbott (eds.), *The trauma of war: Stress and recovery in Vietnam veterans* (pp. 293–308). Washington, DC: American Psychiatric Press.

38. Turkus, J. A. (1991). Psychotherapy and case management for multiple personality disorder: Synthesis for continuity of care. *Psychiatric Clinics of North America,* **14**, 649–660.

39. Nathanson, D. L. (1992). *Shame and pride: Affect, sex, and the birth of the self.* New York: Norton.

40. Kluft, R. P. (1985). The natural history of multiple personality disorder. In R. P. Kluft (ed.) *Childhood antecedents of multiple personality* (pp. 197–238). Washington, DC: American Psychiatric Press.

41. Lyons-Ruth, K., Dutra, L., Schuder, M. R. and Bianchi, I. (2006). From infant attachment disorganization to adult dissociation: Relational adaptations or traumatic experiences? *Psychiatric Clinics of North America,* **29**, 63–86.

42. Kluft, R. P. (1984). Multiple personality in childhood. *Psychiatric Clinics of North America,* 7, 121–134.

43. Dalenberg, C. J. (2000). *Countertransference and the treatment of trauma.* Washington, DC: American Psychological Association.

44. Sands, S. H. (1994). What is dissociated? *Dissociation,* 7, 145–152.

45. Kluft, R. P. (2007). Applications of innate affect theory to the understanding and treatment of dissociative identity disorder. In E. Vermetten, M. Dorahy and D. Spiegel (eds.), *Traumatic dissociation* (pp. 301–316). Washington, DC: American Psychiatric Press.

46. Lewis, H. B. (1990). Shame, repression, field dependence, and psychopathology. In J. L. Singer (ed.), *Repression and dissociation: Implications for personality theory, psychopathology, and health* (pp. 233–257). Chicago, IL: University of Chicago Press.

47. Braun, B. G. (1988). The BASK (behavior, affect, sensation, knowledge) model of dissociation. *Dissociation,* **1**, 4–23.

48. Kluft, R. P. (1986). Personality unification in multiple personality disorder: A follow-up study. In B. G. Braun (ed.), *Treatment of multiple personality disorder* (pp. 29–60). Washington, DC: American Psychiatric Press.

49. Kluft, R. P. (1988). The postunification treatment of multiple personality disorder: First findings. *American Journal of Psychotherapy*, **42**, 212–228.

# Chapter 25

# Cognitive-behavioral treatments for post-traumatic stress disorder

Kathleen M. Chard and Amy F. Buckley

Numerous studies have documented the impact of traumatic events and the resulting post-traumatic stress disorder (PTSD) on physical health, including chronic disorders of the circulatory, digestive, musculoskeletal, endocrine, respiratory and reproductive systems. Initial studies have yielded inconclusive findings regarding the relationship between a decrease in PTSD symptoms and improvement on measures of physical health [1]. For many years, therapists maintained that trauma survivors require years of treatment to reach symptom improvement, but since the early 1990s substantial research has emerged suggesting that brief cognitive-behavioral treatments (CBT) interventions can yield long-term gains in patients' psychosocial, psychological and even physical function. In fact, recent studies have shown that 12–20 sessions of CBT appear to be effective in helping patients to manage their distress not only during treatment but also for up to 5 years after completing therapy [2,3].

Cognitive-behavior therapy is a broad classification that incorporates specific interventions for the treatment of PTSD and related symptoms that can be used alone or in combination with one another. The purpose of this chapter is to review the literature regarding the efficacy of CBT interventions on PTSD and related symptoms. General standards of CBT and efficacy-based treatment research are discussed, although the primary focus of the chapter is an exploration of specific trauma-based therapies.

## Core concepts of cognitive-behavior therapy

A key tenet underlying all CBT models is that individuals' thoughts, attitudes and perceptions about themselves and others influence their interpretation of an external event, which can, in turn, influence subsequent emotions and behaviors. Although integrative models to explain the intricate relationship among thoughts (cognitions), emotions (affect) and behaviors have only recently emerged in the research literature [4], factors such as personality, learned history, and access to internal (e.g., coping strategies) and external (e.g., social support systems) resources have been previously shown to moderate the valence of an experience. In this regard, cognitive therapists maintain that it is not an event itself but rather the *cognitive interpretation* of the event that establishes the probability for a given affect or behavior. Furthermore, the relationship among cognitions, affect and behaviors is viewed as reciprocal rather than linear. Consequently, given this interaction, both cognitions and behaviors are simultaneously targeted in CBT. Cognitive-behavior therapy seeks to enhance individuals' awareness of their cognitive misperceptions (i.e., distortions) and of the behavioral patterns that reinforce and are reinforced by these distortions. It is to be emphasized that not every distortion is targeted for therapy – everyone distorts some aspects of reality in some way. Only those cognitive distortions that are creating the most distress to the individual and his or her significant others are targeted. The essential goal of CBT is for the individual to acquire adaptive coping strategies as well as improve awareness, introspection and evaluation skills [5].

## History of research in post-traumatic stress disorder

In creating the first treatment manuals for PTSD, researchers historically applied approaches that had been shown to be successful for depressive and anxiety disorders (e.g., CBT interventions). These original studies did not meet today's rigorous standards for efficacy-based studies, but they provided a groundwork for the development of more specialized intervention packages and the requisite randomized controlled trials that continue to inform care today. Initially, research on PTSD involved case studies before evolving into wait-list and then comparison designs. More recently, researchers have turned to studies of prediction, dismantling and comparisons with treatments that contain the non-specific elements of therapy, in order to help to ascertain which components of the treatments are most effective and for which types of patient [6].

The International Society for Traumatic Stress Studies (ISTSS) has published practice guidelines for PTSD [7], including assessment and treatment suggestions. The guidelines also review the methodological considerations that should be taken into account when conducting a clinical trial. Foa and Meadows [8] outlined the seven "gold standards" that can be used to evaluate the methodological rigor of PTSD treatment studies: (1) clearly identified target symptoms; (2) reliable and valid measures; (3) use of blind evaluators; (4) assessor training; (5) manualized, replicable, specific treatment protocols; (6) unbiased assignment to condition; and (7) treatment adherence [8]. More recently, Harvey et al. [9] expanded on these standards suggesting (1) the use of independent evaluators; (2) blind assessors to guess at the condition of each participant; (3) the investigator to be blind to random assignment; and (4) evidence to be provided indicating that the treatment was administered in its pure form without the influence of other treatments and was received by the client and applied outside of the session. By using these criteria we can evaluate the clinical trials that have been conducted to date to help to determine the efficacy of various treatments for PTSD.

## Efficacy data

Since the early 1990s, there has been a significant increase in the number of quality studies examining the efficacy of CBT manuals. The ISTSS guidelines support the use of CBT interventions based on existing research data. Typically, PTSD treatments incorporate psychoeducation, basic CBT principles (e.g., collaborative empiricism, socratic questioning) and the addition of one or more trauma-focused CBT techniques such as exposure, cognitive restructuring, written narrative or imagery rehearsal. Treatment-controlled studies have shown that trauma-focused treatments are more efficacious than wait-list conditions, and comparison studies of CBT have yielded commensurate results. More recent attempts to control for the non-specific elements of therapy have largely supported active trauma treatments [10,11] (i.e., those models that address the trauma explicitly), although a large 10-site clinical trial comparing trauma-focused group therapy with present-centered group therapy did not yield statistically significant differences [12].

Several authors have investigated the use of cognitive therapy interventions (e.g., cognitive restructuring) in the treatment of PTSD. For example, studies have included cognitive restructuring for individuals with severe mental illness and PTSD [13], imagery rescripting and reprocessing following industrial injury [14], CBT for acute stress disorder [15] and CBT for disaster workers [16]. While promising, many of these initial studies have not included a comparison group, and further randomized trials are needed to demonstrate the efficacy of these techniques with other populations. Two CBT treatments that have established efficacy are exposure therapy and cognitive-processing therapy (CPT), and they provide evidence that exposure and direct cognitive challenging may not necessarily need to be linked in order to be effective. Research on exposure therapy provides data suggesting that patients who are exposed to the traumatic experience through mental imagery but are not challenged on their cognitive distortions still report an increase in adaptive thought patterns after treatment [7]. Additionally, CPT studies demonstrate that patients who are offered cognitive restructuring without direct trauma reprocessing have faster and equally lasting treatment gains when compared with those who are offered a combination of both [2].

## Exposure techniques

Numerous studies have supported the use of exposure techniques, both alone and in combination with other CBT interventions, for the treatment of PTSD related to different types of trauma, including interpersonal violence [7] and child sexual abuse [17]. Exposure is typically conducted in 9 to 12 sessions lasting 90 minutes each. Although frequently offered in individual sessions, group prolonged exposure (PE) has also been found to be effective with some populations [12].

Prior to exposure therapy, clients rate their initial or "baseline" level of distress to their trauma cues from 0 to 100 using the Subjective Units of Distress Scale (SUDS). Through imagery and/or in vivo exercises, the client is gradually exposed to anxiety-evoking stimuli for longer periods of time. Imaginal exposure typically takes place in the therapist's office, with the client imagining he or she is interacting with the stimuli. During each session, clients are taught to monitor their SUDS rating and to stay in the exposure until their rating drops to some predetermined level. In vivo exposure teaches the client that the stimuli will not hurt them and that they can become safely accustomed to interacting with the stimuli [18]. Imaginal exposure is often compared to systematic desensitization, although it does not require that the client be taught relaxation skills first; systematic desensitization exposures are typically conducted only after the client has been fully relaxed prior to the exposure.

After educating the patient about PTSD and the treatment rationale, the therapist repeatedly asks the patient to verbally recall the trauma(s) as if the events were presently occurring. This exposure to the traumatic event extends for 45 to 60 minutes. The therapist does not necessarily need to challenge any distorted cognitions the patient may have about the event (e.g., "I am to blame for the rape" or "No one can be trusted"). During the exposure, the therapist frequently asks the patient for ratings of his/her distress. These SUDS ratings are used to determine "hot spots" in the account that should be repeated again.

Researchers have hypothesized that exposing the patient to traumatic memories stimulates the brain's "fear network." The fear network can be described as consisting of fear structures that involve an excessive response to a fear, often pairing non-threatening stimuli with the fear response (e.g., fearing a gas station because of traumatic links to diesel fuel from being in the Gulf War). Continued exposure allows the patient to habituate to this network, with subsequent extinction of fear and anxiety reactions. Foa and colleagues [19] found that mentally re-experiencing a traumatic event helps patients to organize and integrate previously incompatible memory cues about the traumatic event, which, in turn, encourages cognitive restructuring of the trauma.

The PE form of exposure therapy has been shown to enhance the survivor's self-control and personal competence and to decrease generalization of fear to non-assault stimuli [19]. For example, many war veterans report fear of being in situations that may bring back memories tied to the traumatic event, such as going to the beach (Iraq) or into the woods (Vietnam), and many child trauma survivors will report becoming distressed when they see someone who even remotely resembles their abuse perpetrator. Their fears may prevent them from taking part in common activities, such as taking a walk in a park, or special events such as family vacations. Through in vivo exposure, these patients face associations between environmental cues and the trauma. As they learn to modify the fears associated with these cues, their personal and social functioning improves.

According to Foa and Kozak's emotional processing theory [20], in order to produce a reduction in fear through PE, two things must occur. First, the fear structure or network, which is hypothesized to reside in memory, must be activated. Second, incompatible information must be incorporated or combined into this fear structure. Thus, repeated and prolonged exposure to the feared stimulus serves to reduce fear. Furthermore, Foa and Kozak noted three primary indicators that effective emotional processing of fear has occurred: activation of the fear network (emotional engagement), reduction of fear after exposure to the feared stimulus (within-session habituation) and reduction of fear across repeated exposures to the feared stimulus (between-session habituation).

Exposure interventions have been found to be very successful for those who complete therapy, but the treatment dropout rate has varied depending on the study, with reported numbers ranging from 8 to 41% [7]. Some therapists have found success in reducing dropout rates by combining exposure with cognitive restructuring or other techniques that help to stabilize and build patients' coping skills [17]. In addition, some evidence suggests that exposure may work better for individuals whose primary response to the trauma is fear, rather than those whose emotional response is anger [21]. Furthermore, PE may also work better for individuals who are able to experience emotional engagement with their trauma memories during the exposure sessions. Jaycox et al. [22] found that individuals diagnosed with PTSD who experienced both emotional engagement (i.e., activation of the fear network) and habituation across (but not within) sessions showed the most improvement in functioning post-treatment. In fact, highest functioning at end of treatment was not related to habituation within sessions but was associated with both emotional engagement and habituation across sessions. This is important to note because symptoms characteristic of a lack of emotional engagement (e.g., dissociation and numbing) may significantly interfere with trauma processing, thus reducing the effectiveness of PE. This may be particularly relevant for patients with prolonged histories of childhood abuse since they often experience significant dissociative pathology [23,24].

## Cognitive-processing therapy

Cognitive-processing therapy was created as a manualized cognitive behavioral protocol to treat PTSD and related symptoms in rape survivors [25]. In the past, there has been some confusion that CPT is an exposure therapy, because it includes a written narrative component, but the abbreviated nature of the written narrative component and a dismantling study by Resick and colleagues [2] suggest that CPT relies on cognitive restructuring rather than exposure as an agent of change. Randomized controlled trials of CPT have shown the treatment to be effective in the treatment of PTSD from rape, assault, child sexual abuse and combat [25–27].

The original CPT treatment comprised 12 weekly sessions, although versions lasting up to 17 weeks have been developed for adult survivors of child sexual abuse. Therapy is based on cognitive behavioral and information processing theories, with the latter suggesting that as people access a traumatic memory they experience and extinguish emotions attached to the event. Guided by the therapist, the patient identifies and challenges distortions created from the trauma in three cognition domains: the self, others and the world. Patients learn to replace or change these cognitive distortions with more adaptive and healthy beliefs through the examination of beliefs using Socratic Dialogue and Challenging Beliefs worksheets. Disruptive or dysfunctional beliefs are often referred to as "stuck points," making them more concrete and thus more challengeable. Common byproducts of traumatic experiences include feeling out of control or feeling hopeless. Therefore, CPT focuses on personal safety, trust, power/control, esteem and intimacy within each of the three domains. Modules on assertiveness, communication and social support can also be added. Research has shown that CPT can be effectively offered in group, individual or combined formats, depending on the needs and resources of the patients and clinic. Further analysis of existing studies indicates that patients whose trauma experience is heavily dominated with thoughts of blame and emotions of shame and guilt may perform better in CPT than patients who tend to focus on their fear or anxiety [28].

## Combined treatments

In addition to the cognitive and behavioral treatments of PE and CPT, researchers have examined whether CBT combined with social skills training is effective in treatment of PTSD, particularly PTSD resulting from childhood trauma. The effective treatments for PTSD described above were developed for adult rape, with relatively little research to date focused specifically on PTSD that develops as the result of child trauma. Most recent data suggest that almost one million children are abused each year worldwide [29], with close to 10% of these children experiencing sexual abuse. Given that many states/countries do not require mandatory reporting of child abuse, this figure is likely a gross underestimate. These numbers highlight the need for effective treatments geared toward early life trauma, particularly since early childhood traumas are associated with neurobiological changes in the brain including reduced hippocampal volume and impact on the corticotropin-releasing factor system [30]. To date, few studies have examined whether specific treatments for PTSD resulting from childhood sexual abuse are effective. Cloitre and colleagues [17,31] have found that adults with PTSD resulting from child abuse not only have difficulties with arousal, reexperiencing and avoidance symptoms characteristic of PTSD, but also with interpersonal interactions and emotional regulation. In fact, a more recent study by Cloitre *et al.* [32] found that interpersonal difficulties and dysregulation of emotion were significant *independent* predictors of functional impairment in adult survivors of child abuse, beyond what was accounted for by symptoms of PTSD (arousal, avoidance, reexperiencing). Cloitre and colleagues [17] developed a two-phase approach to target disruption of interpersonal functioning and emotion regulation. The first phase of treatment, Skills Training in Affective and Interpersonal Regulation (STAIR), was designed specifically to address the problems in affect regulation and interpersonal functioning that are prevalent in individuals with early life trauma. This phase of treatment is designed to be delivered across 8 weeks of skills-based training, with the second phase of treatment being the more standard prolonged exposure developed by Foa *et al.* [7]. Cloitre *et al.* [17] reported a significant improvement in both interpersonal functioning and affect regulation, in addition to improvement in PTSD symptoms, in a group of 58 women with PTSD who completed STAIR-PE, relative to a wait-list control group. Furthermore, these gains were maintained up to 9 months after treatment.

# Eye movement desensitization and reprocessing

Similar to other PTSD treatments such as PE, eye movement desensitization and reprocessing (EMDR) is based on an "accelerated information-processing" model [33]. Because it also incorporates dissociation and non-verbal representation of traumas (such as visual memories), EMDR is often classified as a cognitive treatment. However, the ISTSS practice guidelines [7] present it as a separate category. Originally EMDR protocols necessitated eye movements as a way to inhibit stress, based on the knowledge that individuals with PTSD often have disrupted REM sleep (identified by frequent eye movements). As the stress is inhibited, the patient is more able to freely access the memory network and thus process the disturbance. More recently, EMDR researchers have posited that auditory cues or hand taps may work just as well as eye movements, although future research needs to be conducted using these techniques.

Although some studies report positive changes after three to six sessions, EMDR is often conducted in 12 to 15 sessions. After obtaining a patient history, establishing rapport and providing education about the treatment, the therapist asks the patient to identify (a) visual images of the trauma, (b) affective and physiological responses to the trauma, (c) negative self-representations created by the trauma, and (d) positive alternative self-representations. The therapist then asks the patient to focus on an image most proximal to the trauma and the associated affective and biological reactions. While the patient is holding these in mind, the therapist introduces distraction stimulation – such as hand movements, auditory tones or hand taps – based on the assumption that concentrating on the distraction will help the patient to access and process the memory. After a set number of eye movements (typically 20 bilateral movements), the therapist asks the patient to "let go" of the memory and discusses any new reactions to the trauma. As patients become less distressed in response to the trauma, they are asked to focus increasingly on alternative positive cognitions while they are imagining the trauma [33].

EMDR has been effective in treating male war veterans, rape victims and other trauma patients [7]. Initial dismantling studies and meta-analyses have suggested that eye movements (or other distracting cues) might not be essential for trauma reprocessing, calling into question the mechanisms thought to create change in EMDR [34]. Studies with larger samples comparing EMDR with other CBT models (especially exposure) are needed to assess EMDR's efficacy for trauma survivors, as initial studies have been inconsistent in their findings [6].

# Comparative studies of therapeutic approaches

Over the last several years a number of studies directly compared the relative efficacy of CBTs (primarily exposure-based treatments) with EMDR. A review of the literature found that the majority of those studies comparing EMDR with CBT consisted of mixed trauma samples including both childhood-onset and adult-onset traumas. The study of Rogers et al. [35] was the one exception. These researchers compared EMDR with exposure therapy in a small sample of Vietnam War veterans, although their study consisted of only 12 participants completing one session of either treatment. Despite this and some other methodological problems, including low sample sizes across most of the studies, limited number of sessions and lack of assessment of treatment integrity, the overall results suggested that CBT and EMDR were both are equally efficacious (Table 25.1 has a more comprehensive review of these studies) [36–42]. However, as noted previously, dismantling studies and meta-analyses provide compelling evidence that the addition of eye movements is unnecessary, calling into question whether the bona fide mechanism of action in EMDR is actually exposure to the distressing or traumatic memories [43].

# Applications for children and adolescents

Many of the CBT interventions described above have also been used for adolescents experiencing the same conditions. In some respects, application of CBT to adolescents may be relatively easier than to young children, given that adolescents have developed abstract thinking abilities, social problem solving and level of insight that would allow for a deeper exploration of cognitive distortions, dysfunctional attitudes and beliefs, and maladaptive behaviors. Depending on the study, it is estimated that 15% to 43% of children will be exposed to a traumatic event, with 3% to 15% of girls

**Table 25.1** Comparison of cognitive-behavioural therapy and eye movement desensitization and reprocessing in treatment of post-traumatic stress disorder

| Study | Treatment comparison | No. enrolled (completed) | Type(s) trauma | Findings/conclusions[a] |
|---|---|---|---|---|
| Devilly and Spence (1999) [36] | EMDR vs. CBT (SIT+PE+CR) | (32)23 | Various traumas | CBT > EMDR, 3-month follow-up ($p < 0.007$) |
| Ironson et al. (2002) [37] | EMDR vs. PE | (22) | Various traumas | PE =EMDR (ns) |
| Lee et al. (2002) [38] | EMDR vs. SIT+PE | 27(24) | Various traumas | EMDR = SIT + PE (ns) |
| Power et al. (2002) [39] | EMDR vs. E+CR vs.WLC | 105(72) | Various traumas | EMDR > E+CR (ns); EMDR > WLC ($p < 0.05$); E + CR > WLC ($p < 0.05$) |
| Rogers et al. (1999) [35] | EMDR vs. PE | 12 | Vietnam veterans | EMDR > PE (ns) |
| Rothbaum et al. (2005) [40] | EMDR vs. standard PE vs. WLC | 74 (60) | Sexual assault (child/adult) | PE > WLC ($p < 0.001$); EMDR > WLC ($p < 0.001$); PE > EMDR (ns) |
| Taylor et al. (2003) [41] | EMDR vs. PE vs. REL | 60 (45) | Chronic PTSD, various traumas | PE > EMDR (ns); PE > REL ($p < 0 < .02$); EMDR > REL (ns) |

CBT, cognitive-behavior therapy; CR, cognitive restructuring; EMDR, eye movement desensitization reprocessing; PE, prolonged exposure; REL, relaxation; SIT, stress inoculation training; WLC, wait-list control; ns, not significant ($p > 0.05$).

[a] Computed effect sizes (Cohen's d).

and 1% to 6% of boys experiencing heightened psychological distress, typically in the form of PTSD [44]. In recent years, there have been significant gains in the treatment of children exposed to traumatic events, primarily by adapting adult treatments for children and youth. Trauma treatments typically involve the non-offending caregivers and other family members, if at all possible, to avoid the implication that the child is at fault and to ensure positive changes for the family. A growing body of research studies support the use of CBT interventions with preschool children and school-aged children upto 18 years [45,46]. Cognitive-behavioral treatments for children typically include one or more of the following: (a) exposure to the traumatic material, (b) cognitive reprocessing and reframing, (c) stress management, and (d) parent treatment. Exposure techniques for children can vary from talking about the traumatic event, drawing pictures about the trauma, writing about the trauma events or recounting the events into a tape recorder. Although exposure to the traumatic memory is the therapeutic norm, therapists should note that not all children need to process the trauma overtly, and instead some may find that going over the trauma is either boring or so anxiety provoking that it is counter to therapeutic gain.

Parent interventions for traumatized children also parallel what is conducted in individual sessions [46,47]. Parents are often asked to go through an exposure phase where they discuss their thoughts and feelings about the child's traumatic event and perhaps recount the details about finding out about the trauma and dealing with its aftermath. In the cognitive processing phase that follows, the therapist uses cognitive restructuring techniques to address the parents' distorted cognitions (usually around the areas of self-blame or in some cases blaming of the child). Finally, stress management is taught to the parents both for their own use and to model healthy reactions to the traumatized child and other children in the household. Parents are also taught behavioral management strategies, where the traumatized child is neither singled out as being "damaged" and needing extra leniency, nor punished when the trauma was thought to have been caused by the child. Instead, parents are taught normal child developmental stages and are encouraged to treat the child with sympathy but also with an expectation that the child will behave in an age-appropriate manner.

## Group interventions

There are many advantages to using CBT in a group setting, including (a) the ability to experience real-world interactions with other people, (b) the possibility of practicing newly learned behaviors in session under the guidance of a therapist before trying them in the non-therapy environment, (c) the potential for role plays where the therapist can be the observer instead of a participant, and (d) the ability for clients to test the hypotheses surrounding their beliefs using feedback from other group members' experiences.

The disadvantages of CBT in a group setting are similar to those found in any group treatment modality. For example, clients in group therapy may feel that they do not receive enough one-on-one individualized care and that they cannot probe deep enough into their own belief structure for fear of monopolizing the group. In addition, group dynamics can sometimes get in the way of the client's ability or willingness to share his or her true thoughts. This may be especially the case among youth, where impression management and social desirability may be more pronounced than in adults (especially given that many youth are referred by teachers and parents as opposed to self-referred). Strategies to reduce these disadvantages include explaining the purpose and role of group therapy to all clients before the group starts, conducting thorough screenings of group members, asking the clients to create group rules that will make the group safe and productive for all group members and offering individual therapy in conjunction with the group for those who require it.

## Predictors of treatment outcome

As the body of literature on empirically based treatments expands, it is becoming more feasible to examine predictors of positive treatment outcome. Variables that have been shown to predict poorer treatment response include a hostile or critical family, substance use disorders, greater pain severity, lower global functioning, pain-related interference in daily activities and use of benzodiazepines during treatment [6]. For example, Brady and colleagues [48] found a dropout rate over 50% in an open trial of PE plus relapse prevention in a study of individuals with PTSD and comorbid cocaine dependence.

Trauma event-based characteristics that have been shown to negatively influence treatment outcome include a history of child sexual abuse or physical violence as part of the index trauma [49]. Some clinicians have conjectured that age or time since trauma may affect treatment outcome, but initial research has shown that age does not seem to have an effect on treatment outcome, and research on length of time since trauma has yielded conflicting findings [50–52]. One study comparing EMDR with fluoxetine or pill placebo found that participants in the EMDR group who had experienced later-life trauma (i.e., after 18 years

of age) showed significantly higher treatment response than those participants in the EMDR group who had experienced childhood-onset trauma [53]. In contrast, there were no differences in improvement based on onset of trauma in either the fluoxetine or pill placebo group. Finally, with the increasing attention turning to the combined effects of traumatic brain injury and PTSD, increased research will be needed to determine the impact that this physical disorder may have on the treatment of PTSD and vice versa.

## Conclusions

Current research has demonstrated that CBT interventions are effective in the treatment of PTSD and related symptoms. As these treatments continue to evolve and are applied to new populations, it will be possible to examine the effects of individual and combined models on very specific individual characteristics to improve therapy–client matching. It is important to note that in a meta-analysis of PTSD treatment studies, Bradley and colleagues [54] remarked that many PTSD studies exclude individuals with comorbid diagnoses such as medical conditions or substance use disorders, and that there is a need for more research on the individuals who present with a more complex diagnostic picture, which is often associated with childhood abuse. As clinicians continue to see overlap between PTSD and illnesses related to physical health, substance use, pain and depression, it will be essential to explore new interventions that can be paired with existing models to improve outcomes for these groups [55]. In addition, continued research on CBT should focus on specific interventions that may be more effective for one type of symptom presentation over another. Researchers are exploring promising integrated CBT models (e.g., couples-based CBT, mindfulness meditation, acupuncture) that may prove to be more beneficial for certain patient groups. Having multiple treatment options available for clinicians will make it easier to find a best fit for the wide variety of symptom presentations that can develop in response to early life trauma.

## References

1. Schnurr, P. P., Green, B. L. and Kaltman, S. (2008). Trauma exposure and physical health. In M. Friedman, T. Keane and P. Resick (eds.), *Handbook of PTSD* (pp. 406–424). New York: Guilford.
2. Resick, P. A., Galovski, T. E., Uhlmansiek, M. O. *et al.* (2008). A randomized clinical trial to dismantle components of cognitive processing therapy for

posttraumatic stress disorder in female victims of interpersonal violence. *Journal of Consulting and Clinical Psychology*, **76**, 243–258.

3. Tarrier, N. and Sommerfield, C. (2004). Treatment of chronic PTSD by cognitive therapy and exposure: 5-year follow-up. *Behavior Therapy, 35*, 231–246.

4. David, D. and Szentagotai, A. (2006). Cognitions in cognitive-behavioral psychotherapies: Toward an integrative model. *Clinical Psychology Review, 26*, 284–298.

5. Beck, A. T. (1967). *Depression: Clinical, experimental and theoretical aspects.* New York: Harper & Row.

6. Resick, P. A., Monson, C. M. and Gutner, C. (2008). Psychosocial treatments for PTSD. In M. Friedman, T. Keane and P. Resick (eds.) *Handbook of PTSD,* Ch. 17. New York: Guilford.

7. Foa, E. B., Keane, T. M. and Friedman, M. J. (eds.) (2000) *Effective treatments for PTSD: Practice guidelines from the international society for traumatic stress studies.* New York: Guilford.

8. Foa, E. B. and Meadows, E. A. (1997). Psychosocial treatments for posttraumatic stress disorder: A critical review. *Annual Review of Psychology, 48*, 449–480.

9. Harvey, A. G., Bryant, R. A. and Tarrier, N. (2003). Cognitive behavior therapy for posttraumatic stress disorder. *Clinical Psychology Review, 23*, 501–522.

10. Blanchard, E. B., Hickling, E. J., Devinei, T. *et al.* (2003). A controlled evaluation of cognitive behavioral therapy for posttraumatic stress in motor vehicle accident survivors. *Behaviour Research and Therapy*, **41**, 79–96.

11. Schnurr, P. P., Friedman, M. J., Engel, C. C. *et al.* (2007). Cognitive behavioral therapy for posttraumatic stress disorder in women; a randomized controlled trial. *Journal of the American Medical Association*, **297**, 820–830.

12. Schnurr, P. P. Friedman, M. J., Foy, D. W. *et al.* (2003). Randomized trial of trauma-focused group therapy for posttraumatic stress disorder: results from a Department of Veterans Affairs cooperative study. *Archives of General Psychiatry*, **60**, 481–489.

13. Mueser, K. T., Rosenberg, S. D, Haiyi Xie, M. *et al.* (2008). A randomized controlled trial of cognitive-behavioral treatment for posttraumatic stress disorder in severe mental illness. *Journal of Consulting and Clinical Psychology*, **76**, 259–271.

14. Grunert, B. K., Weis, J. M., Smucker, M. R. and Christianson, H. F. (2007). Imagery rescripting and reprocessing therapy after failed prolonged exposure for post-traumatic stress disorder following industrial injury. *Journal of Behavior Therapy and Experimental Psychiatry*, **38**, 317–328.

15. van Emmerik, A. A. P., Kamphuis, J. H. and Emmlekamp, P. M. G. (2008). Treating acute stress disorder and posttraumatic stress disorder with cognitive behavioral therapy or structured writing therapy: A randomized controlled trial. *Psychotherapy and Psychosomatics*, **77**, 93–100.

16. Difede, J., Malta, L. S., Best, S. *et al.* (2007). A randomized controlled clinical treatment trial for World Trade Center attack-related PTSD in disaster workers. *Journal of Nervous and Mental Disease*, **195**, 861–865.

17. Cloitre, M., Koenen K. C., Cohen, L. R. and Han, H. (2002). Skills training in affective and interpersonal regulation followed by exposure: A phase-based treatment for PTSD related to childhood abuse. *Journal of Consulting and Clinical Psychology*, **70**, 1067–1074.

18. Nezu, A. M., Nezu, C. M. and Lombardo, E. (2004). *Cognitive-behavioral case formulation and treatment design: A problem solving approach.* New York: Springer.

19. Foa, E. B., Hembree, E. A., Cahill, S. E. *et al.* (2005). Randomized clinical trial of prolonged exposure for posttraumatic stress disorder with and without cognitive restructuring: Outcome at academic and community clinics. *Journal of Consulting and Clinical Psychology*, **73**, 953–964.

20. Foa, E.B. and Kozak, M. J. (1986). Emotional processing of fear: Exposure to corrective information. *Psychological Bulletin*, **99**, 20–35.

21. Rothbaum, B. O., Meadows, E. A., Resick, P. and Foy, D. W. (2000). Cognitive-behavioral therapy. In E. B. Foa, T. M. Keane and M. J. Friedman (eds.), *Effective treatments for PTSD: Practice guidelines from the international society for Traumatic Stress Studies* (pp. 60–83). New York: Guilford.

22. Jaycox, L. H., Foa, E. B. and Morral, A. R. (1998). Influence of emotional engagement and habituation on exposure therapy for PTSD. *Journal of Consulting and Clinical Psychology*, **66**, 185–192.

23. van der Kolk, B. A., Pelcovitz, D., Roth, S. *et al.* (1996). Dissociation, somatization, and affect dysregulation: the complexity of adaptation of trauma. *American Journal of Psychiatry, 153*, 83–93.

24. Stovall-McClough, K. C. and Cloitre, M. (2006). Unresolved attachment, PTSD, and dissociation in women with childhood abuse histories. *Journal of Consulting and Clinical Psychology, 74*, 219–228.

25. Resick, P. A. and Schnicke, M. K. (1992). Cognitive processing therapy for sexual assault victims. *Journal of Consulting and Clinical Psychology, 60*, 748–756.

26. Chard, K. M. (2005). An evaluation of cognitive processing therapy for the treatment of posttraumatic stress disorder related to childhood sexual abuse. *Journal of Consulting and Clinical Psychology, 73*, 965–971.

27. Monson, C. M., Schnurr, P. P., Resick, P. A. *et al.* (2006). Cognitive processing therapy for veterans with military-related posttraumatic stress disorder. *Journal of Consulting and Clinical Psychology, 74*, 898–907.

28. Resick, P. A., Monson, C. M. and Chard, K. M. (2008). *Cognitive processing therapy: Veteran/military treatment manual.* Boston, MA: Veteran's Administration of the US Department of Health and Human Services.

29. US Department of Health and Human Services, Administration on Children, Youth and Families (2008). *Child maltreatment 2006.* Washington, DC: US Government Printing Office.

30. Nemeroff, C. B. (2004). Neurobiological consequences of childhood trauma. *Journal of Clinical Psychiatry,* **65,** 18–28.

31. Cloitre, M., Scarvalone, P. and Difede, J. (1997). Post-traumatic stress disorder, self- and interpersonal dysfunction among sexually retraumatized women. *Journal of Traumatic Stress,* **10,** 435–450.

32. Cloitre, M., Stovall-McClough, M. K. C. and Han, H. (2005). Beyond PTSD: Emotion regulation and interpersonal problems as predictors of functional impairment in survivors of childhood abuse. *Behavior Therapy,* **36,** 119–124.

33. Shapiro, F. (1995). *Eye movement desensitization and reprocessing: Basic principles, protocols, and procedures.* New York: Guilford.

34. Seidler, G. H. and Wagner, F. E. (2006). Comparing the efficacy of EMDR and trauma-focused cognitive-behavioral therapy in the treatment of PTSD: A meta-analytic study. *Psychological Medicine,* **36,** 1515–1522.

35. Rogers, S., Silver, S. M., Goss, J. *et al.* (1999). A single session, group study of exposure and eye movement desensitization and reprocessing in treating posttraumatic stress disorder among Vietnam War veterans: Preliminary data. *Journal of Anxiety Disorders,* **13,** 119–130.

36. Devilly, G. J. and Spence, S. H. (1999). The relative efficacy and treatment distress of EMDR and a cognitive-behavior trauma treatment protocol in the amelioration of posttraumatic stress disorder. *Journal of Anxiety Disorders,* **13,** 131–157.

37. Ironson, G., Freund, B., Strauss, J. L. and Williams, J. (2002). Comparison of two treatments for traumatic stress: A community-based study of EMDR and prolonged exposure. *Journal of Clinical Psychology,* **58,** 113–128.

38. Lee, C., Gavriel, H., Drummond, P., Richards, J. and Greenwald, R. (2002). Treatment of PTSD: Stress inoculation training with prolonged exposure compared to EMDR. *Journal of Clinical Psychology,* **58,** 1071–1089.

39. Power, K., McGoldrick, T., Brown, K. *et al.* (2002). A controlled comparison of eye movement desensitization and reprocessing versus exposure plus cognitive restructuring versus waiting list in the treatment of posttraumatic stress disorder. *Clinical Psychology and Psychotherapy,* **9,** 299–318.

40. Rothbaum, B., Astin, M. C. and Marsteller, F. (2005). Prolonged exposure versus eye movement desensitization and reprocessing (EMDR) for PTSD rape victims. *Journal of Traumatic Stress,* **18,** 607–616.

41. Taylor, S., Thordarson, D. S., Maxfield, L. *et al.* (2003). Comparative efficacy, speed, and adverse effects of three PTSD treatments: Exposure therapy, EMDR, and relaxation training. *Journal of Consulting and Clinical Psychology,* **71,** 330–338.

42. Spates, C.R., Koch, E., Cusack, K., Pagoto, S. and Waller, S. (2009). Eye movement desensitization and reprocessing. In E. B. Foa, T. M. Keane, M. J. Friedman and J. C. Cohen (eds.), *Effective treatments for PTSD: Practice guidelines from the International Society for Traumatic Stress Studies* (pp. 279–305). New York: Guilford Press.

43. Davidson, P. R. and Parker, K. C. H. (2001). Eye movement desensitization and reprocessing (EMDR): A meta-analysis. *Journal of Counseling and Clinical Psychology,* **69,** 305–316.

44. American Academy of Child and Adolescent Psychiatry (1998). Practice parameters for the assessment and treatment of children and adolescents with posttraumatic stress disorder. *Journal of the American Academy of Child and Adolescent Psychiatry,* **37,** 4S–26S.

45. Stallard, P. (2006). Psychological interventions for post-traumatic reactions in children and young people: A review of randomized controlled trials. *Clinical Psychology Review,* **26,** 895–911.

46. Cohen, J. A., Mannarino, A. P., Berliner, L. and Deblinger, E. (2000). Trauma-focused cognitive behavioral therapy for children and adolescents: An empirical update. *Journal of Interpersonal Violence,* **15,** 1202–1223.

47. Cohen, J. A., Deblinger, E. E., Mannarino, A. P. and Steer, R. A. (2004). A multisite, randomized controlled trial for children with sexual abuse-related PTSD symptoms. *Journal of the American Academy of Child and Adolescent Psychiatry,* **43,** 393–402.

48. Brady, K. T., Dansky, B. S., Back, S. E., Foa, E. B. and Carroll, K. M. (2001). Exposure therapy in the treatment of PTSD among cocaine-dependent individuals: Preliminary findings. *Journal of Substance Abuse Treatment,* **21,** 47–54.

49. Hembree, E. A., Street, G., P., Riggs, D. S. and Foa, E. (2004). Do assault-related variables predict response to cognitive behavioral treatments for PTSD? *Journal of Consulting and Clinical Psychology,* **72,** 531–534.

50. Ehlers, A., Clark, D. M., Hackmann, A., McManus, F. and Fennell, M. (2005). Cognitive therapy for post-traumatic stress disorder: Development and evaluation. *Behaviour Research and Therapy,* **43,** 413–431.

51. Duffy, M., Gillespie, K. and Clark, D. M. (2007). Post-traumatic stress disorder in the context of terrorism and

other civil conflict in Northern Ireland: Randomized controlled trial. *British Medical Journal*, **334**, 1147–1150.

52. Wild, J. and Gur, R. C. (2008). Verbal memory and treatment response in post-traumatic stress disorder. *British Journal of Psychiatry*, **193**, 254–255.

53. van der Kolk, B. A., Spinazzola, J., Blaustein, M. E. *et al.* (2007). A randomized clinical trial of eye movement desensitization and reprocessing (EMDR), fluoxetine, and pill placebo in the treatment of posttraumatic stress disorder: Treatment effects and long-term maintenance. *Journal of Clinical Psychiatry*, **68**, 37–46.

54. Bradley, R., Greene, J., Russ, E., Dutra, L. and Westen, D. (2005). A multidimensional meta-analysis of psychotherapy for PTSD. *American Journal of Psychiatry*, **162**, 214–227.

55. Schnurr, P. P. and Green, B. L. (eds.) (2004). *Trauma and health: Physical health consequences of exposure to extreme stress*. Washington, DC: American Psychological Association.

# Chapter

# 26

# Emotions and emotion regulation in the process of trauma recovery: implications for the treatment of post-traumatic stress disorder

Anthony Charuvastra and Marylene Cloitre

## Introduction

Clinicians and researchers are increasingly interested in the emotional basis of post-traumatic stress disorder (PTSD). Specifically, an individual's inability to adequately modulate intense emotions appears to be a core element of this disorder, reflected in symptoms of re-experiencing, hypervigilance and, ultimately, avoidance and numbing [1]. Successful treatment models have stemmed from a view of PTSD as a fear-based disorder in which many of the symptoms result from conditioned fear responses to trauma-related stimuli including internal images, sensations and objects in the physical environment [2]. Experimental studies derived from the principles of fear learning and fear extinction, using both animals and humans, suggest that disturbances in the neural circuitry of fear regulation are indeed associated with PTSD [3,4]. A more precise taxonomy of the physiological and psychological elements of fear regulation may continue to emerge from this approach to PTSD.

However, the emerging science of emotion recognizes that emotions such as fear do not exist in a pure or platonic form but are experienced and directed within the social context. Considering how emotion and emotion regulation inform and direct goals in social contexts, and how social context shapes emotion regulation, allows us to expand upon the fear-based model of PTSD in clinically important ways. A substantial body of research literature indicates that childhood trauma, and in particular trauma in the context of the attachment relationship, can disrupt the development of emotion regulation and social competency. We have in previous work proposed that emotion regulation

disturbances create risk for PTSD and other pathological fear reactions and, conversely, that improvement in emotion regulation can facilitate recovery from fear-based and other affective disorders [5]. We have also highlighted the role of social context, from the attachment relationship through peer/community/ social networks to the therapeutic relationship, in the organization and evolution of emotion regulation capacities. This chapter defines and characterizes emotion regulation in the context of normative human development and reviews some of the literature on childhood maltreatment to illuminate critical components of emotion regulation as they are affected by early traumatic exposure. The chapter continues by describing a developmentally informed evidence-based treatment for PTSD related to childhood abuse in which both the interventions and the principles on which they are based emphasize the centrality of emotion regulation in recovery from trauma.

## Emotion and emotion regulation serve adaptation

From a clinical standpoint, we are interested in how an individual responds to his or her feelings and to the emotional expressions of others; how he or she expresses feelings to others; and how he or she learns to recognize that their own emotional expressions influence reciprocal emotional expressions from others. We describe ways in which a patient can successfully modify and modulate emotional states through cognition, self-directed action and social behavior. In addition, we propose that some of the benefits of traditional trauma processing models can

*The Impact of Early Life Trauma on Health and Disease: The Hidden Epidemic*, ed. Ruth A. Lanius, Eric Vermetten and Clare Pain. Published by Cambridge University Press. Copyright © Cambridge University Press 2010.

be understood as resulting from an experience of learned emotion regulation.

Before proceeding, some definitions are necessary. Being precise about how we speak of emotion is important clinically, because educating patients about emotion is a core component of all treatments that seek to improve emotional regulation. From birth, emotional processes involve, and in many ways bridge, bodily functions, mental activities and social relationships [6]. Emotions are necessary for goal-directed activity and motivated choice [7,8]. Campos *et al.* [9] persuasively argue that because emotions function to promote adaptation it is impossible to consider a person's emotional processes without simultaneously considering that person's context and their construal (e.g., the meaning) of that context. Therefore, a given behavior, such as gaze aversion or intense crying, may reflect shame, joy, sadness or fear depending on what is happening and what the subject perceives or believes to be happening.

Emotions are best understood as physiological and mental processes that assist an individual in achieving some goal. The very act of directing emotional expression towards the attainment of some goal requires that the individual fit the emotion to some specific context. Emotion regulation is the process whereby emotions are modulated in the service of some goal for the individual. Consequently, we do not come across "pure" emotions in the platonic sense, but always some form of regulated emotion. For any given emotional process, whether it is felt as sadness, anger, joy or excitement, emotion regulation will reduce or increase the intensity or duration of the emotion, while changing or sustaining the quality.

In communicating about emotional processes and educating patients about emotions, it is important to highlight that knowledge of emotions, in ourselves and others, is always inferential. The term *feeling* refers to the private mental experience of emotion. Subjectively, we become aware of our own emotions through feelings, and feelings are how we communicate with ourselves about our own emotional experience. Feelings are one way we can monitor ourselves as we react emotionally to events around us; feelings may include states such as anger, sadness or joy [10]. While it is still not fully clear how feelings are produced, it is well documented that feelings inform and influence higher cognitive processes, and an essential aspect of emotional development is being able to label feeling states [8]. We communicate our emotions to others by a variety of expressive behaviors, including words

("I'm feeling sad"), pragmatic aspects of language such as sarcasm (e.g., "I feel *fine*"), facial expressions, body posture and movement, and social behavior (e.g., avoidance, approach, gestures).

Finally there are aspects of emotional experience that are not apparent to ourselves (intrasubjectively) or to others (intersubjectively) but which are nonetheless measurable. These include skin conductance, heart rate or heart rate variability and activation of certain subcortical areas of the brain. Multiple research paradigms have consistently demonstrated that emotional processes are always active, responding to social stimuli and often influencing our behavior, but that we are often only selectively aware of them. During settings that would typically elicit negative feelings, individuals who use "deactivating" or "suppressive" emotional strategies deny experiencing negative feelings yet they show significant increases in the skin conductance, indicating a physiological arousal in the absence of subjectively felt feelings [11]. In a neuroimaging study of "good–bad" evaluations of morally provocative topics (e.g., murder, abortion, welfare), the amygdala was always active in proportion to subsequent conscious reports of the emotional intensity associated with each topic, even when subjects were not consciously making evaluations of these words [12]. During the viewing of an emotional film, women with borderline personality disorder showed diminished parasympathetic tone compared with controls, implicating autonomic outflow as yet another facet of emotional life that occurs beneath the level of conscious awareness and is altered in conditions where emotion self-regulation is impaired [13].

Studies of normal emotional development highlight how interpersonal communication between a young child and the child's attachment figures is essential for the emergence of emotional skills required for emotion regulation. Mothers and infants engage in a dyadic process where they synchronize their emotional expressions and reactions, amplifying or suppressing emotional expressions and reactions in a way that maintains the relationship in an optimal way. This dyadic coregulation has been observed in parent interactions with toddlers and preschoolers [14,15]. The quality of dyadic emotion regulation, as reflected in mother–infant synchrony, predicts later toddler self-control [16]. Synchrony of this kind requires matching of positive emotions and repairing of negative or mismatched emotions [17], indicating that maternal–infant synchrony and subsequent childhood emotional development is critically dependent on the mother's (or other attachment figure's) capacities for emotion identification, regulation and expression.

The capacity to identify and label emotional experiences and then integrate this knowledge into an understanding of events seems to emerge from many iterations of emotional communication between an infant and their attachment caregivers, a process termed social biofeedback [18]. By selectively exaggerating and mirroring a child's emotional expressions, the parent helps to shape the expressions into more regular patterns and enables the child to match the feedback from his or her emotional expressions to his or her feelings states. As children mature, they move away from coregulation and increasingly towards self-regulation, although it is likely that coregulation occurs to some degree through much of childhood. Furthermore, this early experience of coregulation seems necessary to develop a capacity to understand the minds of other people as part of a coherent narrative of emotions, expectations and goals [19].

Awareness of the emotions of others is clearly necessary for the development of social competence, and an individual's awareness of the emotions of others depends on his or her ability to integrate a whole range of expressive behaviors into a coherent picture or narrative of another person. This inferential ability about the emotional states of others depends on the richness of our understanding of our own emotional experience. In this way, children or adults who lack emotional awareness about themselves will also have difficulty understanding the emotional expressions of others. The social biofeedback model suggests how having an absent or frightening caregiver early in life can result in profound deficits of emotional understanding of oneself and of others. The quality of early interactions with caregivers provides the scaffolding for later refinements of an emotional understanding of the self and others, as well as for the emergence of self-regulation, as children acquire an expanding repertoire of cognitive, linguistic and motor capabilities. The necessity for an emotionally competent caregiver to enable the development of a child's emotional capacities makes it clear how childhood maltreatment can cause such profound disruptions in emotional awareness and capacities for emotion regulation.

Adaptive emotional regulation thus involves several features: the capacity to be aware of what one is feeling and how this feeling relates to a narrative of past events, perception of current events and predictions of future events; the capacity to be aware of one's goals and to recognize whether the action tendencies associated with a feeling will promote or retard one's goals; and finally to have emotional modulation, or the capacity to either sustain or modify a feeling depending on whether this will help or hinder the attainment of the goal. A degree of behavioral inhibition is needed both to appraise one's feelings and one's context and to allow oneself an opportunity to recruit internal and external resources for either changing or maintaining an emotional state to the one most optimal for current functioning. Maladaptive behavior emerges if any component of this process is somehow deficient or disordered, indicating that the impaired capacity for emotional modulation is only one part of what we call emotional dysregulation, or the disordered use of emotion. Inherent in this conceptualization is the idea that adaptive emotional regulation requires flexibility but also control.

## Childhood trauma and maltreatment influence emotion regulation

Childhood maltreatment disturbs emotional processes in multiple ways. Compared with peers who were not maltreated, maltreated children show rigid and situationally inappropriate affective displays, diminished emotional self-awareness, difficulty in modulating excitement in emotionally arousing situations, difficulty recovering from frustration or distress, and mood lability. Furthermore, maltreated children are more likely to isolate themselves or withdraw during times of conflict, and they are less likely to initiate social engagement with adults and with their peers. They expect little help under stressful circumstances and tend to interpret the ambiguous or even supportive efforts of others as hostile [20]. Compared with their peers, adolescents with histories of abuse are more likely to attempt suicide and to develop alcohol and substance abuse problems (Nooner K. and Cloitre M. 2008, unpublished data), phenomena which have been attributed to efforts, sometimes desperate, to modulate intensely painful emotional states.

Consistent with the view that emotional and social competencies are integrally linked, maltreated children show substantial social difficulties, particularly in situations of high affect. Compared with their peers, abused children have difficulty with conflict negotiation because of discomfort with high levels of expressed emotion and an inability to recruit adults to assist with conflict resolution [21,22]. In adolescent years, these children are more likely than their peers to drop out of school, engage in deviant or delinquent behaviors and experience interpersonal violence as both perpetrators and victims [23].

Adults with histories of childhood abuse show similar difficulties in emotional and social competencies, including having problems with modulating feeling states, high levels of hostility and anxiety compared with other clinical samples, and chronic problems with anger management. In clinical samples, adults with histories of childhood abuse show low levels of emotion understanding and impaired capacity for negative mood regulation. Interpersonal and social difficulties are reflected in reported problems with sensitivity to criticism, hearing other viewpoints, difficulty standing up for themselves, and a tendency to quit jobs and relationships without negotiation. Adult survivors of childhood abuse expect little by way of comfort, reassurance or assistance from others in times of need, and perceive lower levels of social support than other individuals with psychiatric illness (reviewed by Cloitre et al. [20]). The inability to recruit support from members of a social network creates a higher risk for subsequent psychiatric and physical impairment, and it contributes to social disengagement [5]. Indeed, among women with child-abuse-related PTSD, difficulties with emotion regulation and interpersonal functioning have been found to account for as much functional impairment as PTSD symptoms themselves [24]. Thus, for survivors of childhood trauma, fear as represented in PTSD symptoms remains a core pathological process, but more broadly defined emotional regulation processes above and beyond those associated with PTSD symptoms contribute to substantial impairment in daily life in a variety of domains.

The combination of interpersonal difficulty, general social dysfunction and low emotional competence possessed by children and adults with maltreatment histories make it difficult to engage them in structured psychological treatment, which requires consistency with and trust of a clinician. For many patients who have experienced childhood trauma, it is essential to find ways to help them to join a treatment frame, create and sustain a therapeutic relationship with a therapist and tolerate the emotional experience of therapy without quitting.

## Emotion regulation in clinical settings

There is a convergence of interest in the role of emotion and emotional regulation in psychiatric illness

(reviewed by Mennin [25]). From a clinical standpoint, some mood and anxiety disorders may be characterized by the "overregulation" (underexpression) of emotions as a result of "affect phobias" or reinforced patterns of avoidance of painful negative emotional states such as fear or sadness. Post-traumatic stress disorder is an emotional disorder of particular interest because it involves contextually inappropriate over- and under-expressions of emotion. Emotional hyperreactivity is represented in the re-experiencing and hypervigilant clusters, which are associated with anger, aggression and impulsive behaviors, while social and emotional withdrawal are associated with the avoidance cluster of symptoms, which involves subjective feelings of emotional numbing as well as an inability to face powerfully felt emotions or emotion eliciting situations.

The sequential phase-based treatment model [26] described here expands on traditional fear-based models of intervention for PTSD by incorporating interventions that address emotion regulation and social difficulties and highlight their role in exacerbating or facilitating resolution of PTSD symptoms. The first phase of treatment, "skills training in affect and interpersonal regulation" (STAIR) comprises of interventions that address difficulties typical of PTSD relating to emotion regulation and interpersonal functioning. The second phase of treatment focuses primarily on the working through and meaningful reorganization of traumatic memories, which is supported by and reinforces the emotion regulation skills work completed in the first phase. The often-stated mechanism of action attributed to the success of trauma memory processing in reducing PTSD symptoms is the extinction of the fear response associated with the traumatic memory, which, in turn, allows access to and reorganization of the memory. An alternative and complementary proposal is that trauma memory processing is an activity that recruits, reinforces and consolidates emotion regulation capacities and allows exploration and meaningful reworking of highly charged emotional memories. This interpretation provides an explanation for the sometimes observed effective resolution of trauma-related emotional disturbances in single sessions or single life experiences ("catharsis").

## Treatment goals

The treatment goals and associated interventions in the STAIR phase include (a) enhancing emotional awareness through directed attention and description of feelings as they emerge in daily activities; (b) learning to sustain, modify or modulate feeling states through training in sustained online emotional awareness and affective expression through actions, words and thoughts; (c) learning the adaptive use of emotions to achieve social goals; (d) learning to identify adaptive and achievable social goals in different kinds of relationship; and (e) attaining a sense of emotional and social self-efficacy and self-acceptance that facilitates living in the world with compassion and empathy.

It is a cardinal principle of trauma therapy that the first and enduring goal of the treatment is to help the patient to experience a sense of safety. The experience of safety resulting from the therapeutic process can be viewed as an "antidote" to the fearful state in which the patient lives and the fearful attitude with which the patient regards the world. We suspect that an underlying mechanism of change in any effective trauma treatment is the experience of safety. However, how a sense of safety is developed in a treatment is rarely described. We speculate about its emergence through interventions focused on the development of skills in emotional awareness, emotion regulation and emotionally engaged living.

The therapeutic process involves two distinct components: therapy techniques that teach patients about emotion and emotion regulation, and the therapist's creation of an environment in which a person is able to learn new emotional skills. The former includes, for example, exercises in monitoring the body, behavior, beliefs and feelings, and increasing precision in identifying and discriminating among feelings. As with any kind of learning, there is no substitute for practice. An individual can learn the principles of doing a somersault dive, but actually to be good at it requires feeling confident enough to go and try it, over and over again. Skills-teaching techniques will not be effective without the therapist's ability to respond positively with focused interest in, curiosity about and acceptance of the patient's efforts. These types of response create a feeling of safety that facilitates the patient's interest in and expression of their own unique emotional experience. The therapist's role is to cultivate a shared sense of positive curiosity about emotional phenomena related to the patient's difficulties and how they may be resolved.

## Identifying and expressing feelings

The first several sessions of STAIR focus on eliciting, tracking, reflecting and expressing interest in and enthusiasm for the patient's emotional life. Patients with histories of childhood abuse have often experienced invalidation, neglect or punishment in response to expression of emotions that would normally be adaptive, such as anger, fear, sadness or yearning for attachment. Consequently, the expression of emotions often elicits fear and anxiety in the patient, as such experiences have been associated with emotional, physical or even sexual injury. In addition, environments that neglect, punish or invalidate emotional expression often corrode the individual's sense of emotional agency because the expression of feelings does not lead to consistent or desired outcomes. The therapist's response of interest in the patient's emotional experience, regardless of its nature (fear, anger, hatred) is counter to the patient's expectations. It creates the potential for a corrective experience inviting awareness that the expression of feelings can have positive rather than negative consequences. The therapist's response provides an interpersonal event that is incompatible with some of the patient's cognitive schemata that drive avoidance of emotionally expressive behaviors (e.g., "I will be rejected if I show that I am hurt"). When therapy begins, there is no reason for patients to trust the therapist with their feelings and it takes a certain leap into the unknown for patients to do so. A patient's tasks in the first sessions of therapy are to practice and become more accurate in the identification and discrimination of their feelings. The therapist's positive response creates a sense of safety that lays the foundation for patients to take more risks in the treatment and explore more of their emotional world.

## Emotional expression and emotion regulation

The exploration of feelings and their gradual modification and modulation in the service of effective living requires the elicitation of authentic emotion [29]. This, in turn, requires an attitude of acceptance of the real feelings. Conveying to the patient a genuine sense of curiosity facilitates acceptance by demonstrating to the patient that the therapist is accepting whatever emotions the patient has. Cultivating curiosity in the patient is probably closely related to approaches that teach patients mindfulness. With acceptance of authentic emotion, the patient is able to freely and more effectively work on elements of thoughts and behavior that he or she would like to change. Various strategies are introduced (cognitive reappraisals, breathing techniques, distress tolerance), and those that best match the patient's temperament and needs are selected for skills development and strengthening.

## Expanding the interpersonal and social repertoires

The STAIR interventions progress to exploration of the patient's emotional–behavioral habits in interpersonal and social settings, particularly those that are maladaptive, frightening or challenging. Role-playing of commonly encountered relationship dynamics (e.g., assertiveness, control, flexibility) creates opportunities to practice taught skills (e.g., cognitive reappraisals) and thus experience emotions in a modulated way. The therapist acts as modulator of the patient's emotions, pulling for the contextually salient emotions if needed during the role-play, helping the patient to sustain or reduce emotional intensity if indicated by the context of the role-play, and helping the patient to identify alternative emotions (e.g., joy or sadness, instead of guilt or shame) through the use of collaborative exploration.

The therapist's affective approach and response to these exercises, particularly expressions of curiosity and playfulness, can shape the meaning of these experiences to the patient. Playfulness and humor are incompatible with feelings of fear, and their presence in skills practice such as role-plays conveys the idea that the patient can explore, or "try on for size," feelings and attitudes that approximate and finally represent a skilled presentation of the message the patient wishes to give. Playfulness also involves recognition that there is both a pretend and a real aspect to role-playing. In the pretend aspect, the emotional experience is not as intense because the context does not elicit it (e.g., "I am just pretending to be angry at you, but you are not really my boss"), while the real aspect pulls for a more genuinely felt emotion (e.g., "If I really imagine you are my boss, it is scary to feel this much anger sitting here in your office"). Playfulness involves humor, irreverence and invention, and it creates a sense of equality between therapist and patient. With sensitivity and tact, the therapist can use playfulness to shift the role-play along the pretend–reality spectrum in order to vary the emotional intensity to that which the patient is capable of handling and to facilitate practicing of certain emotional skills. The goal is to give the patient an authentic emotional experience in which they experience self-efficacy, and acceptance by the therapist even as they struggle to practice their new emotional skills. Such practice elicits genuine emotional arousal and facilitates the gradual acceptance of intense emotions as emotion regulation skills improve,

but in a way that continuously allows the patient to feel in control and safe.

## Trauma memory processing and the uses of narration

The interventions in the first phase of treatment focus on everyday life with the goal of improving quality of life and functional capacity. The second phase of treatment focuses on working through the traumatic past. The emotional awareness and emotion regulation skills that have been applied to everyday life in the first phase are implemented in the second phase in the service of helping the patient to explore traumatic memories. In addition, the experience with the therapist in the titration of emotions during role-play and discussion of emotional daily-life matters reinforces confidence in the working relationship.

Emotional awareness and engagement in feelings associated with the trauma are elicited through explicit verbalization and description of the memories and associated feelings. The telling of these feelings and memories is organized within the structure of a narrative with a beginning, middle and end. The use of autobiographical narration and its inherent structure help support, reinforce and consolidate important self-regulatory activities. In the telling of a narrative, the patient (a) learns to regulate the flow of emotion as the narrator of the story; (b) experiences directed, contained and goal-oriented emotional expression through the presence of an explicitly defined narrative structure (beginning, middle, end); and (c) strengthens metacognitive functioning and self-awareness, as he or she is both in the story as its subject but also removed from the story as its narrator.

As introduced by Foa et al. [2], the narrative is tape recorded. The patient and therapist listen to it and engage in an analysis that explores the meaning of the event as experienced at the time as well as a revision of its meaning through the incorporation of new information gleaned from the therapy work so far. These reappraisals often involve the recognition that the chronic fear experienced in the present belongs to an event in the past that can no longer harm the person, that the chronic shame or guilt experienced about the event is misplaced, and that the loss intrinsic to the experience (of a person, a sense of worth, a capacity to relate to others) can be purposefully reworked and transformed in the present.

In this phase of work, the therapist moves from coach and teacher to listener, witness, and, sometimes, co-creator of the new meaning of the trauma. Despite some change in role, the centrality of the positive relationship of the therapist to the patient should be reiterated. Evidence from the psychotherapy process literature indicates that emotional arousal is a substantial contributor to positive change in the treatment of many disorders, but only in the presence of a strong therapeutic alliance (reviewed by Whelton [28]). Process research of this phase-based treatment suggests that a positive therapeutic alliance can be forged from effective work in skills development in the initial phase of treatment, and that this, in turn, contributes to the effective use of emotion regulation skills during the memory processing phase. Specifically, the therapeutic alliance established early in treatment reliably predicts emotion regulation capacity during the memory processing phase of the treatment, which, in turn, predicts good outcome at post-treatment as measured by reduction of PTSD symptoms [29].

## Conclusions

Exposure to and emotional engagement with feared trauma memories play an important role in recovery from traumas. In this context, the experience and impact of trauma can be reflected upon and incorporated into the person's life in a way that provides meaning and facilitates ongoing integration to a world governed by the rule of law and respect for persons. Improved emotion regulation helps patients in this process [26]. However, improved emotion regulation skills provide a benefit beyond therapy. We believe that by helping patients to appreciate the deeply interpersonal nature of emotional life, and conversely the deeply emotional nature of relationships, they will leave therapy with a greater sense of connection, compassion and empathy for other people in the world. The ultimate recovery from a childhood marked by abuse, neglect and the perversion of meaning so often found in these situations must be a person's ability to join their communities as a loving, working and generative human being.

## References

1. Frewen, P. A. and Lanius, R. A. (2006). Toward a psychobiology of posttraumatic self-dysregulation: Reexperiencing, hyperarousal, dissociation, and emotional numbing. *Annals of the New York Academy of Sciences,* **1071**, 110–124.

2. Foa, E. B., Keane, T. M. and Friedman, M. J. (2004). *Effective treatments for PTSD: Practice guidelines from the International Society for Traumatic Stress Studies.* New York: Guilford.

3. Phelps, E. A. and LeDoux, J. E. (2005). Contributions of the amygdala to emotion processing: From animal models to human behavior. *Neuron, 48*, 175–187.

4. Shin, L. M., Rauch, S. L. and Pitman, R. K. (2006). Amygdala, medial prefrontal cortex, and hippocampal function in PTSD. *Annals of the New York Academy of Sciences,* **1071**, 67–79.

5. Charuvastra, A. and Cloitre, M. (2008) Social bonds and posttraumatic stress disorder. *Annual Review of Psychology,* **59**, 301–328.

6. Davidson, R. J., Scherer, K. R. and Goldsmih, H. H. (eds.), (2003). *Handbood of affective sciences.* New York: Oxford University Press.

7. Bechara, A., Damasio, H. and Damasio, A. R.. (2000). Emotion, decision making and the orbitofrontal cortex. *Cerebral Cortex Cerebral,* **10**, 295–307.

8. Damasio, A. (2000). *The feeling of what happens: Body and emotion in the making of consciousness.* New York: Harcourt Brace.

9. Campos, J. J., Frankel, C. B. and Camras, L. (2004). On the nature of emotion regulation. *Child Development, 75,* 377–394.

10. Hoeksma, J. B., Oosterlaan, J. and Schipper, E. M. (2004). Emotion regulation and the dynamics of feelings: a conceptual and methodological framework. *Child Development, 75,* 354–360.

11. Dozier, M. and Kobak, R. R. (1992). Psychophysiology in attachment interviews: Converging evidence for deactivating strategies. *Child Development, 63,* 1473–1480.

12. Cunningham, W. A., Raye, C. L. and Johnson, M. K. (2004) Implicit and explicit evaluation: FMRI correlates of valence, emotional intensity, and control in the processing of attitudes. *Journal of Cognitive and Neuroscience, 16,* 1717–1729.

13. Austin, M. A., Riniolo, T. C. and Porges, S. W. (2007). Borderline personality disorder and emotion regulation: insights from the Polyvagal Theory. *Brain and Cognition, 65,* 69–76.

14. Field, T. (1994). The effects of mother's physical and emotional unavailability on emotion regulation. *Monographs of the Society for Research in Child Development, 59,* 208–227.

15. Cole, P. M., Teti, L. O. and Zahn-Waxler, C. (2003). Mutual emotion regulation and the stability of conduct problems between preschool and early school age. *Developmental Psychopathology, 15,* 1–18.

16. Feldman, R. (2007). Parent–infant synchrony and the construction of shared timing: Physiological precursors, developmental outcomes, and risk conditions. *Journal Child Psychology and Psychiatry, 48,* 329–354.

17. Tronick, E. Z. and Cohn, J. F. (1989). Infant–mother face-to-face interaction: Age and gender differences in coordination and the occurrence of miscoordination. *Child Development*, **60**, 85–92.

18. Gergely, G. and Watson, J. S. (1996). The social biofeedback theory of parental affect-mirroring: The development of emotional self-awareness and self-control in infancy. *International Journal of Psycho-Analysis,* **77**, 1181–1212.

19. Fonagy, P., Gergely, G., Jurist, E. and Target, M. (2002). *Affect regulation, mentalization, and the development of the self.* New York: Other Press.

20. Cloitre, M., Cohen, L. and Koenan, K. C. (2006) *Treating survivors of childhood abuse: Psychotherapy for the interrupted life.* New York: Guildford.

21. Cummings, E. M., Hennessy, K., Rabideau, G. and Cicchetti, D. (1994). Responses of physically abused boys to interadult anger involving their mothers. *Developmental Psychology*, **6**, 31–41.

22. Schwartz, D. and Proctor, L. J. (2000). Community violence exposure and children's social adjustment in the school peer groups: The mediating roles of emotion regulation and social cognition. *Journal of Consulting and Clinical Psychology*, **68**, 670–683.

23. Kilpatrick, D. G., Ruggiero, K. J., Acierno, R. *et al.* (2003). Violence and risk of PTSD, major depression, substance abuse/dependence, and comorbidity: Results from the National Survey of Adolescents. *Journal of Consulting and Clinical Psychology*, **71**, 692–700.

24. Cloitre, M., Miranda, R., Stovall-McClough, C. and Han, H. (2005) Beyond PTSD: Emotion regulation and interpersonal problems as predictors of functional impairment in survivors of childhood abuse. *Behavior Therapy*, **36**, 119–124.

25. Mennin, D. and Farach, F. (2007) Emotion and evolving treatments for adult psychopathology. *Clinical Psychology and Science Practice*, **14**, 329–352.

26. Cloitre, M., Koenen, K. C., Cohen, L. R. and Han, H. (2002) Skills training in affective and interpersonal regulation followed by exposure: A phase-based treatment for PTSD related to childhood abuse. *Journal of Consulting and Clinical Psychology*, **70**, 1067–1074.

27. Greenberg, L. (2006) Emotion-focused therapy: A synopsis. *Journal of Contempory Psychotherapy.* **36**, 87–93.

28. Whelton, W. J. (2004). Emotional processes in psychotherapy: Evidence across therapeutic modalities. *Clinical Psychology and Psychotherapy*, **11**, 58–71.

29. Cloitre, M., Stovall-McClough, C., Miranda, R. and Chemtob, C. M. (2004) Therapeutic alliance, negative mood regulation, and treatment outcome in child abuse-related posttraumatic stress disorder. *Journal of Consulting and Clinical Psychology*, **72**, 411–416.

# Psychodynamic psychotherapy: adaptations for the treatment of patients with chronic complex post-traumatic stress disorder

Clare Pain, Ruth A. Lanius, Pat Ogden and Eric Vermetten

## Introduction

This chapter proposes that patients with chronic complex post-traumatic stress disorder (PTSD) are unable to fully take advantage of brief models of empirically validated manual-based therapy. It suggests that psychodynamic psychotherapy (PDPT) provides an evidence-based model and intervention strategy flexible enough for therapists to understand and assist patients with complex trauma to recover, while recognizing the therapeutic relationship as central to the resolution of traumatic sequalae. However, because of certain general features shared by patients with chronic trauma, some adaptation to PDPT is required to address elements of their condition that elude both the brief therapy-specific approach and PDPT unadapted to trauma. These adaptations are illustrated with a case history describing the treatment of a patient with complex trauma. First, however, the differences between simple and complex PTSD will be identified together with some of the limitations of brief models of PTSD therapy treatment.

## Simple and complex post-traumatic stress disorder

Judith Herman [1] suggested that many patients with PTSD are better described as having a chronic complex trauma disorder following early or prolonged traumatic experiences. Comorbidity is common in these patients, as are a range of psychological problems and inhibitions. Following extensive field trials, a syndrome was identified [2,3] that was named disorder of extreme stress not otherwise specified (DESNOS), with six categories of symptoms: alterations in

regulating affect, attention or consciousness; the frequent co-occurrence of somatization; changes in the patient's self-perception; change in the patient's systems of meaning and in their relationships with other people. The identification of DESNOS was an attempt to put diagnostic predictability and order into what is otherwise an apparently unrelated mixed array of axis I and II diagnoses that almost inevitably accompany chronic PTSD.

## Limited efficacy of brief models of post-traumatic stress disorder therapy

With the increasing recognition of how frequently PTSD constitutes a disorder requiring treatment, there has been a parallel increase in research concerning the best methods of treatment. Research on the treatment of PTSD has usually focused on brief therapies such as cognitive-behavioral therapy (CBT), trauma-focused CBT, prolonged exposure and so on. Results are encouraging, but even in very well-executed research trials fewer than 50% of patients with simple PTSD show substantial improvement [4–8]. There is also a growing literature on the limitations of these treatments in securing full symptom remission and full functional restoration [7,8]. Although it has been generally found that imaginal or actual exposure of the patient to their traumatic material is an essential component of recovery, there are also some data suggesting that exposure or desensitization can be detrimental to some patients [5,9–13], as evidenced by high drop out rates, symptom exacerbation, and compliance problems. It has been suggested that the ability to help patients to face their past usefully, to know the defenses they have used to manage it and the meaning it has for them, is dependent on the experience and skills of the therapist [14,15]. It is to the skill or "art" of therapy, rather than the science of therapy, that this chapter on PDPT for complex trauma patients is directed.

As well, empirically supported therapies are essential for the development of effective psychotherapy treatments, although they usually exclude patients on the basis of a number of factors including comorbidity, concurrent personality disorder, substance misuse/abuse/dependence/suicidality and/or self-harm [16]. Yet it is these patients with complex trauma who commonly present to community psychotherapists, many of whom rely on PDPT to assist them in understanding the complexity of their patients [17]. Although it is easier to do research on brief models of therapy, evidence exists to support long-term PDPT as being effective for patients with complex mixtures of axis I and II disorders [7,18–20].

## The need to adapt psychodynamic psychotherapy

This chapter uses the quotation of Gunderson and Gabbard [21] given by Leichsenring and Rabung [20] to define long-term PDPT as "a therapy that involves careful attention to the therapist–patient interaction, with thoughtfully timed interpretation of transference and resistance embedded in a sophisticated appreciation of the therapist's contribution to the two-person field" (p. 685).

In Ch. 23, Allen *et al.* note that unmodified psychodynamic psychotherapy can make the traumatized patient worse [22] and lead to a protracted therapy [23], or it can, when adequately adapted, point in the direction of more favorable outcomes [24], as indeed does the adaptation called mentalizing-based psychotherapy (MBP) described by Allen *et al.* (Ch. 23) [25,26].

Allen *et al.* in Ch. 23 note differences between the MBP and PDPT. For example, MBP takes a here-and-now stance, favors process over content and discourages free associations. Chapter 23 also describes concomitant attention to the therapist's own ability to bear the patient's mind in the therapist's mind. The therapist's own stance and interventions effectively model his or her capacity to mentalize the patient, ultimately enabling the patient to adequately mentalize self and others. Allen *et al.* (Ch. 23) write that the goal of the MBT is to "help the patient to think, feel, and talk about traumatic experiences....we promote mentalizing in relation to the trauma in the context of an attachment relationship, on the assumption that lacking the opportunity to mentalize in the course of the traumatic events constitutes the core of the trauma." Although we share this concept of the goal of trauma treatment and we focus on a therapeutic stance of mentalizing, we include more attention to the need to deal with the patient's memories, their chronic dissociation and fear states and the patient's free associations to guide this process.

## Common attributes of chronic complex post-traumatic stress disorder and suggested adaptations to psychodynamic psychotherapy

There are several common attributes of chronic complex patients with PTSD, summarized in the six categories of symptoms in DESNOS, that warrant special consideration and management from the psychodynamic therapist (Table 27.1). These are deeply intertwined and make up the double binds of trauma and recovery for the patient.

### The ubiquity of fear

The emotion of fear is pervasively central to the experience of chronic complex trauma. The immediacy of the fear of the trauma persists for as long as the event is too frightening and distressing to be thought about, to find words for, to explore and to untangle its meaning. We know that the most pernicious trauma is at the hands of another person, and that the unavailability of adequate support following the traumatic event(s) is a major factor in the development of PTSD [27]. The traumatized patient has discovered that another person – usually one entrusted with their care – that can be dangerous and then experienced a subsequent lack of appropriate help. It is this two-part betrayal experience that makes coming into therapy particularly difficult. Therapy raises both the fear of the trauma and the experience of feeling vulnerable to someone who should, but cannot, be trusted, and whom the patient expects to agree with his or her own self-assessment of being despicable, weak, bad and less than human.

### Dissociation

Patients raised in sufficiently invalidating environment are frequently alexithymic, which has been associated with increased use of dissociative defenses in adulthood [28,29]. Brothers [30] has stated succinctly that "trauma goes hand in hand with dissociation." She recognizes

**Table 27.1** Common attributes of patients with chronic complex post-traumatic stress disorder that warrant special consideration and management in psychodynamic psychotherapy

| Common attributes | Suggestions for adaptation |
|---|---|
| General | Overall focus on a mentalizing therapeutic stance |
| The ubiquity of fear | Address the patient's fear early in therapy and often |
| Chronic mistrust of relationships | Give a "therapeutic map" early in the course of treatment and as often as necessary as treatment progresses, so that the patient can "read" the therapeutic intent |
| Fragmentation of memory and chronic dissociation | Work with the patient to discard dissociation as a defense; adhere to the three phases of trauma treatment:<br>• stabilization and symptom reduction: stabilize and ground as necessary<br>• memory work: pace memory work within the window of tolerance, promote patient's recognition of his or her changes in state using safe place guided imagery, affect managing strategies (e.g., the screen technique, and sensorimotor psychotherapy methods to "tune into the body")<br>• rehabilitation, reintegration: observe and foster the patient's development of new relationships and activities |

that following trauma "the subject reflexly attempts some kind of psychological restoration of the self." This involves keeping the traumatic experience out of mind, which requires a variety of avoidant, dissociative and cognitive strategies. Dissociation modifies the emotional weight and acute distress of the experience by keeping it separate or at a distance from daily experience. This defensive strategy simplifies the implications of meaning, and complexity is replaced by the need to cling to a rigidity of thinking and self-organization [30]. The malignant intent or motivation of the abuser is too terrifying to contemplate, so the victim defensively turns off the ability to reflect on the intentionality of others. The capacity to read another's and importantly one's own mind – the essence of mentalizing – is "decoupled" [31]. Allen [31] wrote "Trauma provokes extreme distress and simultaneously undermines the development of capacities to regulate it." Thus the patient has little insight or understanding of the origins and reasons for their difficulties and remains vulnerable to traumatic reminders, which out of nowhere rekindle their fear and cognitive disorganization.

## Self-blame and self-loathing

Lerner [32,33] and Rubin and Peplau [34] have proposed that, in general, people (and we would add children in particular) believe in a "just world theory" in which the world is a fair place and people get what they deserve; good things come to good people and conversely bad treatment only happens to bad people. This defense seems particularly pervasive in adult survivors of childhood sexual abuse, who are unusually cruel and dismissive of the abused child that they were. Although they would not use this explanation for another abused person, they blame themselves for their abuse and frequently believe that they not only brought the abuse upon themselves but they also deserved it, otherwise they themselves or someone else would have stopped it. They judge themselves to be dirty and despicable and rigidly adhere to this explanation as a reason to dismiss the suffering of the vulnerable child they were, and whom they despise. The ability of the patient to learn to mentalize his or her own distress as an abused child constitutes one of the objectives of therapy. This becomes possible as the therapist shares his or her own compassionate thoughts about the child's frightening predicament and notes accurately the strengths which the child drew upon to survive.

## Address safety early in treatment

It is the double bind of fear and dissociation, the failure of previous relationships to provide sufficient safety or structure to assist recovery, and the patient's negative self-appraisal that makes engaging in therapy difficult. When asked, the patient is usually aware of being afraid most of the time, but PDPT therapists may be unfamiliar with the magnitude and omnipresence of their patients' chronic fear and dissociation and their own need to enquire about it. Often, the trauma-naive therapist in the presence of such a patient feels her or his own sense of non-engagement or even boredom during the session. It can be difficult for a therapist to believe the patient is experiencing him or her as frightening. Is the patient afraid of the therapist physically or afraid the therapist will emotionally abuse or take sexual advantage? It is helpful for the therapist to ask and explore these questions, stating clearly that he or she will neither physically harm nor take sexual advantage of the patient. If inadvertently the therapist hurts the patient with his or her words, feedback is both helpful and necessary. Usually the simple exploration of this issue demonstrates that the therapist is attuned to the patient's fundamental lack of a sense of safety, and assists in the formation of an early therapeutic alliance.

Before proceeding further we will use a clinical case – "Sandy"– to further illustrate both the common attributes of a patient with chronic trauma and their unique portrayal, as well as specific adaptations to PDPT.

Sandy is an attractive 39-year-old single woman who has been in therapy (with one of the authors) for a number of years. She now has a meaningful job in the area of human rights and is well loved by her many friends. However, she has never had a romantic sexual relationship, and despite wanting to marry and have children, she drops any man whom she begins to feel attracted to, overwhelmed with fear and disgust.

When Sandy was 7 years old her mother was diagnosed with cancer and she was left in her grandparents' care when her parents drove to the city for her mother's innumerable medical appointments. Her mother died when Sandy was 15 years old, and her father remarried within the year to a difficult and controlling woman. Sandy moved out at 17 years of age to a friend's parent's home.

During the time she was 7–14 years of age, her grandfather sexually and physically tortured her during the weekends when she was in his house. She never told her parents (or anyone else prior to therapy), and they never apparently noticed or commented on her state following the visits, despite the fact that her grandfather was unpopular and feared in the family, and his wife was a shadowy woman thoroughly under his influence.

Sandy did well at school, loved sports and made friends easily, although she described this as "making nice" for fear of being alone and unprotected. She allied with strong people who she secretly felt dependent on. Initially, she said it had been difficult to hold on to good feelings, that there were "holes" in her, and that "there is something dark and disgusting inside" her which she wanted to push away. At the time she started therapy she felt anxious most of the time, suffering from panic attacks, difficulty in sleeping, nightmares and

intermittent "attacks of shaking." Although she had traveled and worked abroad, she had little pleasure or joy in her life and seldom felt fully present. When she started therapy, she had been experiencing more and more intrusive flashbacks of "stuff that happened as a kid" and "body memories and flashes" that implicated her grandfather, although she would call herself "a liar" and "a drama queen" every time she thought this. These perceptions occurred for a few minutes, after which she was barely able to function for the next two or more days. Identifying this as "the flu," she would take time off work to recover. She sought treatment for what she wondered might be memories of sexual abuse.

## Sharing a map

Because of the inherent mistrust and fear that a patient with chronic trauma has of the therapist, and the patient's self-denigrating denial of own suffering as a child, it is helpful for the therapist to convey short portions of his or her ideas about healing and therapeutic intent. This is useful intermittently throughout therapy, but particularly so at the beginning. It provides an early basic map that spells out to the patient how the therapist is thinking. For instance, in the case history, this was co-created by therapist and patient (see below).

Sandy brought to her sessions almost overwhelming experiences of emotional distress connected to somatosensory fragments related to her childhood sexual abuse. She was easily triggered into acute distress and re-experiencing by various abuse-related reminders. She had kept her past outside of her thoughts, and she was afraid of what she would discover if she could think about or know what caused this distress. However, therapist and patient agreed that as an adult she had built a safe life without physical, sexual or verbal abuse. They agreed to go slowly and simply discover what she had on her mind so eventually she would not have to fear her own thoughts. Sandy developed a metaphor of opening her mind up to the light of day, like a house with all its windows open to the fresh spring air after winter.

## The fragmentation of memory and chronic dissociation

Following the three-stage model of treatment: stabilization and symptom reduction; memory work, and rehabilitation and reintegration [2,35], Sandy stabilized relatively quickly. She got a better job and stopped binge drinking. Many of the early sessions involved Sandy trying to talk about her memories of abuse, within her capacity to function at work and home. She experienced a variety of distorted perceptual experiences and struggled to stay adequately present in therapy. Her speech would become extremely fragmented, and her grammar and syntax deteriorated. A segment of her therapy illustrates this. The immediate preceding association was of a man she met socially.

> There is a guy I thought was cool – I didn't feel 16, it was, it was kinda a fear – every time I catch myself – I don't know if its metaphysical but I have a fear of being hit, slapped across the side of my head hard. New flash, I want to throw up, I want to go away now. Oh God, I feel quite nauseous and sea sick like I always get. Oh shit, uh the image uh that passed through my head was (of) being hit and, there're just words, it's just an image. Um I don't know really. My mind's playing a lot of games – its calling me a liar, that I'm just doing this for dramatic effect. Oh God. Being hit then being, oh God, peed on – on my body, naked, oh God, its so degrading. I've always hated the sound of a man peeing in the bathroom, even if it's the most benign man in the world, like my brother. The sound, because it's followed by something else – a gut reaction. Err something about my mouth too – err I don't know if it's associated with that. Vivid images, visual and other images – you can um say feeling images – that's bothering me and smells. It evokes a very subdued anger, it's so gross. The err image, I need to separate it, so I'm going to talk in the third person and pretend it's (on) a screen. So the person is being peed on the head and body, then the image is very close not necessarily just visual at all. She smells penis and pubic hair in the mouth and all other things associated with that. I want them to go away. I hate him, she sees him breathing hard, flaring nostril, oh God I hate him, its so messed up. He's making her feel it's her fault. No. He says my mother won't love me if she knew, he always made it like we were in it together, like I was his, a little secrete relationship. He was so unpredictable, he'd take me on the subway and everyone would think what a nice relationship between grandfather and grandchild and he'd act all nice. Somehow he'd make me feel, him and I, and there was the rest of my family, I wasn't part of it.

## Guided imagery, screen technique and sensorimotor psychotherapy

Because most patients with chronic trauma are to a greater or lesser degree dissociating much of the time with the stress of startng therapy, it is difficult for the therapist to gauge how present the patient is in the sessions. For therapy to be effective, the patient needs to be fully present in the here and now. Negotiating this forms a useful place of collaboration between therapist and patient. We have found that relaxation techniques

have a paradoxical effect, precipitating acute anxiety in the patient rather than promoting a sense of calm. Instead, incorporating aspects of hypnosis – guided imagery and screen technique – more reliably modify emotional states and are valuable additions to PDPT. The former technique is useful to assist the patient to learn to move out of chronic fear and dissociative states and find a reliable imaginary safe place where their self-state is calm and comfortable. The screen technique is a way of helping the patient to distance from a difficult memory by "putting the experience on a video screen." It can reduce overwhelming arousal levels and promote an improvement in affect regulation [36].

As well, we incorporate two basic techniques from sensorimotor psychotherapy [37].. In this model, the patient's body is understood to hold and express the as yet unsymbolized non-verbal complexity of their traumatic experience. As part of their dissociative response, patients with chronic trauma have usually significantly "shut off" data that comes from their body in an attempt to manage their unresolved past and the affect dysregulation that accompanies it. But without tuning into the somatic experience which accompanies their emotions, the relationship between their thoughts, emotions and bodily sensations is compromised [38]. Interventions to help the patient to reestablish this awareness and interest in their inner physical experiences promote a more integrated knowledge of their response to past traumatic events and their current emotions, and decreases psychological and physical dysregulation. Sensorimotor psychotherapy uses the patient's bodily experiences in the session to engage the patient's attention and curiosity concerning the processing of therapeutic material. Such interventions within the context of a relationally attuned therapy help to build a stronger sense of self-awareness, and self-confidence in the patient's own judgment.

In therapy a way of working was developed that held Sandy more fully in the present with "just a toe in the past." To distance herself from its full impact, she would "put the experience on a screen" and describe what was happening in the third person. It was agreed that 90% or more of her needed to be "in the room" during therapy, and if this slipped she learned to stop and ground herself. It was as though she had to experience a little of the lived past to be able to try and think about it – but only a little. Guided imagery of a safe place was used to combine a number of beautiful places she liked. To her surprise, no matter how distressed she was, she learned to switch into a calm, safe comfortable state of mind.

During this early stage of therapy, she put into words for the first time the known but unspoken-of traumatic experience, recognizing how impossible it had been to think about her past by herself. Her chronic dissociative state lessened occasionally and she had moments of feeling better. However she also said, "I can't think about it a lot, I, I pay, its very painful sometimes, it feels dying is easier." Her previously repetitive thoughts about herself as a slut and a prostitute, and a less than human being, started making sense to her.

## Tuning into the body

While PDPT depends primarily on a patient's verbal descriptions of their inner state to guide the therapeutic process, therapists cannot rely on this capacity in patients with chronic complex trauma. The ability to find salient and nuanced words to describe somatic experiences and relate them to emotional states is a skill learned over time and an outcome of successful treatment. It requires the patient to tune in and observe their physical experience, which has been defensively tuned out, numbed, minimized or ignored in an attempt to provide distance from distress.

With Sandy, who early in treatment experienced both dissociation and hyperarousal states, helping her tune into her somatic experience was crucial. It was as though she did not really recognize how very upset she was but asking Sandy how her body felt only increased her distress from the body memories of rape. At first, the therapeutic question had to be more specific, such as "please can you 'look inside your body' and tell me what your heart feels like?" She was surprised to find that her heart was "racing". Over time, she learned how to identify the subtle fluctuations of her inner sensations in texture, quality and intensity. She began to differentiate between words that described emotional states, such as panic and terror, from words that described bodily sensations, such as hot, frozen, churning, heavy and so on. Through cultivating the ability to form accurate verbal descriptions of her physical feelings, she expanded her perception and processing of physical sensations in much the same way that familiarity with a variety of words describing emotion will aid in the perception and processing of emotions.

The careful, mindful observation of the patient's body by the therapist and the engagement of the patient's awareness of his or her own body also sheds light on the connections between the body and emotions and beliefs. For instance, Sandy could notice how her belief "I'm a bad person" increased when she put her hands together as though they were still bound by her grandfather, and decreased when she crossed her knees and put her hands by her sides. This recognition helped Sandy to use data from her body as a means to gain more control over her distress than she had realized was possible, and to recognize that her belief that she was bad was more about how she survived the abuse as a child than a real fact about herself.

The second technique borrowed from sensorimotor psychotherapy and incorporated into PDPT is an extension of the patient's ability to observe his or her own inner physical state. It helps in pacing the amount of material that is distressing for the patient. The therapist's task is to help "hold" the patient's arousal level within his or her "window of tolerance." This is understood to be the extent of the patient's capacity to feel and think and understand what is happening to in the present [39]. Thus the patient accesses enough traumatic material to process, but not so much that the window of tolerance is exceeded. When arousal neared either extreme of hyper- or hypoarousal, Sandy was asked to temporarily drop all thoughts and images and disregard her emotions, and instead follow the development of her physical sensations and movements in detail until these sensations settled and a physiological baseline resumed. At this point, she could return again to the memories. In this way, she learned to limit the amount of information she could attend to at any given moment, which prevented the experience of feeling flooded by an overload of information coming from within.

With the use of this combination of adaptations to PDPT, Sandy had an increased ability to find words for what had happened, and she was no longer hijacked by a particular trigger and memory in the same way. With this increased tolerance to knowing and a growing ability to symbolize verbally the memories of her abuse, Sandy could make links and was able to achieve a growing degree of synthesis. She began to know the contents of her own mind.

## The return of complexity

Sandy realized she had believed her grandfather's words when he told her she wanted and deserved his brutality. She had also believed that she caused her mother's cancer and that bearing the abuse was necessary to lessen her mother's suffering. These beliefs protected her from feeling anger towards her mother for failing to protect her and for ultimately abandoning her by dying. Superficially, she idealized her "golden" mother, longed for her good opinion while fearing she herself was unlovable and unworthy. Because the abuse occurred without her mother's censor, she "knows" she both deserved it and was "disposable."

Sandy's dawning awareness of her anger and simultaneous defensive "grateful compliance" suffused the therapy sessions. The therapist began to notice that Sandy's abuse memories and their accompanying, now milder, physical reactions, tended to occur in response to her anticipation of breaks in the therapy, or her nascent ability to acknowledge her disappointment in her mother or therapist. Sandy found it difficult to stay with her irritation and she would slip more readily into a fear state of half-dissociated, half-remembered experience of the basement with her grandfather again. The fear that her abuse precipitated saved her in the sessions from recognizing how angry and disappointed she was with the therapist/her mother for failing to protect her and then abandoning her. Feeling anger or irritation was an unfamiliar luxury she has never been able to risk. Sandy said it was as though by developing cancer, her mother had trumped her right to be angry and filled her with both despair, which she managed by more or less denying her mother's death, and fear that she had killed her.

The therapeutic space provided her with some room to let her mind associate her defenses with knowing what happened with her grandfather. Into this space, fragments of her unsymbolized childhood abuse became available for her to recognize and name. Her mother failed to protect her or recognize that she had been abused. With no parental mind for Sandy to use as a safe and empathic container, she was unable to adequately symbolize, integrate and synthesize the experience. Her dissociation, avoidance and self-denigrating cognitive tricks (calling herself a liar and drama queen), used to distance herself from her experience, enabled her to accept her mother's implied blame and take full responsibility for the abuse, and know herself as bad.

## Mentalizing oneself

Although Sandy has good judgment, an intelligent reflective thoughtfulness, and an easy and accurate understanding of others, she remained harsh and unforgiving of the child she had been. Therapy had progressed well, but it was evident that her inability to acknowledge her desire for a romantic partner was in part connected to her incapacity to empathize reliably with herself as the tortured child of her past. When asked to look within at the child she was, she could report, "The child is frightened and alone, dirty

and hurting." For years she had rejected and despised this aspect of herself. Recently, she noted about her abuse, "It's like a crazy news story." It shocks her over and over again as she digests the fact that her abuser was her grandfather and she was a child. Her recognition that "bearing things silently did not save anything" has also been a painful and fluctuating realization. She knows that her defensive ability to be "tough, stoic and suck it up" reinforces her avoidance and inhibition of her sexuality, successfully keeping many of her fears about herself at bay. For as long as she keeps the topic of dating absolutely out of her imagination she does not have to separate the sexually abused child from the adult woman she is, capable of sexual desire.

As her overall stability and function improved, her increased ability to engage with the world recruits more integration of her past. Recently, and for the first time, she bought herself a new bed. She had taken time to find a bed she really liked. Although the new white bed had a head board that "someone could tie you to" and precipitated discomfort, it did not trigger dissociated abuse flashbacks as it would have earlier in therapy. Nevertheless, with this purchase she remembered her grandfather had started doing "weird things" to her in her own bed at home. Then there had been an invitation to his home for a "special week-end" and the abuse started. She remembered now clearly how he told her she was a slut and liked and wanted sex, and how he would inflict pain to negotiate her silence. In response to these memories, which are indeed more memory than reliving experiences, Sandy is easy to coach into checking in with her body and with the child she had been. The therapist asks: "Did that child want what he said she wanted?" "What was her body telling her?" "If she was not tied up what would she have done? What do her legs tell her? Her arms?" It seemed increasingly clear to Sandy, based on tuning into her body, that she would have run far away from her grandfather had this been possible. As a child she had managed the pain and assaults and degradation as best she could – but if she imagined a choice she would have fled. She feels the shift and reports that the child in her is calm and asleep for the first time on her bed.

## Conclusions

We have invoked and included many of the ideas of Allen et al. (Ch. 23) [31] about mentalizing into our considerations for modified PDPT, in particular the therapeutic stance, the goals of trauma treatment and the specific double bind of fear for the patient coming into therapy induced by "trauma-related affects," which "stimulate attachment needs." These attachment needs, unmet in the patient's past, promote the persistence and toxicity of the multifaceted defenses used by patients to manage their traumatic history. In so far as therapy mimics this situation, the patient is unable to feel reliant upon the therapist, dissociates as a defensive "solution" and the traumatic experience is once again inevitably rendered unthinkable. We have suggested, using a long case description as a unique example of these common problems, adapted PDPT is the most useful current treatment for patients with chronic complex PTSD. With small changes in focus and emphasis, and by including some techniques derived from hypnosis and sensorimotor psychotherapy, a PDPT therapist can address the ubiquity of the fears and mistrust of a patient with chronic complex trauma, and the affective and cognitive disruptions that prevent a patient knowing his or her own mind and body.

We have placed special emphasis on the conviction that the patient's body is not only the combat zone on which the abuse occurred, but it also is a source of knowledge and veracity that is defensively tuned out by the patient. Including some simple sensorimotor psychotherapy methods provides the basis from which a patient can ultimately hold their own past self in mind, compassionately recognizing the fear and distress of the child they were. The endeavor of creating symbolic representations of terrifying experiences [40], to make sense of the past in the mindful presence of the mentalizing therapist, holds out the possibility for the patient of building a life worth living.

It is difficult to do research on therapy that is not contained in a manual, relies on a long apprenticeship and is better described as an art or craft than a science, but it is nevertheless necessary. How else can we find ways to be more effective and reduce the time therapy takes to restore a patient to adaptable functioning in the present?

# References

1. Herman, J. L. (1997). *Trauma and recovery: The aftermath of violence from domestic abuse to political terror.* New York: Basic Books.

2. Herman, J. L. (1992). Complex PTSD: A syndrome in survivors of prolonged and repeated trauma. *Journal of Trauma and Stress,* **5**, 377–391.

3. Pelcovitz, D., van der Kolk, B. A., Roth, S. *et al.* (1997). Development of a criteria set and a structured interview for disorder of extreme stress (SIDES). *Journal of Trauma and Stress,* **10**, 3–16.

4. Marks, I., Lovell, K., Noshirvani, H. *et al.* (1998). Treatment of posttraumatic stress disorder by exposure and/or cognitive restructuring: A controlled study. *Archives of General Psychiatry,* **55**, 317–325.

5. Tarrier, N., Pilgrim, H., Somerfield, C. *et al.* (1999). A randomized trial of cognitive therapy and imaginal exposure in the treatment of chronic posttraumatic stress disorder. *Journal of Consulting and Clinical Psychology,* **67**, 13–18.

6. Foa, E. B., Dancu, C. V., Hembree, E. A. *et al.* (1999). A comparison of exposure therapy, stress inoculation training, and their combination in reducing posttraumatic stress disorder in female assault victims. *Journal of Consulting and Clinical Psychology,* **67**, 184–200.

7. Schottenbauer, M. A., Glass, C. R., Arnkoff, D. B. *et al.* (2008). Contributions of psychodynamic approaches to treatment of PTSD and trauma: A review of the empirical treatment and psychopathology literature. *Psychiatry,* **71**, 13–34.

8. Feeny, N. C., Zoellner, L. A. and Foa, E. B. (2002). Treatment outcome for chronic PTSD among female assault victims with borderline personality characteristics: A preliminary examination. *Journal of Personality Disorders,* **16**, 30–40.

9. Burnstein, A. (1986). Treatment noncompliance in patients with posttraumatic stress disorder. *Psychosomatics,* **27**, 37–40.

10. Pitman, R. K., Altman, B., Greenwald, E. *et al.* (1991). Psychiatric complications during flooding therapy for post-traumatic stress disorder. *Journal of Clinical Psychiatry,* **52**, 17–20.

11. Scott, M. J. and Stradling, S. G. (1997). Client compliance with exposure treatments for posttraumatic stress disorder. *Journal of Traumatic Stress,* **10**, 523–526.

12. Tarrier, N. (2001). What can be learned from clinical trials? [reply to Devilly and Foa]. *Journal of Consulting and Clinical Psychology,* **69**, 117–118.

13. Devilly, G. R. and Foa, E. B. (2001). The investigation of exposure and cognitive therapy: Comment on Tarrier *et al.* (1999). *Journal of Consulting and Clinical Psychology,* **69**, 114–116.

14. Allen, J. G. (2008). Psychotherapy: The artful use of science. *Smith College Studies in Social Work,* **78**, 159–187.

15. Herman, J. L. (2008). Craft and science in the treatment of traumatized people. *Journal of Trauma & Dissociation,* **9**, 293–230.

16. Western, D., Novotny, C. and Thompson-Brenner, H. (2004). The empirical status of empirically supported psychotherapies: Assumptions, findings and reporting in controlled clinical trials. *Psychological Bulletin,* **130**, 631–663.

17. American Psychiatric Association (2004). Practice guidelines for the treatment of patients with acute stress disorder and posttraumatic stress disorder. *American Journal of Psychiatry*, **161**(Suppl.), 3–31.

18. Doidge, N. (1997). Empirical evidence for the efficacy of psychoanalytic psychotherapies and psychoanalysis: An overview. *Psychoanalytic Inquiry*, Supplement, 102–150.

19. Miller, N. E., Luborsky, L., Barber, J. P. *et al.* (eds.) (1993). *Psychodynamic treatment research*. New York: Basic Books.

20. Leichsenring, F. and Rabung, S. (2008). Effectiveness of long-term psychodynamic psychotherapy: A meta-analysis. *Journal of the American Medical Association*, **300**, 1551–1564.

21. Gunderson, J. G. and Gabbard, G. O. (1999). Making the case for psychoanalytic therapies in the current psychiatric environment. *Journal of the American Psychoanalytic Association*, **47**, 679–704.

22. Fonagy, P. and Bateman, A. W. (2006). Progress in the treatment of borderline personality disorder. *British Journal of Psychiatry*, **188**, 1–3.

23. Stone, M. H. (1990). *The fate of borderline patients: Successful outcome and psychiatric practice*. New York: Guilford.

24. Zanarini, M. C., Frankenberg, F. R., Hennen, J. and Silk, K. R. (2003). The longitudinal course of borderline psychopathology: 6-year prospective follow-up of the phenomenology of borderline personality disorder. *American Journal of Psychiatry*, **160**, 274–283.

25. Bateman, A. W. and Fonagy, P. (1999). Effectiveness of partial hospitalization in the treatment of borderline personality disorder: A randomized controlled trial. *American Journal of Psychiatry*, **156**, 1563–1569.

26. Bateman, A. W. and Fonagy, P. (2001). Treatment of borderline personality disorder with psycho-analytically oriented partial hospitalization: An 18-month follow-up. *American Journal of Psychiatry*, **158**, 36–42.

27. Brewin, C. R., Andrews, B. and Valentine, J. D. (2000). Meta-analysis of risk factors for posttraumatic stress disorder in trauma-exposed adults. *Journal of Consulting and Clinical Psychology*, **68**, 748–766.

28. Frewen, P. A., Pain, C., Dozois, A. and Lanius, R. (2006). Alexithymia in PTSD psychometric and FMRI studies. *Annals of New York Academy of Sciences*, **1071**, 397–400.

29. Lyons-Ruth, K. (2003). Dissociation and the parent-infant dialogue: A longditudinal perspective from attachment research. *Journal of the American Psychoanalytic Association, * **3**, 883–911.

30. Brothers, D. (2009). Trauma centered psychoanalysis transforming experiences of unbearable uncertainly. *Annals of New York Academy of Sciences, * **1159**, 51–62.

31. Allen, J. G. (2001). *Traumatic relationships and serious mental disorders*. Chichester, UK: Wiley.

32. Lerner, M. J. (1970). The desire for justice and reactions to victims: Social psychological studies of some antecedents and consequences. In J. Macauley and L. Berkowitz (eds.), *Altruism and helping behaviors* (pp. 205–229). New York: Academic Press.

33. Lerner, M. J. (1980). *The belief in a just world: A fundamental delusion*. New York: Plenum.

34. Rubin, Z. and Peplau, L. A. (1975). Who believes in a just world? *Journal of Social Issues*, **31**, 65–90.

35. van der Hart, O., Brown, P. and van der Kolk, B. A. (1989). Pierre Janet's treatment of post-traumatic stress. *Journal of Traumatic Stress Studies*, **2**, 379–395.

36. Maldonado, J. R. and Spiegel, D. (1998). Trauma, dissociation and hypnotizability. In J. D. Bremner and C. M. Marmar (eds.), *Trauma memory and dissociation* (pp. 57–106). Washington, DC: American Psychiatric Press.

37. Ogden, P., Minton, K. and Pain, C. (2006). *Trauma and the body: A sensorimotor approach to psychotherapy*. New York: Norton.

38. Damasio, A. (1999). *The feeling of what happens: Body and emotions in the making of consciousness*. New York: Harcourt.

39. Siegel, D. (1999). *The developing mind*. New York: Guilford.

40. van der Kolk, B. A. (1994). The body keeps the score: Memory and the evolving psychobiology of post traumatic stress. *Harvard Review of Psychiatry*, **1**, 253–265.

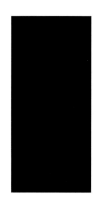

# Part 6 synopsis

Tal Astrachan, Carla Bernardes and Judith Herman

## Overview

Successful treatment of the psychological effects of early life trauma requires attention not only to what happened to the survivor but also to what did not happen. Early life trauma involves prolonged, recurring abuse, which is generally coupled with neglect. The survivor must try to contend with the impact of the abuse, while lacking the developmental learning that comes from having had a secure attachment figure.

The chapters in this part describe five approaches to treating the complex traumatic disorders that result from childhood abuse and neglect. At first glance, all approaches are specialized, using unique language to describe their theoretical frameworks and therapeutic techniques. Nevertheless, despite the specificity of each treatment model, the chapters share a number of common themes that are interpersonal and affect focused in nature. How does the therapist help to create a sense of safety, when it is paradoxically both a prerequisite and an anticipated outcome of successful treatment? What is the affective core of trauma-related pathology and how should this be addressed in treatment? How can therapist and patient together create a relational framework within which traumatic memories can be addressed?

## Safety

Childhood trauma disrupts the developmental trajectory of attachment. Not surprisingly, many chronically abused individuals develop disorganized and insecure attachment styles [1], which have been associated with the development of dissociative disorders as well as other psychiatric disorders in adulthood [2]. Disruption of safe attachment leaves the survivor feeling profoundly unsafe in the world. Consequently, the first step in treating survivors of childhood trauma

must be to establish of a sense of safety within the therapeutic relationship. Without achieving some level of safety and trust, it may be impossible to achieve any other treatment goals.

Several authors note the paradox that psychotherapy creates for survivors of childhood trauma. Survivors come to psychotherapy with a variety of symptoms related to disorganized attachment, and yet they are asked, as the foundation for treatment, to try to form a safe attachment to a therapist. They have been deeply hurt in dependent relationships, and yet they are asked to enter into a dependent relationship in order to heal. Creating a sense of safety in psychotherapy is, therefore, both a complicated and an essential task for the therapist. Each of these authors offers some description of what they do to help to create a sense of safety in the treatment.

In their mentalization-based therapy (MBT), Allen *et al.* (Ch. 23) adopt a "mentalizing stance" that encourages exploration of mental states with an open, curious attitude, rather than providing interpretations of the patient's internal experience. This helps to create a sense of safety by allowing the patient a sense of burgeoning agency in understanding self and others, rather than replicating the experience of childhood trauma, in which perpetrators often provide a heavily distorted and yet definitive understanding of what they are doing and how this feels for the child.

Charuvastra and Cloitre (Ch. 26) suggest that "an underlying mechanism of change in any effective trauma treatment is the experience of safety." They, too, believe that the therapist's attitude of curiosity and acceptance of the patient's emotional experience are essential in creating a sense of safety in treatment. As the patient feels the therapist's acceptance of his or her emotions, the patient's own ability to name, understand and accept emotions is enhanced. The authors

*The Impact of Early Life Trauma on Health and Disease: The Hidden Epidemic*, ed. Ruth A. Lanius, Eric Vermetten and Clare Pain. Published by Cambridge University Press. Copyright © Cambridge University Press 2010.

argue that the therapist's stance is particularly import-ant in the early sessions of their "skills training in affect and interpersonal regulation" (STAIR) treatment, as an alliance is being built with the patient. The goal is to create an experience counter to the common experi-ence of childhood trauma survivors, in which the expression of emotion has often been met with invali-dation, neglect or punishment, and at the same time to introduce an experience in which the expression of emotion can be adaptive and positive.

Pain *et al.* (Ch. 27) also stress the importance of addressing safety early in treatment. Developing trust is especially problematic in a relationship where there is a power differential, and where one of the parties, the therapist, has the advantage of professional knowledge and expertise. To the patient, this relationship will be all too reminiscent of the experience as a victim of abuse. These authors suggest a frank discussion of the patient's potential fears of the therapist, recognizing these fears as an understandable result of a traumatic past. They recommend making an explicit statement that the therapist will not physically harm or take advantage of the patient sexually. They also suggest that the therapist share with the patient a basic "map" of therapy, including some of the therapist's notions of how healing happens, so as to make the thought proc-ess of the therapist more transparent and accessible to the patient.

Loewenstein and Welzant (Ch. 24) stress the importance of attending to "basic life and health" needs as a prerequisite for safety. It is clearly impossi-ble to achieve safety and trust in a therapeutic relation-ship when a patient's basic needs, such as lack of food, housing or access to medical care, are not being met. Similarly, risky behavior, such as substance use, unsafe sex and compulsive self-harm, needs to be addressed if a sense of safety and trust is to develop in the therapy relationship. Trust, after all, is a two-way street, and a well-developed therapy relationship trends towards mutuality. Patients' motivation to take care of them-selves is often enhanced when they wish to gain or maintain the therapist's trust.

Once the patient has established some stability in daily life, safety issues take on a new form. Loewenstein and Welzant highlight the importance of attending to safety in the processing of traumatic memory. Invoking a stage-based model of treatment [3], they argue that the therapist must work to make this stage of treat-ment as predictable and planful as possible, in con-trast to the original experience of trauma as inherently

unpredictable and uncontrollable. They suggest that an explicit plan should be made as to the content, pac-ing and ways of coping with memory processing before it begins. During the sessions, the therapist must be active, structuring and containing as memory work proceeds. Possible reactions after the sessions should also be anticipated, and coping strategies should be reviewed.

## Fear, shame and emotional dysregulation

Several of the authors suggest that the conceptualiza-tion of the affective core of trauma-related pathology should be expanded from fear alone to include other core affective responses to trauma, particularly shame. Moreover, survivors of childhood trauma may often be best understood as suffering from pervasive dif-ficulties in emotional regulation rather than a simple anxiety disorder such as post-traumatic stress disorder (PTSD). Most of these authors invoke the concept of complex PTSD [4] to describe the multiple domains of symptomatology in survivors of childhood trauma.

To Charuvastra and Cloitre (Ch. 26), the effective-ness of processing traumatic memories in resolving PTSD does not result simply from habituation to the fear response associated with traumatic memories. Instead, they maintain that processing memories within the safe context of a relationship "recruits, rein-forces and consolidates" the capacity for emotional regulation. Their STAIR treatment model is based on the premise that survivors of complex trauma have broad difficulties in emotional regulation that extend well past fear-based pathology. Having found that in women with child-abuse-related PTSD, difficulties in emotional regulation and interpersonal function-ing account for as much functional impairment as do PTSD symptoms [5], they argue for the importance of addressing these broader difficulties in emotional regulation when treating survivors of childhood abuse. Trauma survivors must learn to tolerate a range of feelings, avoiding the extremes of hyperarousal (e.g., hypervigilance, panic, emotional reactivity, intru-sive thoughts, disorganized cognitive processing) or hypoarousal (e.g., numbing of emotions, absence of sensations, avoidance of triggers, reduced physical movement, and hopelessness).

Allen *et al.* (Ch. 23) make a similar point, arguing that the concept of desensitization or habituation is inadequate to describe the change process resulting from exposure to traumatic memories that occurs in all trauma treatments. Instead, they suggest that this is a process of active mastery, building the capacity for emotional regulation in the context of a relationship. Patients learn not only how to integrate specific traumatic memories but also how to understand and bear with emotions, both in themselves and in other people. In this manner, they develop their potential for relationships based upon mutual regard and mutual empathy rather than dominance and subordination. While the process of controlled exposure to traumatic memories is focused on the past, the capacity to name, accept and regulate emotions widens the patient's horizons toward the present and the future.

In their review of cognitive-behavioral treatment for PTSD, Chard and Buckley (Ch. 25) do not specifically address the sequelae of childhood trauma, except to note that "to date, few studies have examined whether specific treatments for PTSD resulting from childhood sexual abuse are effective." However, they, too, recognize the role of multiple emotional states as variables affecting treatment outcome for trauma survivors. They note that prolonged exposure treatment may lead to better treatment outcomes for patients who primarily experience fear rather than anger in reaction to trauma [6]. In addition, patients who struggle with higher levels of emotional overregulation, such as dissociation and numbing symptoms, and who are, therefore, less emotionally engaged during exposures, may experience poorer outcomes in exposure-based treatment. Moreover, some treatments may be better suited to particular dominant affective states than others. For example, patients who primarily struggle with shame, guilt and self-blame may have better treatment outcomes in cognitive processing therapy (CPT) than those who primarily struggle with fear or anxiety [7].

Loewenstein and Welzant (Ch. 24) emphasize the pervasive role of shame in responses to complex trauma, and they argue that shame is often insufficiently noticed. They argue that a crucial early task in treatment is helping patients to decipher the ways in which many of their emotional, relational and behavioral difficulties may be understandable adaptations that developed in the context of their trauma histories. This process can go a long way toward reducing the overwhelming feelings of shame that many trauma survivors experience. They recommend explicit psychoeducation about shame and its impact, which in turn may open the door to exploration of the many manifestations of shame in patients' lives. Addressing the delicate issue of shame in the therapy relationship can also be extremely helpful.

These chapters highlight how successful treatment for complex trauma-based pathology requires attention to a wide range of affective experiences in addition to fear. Pathological shame is a particularly common core affective experience for survivors of complex trauma. More broadly, the frequently pervasive difficulties in emotional regulation that arise in the aftermath of complex trauma need to be addressed as an integral element of successful treatment. Although each chapter presents a specific therapeutic model, the objectives are similar: to help patients to manage dysregulated arousal states within a relational context. In this manner, the deficiencies resulting from insecure attachment in childhood may be remediated.

## Future directions

In reading these chapters, clear commonalities emerge, particularly on the level of technique. It would seem particularly important not to get too attached to one particular set of concepts or language, which can lead one to overlook the utility of other treatment models. We are still very early in the process of discovering effective treatment for survivors of complex trauma [8].

While all of the authors in the present volume recognize the primarily interpersonal nature of complex trauma, as well as its impact on the interpersonal lives of trauma survivors, surprisingly, with the exception of Chard and Buckley (Ch. 25), none of the authors pays particular attention to the healing potential of groups. Chard and Buckley cite a number of advantages offered by groups, but unfortunately they do not elaborate on these points; the one study they cite [9], a 10-site randomized controlled trial comparing trauma-focused with present-focused groups for combat veterans with PTSD, found no difference between the two types of treatment. This particular study, unfortunately, made no attempt to match the type of treatment to the patient based on the patient's stage of recovery, and thereby it may have missed an important opportunity to advance our knowledge of effective treatments.

Yet there are many reasons to suppose that group psychotherapy might be a treatment of choice for survivors of complex trauma. Friendship and peer support has been shown to have a protective role in the psychological development of children who have suffered abuse and neglect [10,11]. Group therapy provides the survivor of interpersonal violence with unparalleled opportunities to combat social isolation, connect with sources of resilience and self-esteem, and rebuild relational capacities. A number of group treatment models specifically for this population have been published in recent years [12–14]. Peer interaction in a day-treatment milieu, followed by group treatment, is at the heart of a mentalization-based treatment program for patients with borderline personality disorder that has demonstrated its effectiveness in an extraordinary 8-year follow up study [15]. These same authors mention groups only in passing in the current volume (Ch. 23), but they quote a vignette from a group interaction that elegantly sums up the wisdom of group treatment: "A patient in one of our psychoeducational groups brilliantly epitomized trauma therapy…when the leader proposed that 'the mind can be a scary place,' she exclaimed, 'Yes, and you wouldn't want to go in there alone!'"

One of the important goals of treatment for complex childhood trauma-based pathology is to help survivors to learn how to have mutually rewarding and freely chosen relationships. This goal is especially well suited to group treatment. Groups provide survivors with an experience of commonality and belonging, and can reduce feelings of isolation and alienation [3]. By providing a felt experience of reciprocal relationships marked by caring and compassion, group therapy can empower survivors to seek out safe and affirming relationships in their lives outside of group [16], functioning as an "ecological bridge to new community" (p. 227).

At the Victims of Violence Program, our home base in the Department of Psychiatry at Cambridge Health Alliance, groups specifically designed for three different stages of recovery are mainstays of our treatment program. While groups for early recovery focus on coping in the present, trauma-focused groups are most appropriate for those survivors who have established safety and self-care in their present lives, and survivors who have come to terms with their traumatic past still may benefit from more heterogeneous groups focused on the dynamics of interpersonal relationships. A treatment guide to our trauma-focused group model has just been completed [17]. Hopefully this may lead to widespread replication and rigorous testing of the model by other researchers in the future.

Effective, nuanced treatment of complex childhood-trauma-related pathology has the potential to help trauma survivors to have a dramatically different experience of life. In the words of one survivor who engaged in treatment at the Victims of Violence Program:

> Yeah, it's like I've been under water, I described it like I was watching my life from up in the clouds, just like on autopilot. I felt very detached from my own life and now I'm feeling like it's okay to reconnect and be present every day. That's really it for me. It feels very new to me but it's really good.

# References

1. Baer, J. C. and Martinez, C. D. (2006). Child maltreatment and insecure attachment: A meta-analysis. *Journal of Reproductive and Infant Psychology*, **24**, 187–197.

2. Lyons-Ruth, K., Dutra, L., Schuder, M. R. and Bianchi, I. (2005). From infant attachment disorganization to adult dissociation: Relational adaptations or traumatic experiences? *Psychiatric Clinics of North America*, **29**, 63–86.

3. Herman, J. L. (1992). *Trauma and recovery.* New York: Basic Books.

4. Herman, J. L. (1992). Complex PTSD: A syndrome in survivors of prolonged and repeated trauma. *Journal of Traumatic Stress*, **3**, 377–391.

5. Cloitre, M., Miranda, R., Stovall-McClough, C. and Han, H. (2005). Beyond PTSD: Emotion regulation and interpersonal problems as predictors of functional impairment in survivors of childhood abuse. *Behavior Therapy*, **36**, 119–124.

6. Rothbaum, B. O., Meadows, E. A., Resick, P. and Foy, D. W. (2000). Cognitive-behavioral therapy. In E. B. Foa, T. M. Keane and M. J. Friedman (eds.), *Effective treatments for PTSD: Practice guidelines from the international society for traumatic stress studies* (pp. 60–83). New York: Guilford.

7. Resick, P. A., Monson, C. M. and Chard, K. M. (2008). *Cognitive processing therapy: Veteran/military treatment manual.* Boston, MA: Veteran's Administration.

8. Herman, J. L. (2008). Craft and science in the treatment of traumatized people. *Journal of Trauma & Dissociation*, **9**, 293–300.

9. Schnurr, P. P. Friedman, M. J., Foy, D. W. *et al.* (2003). Randomized trial of trauma-focused group therapy for posttraumatic stress disorder: Results from a Department of Veterans Affairs cooperative study. *Archives of General Psychiatry*, **60**, 481–489.

10. Werner, E. and Smith, R. S. (2001). *Journeys from childhood to midlife: Risk, resilience and Recovery.* Ithaca, NY: Cornell University Press.

11. Powers, A., Ressler, K. J. and Bradley, R. G. (2008). The protective role of friendship on the effects of childhood abuse and depression. *Depression and Anxiety*, **26**, 46–53.

12. Harris, M. (1998). *T.R.E.M. trauma recovery and empowerment: A clinician's guide to working with women in groups*. New York: The Free Press.

13. Westwood, M. and Wilensky, P. (2005). *Therapeutic enactment: Restoring vitality through trauma repair in groups*. Vancouver: Group Action Press.

14. Lubin, H. and Johnson, D. R. (2008). *Trauma-centered group psychotherapy for women*. New York: Guilford.

15. Bateman, A. and Fonagy, P. (2008). 8-year follow-up of patients treated for borderline personality disorder: Mentalization-based treatment versus treatment as usual. *American Journal of Psychiatry*, **165**, 631–638.

16. Mendelsohn, M., Zachary, R. and Harney, P. (2007). Group therapy as an ecological bridge to a new community. *Journal of Aggression, Maltreatment and Trauma*, **14**, 227–243.

17. Mendelsohn, M., Herman, J. L., Schatzow, E. *et al.* (2010). *The trauma recovery group: A treatment guide.* New York: Guilford, in press.

# Epilogue

The psychological effects of childhood trauma have been recognized, albeit intermittently, for centuries. In 1998, Felitti, Anda and their group at the Center of Disease Control in Atlanta published a series of landmark studies which linked the effects of adverse childhood experience (ACE) with early physical morbidity and mortality, elegantly and powerfully demonstrating for the first time the link between childhood trauma and its broad and profound effects on health [1]. Hence Felitti's poetic and poignant introduction to this book: *"Traumatic events of the earliest years of infancy and childhood are not lost but, like a child's footprints in wet cement, are often preserved life-long. Time does not heal the wounds that occur in those earliest years; time conceals them. They are not lost; they are embodied."*

In this book, we have invited many leading scientists and clinicians to address not only the biological and psychological sequalea of early life trauma, but also the social and cultural effects and repercussions it engenders. Despite the extraordinarily strong evidence pointing towards the devastating biological, psychological, and physical effects of early life adversity, the problem of childhood trauma in society as a whole has remained a hidden epidemic. McFarlane's comment in the first synopsis of this book is sadly and powerfully true. *"Clinicians and researchers continue to struggle with the broad challenges and tensions within society. The demand for idealization and social harmony erodes a willingness within the community at large to acknowledge and understand the brutality and exploitation that can sit behind the tidy gardens of suburbia. There is probably no other field that more challenges the reluctance of individuals to have their illusions shattered and face the capacity for inhumanity that pervades many people's lives than the area of childhood abuse."*

McFarlane speaks in part to a mechanism that reinforces our apparent denial of the extent of the problems that early life trauma present; he notes *"History highlights how in many ways clinicians' capacities for observation and description of patients' predicaments are more determined by the models of psychopathology they adhere to, than the history presented to them by the patient … Ultimately, the ability of a clinician to see and understand what a patient describes is as determined by the imposed attitudes and beliefs from the broader society, as it is from the reality of what the patient tells. Hence, clinicians practice in an environment where prevailing professional practice can blind their observation."*

The pervasive societal denial of the importance of sexual abuse persisted for the majority of the twentieth century. Was this related to the popular idea that Freud renounced his early belief that childhood abuse significantly affected the individual, in favor of the role of phantasy? Although this question continues to cause disagreement, it is problematic to use it to explain over 50 years of silence concerning the adverse effect of child abuse.

The polemic is set up in part by the use of the word phantasy, which implies "false belief," but Freud used the word phantasy to mean the complex of often unconscious or preconscious thought, interweaving of memories, ideas, defenses, wishes, and even transferences. He wrote that phantasies were often the best path to gaining access to previously suppressed, or otherwise inaccessible scenes and memories. Thus an analytic concern with phantasies does not imply a disinterest in reality; rather, by following a phantasy, a distant occurrence or a suppressed reality can be explored. A child who is abused, and who then develops the phantasy, "it happened because I was bad" is, in psychoanalytic terms, having a phantasy, which should indeed form a focus of treatment.

Certainly Freud's own private deliberations to Fleiss could have had little effect on the failure of society to recognize the suffering of abused children, because they were only published in German in 1950 and in English in 1954. Similarly, Masson's work was published much later still in 1985. What is clear is that, throughout Freud's published writings until he died in 1939, he reasserted the importance of sexual abuse and its etiological significance in mental illness. (Norman Doidge, personal communication, 2010).

A further present-day complexity is the definition of trauma in the DSM IV which remains unsatisfactory. As Lieberman states in the second synopsis, *"The definition of trauma is still subject to debate as is evident in the range of conditions (such as maternal depression and child affective dysregulation) that are encompassed within the umbrella of trauma in many of the chapters."* In addition, we have yet to develop an approach to the diagnosis of trauma that goes beyond co-morbidity and grapples with the complications of traumatic responses. She continues *"the diagnosis of multiply traumatized children lacks parsimony and etiological clarity and may interfere with a case formulation leading to a comprehensive treatment approach by focusing attention on discrete aspects of the child's and adults symptomatology rather than on the impact of trauma as the organizing substrate for the child's seemingly unrelated symptoms."* Without the establishment of a clear diagnostic category that embraces the complexity of response to early life trauma both from a psychological and physical perspective, research examining the pathogenesis and treatment outcome of this population will never be able to reach its full potential. This lack will prevent an understanding of trauma as an integrated system's response that is at the core of its many psychological and physical symptoms. This is particularly important in light of an overwhelming body of research examining the biological basis of psychological trauma that has emerged over the last decade. Studies have moved from solely examining the effects of physical or sexual abuse, to the stressors resulting from dysfunctional attachment relationships between child and caregivers. We now have accumulating evidence for the mechanism by which early life attachment difficulties alter the developmental trajectory of stress and affect regulation across the life span, and predisposes toward significant mental health problems following later traumatic live events. *"This work is relevant to the fundamental problem of the intergenerational transmission of relational trauma and the early pathogenesis of later-forming psychiatric disorders."* (Schore, third synopsis, this volume)

This book has also summarized the intricate relationships of genes, environment, and development. We have given the floor to authors acknowledging the biological, developmental, and cognitive processes that can result from exposure to adverse environments. This approach is reinforced by Lupien in the fourth

synopsis who states *"future studies assessing the intricate relationship between genes and environment in the development of mental health disorders in response to early adversity will have to include the developmental stage of the individual exposed to the adverse event into the equation."* Future research taking a developmental psychopathological perspective will have significant implications for early diagnosis and for knowing when an intervention is most effective in reversing the developmental trajectory of the early life insult. As Schore notes *"This perspective clearly implies that early intervention will be more successful in re-establishing a more normal developmental trajectory if we can more deeply understand the developmental stage-dependent expressions of various emotional disorders."*

This need continues throughout the life span, and Judith Herman writes (synopsis 6) in relation to the treatment of adults with early life trauma, *"the frequently pervasive difficulties in emotional regulation that arise in the aftermath of complex trauma need to be addressed as an integral element of successful treatment."* She stressed the importance of *"helping patients to manage dysregulated arousal states within a relational context. In this manner, the deficiencies resulting from insecure attachment in childhood may be remediated."*

The chapter by Heidenrich, Ruiz-Casares, and Rousseau supports Herman and Schore's remarks in their synopses by addressing the important and often overlooked issue of culture. They emphasize the need to take into account the age of the child when traumatized, but also the specificity of the cultural context of the early life trauma as well as the family system intimately connected to the developing child. They emphasize in their conclusion that there is no simple linear model connecting exposure to organized violence in children and outcomes, and suggest that *"clinicians and researchers have to be aware of the possibility of paradoxical reactions and of the diversity of outcomes as a function of the complex interactions of collective and individual factors. The importance of both culture and context when it comes to the impact of organized violence on children requests a systemic and interdisciplinary appraisal in order to adopt interventions and innovate in terms of prevention."*

Lieberman makes a compelling case for *"The most urgently needed direction in the field of trauma … involves the search for and implementation of effective treatments for multiply traumatized children. The routine experience of violence in the home, the school, the street, and the community at large has grown to epidemic proportions for large sectors of the population – precisely those sectors most bereft of protective factors that may moderate both the incidence and the impact of violence, such as adequate housing, education, income, and healthcare.* As quoted by Lieberman in her synopsis, Steven Sharfstein stated that *"interpersonal violence, especially violence experienced by children, is the largest single preventable cause of mental illness. What cigarette smoking is to the rest of medicine, early childhood violence is to psychiatry."* And Lieberman further suggests …*"there is a persistent discrepancy between the availability, efficacy, and effectiveness of treatment available to multiply traumatized children and the scope of the need."* She co-wrote a paper in which the term "supraclinical," (meaning over and above clinical understandings and interventions) was used to describe the nature of the interventions needed to address the sequelae of multiple trauma in the context of poverty and inter-generational transmission of maladaptive patterns of adaptation, including the overlap of different forms of trauma [2].

As a scientific and clinical community, we have come a long way from ignoring the effects of trauma or blaming the victim for their difficulties in psychological and social functioning. As Spiegel highlights in his Synopsis *"the strength required to survive the aftermath of trauma may exact a high cost in cognitive function, affect management, identity development, and relationship growth."* But we have not come far enough in ensuring all students of health care and mental health are taught the findings noted in this edited book and learn to operationalize them in their assessment and treatment of all those who become patients. If we teach our students adequately, their role as advocates lobbying at all levels of the health system for the

protection of the child would be a fundamental result of training in all of the health disciplines.

The evidence presented throughout this book points toward the need for a paradigm shift that recognizes that the etiology of the complex response to traumatic stress is the arbitrary, and sometimes purposeful, maltreatment of children. The final common pathway of neglect and abuse, and unresolved psychological trauma is indeed in the domain of mental and physical health – but the prevention of early life trauma reaches into changing the social determinants of health and lies well outside the capacity of medicine to deliver.

The goal and moral imperative of the next decade must be to mitigate the effects of early life trauma through a major public health response that focuses on prevention and effective intervention. If successfully accomplished, this will be a major public health advance of our time and alleviate the tremendous suffering and costs associated with the devastating effects of adverse childhood experience. Nelson Mandela said "Education is the most powerful weapon you can use to change the world." We are idealistic enough to believe he is right!

# References

1. Felitti, V. J., Anda, R. F., Nordenberg, D., Williamson, D. F., Spitz, A. M., Edwards, V., Koss, M. P. and Marks, J. S. (1998). Relationship of childhood abuse and household dysfunction to many of the leading causes of death in adults. The Adverse Childhood Experiences (ACE) Study. *Am J Prev Med.* **14**(4):245–58.

2. Harris, W. W., Lieberman, A. F. and Marans, S. (2007). In the best interests of society. *J Child Psychol Psychiatry.* **48**(3–4):392–411.

# Index

abuse
  ACE study reference category 78–79
  barriers to recognition 43–44
  data-gathering methods 152–153
  definition 18–19
  early life stress 124
  evaluation of related factors 153
  minimizing 45
  prevalence 58, 157–158
  recording 45
  transmission 38
  unawareness of 220
  *see also* general abuse outcomes;
      physical abuse; sexual abuse
ACE study *see* Adverse Child
      Experiences study
ACTH *see* adrenocorticotropic
      hormone
acting out behaviors 211
adaptation, positive to previous
      adversities 40
addictive behaviors 211
adjustment, sexual abuse impact 27
adolescents, CBT applications
      272–273
adoption, overseas 136
adrenocorticotropic hormone
      95, 96
  depressive disorders 159
  HPA axis 158
  stress response 125
Adult Attachment Interview (AAI)
      211–212
adults
  affect regulation 211
  assessment of childhood trauma
      effects 207–213
    approach 208–209
    measures 211–213
  complex outcomes 208
  disrupted attachment effects
      210–211
  dissociation 210
  early childhood trauma 207–208
    outcomes 208, 210–213
  general abuse outcomes 208–210

generic measures 209
identity 210–211
late childhood trauma 207–208
medical disease 77–78
  ACE study 82–83
  early life stress 133–138
psychiatric disease 77–78, 89
  ACE study 79–80
psychiatric morbidity 50–51
psychological disturbance 207
relatedness 211
symptoms of childhood abuse 208
trauma-specific measures 209–210
Adverse Child Experiences (ACE)
      study 77–78, 89–90
  data processing 85
  findings 79–84
  health risks 80–82
  healthcare implications 84–86
  outline 78–79
  psychiatric disease 79–80
  reference categories 78–79
  setting 78–79
  treatment implications 85–86
  weight program 77, 80
affect dysregulation 211
  borderline personality disorder 249
  childhood interpersonal trauma 62
affect regulation, complex PTSD 260
afferent input of fear-producing
      events 166
age
  exposure to potentially traumatic
      events 17
  prevalence of abuse 19
  trauma exposure risk 20
aggression measures 209
alarm states 59
  continuous 59
alcohol use, ACE study 80–82
alexithymia 59, 171
amnesia
  ACE study 80
  dissociation 244
  dissociative 167, 229
  functional 244

infantile 229–230
traumatic 243–244
amygdala
  childhood adversity 113–114
  deactivation in dissociative states 183
  defensive behaviors 179
  development 145
  fear processing 167
  function in PTSD 245
  functional activity 150–151
  inhibition by prefrontal cortex
      150–151, 168
  lateralization of function 146
  learning processes 185
  neural circuitry of stress 170
  stress response 125
analgesia 180
  emotional responses 180
anterior cingulate 145
  emotional responsiveness
      modulation 168
antisocial behavior, neglect 126
anxiety/anxiety disorders 95
  corticotropin-releasing factor
      149–150, 160
  early life stress 160
  emotional expression 282
  gender 98–99
  HPA axis 149–151
  *5-HTTLPR* polymorphisms 149
  juvenile stress-induced 97–98
  neglect 124
  onset 97
  resilience 149–151
  risk 149–151
  symptoms in childhood 98
arousal modulation, childhood
      interpersonal trauma 64
associative processes, fear
      conditioning 167
attachment 39–40
  behavior patterns 49
  bond with primary caregiver 49
  brain development 144–145
  classification 211
  complex PTSD 260–261

attachment (*cont.*)
  disorganized 40, 49, 145, 249
    *DRD4* 7-repeat allele 52
    psychiatric morbidity in adults
      50–51
  disrupted effects 210–211
  early trauma 243
  HPA axis dysregulation 50
  *5-HTTLPR* polymorphisms 52
  infancy as sensitive period
    48–49
  infant security 49
  insecure 145, 211, 248–249
  insecure-ambivalent 49
  insecure-avoidant 49
  measures 211–212
  mentalizing
    insecure 248–249
    secure 248
    transgenerational transmission of
      relationship 248–249
    treatment for attachment trauma
      247–253
  relational trauma 145–146
  right brain 144–145
  secure 49, 248, 249
  self-report measures 212
  transgenerational transmission
    of mentalizing relationship
    248–249
  traumatic 145–146, 252
attachment dysregulation 48–53, 88
  borderline personality disorder
    249–250
  institutionalized infants 124
attachment figures, war situations
  235
attachment theory of Bowlby 49
attachment trauma/abuse 39
  mentalizing role in treatment
    247–253
attention
  disturbances in childhood
    interpersonal trauma 62
  impaired capacity for effortful
    control 249
attention-deficit hyperactivity disorder
  (ADHD) 151
  maltreated children 159
autobiographical memory 179,
  219–222, 265
  impoverished 220–222
autoimmune disease, ACEstudy 83
autonomic buffering 40
autonomic nervous system
  stress response 190–191
  traumatic attachments 145

babbling, infant 109
Babinski, Joseph, simulation
  model 6
Bartholomew and Horowitz's
  Relationship Questionnaire
  (RQ) 212
battered child syndrome 7
  historical aspects 7
behavioral characteristics, trauma
  exposure risk 20
beliefs, dysfunctional/disruptive 271
Bell Object Relations and Reality Testing
  Inventory (BORRTI) 212
betrayal trauma theory 220, 245
biological dysregulation, childhood
  interpersonal trauma 62
biological stress response systems 124,
  125
  fight or flight or freeze reaction
    125
  immune system effects 126
biological system disruption, childhood
  interpersonal trauma 63
black children, Family Mosaic Program
  36
body
  stressor responses 124
  tuning into in psychodynamic
    psychotherapy 291
borderline personality disorder 179
  affect dysregulation 249
  amygdala deactivation 183
  analgesia state 180
  attachment dysregulation 249–250
  conditioned stimulus 185
  impaired capacity for effortful
    control of attention 249
  mentalizing 247, 249–250
    interventions 250–253
    treatment 247
  parenting quality 249–250
  pre-mentalizing modes of
    experience 250
  pretend mode 250
  psychic-equivalence mode 250
  startle response 185
  teleological mode 250
Bowlby, John 33–34
  attachment theory 49
  trauma concept 38
brain
  activity in childhood interpersonal
    trauma 59
  asymmetry for emotional processing
    103
  childhood interpersonal trauma
    regional effects 63

compromised integrity in
    impoverished autobiographical
    memory 220
default mode network 170–171
development
  adverse 127
  attachment 144–145
  gender effects 128
  healthy childhood 126–127
  PTSD 127–128
  sexual abuse 116
  stress 146
emotional 144
fear network 270
lateralization of function 103, 109
maturation investigations in neglect
    127–128
neglect
  development 127
  maturation investigations
    127–128
remodeling 96–97
sensitive periods for childhood
    adversity 116
stress effects 96–97, 220
stressor responses 124
structural changes with threats
    189–190
volume
  PTSD 128
  stress response 190
*see also named regions of brain*
brain-derived neurotrophic factor
  (BDNF)
  hippocampal activity 170
  polymorphisms and depressive
    disorders 163
Briquet, Paul 4

care quality
  child genetic predisposition
    expression 52–53
  disorganization 51
  HPA axis 143
  psychiatric morbidity in adults
    50–51
  unresponsive for infants 48, 59
caregiver
  education and exposure to
    potentially traumatic events
    18
  primary 49
    disruption with foster care
    133–134
  therapeutic interventions after early
    life stress 137–138
  *see also* parent(s); parental *entries*

causation, neurobiology studies
171–172
CBT *see* cognitive-behavioral therapy
central benzodiazepine receptors,
stress 113–114
cerebral cortex
brain development 126–127
childhood adversity 114–115
parietal and motor response to
threats 168
volume in PTSD 128
*see also* prefrontal cortex
cerebral hemispheres *see* hemispheric
development
Charcot, Jean Martin 4–5
Child Abuse Prevention and
Treatment Act 1988 19
Child Behavior Checklist (CBCL) 39
child protection services 45–46
child soldiers 236, 242
PTSD 236
childhood adversity 112
amygdala effects 113–114
cerebral cortex effects 114–115
corpus callosum effects 112–113
hemispheric development 114
hemispheric integration 112–113
hippocampus effects 113
neurobiology 112–120
sensitive periods 116
verbal abuse neuropsychiatric
effects 116–117
voxel-based morphometry 115–116
childhood interpersonal trauma 57–65
affect dysregulation 62
arousal modulation 64
attention disturbances 62
biological dysregulation 62
biological system disruption 63
brain activity effects 59
brain region impact 63
clinical assessment 63–64
cognition disturbances 62
comorbidities 58, 63
consciousness disturbances 62
co-occurring symptoms 62–63
effective action taking 64
impulse dysregulation 62
interoception capacity increase 64
interpersonal difficulties 62
regulation of self 64
self-experience 59
self-perception distortion 62
social functioning 59
somatization dysregulation 62
source of developmental trauma
disorder 63

stress hormone reactivity 63
symptomatology 62–63
systems of meaning distortion 62
treatment 63–64
childhood traumatic victimization
adverse outcomes 69–70
current knowledge limitations
70–72
psychobiological functioning 71–72
resilience 72
socioeconomic status 71
timing 70–71
childrearing
inadequate 5
modes 3
chronic obstructive pulmonary
disease, ACE study 83
circa-strike defense 180
clarification interviews
false memory 228
recovered memory 228
classical conditioning, borderline
personality disorder 185
clinician-administered PTSD scale
(CAPS) 210
cognition disturbances, childhood
interpersonal trauma 62
cognitive appraisal of threats 166–167
cognitive-behavioral therapy (CBT)
252, 297
applications for children/
adolescents 272–273
children traumatized by organized
violence 238
combined treatments 271–272
core concepts 268
efficacy data 269
exposure techniques 269–271
children 273
parents of traumatized children
273
prolonged 270, 271–272,
286–287
eye movement desensitization and
reprocessing, comparison 272
group interventions 273–274
imagery 269–270
predictors of treatment outcome
274
prolonged 270
PTSD 268–274, 286–287
cognitive capacity
early life stress 136
neglect 127
non-verbal 59
cognitive distortion
complex PTSD 264

measures 209
cognitive flexibility 194–195
cognitive processes
active inhibitory 220–221
autobiographical memory 220–221
cognitive-processing therapy (CPT)
271, 297
combined with prolonged exposure
271–272
communicative gestures, lateral
asymmetries in infants
103–109, 143–144
ISOG coding system 105–106
study 105–109
community factors, trauma exposure
risk 21–22
complex post-traumatic stress disorder
(CPTSD) 208, 210, 286
affect regulation 260
attachment 260–261
attributes of patients 287–292
clinician issues 258
cognitive distortions 264
coping strategies 265
counter-transference reactions 258,
260–261
disruptions in life 258
dissociation 287–288
chronic 289–290
fear 287
flashbacks 259
guided imagery 290–291
historical aspects 257
map sharing 289
memory fragmentation 289–290
memory processing 296
session 263–264
phasic trauma treatment 259–262
policy issues 258
psychodynamic psychotherapy
286–293
adaptation 287–292
psychotherapeutic interventions
259
safety in therapy 259, 288–289
screen technique 290–291
self-blame/loathing 288
self-destructive behaviors 259–260
sensorimotor psychotherapy
290–291
shame 261–262
social factors 258
stability 259
suicidal ideation 260
therapeutic alliance 260–261
trauma focus 260–259
traumatic transference 260–261

complex post-traumatic stress disorder
(CPTSD) (cont.)
treatment 257–265
approach 258
informed consent 258, 262
stage 2 262–264
stage 3 264–265
tuning in to the body 291
conduct disorder 151
consciousness
altered 178–179
disturbances in childhood
interpersonal trauma 62
coronary artery disease, ACE study 83
corpus callosum
brain development 126–127
childhood adversity effects 112–113
neglect 127–128
PTSD 127–128
cortex see cerebral cortex; prefrontal
cortex
corticolimbic inhibition
excessive 182–183, 184
failure 181–182
versus excessive 180–181, 184
corticosterone 96, 99
corticotropin-releasing factor (CRF)
50, 95
anxiety disorders 149–150, 160
depressive disorders 149–150,
159–160
early life stress 135, 160–161
extrahypothalamic system 158–159
HPA stress response 191
neurons 158–159
neurotransmission impact of stress 96
sexual abuse 162
stress response 125
corticotropin-releasing factor (CRF)
receptors 158–159
HPA stress response 191
cortisol production 50
childhood interpersonal trauma 63
early adoption 136
early life stress 135, 136, 162
emotional stimuli response 146
HPA stress response 191
neglect 126, 143
sexual abuse 162
counter-transference reactions
complex PTSD 258, 260–261
dissociation 258
country/nation factors, trauma
exposure risk 22
CRF see corticotropin-releasing factor
culture, organized violence 235–236,
238, 242

"dealing but not feeling" 59
Deese–Roediger–McDermott (DRM)
paradigm 228, 244
defense responses, animal models
179–180
dehydroepiandrosterone 191
depersonalization 182
depersonalization disorder 183,
257–258
neural correlates 184
depression/depressive disorders
ACTH levels 159
adult
ACE study 79–80
impact of maternal on infants
48–49
amygdala functional activity
150–151
BDNF polymorphisms 163
childhood 98
maltreated children 159
offspring and parenting quality 51
corticotropin-releasing factor 149–
150, 159–160
early life stress 159–160, 163
HPA axis 159
5-HTTLPR polymorphisms 163, 193
neuroendocrine system 163
derealization 182
desensitization, PTSD treatment
185
detailed assessment of post-traumatic
stress (DAPS) 209, 210
developing world, trauma exposure
risk 22
development of children 242
developmental disorders 144
institutionalized infants 124
developmental neurobiological models
148–154
developmental neuroscience 144
developmental trauma disorder (DTD)
88–89
characteristics 220.10,
childhood interpersonal trauma as
source 63
diagnosis impact on treatment
outcome 63
need for diagnosis 59–61
rationale for diagnosis 220.10,
symptom spectrum 62–63
developmental traumatology 124
Diagnostic and Statistical Manual of
Mental Disorders (DSM) 39
third edition (DSM-III), PTSD 45
fourth edition (DSM-IV), stressor
criterion 45

diffusion tensor imaging
peer verbal bullying 118
white matter tract effects of parental
verbal abuse 117
disorders of extreme stress not
otherwise specified (DESNOS)
69–70, 208, 210, 213, 257
diagnostic value 286
symptom categories 286, 287–292
disorganization
care quality 51
in infancy 40, 49
psychiatric morbidity in adults
50–51
dissociation 178, 202
adults 210
affect dysregulation 211
amnesia 167, 229, 244
amygdala deactivation 183
analgesia 180
animal defense responses as model
179–180
attention conditions 219
autobiographical memory
impoverishment 221–222
chronic 289–290
circa-strike defense 180
complex PTSD 287–288
corticolimbic inhibition 180–181
failure 181–182
counter-transference reactions
258
defensive strategy 288
depersonalization disorder 183
depersonalization/derealization
182
temporal lobe activation 184
distress 288
explicit memory 218–219
false memory acceptance
227–228
fear stimuli 182–183
forms 179
freezing response 180
learning impact 185
limbic system hyperinhibition 183
measures 210
neurologic etiology 180–184
primary 181, 202
protective factor 202
PTSD 181, 245
recovered memory 228–229
resilience 202
secondary 181, 185, 202
temporal lobe 184
traumatic early life-associated
178–185

dissociative disorder not otherwise specified (DDNOS) 179, 258
dissociative disorders 257–258
  clinician issues 258
  memory-processing session 263–264
  treatment
    stage 2 262–264
    stage 3 264–265
Dissociative Experiences Scale (DES) 210
dissociative identity disorder (DID) 179, 257–258
  coping strategies 265
  neural correlates 184
  self-states 259, 261, 262
    treatment 263
    unknown 263
  treatment 259, 263
distress, dissociative states 288
divorce impact, long-term outcomes 38–39
DNA methylation 150
domestic violence 39
  witnessing
    IQ impact 128–129
    white matter tract effects 118
dopamine
  early life stress 162
  externalizing disorder 151–152
  neural circuitry of stress 170
dopamine D$_2$ receptor
  DRD2 allele 192–193
dopamine D$_4$ receptor 52, 151–152
  DRD4 7-repeat allele 52, 151–152
dopamine transporter
  DAT allele 151, 192–193
dopaminergic system, mesofrontal 170
dyadic therapy 238

early trauma outcomes 208, 210–213
eating disorder measures 209
education level, maternal and trauma risk exposure 21
ego strength 40
emotion(s)
  adaptation 278–280
  awareness of others' 280
  communication 279–280
  coregulation 280
  cortisol production 146
  definition 279
  early life trauma 144
  feelings 279
    identifying and expressing 282
  lateralization 104, 146
  mentalizing 248

self-regulation 280
social context 278
trauma recovery 278–284
emotional awareness 171, 283–284
emotional brain 144
emotional competence 280–281
  social competence 280–281
emotional development 279–280
emotional environment
  growth-facilitating 145
  parental care impact 135
emotional expression 280, 282–283
  directing 279
  fear and anxiety eliciting 282
  PTSD 281
emotional maltreatment, co-occurrence with neglect 133
emotional memory 167
  suppression 183
emotional neglect 7
  long-term outcome studies 35
emotional processes, not apparent 279
emotional processing
  brain asymmetry 103
  theory 270
emotional regulation 211, 296–297
  adaptive 278–280
  clinical settings 281
  definition 279
  impaired in PTSD 182
  interpersonal difficulties 281
  learned 278–279
  maltreatment influence 280–281
  narration use 283–284
  sensitivity of system to stress 135
  social competence 280–281
  social dysfunction 281
  therapy 282–283
  trauma influence 280–281
  trauma memory processing 281, 283–284
  trauma recovery 278–284
  see also Skills Training in Affective and Interpersonal Regulation
emotional responses, analgesia 180
emotional responsiveness modulation 167–168
emotional undermodulation 181
emotionally valenced word retrieval 168
environment, definition 152–153
epidemiology of early life trauma 13–22
  role 45
  study populations 45

epigenetic processes, HPA axis control 150
epinephrine 162, 191
episodic memory 179
ethnicity see race/ethnicity
executive cognitive function 136
Experiences in Close Relationships–Revised (ECR-R) 212
exposure techniques of CBT 269–271
  children 273
  dropout rate 270–271
  parents of traumatized children 273
  prolonged 270, 286–287
    combined with cognitive-processing therapy 271–272
expressive gestures
  asymmetrical organization 104–105
  FFSF paradigm 104–105
  modalities 108
  other-directed 104–105
  self-directed 104–105
expressive language, trauma impact 46
expressive systems, linking 108
externalizing behavior problems 69
  dopamine 151–152
  monoamine oxidase A 151–152
  neglect 126
  risk/resilience 151–152
  see also attention deficit hyperactivity disorder; conduct disorder
extrapyramidal motor system, motor response to threats 168
extreme events, recovered memory 29–30
eye movement desensitization and reprocessing (EMDR) 272
  CBT comparison 272

face-to-face still-face (FFSF) paradigm 103, 143–144
  expressive gestures 104–105
  time of gestures performed with right or left hemibody 106
false memory 127.10225–231, 243
  acceptance correlation with dissociation 227–228
  anecdotes 226
  clarification interviews 228
  complex studies 230
  criticisms 225
  extreme events 29–30
  individual case deep studies 231
  mechanisms 227–228
  misunderstandings among researchers 30–31
  professional consensus 25

false memory (*cont.*)
  publications 30
  recovered memory corroboration
    226–227
  research 27–28
  Rind study 27–28
  zealotry 26
  *see also* recovered memory
False Memory Syndrome Foundation
    30–31
family composition, trauma risk
    exposure 21
family factors
  refugee children in Western
    countries 236
  trauma risk exposure 21
Family Mosaic Program 36
family resilience 237–238, 242
family therapies, children traumatized
    by organized violence 238
fear 296–297
  brain network 270
  complex PTSD 287
  emotional expression 282
  extinction 194
  processing in amygdala 167
  response 218
  social context 278
  stimuli and dissociation 182–183
fear conditioning 167, 194
  PTSD 194, 218
  resilience 194
  resistance 194
fear state-dependency 229
fear-producing events, afferent
    input 166
"feeling but not dealing" 59
feelings 279
  identifying and expressing 282
  shame 297
FFSF *see* face-to-face still-face
    paradigm
fight or flight or freeze reaction 125
*FKBP5* gene
  polymorphisms 137
  PTSD risk 193
  SNP interactions 150
flashbacks, complex PTSD 259
food shortages, war situations 236
foraging demand, unpredictable
    in primate neuroendocrine
    studies 161–162
forebrain, early life stress 136
forgetting, motivated 229
foster care 133–134
  adult outcomes 133–134
  chronic stress 135

disruption of primary caregiver
    relationship 133–134
  early life stress risk/resiliency
    134–135
  emotional maltreatment
    co-occurrence with neglect 133
  placement for maltreatment
    133–134
  therapeutic intervention 138
fractional anisotropy
  peer verbal bullying 118–119
  verbal abuse 117, 119
freezing response 179, 180, 190
Freud, Sigmund 5
  infantile sexuality theory 43–44
  intrapsychic fantasy model 6
  repetition compulsion 33
  seduction term 5
  sexual etiology of hysteria 5
functioning level
  multiple trauma 38–39
  traumatic experiences 38
fusiform gyrus 115

$GABA_A$ receptors, stress 113–114
galanin 191
gaze aversion, still-face effect 104
gender
  anxiety disorders 98–99
  mood disorders 98–99
  psychological trauma studies 71
  PTSD effects on brain development
    128
  stress effects 98–99
  trauma exposure risk 20
gene–environment interactions 52,
    148–154, 200–201
  abuse data-gathering methods
    152–153
  abuse-related factors 153
  amygdala functional activity
    150–151
  dopamine 151–152
  early life stress 148–149
  environment definition 152–153
  externalizing disorder risk/resilience
    151–152
  monoamine oxidase A 151–152
  outcomes 153–154
  PTSD 163
  resilience to stress 192–194
  risk/resilience research 153–154
general abuse outcomes 208–210
  assessment approach 208–209
  generic measures 209
genetic factors
  HPA axis development 134–135

maltreatment sequelae 137
  neglect 128–129
  neuroendocrine system 163
  PTSD 192
  stress 129, 137
genetic predisposition of child,
    expression with care quality
    52–53
girls, organized violence 239
Global Assessment of Functioning
    (GAF) 38
glucocorticoid receptor (GR), HPA
    axis 158
glucocorticoid receptor (GR) gene 150
glucocorticoids 95
  HPA axis 158
gray matter, brain development
    126–127
gray matter volume
  peer verbal bullying 118–119
  PTSD effects 114–115
group therapy 297–298
  CBT 273–274
growth, optimal and maturational
    processes 33–34
guided imagery 290–291

hallucinations, ACE study 80
health
  risks in ACE study 80–82
  trauma exposure risk 20
  war situations 236
healthcare costs 77–78
  ACE study 83
healthcare implications
  ACE study 84–86
  of early trauma 77–86
hemispheric development
  asymmetry 145–146
  attachment 144–145
  childhood adversity effects 114
hemispheric integration in childhood
    adversity 112–113
heritability 192
hippocampus
  childhood adversity 113
  episodic memory 220
  memory dysfunction in PTSD
    169–170
  memory function 190
  neglect effects 128
  plasticity 170
  stress effects 113, 128, 190
  volume reduction 220, 245
Hispanic children, Family Mosaic
    Program 36
histone acetylation 150

historical aspects of early life trauma/
        abuse 3–9
    1850s to 1900 3–6
    1900 to 1960s 6–7
    1960s onwards 7–8
    complex PTSD 257
    neglect 7–8, 123–124
    PTSD research 268–269
    recovered memory 25–31
Holocaust survivors, children of
        237
HPA axis see hypothalamic–pituitary–
        adrenal axis
household dysfunction, ACE study
        reference category 78–79
5-HTTLPR polymorphisms 52
    depression risk 163, 193
    HPA axis 150
    risk/resilience for mood/anxiety
        disorders 149
humor use by therapist using STAIR
        283
hypervigilance 210–211, 217–218
hypothalamic–pituitary–adrenal
        (HPA) axis 95
    care quality 143
    depressive disorders 159
    dysregulation 50
    early life stress 134, 136
        adult outcomes 137
    epigenetic processes in
        control 150
    5-HTTLPR polymorphisms 150
    infant stress reactions 50
    inhibition 191–192
    maternal separation 161
    neglect 126
    parental care effects on
        development 135
    PTSD 171
    regulation
        and quality of care 50
        by right brain 146
    risk/resilience for anxiety/mood
        disorders 149–151
    stress
        effects 96
        sensitivity to 150
    stress response 125, 191–192
        regulation 158
    therapeutic foster care intervention
        138
hypothalamus
    defensive behaviors 179
    stress response 168–169, 190
hysteria 4–5
    sexual etiology 5

identity 210–211
imagery 269–270
    guided 290–291
immune system
    biological stress response systems
        126
    neglect effects 126
    stress 125, 126
impact of event scale 210
impulse dysregulation 62
impulsive behaviors 51
incest 7, 58
    reported prevalence 44
    taboo 26–27
income, trauma risk exposure 21
infancy/infants
    attachment dysregulation 48–53
    babbling 109
    disorganization 40, 49
    institutionalized 123–124, 143
        early life stress 146
    lateral asymmetries of regulatory/
        communication gestures
        103–109, 143–144
        ISOG coding system 105–106
        study 105–109
    maternal depression impact 48–49
    parental care 48, 49
    physiological stress reactions 50
    security of attachment 49
    sensitive period 48–49
    threats 48
    unresponsive early care 48
Infant Self-directed regulatory and
        Other-directed Gestures
        (ISOG) coding system
        105–106
    configurations 105–106
infantile sexuality theory of Freud
        43–44
information inaccessibility
        phenomenon 220
information processing theory 271
    resilience 194–195
informed consent 258, 262
institutionalized infants 123–124, 143
    early life stress 146
insula, peer verbal bullying effects
        118–119
internal working models, altered 211
International Society for Traumatic
        Stress Studies, practice
        guidelines for PTSD 269
interoception capacity increase,
        childhood interpersonal
        trauma 64
interpersonal difficulties 62

emotional regulation 281
    see also childhood interpersonal
        trauma
interpersonal functioning, difficulties
        271–272
interpersonal problem measures 209
interpersonal repertoire expansion 283
intrapsychic fantasy model of Freud 6
intravenous drug use, ACE study
        80–82
Inventory of Altered Self Capacities
        (IASC) 212
invincibility see resilience
IQ, domestic violence witnessing
        128–129
ISOG see Infant Self-directed regulatory
        and Other-directed Gestures
        coding system

Janet, Pierre 5
just world theory 288

language, lateralization of function
        109, 114
lateral asymmetries, infant regulatory/
        communicative gestures
        103–109, 143–144
    ISOG coding system 105–106
    study 105–109
lateralization of function 103
    amygdala 146
    emotion 104, 146
    language 109, 114
    motor 114
learned helplessness 190
learning
    amygdala-based processes 185
    dissociative states 185
legal system 45–46
life expectancy 77–78
    ACE study 84
limbic system
    hyperinhibition 183
    traumatic attachments 145
limbic system checklist 33 (LSCL-33)
        114, 184
lingual gyrus 115
liver disease, ACE study 83
locus ceruleus–norepinephrine
        (LC-NE) system 158
long-term outcomes of childhood
        trauma 33–41
    attachment trauma/abuse 39
    divorce impact 38–39
    emotional neglect studies 35
    Family Mosaic Program 36
    interparent violence 39

long-term outcomes of childhood
    trauma (*cont.*)
  intervention impact 45
  mothers abused as children 35–36
  multiple trauma 38–39
  physical abuse studies 34–35
  studies 34–36
  verbal abuse studies 35
"lost in the mall" (LIM) study 228
low birthweight, trauma exposure
    risk 20

magnetic resonance imaging (MRI),
    brain development 126–127
magnetic resonance spectroscopy
    (MRS), childhood adversity
    effects on brain 114
malingering 231
maltreatment
  emotional 7
  "existence" 8–9
  foster care placement 133–134
  historical aspects 6–8
  professional resistance 8–9
maternal buffering 52–53
maternal deprivation
  preclinical studies 123
  primate studies 161–162
  stress 192
    sensitivity 195
maternal insensitivity 49
maternal sensitivity 49
maturational processes towards
    optimal growth 34
  repetition compulsion integration
    33–34
medical disease, adult 77–78
  ACE study 82–83
  early life stress 133–138
memory 243
  autobiographical 179, 219–222, 265
    impoverished 220–222
  central node/core 264
  controlled exposure 296–297
  disruptions 217–222
  dysfunction in PTSD 169–170,
    217–218, 244–245
  emotional 167
    suppression 183
  explicit
    dissociation 218–219
    PTSD 217–218
  fragmentation 289–290
  hippocampus 190
  impairment for trauma 219
  implicit 218
  meta-awareness changes 221

ordinary 229–230
  retrieval 225
  therapeutic exposure to traumatic 252
  trace formation 167
  verbal 169–170
  *see also* false memory; recovered
    memory
memory processing 296
  session for complex PTSD 263–264
mental health problems
  parental
    prevalence of abuse 158
    trauma risk exposure 21
  refugee children in Western
    countries 236
  trauma exposure risk 20
mentalization-based therapy 250–251
  early intervention 252–253
  intensive outpatient programs 251
  partial hospital program 251
  principles 251
  psychodynamic psychotherapy
    differences 287
  safety 295
  trauma-related interventions 251–252
mentalizing 247–248
  attachment
    insecure 248–249
    secure 248
    transgenerational transmission of
      relationship 248–249
    treatment for attachment trauma
      247–253
  borderline personality disorder 247,
    249–250
    interventions 250–253
  definition 247
  emotion 248
  psychodynamic psychotherapy 292
  transgenerational transmission of
    attachment relationship 248–249
  treatment for attachment trauma
    247–253
meta-awareness changes 221
Millon Clinical Multiaxial Inventory
    (MCMI) 209
Minding the Baby program 252–253
minimizing of neglect/abuse 45
Minnesota Multiphasic Personality
    Inventory (MMPI) 209
monoamine oxidase A 151
  externalizing behavior problems
    151–152
mood disorders 95, 97
  early onset 98
  gender 98–99
  HPA axis 149–151

*5-HTTLPR* polymorphisms 149
  resiliency 149–151
  risk 149–151
mood state-dependency 229
mother–infant synchrony 279–280
mothers abused as children
  long-term outcome studies 35–36
  protective factors 35
motor lateralization 114
Multidimensional Inventory of
    Dissociation (MID) 210
Multidimensional Treatment
    Foster Care for Preschoolers
    (MTFC-P) 138
multiple personality 6
Multiscale Dissociation Inventory
    (MDI) 210
myelin 126

narration, STAIR therapy 283–284
narrative
  individual 46, 283–284
  verbal 46
National Child Traumatic Stress
    Network 58–59
National Comorbidity Study –
    Replication (NCS–R) 13
  age effects 19
  cohort effects 19
  data collection methods 19
  definitions 18–19
  official data 19
  population sampled 19
  prevalence of early trauma 13–18
  prospective reporting 19
  retrospective reporting 19
  self-report data 19
  survey response rates 19
neglect 143
  ACE study reference category 78–79
  adult outcome 208
  antisocial behavior 126
  anxiety 124
  brain maturation investigations
    127–128
  cognitive development 127
  corpus callosum effects 127–128
  cortisol production 126, 143
  definition 18–19, 123
  developmental traumatology 124
  early life stress 124
  emotional 7
    long-term outcome studies 35
  emotional maltreatment
    co-occurrence 133
  externalizing behavior problems 126
  genetic factors 128–129

hippocampus effects 128
historical aspects 7–8, 123–124
HPA axis 126
immune system 126
minimizing 45
neurobiology 112–116, 123–129
neuroendocrine systems 125–126
neurotransmitter systems 125–126
prefrontal cortex effects 127
prevalence 58, 157–158
primate studies 162
PTSD 126
stressor 124
"neither feeling nor dealing" 59
neural systems
alterations with early life stress
135–136
working model for circuitry of
traumatic stress 166–169,
201–202
neurobiology of disorders
causation issues in studies 171–172
early life stress 160–163
disorders related to 159–160
long-lasting effects 166–172
psychosocial moderators of stress/
trauma 189–196
social support in stress resilience
195–196
neurobiology of neglect 112–116,
123–129
neurobiology of trauma/adversity
112–120, 142
amygdala 113–114
cerebral cortex 114–115
corpus callosum 112–113
hemispheric development 114
hippocampus 113
parental verbal abuse
neuropsychiatric effects 116–117
signal strength abnormalities 118
white matter tract abnormalities
117–118
peer verbal bullying,
neuropsychiatric effects
116–117
sensitive periods 116
white matter tract
domestic violence witnessing 118
parental verbal abuse effects
117–118
neurochemistry of resilience 190–192
neuroendocrine system
clinical studies 162–163
depressive disorders 163
early life stress 160–163
early life trauma effects 157–163

genetic factors 163
neglect 125–126
primate studies 161–162
rodent studies 160–161
sexual abuse 162
stress 125–126
stress response regulation 158–159
neurological damage, abused
children 58
neuropeptide Y 191
neuroscience, developmental 144
neurotransmitter systems
neglect 125–126
stress 125–126
neurotransmitters, stress effects 96
nicotine use
ACE study 80–82
adult disease 83
non-accidental injury, documentation
of reality 44
norepinephrine 162, 163, 191
neural circuitry of stress 170
normality 39
not-thinking 230
nutrition, war situations 236

obesity, ACE study 80
organized violence 234–239
countries at war 235–236
culture 235–236, 238, 242
definition 234
gender-based 239
non-Western populations 234–235
paradoxical effects 237–238
policy issues 237
postconflict situations 235–236
protection determinants 235–237
psychological outcomes 235
psychosocial factors 237
PTSD 234, 235
refugee children in Western
countries 236–237
resilience 234, 237–238, 242
risk determinants 235–237
separation 235
social implications 237–238,
242–243
therapeutic interventions 238
transgenerational transmission 237
trauma transmission mechanisms
239
orphans
trauma exposure risk 22
war situations 235
other-directed behaviors 103–104,
106
differential distribution 107–109

gesture lateralization 106
left-sided 108
linguistic 109
other-directedness 210–211
oxytocin 195

pain perception 180
parent(s)
bereavement and trauma exposure
risk 22
frightening/frightened behavior
249
involvement in CBT for children 273
see also maternal entries; mother
entries
parental care
HPA axis development 135
infant physiological stress reactions
50
infants 48, 49
quality and HPA axis regulation 50
sensitivity of stress system 135
war situations 235
parental verbal abuse
neuropsychiatric effects 116–117
signal strength abnormalities 118
white matter tract abnormalities
117–118
parenting quality 49
borderline personality disorder
249–250
depression in offspring 51
parietal cortex, motor response to
threats 168
peer verbal bullying
fractional anisotropy 118–119
gray matter volume 118–119
neuropsychiatric effects 116–117
periaqueductal gray, defensive
behaviors 179
perpetuation of abuse 38
phasic trauma treatment, complex
PTSD 259–262
phenotypic plasticity 52
phenylketonuria 193
physical abuse
long-term outcome studies 34–35
neurobiology 112–116
prevalence 158
primate studies 162
physical disabilities, trauma exposure
risk 20
physical injuries
historical aspects 6–7
structural damage 7
Piaget, Jean 33–34
playfulness, therapist using STAIR 283

postconflict situations, organized
        violence 235–236
post-traumatic disturbance, complex
        212
post-traumatic stress diagnostic scale
        (PDS) 210
post-traumatic stress disorder (PTSD)
    amygdala
        deactivation 183
        function 245
    analgesia state 180
    autobiographical memory
        impoverishment 221–222
    avoidance symptoms 261
    brain
        default network 171
        development 127–128
        volume 128
    brief models of treatment 286–287
    cerebral cortex
        effects 114–115
        volume 128
    child soldiers 236
    childhood traumatic victimization
        69–70
    chronic 69
        psychodynamic psychotherapy
            286–293
        psychodynamic psychotherapy
            adaptation 287–292
    chronic adaptations 257
    CBT 268–274, 286–287
        combined 271–272
        group 273–274
        predictors of treatment outcome
            274
    cognitive-processing therapy 271
    conditioned fear responses 194
    corpus callosum effects 127–128
    corticolimbic inhibition failure
        181–182
    depersonalization/derealization
        dissociative states 184
    desensitization treatment 185
    diagnosis 57
    dissociation 181, 245
    DRD2 allele 192–193
    DSM-III 45
    emotional expression 281
    emotional regulation 278–284
    emotional responsiveness
        modulation 168
    emotionally valenced word retrieval
        168
    emotions in recovery 278–284
    explicit memory 217–218
    exposure techniques of CBT 269–271

    children 273
        parents of traumatized children 273
        prolonged 270, 271–272
    eye movement desensitization and
        reprocessing 272
    fear conditioning 218
    FKBP5 gene 193
        SNP interactions 150
    gene–environment interactions 163
    genetic factors 192
    genetic heterogeneity 193
    hippocampal volume reduction 220,
        245
    hippocampus effects 113
    history of research 268–269
    HPA axis 171
    impaired emotion regulation 182
    implicit memory 218
    incorporation of DESNOS
        (disorders of extreme stress not
        otherwise specified) 70
    maltreated children 159
    measures 210
    memory dysfunction 169–170,
        217–218, 244–245
    memory processing 296
    neglect 126
    neuroendocrine systems 160
    organized violence 234, 235
    practice guidelines from the
        International Society for
        Traumatic Stress Studies 269
    prevalence 45
    prolonged exposure 270, 286–287
        combined with cognitive-
        processing therapy 271–272
    reminders of trauma 252
    simple 286
    trauma memory processing 281
    traumatic attachment 252
    treatment model 281
    verbal memory deficit 169–170
    see also complex post-traumatic
        stress disorder
PTSD see post-traumatic stress
        disorder
post-traumatic symptoms,
        autobiographical memory
        impoverishment 221–222
poverty, trauma exposure risk 21, 22
prefrontal cortex 114
    brain development 126–127
    emotional responsiveness
        modulation 167–168
    inhibitory influence on amygdala
        150–151, 168
    medial 170–171

    motor response to threats 168
    neglect 127
    neural circuitry of stress 170
    stress
        early life 127
        response 125, 190
    preschool children, CBT applications 273
    prescription costs 83
    prevalence of early trauma 13–18, 58,
        157–158
        methodology 18
    prolactin, early life stress 162
    prolonged exposure 270, 286–287
        combined with cognitive-processing
            therapy 271–272
    protective factors, trauma exposure 21
    psychasthenia 5
    psychiatric disease, adult 77–78, 89
        ACE study 79–80
    psychiatric morbidity in adulthood
        50–51
    psychoanalysis 6
    psychobiological self-regulatory
        capacity 69
        childhood traumatic victimization
            71–72
    psychodynamic psychotherapy
        286–293
        adaptation 287
            for complex PTSD 287–292
        chronic dissociation 289–290
        guided imagery 290–291
        map sharing 289
        memory fragmentation 289–290
        mentalization-based therapy
            differences 287
        mentalizing 292
        safety 288–289, 295–296
        screen technique 290–291
        sensorimotor psychotherapy
            290–291
        tuning in to the body 291
        verbal descriptions 291
    Psychological Assessment Inventory
        (PAI) 209
    psychological trauma
        chronic PTSD 69
        complex adult sequelae 69–72
        current knowledge limitations 70–72
        denial of significance 44
        externalizing behavior problems 69
        gender 71
        psychobiological self-regulatory
            capacity effects 69
        PTSD risk 69–70
        race/ethnicity 71
        timing 70–71

psychosis, causes 9
psychosocial factors, organized
    violence 237
psychosocial moderators of stress/
    trauma 189–196
psychotherapy in the kitchen 252
public health, adult disease 83
public policy, early life stress
    interventions 138

race/ethnicity
    exposure to potentially traumatic
        events 16, 18
    Family Mosaic Program 36
    psychological trauma studies 71
    trauma exposure risk 20
rape 40–41
recording of abuse 45
recovered memory 225–231, 243–244
    accuracy 226
    age at trauma 227
    anecdotal evidence 225–226
    bias acknowledgement 230
    clarification interviews 228
    complex studies 230
    concept 225
    content 227
    corroboration 226–227
    dissociation 228–229
    extreme belief 29–30
    extreme events 29–30
    "firewall" between science and
        politics 28–29
    forensic evaluation 231
    fragments 227
    historical aspects 25–31
    individual case deep studies 231
    lay groups 27
    mechanisms 227–230
    misunderstandings among
        researchers 30–31
    motivated forgetting 229
    motivational forces 229
    not-thinking 230
    ordinary memory 229–230
    phenomenology of experiences 227
    professional consensus 25
    publications 30
    repression concept 29, 228–229
    research 26–27
    Rind study 27–28
    science/non-science 28–29
    scientific approaches 26–27
    "scientists" versus "clinicians" 28
    sexual abuse 227
    state-dependency 229
    think/no think procedure 229

timing 227
triggers 227
zealotry 26
refugee children in Western countries
    236–237, 242
    policy issues 237
    resettlement 236–237
    unaccompanied 237
regulation of self see self-regulation
regulatory gestures, lateral
    asymmetries in infants
    103–109, 143–144
    ISOG coding system 105–106
    left-sided 108
    stress 108
    study 105–109
relatedness 211
Relationship Questionnaire (RQ) 212
repetition compulsion 33–34
repressed trauma, diagnosis 26
repression in recovered memory 29,
    228–229
    criteria 228
resettlement, refugee children in
    Western countries 236–237
resilience 40, 189, 202–203
    childhood traumatic victimization
        72
    cognitive flexibility 194–195
    dissociation 202
    family 237–238, 242
    fear conditioning 194
    gene–environment interactions
        192–194
    information processing theory
        194–195
    neurochemistry 190–192
    neurocircuitry 189–190
    organized violence 234, 237–238,
        242
    protective factors 189
    social support 195–196
resilient groups 40
Revised Adult Attachment Scale
    (AAS-Revised) 212
Rind study of false memory 27–28
Rorschach test 209, 213

safety
    complex PTSD therapy 288–289,
        295–296
    mentalization-based therapy 295
    STAIR therapy 295–296
    trauma therapy 282, 295–296
schemata, disrupted 212
screen technique 290–291
secondary gain 4, 6

seduction 40–41
    term 5
    theory 5
seizures, temporal lobe 184
self-blame, complex PTSD 288
self-capacity tests 212–213
self-control 249
self-damaging borderline features 51
self-destructive behaviors
    affect dysregulation 211
    complex PTSD 259–260
self-directed gestures 103, 106
    stress 106–107
self-experience 59
self-loathing, complex PTSD 288
self-perception distortion, childhood
    interpersonal trauma 62
self-regulation 64
    behaviors 103–104
        differential distribution 107–109
    childhood interpersonal trauma 64,
        271–272
    complex PTSD 260
    gestures 103, 106, 107
self-states, dissociative identity
    disorder 259, 261, 262
    treatment 263
    unknown 263
sensorimotor psychotherapy 290–291
separation
    organized violence 235
    primate studies 161–162
    rodent studies 161
    stress 192
        sensitivity 195
    war situations 235
serotonin system, stress response 125
serotonin transporter gene (5-HTTLPR)
    polymorphisms 52
    depression risk 163, 193
    HPA axis 150
    risk/resilience for mood/anxiety
        disorders 149
sex steroids, brain development 127
sexual abuse
    adjustment impact 27
    brain development 116
    corticotropin-releasing factor 162
    cortisol production 162
    definition 18–19
    etiology 8
    gray matter volume reduction 115
    historical aspects 4
    neurobiology 112–116
    neuroendocrine system 162
    prevalence 158
    recovered memory 227

313

sexual behavior 77–78
  ACE study 80, 82
sexual trauma, severity of adult
      outcome 69
shame
  attack other 261–262
  avoidance 262
  complex PTSD 261–262
  feelings 297
  self-attack 261
  withdrawal 262
shock, inescapable 180
simulation model of Babinski 6
Skills Training in Affective and
      Interpersonal Regulation
      (STAIR) 271–272, 281
  emotional expression/regulation
      282–283
  feelings expression/identification 282
  narration use 283–284
  safety 295–296
  social repertoire expansion 283
  trauma memory processing 283–284
  treatment goals 281–282
smoking
  ACE study 80–82, 83
  see also nicotine use
social biofeedback 280
Social Cognition and Object Relations
      Scale (SCORS) 213
social collusion 45
social competence 280–281
social dysfunction 281
social factors, complex PTSD 258
social functioning 59
social isolation 123, 195
social repertoire expansion 283
social support, resilience 195–196
social–emotional development
      impairment 145–146
socioeconomic status
  childhood traumatic victimization
      71
  poverty 21, 22
somatization
  disorders in ACE study 80
  dysregulation, childhood
      interpersonal trauma 62
splanchnic nerve 169
stage-oriented treatment 257–265
STAIR see Skills Training in Affective
      and Interpersonal Regulation
startle response
  borderline personality disorder 185
  PTSD 218
state reexperiencing 181–182

state-dependency, recovered memory
      229
still-face effect 104
stress
  abnormal reactions 95
  brain effects 96–97, 220
  central benzodiazepine receptors
      113–114
  chronic 83
    foster care 135
  corpus callosum effects 127–128
  emotional regulatory system
      sensitivity 135
  fight or flight or freeze reaction 125
  GABA$_A$ receptors 113–114
  gender effects 98–99
  genetic factors 129, 137
  hippocampus effects 113, 128, 190
  HPA axis sensitivity 150
  immune system 125, 126
  inoculation 136, 137, 191–192
  learned helplessness 190
  maternal deprivation 192
  neuroendocrine systems 125–126
  neurotransmitter systems 125–126
  prefrontal cortex effects 127
  psychosocial moderators 189–196
  reactions
    adult disease 83
    physiological in infants 50
  regulatory gestures 108
  regulatory neural system
    foster care therapeutic intervention
      138
    plasticity 137–138
  repeated 190
  self-directed gestures 106–107
  separation 192
    sensitivity 195
  vulnerability 97
  working model for neural circuitry
      166–169
  see also resilience
stress, early life 96
  abuse 124
  adult disease 133–138
  anxiety disorders 160
  brain development 146
  caregiver-based therapeutic
      interventions 137–138
  clinical studies 162–163
  corticotropin-releasing factor
      160–161
  cortisol production 136, 162
  definition 157
  depressive disorders 159–160, 163

developmental neurobiological
      models 148–154
  executive cognitive function 136
  foster care 133–134
  genetic variables 129
  HPA axis 134, 136, 137
  individual differences 137
  institutionalized infants 146
  interventions 138
  neglect 124, 127–128
  neural system alterations 135–136
  neurobiology of disorders 159–163
  neuroendocrine effects 157–163
  neuroendocrine systems 160–163
  prevalence 157–158
  primate studies 161–162
  resiliency 134–135, 136–137,
      148–154
    gene–environment interactions
      149, 153–154
  risks 134–135, 136–137, 148–154
    gene–environment interactions
      149, 153–154
  rodent studies 160–161
  severity 136–137
stress, juvenile 95–99, 142
  anxiety levels 97
  anxious behavior 97–98
  corticosterone levels 99
  long-term exposure 97
  model 96–97
  short-term exposure 97–99
stress hormone see cortisol production
stress response 95
  autonomic nervous system 190–191
  brain structure 190
  brain volume 190
  HPA axis 125, 191–192
    regulation 158
  hypothalamus 168–169, 190
  prefrontal cortex 125, 190
  preparation 168–169
  regulation 158–159
  sympathetic nervous system
      190–191
stress–diathesis theory 193–194
stressor criterion 45
stressors
  body responses 124
  brain responses 124
  early life 96
  HPA axis response 95
  neglect 124
striatum, motor response to threats 168
Structured Clinical Interview for
      DSM-IV dissociative disorders
      (SCID-D) 210

Structured Interview for disorders of extreme stress (SIDES) 70, 212, 213
study populations 45
subdural hematoma
  documentation of reality 44
  historical aspects 6–7
Subjective Units of Distress Scale (SUDS) 269–270
substance abuse
  affect dysregulation 211
  measures 209
suicidal ideation, complex PTSD 260
suicidality
  affect dysregulation 211
  measures 209
sympathetic nervous system, stress response 190–191
Symptom Checklist-90-Revised (SCL-90-R) 209
systems of meaning distortion, childhood interpersonal trauma 62

Tardieu, Ambroise 3–4
temporal lobe
  dissociation 184
  seizures 184
Thematic Apperception Test (TAT) 212, 213
theory of mind 247–248
threats
  afferent input 166
  cognitive appraisal 166–167
  hypervigilance 217–218
  to infants 48
  memory trace formation 167
  motor response 168
  peripheral responses 168–169
  response preparation 168–169
  structural changes to brain 189–190
transgenerational transmission of traumatic experience 237
translational developmental science 138
transmission of abuse 38
trauma
  attachment effects 243
  community level factors 21–22
  definition 13
  destructiveness 44
  developmental effects 242
  directions of study 90–91
  emotion 144

exposure to potentially traumatic events 14, 18
  incidence 95
  measurement 45
  memory processing 281, 283–284
  mentalization-based therapy 251–252
  multiple 38–39
  neurobiology 112–120
  prior 21
  protective factors 21
  psychological 13
  psychosocial moderators 189–196
  risk factors for exposure 19–22
  transgenerational transmission 237
  treatment of sequelae 91
  violent 69
Trauma and Attachment Belief Scale (TABS) 212
trauma disorder diagnosis 57–65
Trauma Symptom Inventory (TSI) 209–210, 212–213
traumatic dissociation, early life related 178–185
traumatic transference, complex PTSD 260–261
treatment 295–298
  caregiver-based after early life stress 137–138
  childhood interpersonal trauma 63–64
  children traumatized by organized violence 238
  complex PTSD 257–265
    stage 3 264–265
  dissociative identity disorder 259
  dissociative states 185
  group 297–298
  implications of ACE study 85–86
  informed consent 258, 262
  mentalizing role for attachment trauma 247–253
  phasic trauma for complex PTSD 259–262
  preventive interventions 137–138
  stage-oriented 257–265
  trauma sequelae 91
  see also cognitive behavioral therapy; mentalization-based therapy; psychodynamic psychotherapy; Skills Training in Affective and Interpersonal Regulation
tuning in to the body 291

uncinate fasciculus 146
undernutrition, trauma exposure risk 22

vagus nerve 169
vasopressin 195
verbal abuse
  fractional anisotropy 117, 118–119
  gray matter volume 118–119
  long-term outcome studies 35
  neuropsychiatric effects 116–117
  signal strength abnormalities 118
  see also parental verbal abuse; peer verbal bullying
verbal memory, deficit in PTSD 169–170
verbal narrative, creation of coherent 46
victimization 89
  adult outcome 208
  adverse outcomes 69–70
  current knowledge limitations 70–72
  externalizing behavior problems 69
  PTSD risk 69–70
  trauma exposure risk 21
  see also childhood traumatic victimization
violence
  interparent 39
  see also domestic violence; organized violence
violent trauma, severity of adult outcome 69
voxel-based morphometry, childhood adversity studies 115–116
vulnerable groups 40

wars
  organized violence 235–236
  psychological effects 44
weight loss 77
white matter tract
  deprivation-induced disorganization 146
  domestic violence witnessing effects 118
  parental verbal abuse effects 117–118
Winnicott, Donald 33–34
withdrawing behavior, parental 51
word formulation, disruption 46

zealotry, recovered/false memory 26